# THE PHARMACOLOGIC MANAGEMENT OF HEART DISEASE

# THE PHARMACOLOGIC MANAGEMENT OF HEART DISEASE


EDITORS

JOEL KUPERSMITH, MD

*Professor and Chairperson, Department of Medicine*
*College of Human Medicine*
*Michigan State University*
*East Lansing, Michigan*

PRAKASH C. DEEDWANIA, MD

*Chief, Cardiology Section, VA Medical Center*
*Fresno, California*
*Clinical Professor of Medicine*
*University of California, San Francisco*
*School of Medicine*
*San Francisco, California*


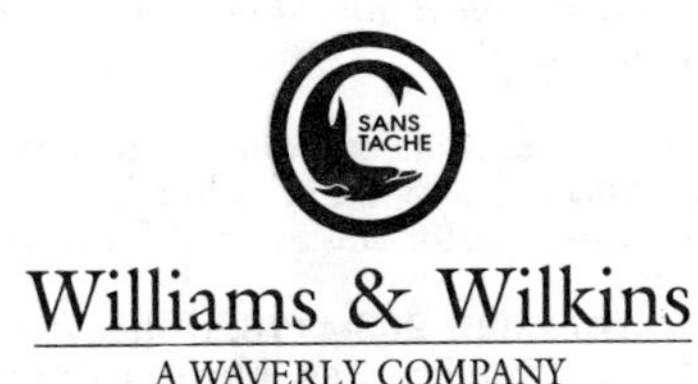



Williams & Wilkins

A WAVERLY COMPANY

BALTIMORE • PHILADELPHIA • LONDON • PARIS • BANGKOK
BUENOS AIRES • HONG KONG • MUNICH • SYDNEY • TOKYO • WROCLAW

*Editor: Jonathan W. Pine, Jr*
*Managing Editor: Molly L. Mullen*
*Production Coordinator: Marette Magargle-Smith*
*Book Project Editor: Robert D. Magee*
*Designer: Norman W. Och*
*Cover Designer: Tom Scheuerman*
*Typesetter: Peirce Graphic Services, Inc.*
*Printer & Binder: Vicks Lithograph & Printing Corp.*



351 West Camden Street
Baltimore, Maryland 21201-2436 USA

Rose Tree Corporate Center
1400 North Providence Road
Building II, Suite 5025
Media, Pennsylvania 19063-2043 USA

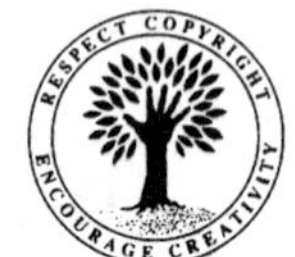




Accurate indications, adverse reactions and dosage schedules for drugs are provided in this book, but it is possible that they may change. The reader is urged to review the package information data of the manufacturers of the medications mentioned.

*Printed in the United States of America*

First Edition,

**Library of Congress Cataloging-in-Publication Data**

The pharmacologic management of heart disease / editors,
Joel Kupersmith, Prakash Deedwania.
p. cm.
Includes index.
ISBN 0-683-04796-5
1. Cardiovascular agents. 2. Heart—Diseases—Chemotherapy.
I. Kupersmith, Joel, 1939– II. Deedwania, Prakash C., 1948–
[DNLM: 1. Heart Diseases—drug therapy. WG 210 H435 1996]
RM345.H4 1996
615′.71—dc20
DNLM/DLC 96-326
for Library of Congress CIP

*The publishers have made every effort to trace the copyright holders for borrowed material. If they have inadvertently overlooked any, they will be pleased to make the necessary arrangements at the first opportunity.*

To purchase additional copies of this book, call our customer service department at **(800) 638-0672** or fax orders to **(800)447-8438.** For other book services, including chapter reprints and large quantity sales, ask for the Special Sales Department.

Canadian customers should call **(800) 268-4178,** or fax **(905) 470-6780.** For all other calls originating outside of the United States, please call **(410) 528-4223** or fax us at **(410) 528-8550.**

***Visit Williams & Wilkins on the Internet:*** **http://www.wwilkins.com** or contact our customer service department at **custserv@wwilkins.com.** Williams & Wilkins customer service representatives are available from 8:30 am to 6:00 pm, EST, Monday through Friday, for telephone access.

97 98 99
1 2 3 4 5 6 7 8 9 10

# DEDICATION

To our wives and children who have been a source of support and encouragement and to the house staff and students who have been a constant source of inspiration.

# PREFACE

Our healthcare system is changing, and amidst these changes new roles emerge for physicians in the treatment of their patients. The primary care physician may find it more difficult to call on the cardiologist for consultative help, a particular problem because patients with heart disease are so common. The subspecialist may find that he or she must now often assume a generalist and primary care role. The trainee must be prepared broadly for the new medical marketplace so that with general knowledge he or she will face a more certain future. The new healthcare system also demands that in all of these roles, the cost-effectiveness of care assumes more importance than ever, although, as always, the quality of care is paramount.

To treat heart disease, physicians must be well prepared with general knowledge and guidance in pharmacologic management. Especially when cost-effective care is a consideration, pharmacologic treatments will often be favored over other forms of therapy. In addition, precise drug therapy is crucial for good therapeutic results. At the same time, fortunately, the relentless march of discovery continues with the appearance of new drugs, new classes of drugs, new facts about old drugs, and new uses for some old drugs while other old drugs fall by the wayside.

"The Pharmacologic Management of Heart Disease" gives physicians who treat patients with heart disease what they need for these changing times. We offer a book that uniquely both covers the field of cardiovascular drug therapeutics and presents an integrated approach that goes beyond the scope of review articles on drug therapies. The book covers the entire spectrum of cardiovascular drug treatments. It begins with an overview of basic pharmacologic principles that are pertinent to the clinician, including the basics of determining cost-effectiveness. This is followed by sections on preventive treatments; ischemic heart disease; thrombolytic, antithrombotic, and anticoagulant treatments; congestive heart failure; and antiarrhythmic treatments. Each section provides basic information on drugs with all the pertinent details for the practicing physician. Special emphasis has been given to describing how to use drugs in practice, how to manage diseases with drugs, and how to avoid pitfalls in therapy. All chapters were written by leading experts, and sections are concise, practical, and authoritative. A serious effort has been made to offer material in a well-coordinated fashion, making this book more than a compilation of individual treatises.

We would like to give special thanks to our prestigious colleagues who have joined us in this effort. It is our sincere hope that this book will help clinicians provide the best possible care for their patients with heart disease.

We would also like to acknowledge Laurie Harrington and Lisa Worgul for their most valuable secretarial assistance.

# FOREWORD

From the 1960s to the 1980s the field of cardiovascular medicine developed remarkable and effective surgical and interventional techniques to deal with the ravages of congenital, valvular, and ischemic heart disease. Even end stage heart failure was approached with cardiac transplantation. During this period, important drug discoveries occurred and new agents had more targeted therapeutic use.

Since the late 1980s and into the mid-1990s, the leading edge of advancement has moved toward effective prevention and management through medication and lifestyle changes. A series of critical clinical trials has demonstrated unambiguous benefit of pharmacologic agents in reducing both the mortality and morbidity of cardiovascular disease. In addition, agents that had previously assumed a role in standard medical management were put to the test of modern standards by cardiovascular investigators. As a result, some frequently used agents were found to be without benefit, whereas others were found to be considerably and broadly effective in large patient populations. Future research for many of these agents will shift from clinical trials alone to effectiveness in broad populations and other health services issues.

At present, these therapeutic advances appear to have reached a point of reflection. The treatment mechanisms that led to the major advances came from epidemiologically established risk factors. They also came from a biochemical understanding of the genesis of these risk factors and of the mechanisms of disease and drug targets. Although advances in therapeutics of this nature will not stop now, it appears more likely that the next series of major advances will come from harnessing the techniques of molecular biology. Either new pharmacologic targets will be identified or new therapeutic strategies will be identified proximal to the gene product. The next steps will probably merge basic cardiovascular biology with that of other disciplines also concerned about cell growth, fundamental immunology, cell injury and death, and inflammation.

In primary and secondary prevention of ischemic heart disease and atherosclerosis, the major advance is the recent final proof of the cholesterol hypothesis. Previous studies of the cholesterol hypothesis did not have sufficient numbers of trial subjects to assess total mortality reduction from cholesterol lowering. Thus, doubts remained as to whether overall mortality would be reduced by lowering cholesterol. In the Scandinavian 4S study (4444 subjects), the cholesterol lowering agent simvastatin significantly reduced total mortality and morbidity in patients with ischemic heart disease. An extensive literature had accumulated in the period before publication of this book, raising questions as to whether mortality from depression, accidents, or cancer was increased by cholesterol lowering. No such excess mortality was found in the 4S study, however. In addition, cardiac morbidity was substantially and significantly reduced by treatment.

Regression of angiographic and ultrasonically detected lesions has also been demonstrated with cholesterol- and lipid-lowering drugs. A major observation within these studies was that acute coronary events appeared to decrease almost immediately on cholesterol lowering, even for individuals with only modestly elevated cholesterol levels. The lower rate of these events is believed to reflect reversal of the adverse effects of elevated cholesterol on vascular physiology and the pathobiology of atherosclerotic plaque. Lowering the level of cholesterol may immediately stabilize lesions, thus reducing their propensity to rupture, particularly within the coronary tree. A reduced occurrence of unstable angina or myocardial infarction is the remarkable result of lowering cholesterol for just 1 or 2 months.

Similarly, in the management of ischemic heart disease, there is broad evidence of the benefits of β-blockers in preventing adverse outcomes in nearly all phases of ischemic heart disease, from silent or asymptomatic ischemia, to acute myocardial infarction and its recovery, to long-term management of chronic stable and unstable angina. What is more, β-blocking drugs appear to have a profound effect on ischemic heart disease even when the stage of markedly depressed myocardial function and congestive heart failure has been entered. Although there is evidence for generalized benefit of β-blocking drugs in all forms of heart failure, the results in the long-term management of patients with ischemic heart disease and heart failure are particularly impressive. Unfortunately, the value of nitrate in ischemic heart disease has not been definitively assessed and proved via trials. However, the immediate benefits of nitrates on angina of effort and various ischemic chest pain syndromes make its use as an acute agent, as well as a preventive, straightforward. Finally, in the last decade, perhaps the greatest disappointment in the area of treatment of ischemic heart disease has been the calcium channel blockers. These agents remain useful as adjunctive agents when medical management is preferred and β-blockers and nitrates are either ineffective or contraindicated. Routine use of the calcium channel blockers is decreasing.

The importance of antiplatelet agents in both immediate and long-term management of acute and chronic ischemic heart disease is now established in several large-scale clinical trials. For chronic ischemic heart disease, the physician must always consider both aspirin and β-blockers as the important therapeutic agents unless there is a definitive reason for withholding their use. Our understanding of the role of these agents is clear and unmistakable. There is also promise for more potent antiplatelet agents on the therapeutic horizon.

Beginning with the definitive Italian multicenter study of 1985, Gruppo Italiano per lo Studio della Sopravvivenza nell'Infarto Miocardico (GISSI-I), thrombolytics have played the major role in treatment of patients with acute myocardial infarction. Their rapid use after the onset of symptoms has been a major focus of public and professional attention over the last decade. It is now established that the open artery hypothesis is correct: the faster a coronary artery occluded by thrombosis is reopened, the lower the mortality, the smaller the infarct size, and the less heart failure and myocardial damage will occur. An open artery perfusing even an infarcted segment is a benefit because a perfused infarct heals with a smaller scar and thicker wall than an aneurysmal ischemic infarct. Open arteries also provide collateral blood flow to other vascular beds. Investigation of these possibilities has been thrust into focus because of randomized trials showing that immediate angioplasty is associated with lower mortality and morbidity than thrombolytic therapy. There is considerable interest in even more rapid administration of higher doses of thrombolytic drugs as well as addition of other agents that may more quickly lead to clot lysis. It is not clear, however, that optimal use of a single thrombolytic drug is insufficient to achieve rapid and consistent meaningful thrombolysis of an infarct-related thrombosis.

Management of congestive heart failure has advanced from digitalis and diuretics as mainstays to regimens in which angiotensin-converting enzyme (ACE) inhibitors and other vasodilators form the most potent initial strategy. Digitalis may be useful in some patients, and definitive large scale studies are ongoing. Diuretics are clearly only symptomatic medications. There is new and major interest in use of β-blockers, as noted, not just in heart failure caused by ischemic heart disease but in heart failure in general, in which they will probably add potently to the therapeutic effects of ACE inhibitors. Moreover, study after study has shown that the use of inotropic agents other than digitalis adversely influences mortality from heart failure.

Finally, for antiarrhythmic drugs, we have had the shock of discovering that routinely employed agents affect mortality adversely. This is true when the goal is suppression of ventricular arrhythmias to prevent sudden death in patients with significant myocardial disease. Amiodarone and sotalol have a role in patients at risk of sudden death; in this situation the rationale is suppression of arrhythmias and prevention of lethal arrhythmias. The beneficial effects of these agents may be related to their crossover effects as β-blockers as well as some specific channel and membrane effects. The use of antiarrhythmic drugs during cardiac arrest and in the setting of atrial arrhythmias has also diminished. It is clear for cardiac arrest that the mainstays of treatment are early defibrillation, cardiopulmonary resuscitation, and use of epinephrine as an α peripheral vasoconstrictor to improve coronary flow. For atrial arrhythmias with normal ventricular function, suppressive antiarrhythmic drugs may be used with little risk and some measurable benefit. The more severe the myocardial disease, the more worrisome become the proarrhythmic effects of these agents in individual patients. The proarrhythmic risk must be weighed against the risk of serious consequences of atrial fibrillation on a patient-by-patient basis.

The volume edited by Kupersmith and Deedwania brings together leaders in the field to present their individual commentaries on the therapeutic advances. The authors are among those who have contributed most of the current generation of cardiovascular investigators. It is a tribute to the field of cardiovascular medicine that so many important areas of clinical interest are supported by presentation of definitive clinical trials. Many of the authors of this book are the individuals who have proposed or carried out the important definitive studies. Most chapters should be of particular interest for the practicing physician involved in management of heart disease. All the chapters provide up-to-date information in their respective areas and important practical guidelines regarding the use of pharmacologic agents. This book should greatly enhance the physician's knowledge and insight.

Myron L. Weisfeldt, M.D.
Samuel Bard Professor and Chair
College of Physicians and Surgeons
Columbia University
New York, New York

# CONTRIBUTORS

Joseph S. Alpert, M.D.
*Head, Department of Medicine*
*University of Arizona Health Science Center*
*Robert S. and Irene P. Flinn Professor of Medicine*
*University of Arizona*
*Tucson, Arizona*

William Virgil Brown, M.D.
*Charles Howard Candler Professor Internal Medicine*
*Director, Division of Arteriosclerosis and Lipid Metabolism*
*Emory University School of Medicine*
*Atlanta, Georgia*

Robert M. Califf, M.D.
*Professor of Medicine*
*Director of CCU*
*Director, Clinical Epidemiology and Biostatistics*
*Department of Medicine*
*Duke University*
*Durham, North Carolina*

Robert J. Cody, M.D.
*The James H. and Ruth J. Wilson Professor of Medicine*
*Assistant Division Director, Research Affairs*
*Division of Cardiology*
*The Ohio State University Medical Center*
*Columbus, Ohio*

Prakash C. Deedwania, M.D.
*Chief, Cardiology Section*
*VA Medical Center*
*Fresno, California*
*Professor of Medicine*
*University of California, San Francisco*
*School of Medicine*
*San Francisco, California*

Laura A. Demopoulos, M.D.
*Assistant Professor of Medicine*
*Department of Medicine/Cardiology*
*Albert Einstein College of Medicine*
*The Bronx, New York*

Gordon A. Ewy, M.D.
*Director, University Heart Center*
*Professor and Chief, Section of Cardiology*
*University of Arizona College of Medicine*
*Tucson, Arizona*

Rodney H. Falk, M.D.
*Professor of Medicine*
*Director of Clinical Cardiac Research*
*Boston University School of Medicine*
*Boston, Massachusetts*

John A. Farmer, M.D.
*Associate Professor of Medicine*
*Department of Internal Medicine*
*Divisions of Atherosclerosis and Cardiology*
*Baylor College of Medicine*
*Houston, Texas*

Richard Gorlin, M.D.
*Senior Vice President and*
*Dr. George Baehr Professor of Clinical Medicine*
*Department of Medicine*
*Mount Sinai School of Medicine*
*New York, New York*

Antonio M. Gotto, Jr., M.D., D.Phil.
*Professor and Chairman*
*Department of Medicine*
*Baylor College of Medicine*
*Chief, Internal Medicine Service*
*The Methodist Hospital*
*Houston, Texas*

Jonathan L. Halperin, M.D.
*Professor of Medicine*
*Director of Clinical Services*
*The Cardiovascular Institute*
*Mount Sinai Medical Center*
*New York, New York*

Karl B. Kern, M.D.
*Associate Professor of Medicine*
*Department of Medicine/Cardiology*
*University of Arizona*
*Associate Director, Cardiac Catheterization*
*University Medical Center*
*Tucson, Arizona*

Jack W. Kinch, M.D.
*Assistant Professor of Medicine*
*Department of Cardiology*
*Boston University*
*Boston, Massachusetts*

Joel Kupersmith, M.D.
*Professor and Chairperson*
*Department of Medicine*
*College of Human Medicine*
*Michigan State University*
*East Lansing, Michigan*

Ngoc-Anh Le, Ph.D.
*Associate Professor of Medicine*
*Department of Medicine - Lipids*
*Emory University School of Medicine*
*Atlanta, Georgia*

Evan Loh, M.D.
*Medical Director,*
*Heart Failure and Cardiac Transplantation Program*
*Assistant Professor of Medicine*
*Cardiovascular Division*
*Hospital of the University of Pennsylvania*
*Philadelphia, Pennsylvania*

Thierry H. LeJemtel, M.D.
*Professor of Medicine*
*Department of Medicine*
*Albert Einstein College of Medicine*
*The Bronx, New York*

Frank I. Marcus, M.D.
*Distinguished Professor of Medicine*
*Department of Medicine*
*Section of Cardiology*
*University of Arizona Health Sciences Center*
*Tucson, Arizona*

Roxana Mehran, M.D.
*Research Fellow, Interventional Cardiology*
*Department of Cardiology*
*Washington Hospital Center*
*Washington, D.C.*

William Parmley, M.D.
*Chief, Cardiology Division*
*Professor of Medicine*
*University of California San Francisco Medical Center*
*San Francisco, California*

Marc A. Pfeffer, M.D., Ph.D.
*Associate Professor of Medicine*
*Harvard Medical School*
*Director, Heart Failure/Transplant Center*
*Brigham and Women's Hospital*
*Boston, Massachusetts*

David G. Robertson, MD
*Assistant Professor of Medicine*
*Emory University School of Medicine*
*Atlanta, Georgia*

Kenneth A. Schwartz, M.D.
*Professor of Medicine*
*Michigan State University*
*East Lansing, Michigan*

Edmund H. Sonnenblick, M.D.
*Olson Professor of Medicine*
*Department of Medicine*
*Albert Einstein College of Medicine*
*Chief of Cardiology*
*The Bronx, New York*

Gary E. Stein, Pharm.D.
*Associate Professor of Medicine and Pharmacology*
*Department of Medicine*
*Michigan State University*
*East Lansing, Michigan*

Myron L. Weisfeldt, M.D.
*Samuel Bard Professor and Chairperson*
*Department of Medicine*
*College of Physicians and Surgeons*
*Columbia University*
*New York, New York*

# CONTENTS

## PART V
## Therapy of Congestive Heart Failure



## PART VI
## Antiarrhythmic Therapy

# PART I

# Basic Concepts

CHAPTER 1

# Principles and Practice of Pharmacotherapy

Gary E. Stein, PharmD, and Joel Kupersmith, MD

Precise drug therapy is crucial to patients with cardiovascular disease. Choosing a drug, administering it, and appropriately evaluating its response comprise a number of programmed steps to achieve maximal efficacy and minimal toxicity. These steps include selecting the desired effect, prescribing the appropriate dose and using standardized methods to measure wanted and unwanted effects in the specific clinical setting (1). In acutely ill patients as well as in those with chronic disease, even the safest, most beneficial medications can be harmful and difficult to apply. Conversely, even in individuals who are relatively healthy, many commonly used cardiac drugs, such as digoxin, have narrow ranges of efficacy to toxicity and require close monitoring.

In this introductory chapter we review the general concepts that form the underpinnings of rational drug therapy and allow for precision in pharmacotherapy. Subsequent chapters address drug properties, use, and monitoring in specific disease states.

## APPLIED PHARMACOKINETICS

A knowledge of pharmacokinetics (what the body does to a drug) and pharmacodynamics (what a drug does to the body) is important in managing patients for any malady. Each patient and each drug has its own individual characteristics, and the reasons that different patients need different doses of a drug are numerous and varied. Differences in absorption, distribution, metabolism, and excretion may lead to plasma level variation obtained with a given dose. Furthermore, even at a given plasma level, variations in response can be caused by changes in the number of available receptors, the development of tolerance, differences in disease severity, and other aspects of the patient's clinical state. It is therefore most important that the clinician have an understanding of the fundamentals of pharmacokinetics.

A drug regimen includes certain basic elements, namely, (1) the dose of the drug, (2) the dosage form, (3) the route of administration, and (4) the dosage interval. These components of the dosage regimen should be based on pathophysiologic and environmental factors in a given patient as well as on the known pharmacokinetics of the drug (2). Using clinical pharmacokinetic principles, the physician can then give each patient the most optimal dosage regimen possible. The discussion of pharmacokinetics in this chapter follows a drug through absorption, distribution, and elimination.

## Absorption and Distribution

With intravenous administration, a drug, of course, passes directly into the blood stream, but with oral administration, a drug must pass through two "stations" before entering the systemic circulation. It must be absorbed from the gastrointestinal tract into the portal circulation and it must pass through the liver.

The total amount of drug absorbed and the rate of drug absorption (in quantitative terms the "half-life" of absorption) are influenced by similar factors. These include the dosage formulation as well as gastric contents, gastric emptying time, and blood flow to gastric and intestinal absorption sites. When the rate of drug absorption is decreased, the time of peak concentration of drug occurs later and the peak concentration is lower. Even if the same overall fraction of drug is absorbed, such an alteration in absorption rate can have clinical consequences. For example, furosemide may not be as effective orally as parenterally in patients with decompensated heart failure due to an altered rate of absorption (3). Sustained-release products are intentionally made to be absorbed more slowly. These include products containing beads, wax matrix, and so forth: for example, ProcanSR (Parke-Davis, Morris Plains, New Jersey) wax matrix; Procardia XL (Pfizer, Inc., New York, New York) osmotic release tablet; and Nitrodur (Key Pharmaceuticals, Kenilworth, New Jersey) acrylic-based polymer.

After absorption, a drug passes through the portal circulation, and it is extracted by the liver and may be metabolized. The extraction ratio varies and for certain drugs may be so high that a significant amount of drug is metabolized on first-pass. For example, about 60–70% of propranolol and diltiazem are metabolized by the liver on first-pass.

Figure 1.1 is a schematic diagram of first-pass metabolism (4). Drugs that exhibit first-pass metabolism have certain features: (1) intravenous doses are much lower than oral, (2) if metabolites formed by the liver on first-pass are pharmacologically active, they play an important role when the drug is used orally and less of a role in intravenous administrations, (3) in a seeming paradox, food may at times and in some patients improve bioavailability. This phenomenon occurs because the increased hepatic blood flow that accompanies the ingestion of food may cause more rapid drug passage through the liver and thus less time for hepatic metabolism. (4) diminished cardiac output reduces elimination of these drugs. After the drug reaches the systemic circulation, there is still a high hepatic extraction ratio, i.e., the liver removes drug from the bloodstream as soon as it is delivered. For this reason, the amount of drug metabolized depends essentially on its delivery to the liver or, in other words, on the hepatic blood

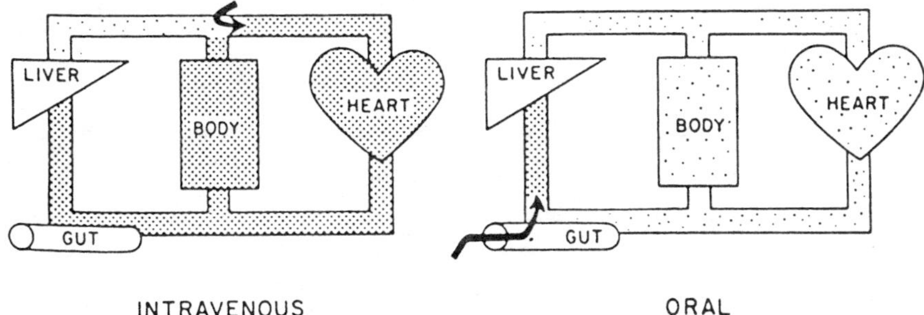


Figure 1.1. First-pass metabolism. *Right,* A drug administered orally passes from the gut to the portal circulation where most of it is extracted and metabolized, leaving a relatively small proportion to enter the body. Thus, bioavailability is low. *Left,* When a drug is administered intravenously, the liver is bypassed, with considerably more drug entering the body. Reprinted from Nies AS, Shand DG. Clinical pharmacology of propranolol. Circulation 1975; 52:6–15 by permission of the American Heart Association, Inc.

flow. If blood flow is reduced, there is less drug delivered and, therefore, less metabolized and eliminated.

*Bioavailability* refers to the proportion of drug that reaches the systematic circulation after absorption from the gastrointestinal tract and passage through the liver. Technically, it is defined as the area under the curve after oral administration divided by the area under the curve after the intravenous administration. If the area under the curve is identical for parental and oral administration, then the oral dose is completely bioavailable (100%) (5). The bioavailability fraction of the drug is influenced by the rate of administration, the dosage form, and the physiologic status of the patient. It is also influenced by the extent of hepatic first-pass metabolism as described earlier; i.e., drugs with extensive first-pass metabolism have low bioavailability.

Once the medication enters the systemic circulation, it undergoes simultaneous distribution to body tissues (compartments) and elimination by organs that clear the drug. The theoretical construct that describes this distribution for most drugs is the two-compartment model (6, 7) (Fig. 1.2), though for some drugs a multicompartment construct is more accurate. In the two-compartment model there is a "central" and a "peripheral" compartment each with its "volume of distribution."

The volume into which a drug is distributed after absorption of the initial dose is the central compartment. It includes blood volume and body tissues that are highly perfused, and it is also the compartment from which direct drug elimination occurs. The drug then is distributed into and equilibrates with the peripheral compartment, which involves the more slowly equilibrating peripheral tissues (Fig. 1.2). The rate of this process is the distributional, or $\alpha$, half-life. Equilibrium is achieved when both of these compartments are "filled" to the extent that they will be at a given dose; at that point drug dose equals its elimination.

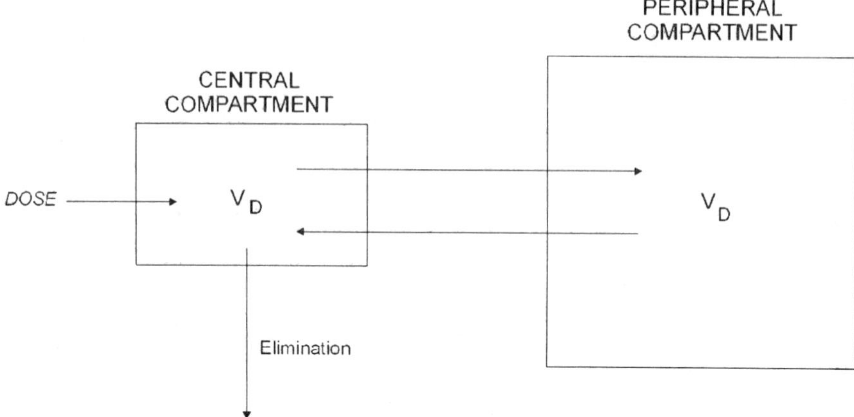


Figure 1.2. Schematic diagram of two-compartment model. This theoretical construct has a central compartment and a peripheral compartment, each with its volume of distribution ($V_D$). The initial volume into which a drug distributes is the central compartment, which generally includes blood volume in the highly perfused body tissues; it is also the compartment from which all drug elimination occurs. From the central compartment the drug may move into a peripheral compartment or be eliminated (*downward arrow).* The peripheral compartment includes the tissues with more slowly equilibrating tissue. The volume of distribution of the peripheral compartment depends in part on how much drug is bound to plasma protein and tissues. Drugs that are highly bound to tissue proteins have a high volume of distribution.

The size of the peripheral compartment's volume of distribution depends on how much of the drug is bound to plasma protein and tissues. A drug that is highly bound to proteins in tissue (e.g., digoxin) has a large volume of distribution. It is slowly removed from the body because most of the drug is inaccessible to blood, which carries it to the eliminating organs. On the other hand, a drug that does not bind extensively to tissues outside the vascular space tends to have a small volume of distribution whether or not it is highly bound to plasma proteins. Examples of drugs with relatively small volumes of distribution are warfarin, heparin, and furosemide. The volume of distribution of the peripheral compartment is important in drug dosing (see below) and factors influencing it are listed in Table 1.1.

In intravenous formulations, the rate of drug distribution ($\alpha$ half-life) can be very important. Some drugs have a rapid distribution phase and concentrations can quickly fall below the minimum effective concentration after the initial dose. This therapeutic problem is best illustrated in the case of lidocaine dosing. When an initial bolus or loading dose is followed by a continuous infusion (such as 2 mg/minute), plasma concentrations may still drop below the therapeutic range within the first hour of initiation of therapy (Fig. 1.3). This pharmacokinetic dip can lead to loss of efficacy and a possible mistaken conclusion that the arrhythmia is resistant to lidocaine therapy. Several dosage regimens have been devised to avoid

**Table 1.1**
**Factors that Alter Drug Volume of Distribution**

| | |
|---|---|
| Age | Drug interactions |
| Obesity | Hypoalbuminemia |
| Uremia | Malnutrition |
| Pulmonary disease | Heart failure |

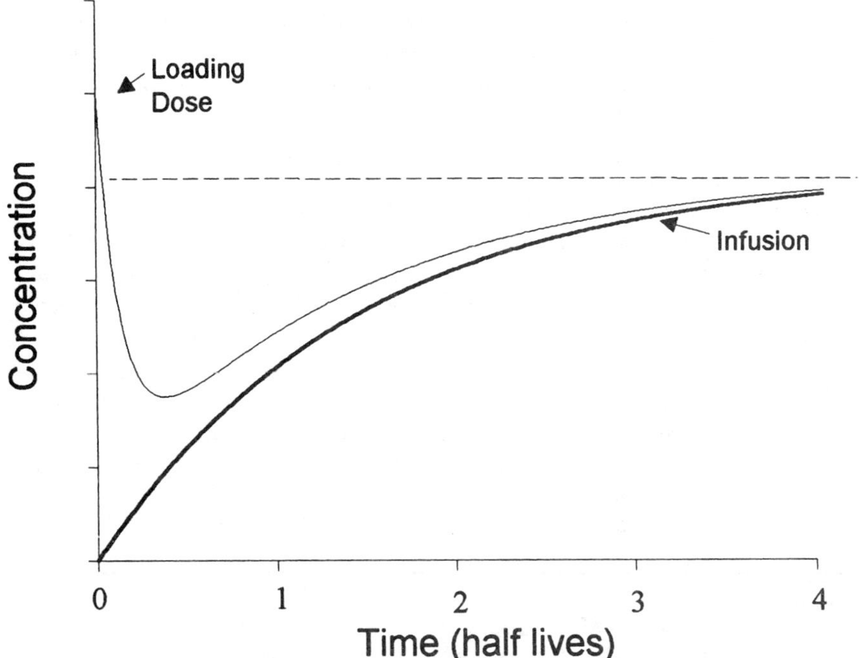


Figure 1.3. Plasma levels of drug with an intravenous loading dose followed by a continuous infusion *(thin solid line)* and continuous infusion alone *(thick solid line)*. Time pips on horizontal axis represent one half-life. A standard infusion will take four half-lives to reach 94% of steady-state therapeutic concentration. Steady-state is arrived at earlier with a loading dose, but there is still dip in serum level that can be avoided with multiple boluses of drug or more rapid continuous infusion. See text for further discussion.

this excessive drop in plasma concentrations. These regimens usually employ one or multiple small bolus injections after the initial loading dose, followed by the constant infusion. At times this method can lead to excessive levels of lidocaine and adverse effects; for this reason it should be performed cautiously (8). Another regimen involves a two-step infusion after the loading dose to maintain therapeutic plasma concentrations (9). This method, though more cumbersome, allows for less variance in lidocaine levels and reduces the risk of dosage errors.

## Elimination

Drugs are eliminated from the body predominantly by the renal route or the hepatic route. Rate of elimination is expressed as the elimination, or β, half-life. The concept used for overall quantification of a drug removal or elimination is *clearance.* Total body clearance of a drug assumes that the body acts as a drug-eliminating system and is defined as the volume of blood that is totally cleared of drug per unit of time. It is calculated by dividing the rate of drug elimination by its average plasma concentration. In regard to drug clearance, a distinction is made between renal and nonrenal (mainly hepatic, but also for some drugs lung, skin, and so forth) clearances. In this discussion, hepatic and renal clearances will be considered separately.

### *Hepatic Metabolism*

For most drugs the liver is the predominant site for transformation (metabolism), which usually results in a compound that is readily excreted into bile or urine, or both. Drugs may be metabolized by phase I (oxidation and reduction) or by phase II (acetylation, sulfation, and glucuronidation) reactions. Drugs are usually metabolized to inactive metabolites, but in some cases they are converted to active compounds, such as procainamide to N-acetylprocainamide (NAPA). Furthermore, some inactive metabolites excreted in bile are susceptible to hydrolysis in the gastrointestinal tract back to the active state, an effect that can lead to reabsorption and enterohepatic circulation of the active drug. Table 1.2 lists factors altering drug metabolism.

**Table 1.2**
**Factors that Alter Drug Metabolism**

| | |
|---|---|
| Age | Drug dosage |
| Gender | Drug interactions |
| Pregnancy | Malnutrition |
| Liver disease | Diet |
| Cardiac output | Smoking |
| Thyroid disease | Alcohol |
| Genetics | Renal disease |

For most drugs, concentrations in the liver are not high enough to saturate enzyme sites after therapeutic doses. However, for some drugs (e.g., phenytoin and aspirin) the number of enzymes available for metabolism is more limited. Here, hepatic clearance is a capacity-limited process whereby drug concentrations can become high enough to saturate enzyme sites. When this level is passed, the rate of metabolism will not increase proportionally to an increase in drug concentration, and increases in administered dose lead to greater than proportional increases in serum drug concentration (See Glossary, *zero order kinetics* and *first order kinetics*). Administration of these drugs must be performed cautiously. Figure 14.7, Chapter 14, shows an example of capacity-limited hepatic metabolism (for propafenone).

### *Renal Elimination*

Renal clearance of drugs and metabolites is variable from drug to drug. It can exceed or be less than filtration rate, depending on whether there is active tubular secretion or reabsorption. Tubular secretion is influenced by a number of factors, including the plasma flow to the proximal tubule, the activity of the secretion carriers, and the fraction of drug unbound in serum. Tubular reabsorption is influenced by urine flow, the concentration gradient of drug compared to blood that surrounds the tubule, and the intrinsic ability of drug to pass through tubular membrane as determined by lipid solubility. Greater lipid solubility of drug leads to greater ability to cross the tubular membranes. Lipid solubility is less for ionized drug. Therefore, the greater the fraction of ionized drug, the less its ability to be reabsorbed through tubular membranes and the greater its renal elimination. Ionization is, in turn, determined by the pH of the tubular fluids. For "acidic" drugs, there is greater ionization at higher pH and vice versa for the "basic" drugs. For example, the renal clearance of salicylate, an acidic drug, can increase at least twentyfold as urinary pH range moves from 5 to 8 due to the consequent greater proportion of ionized moiety.

In chronic renal disease, tubular processes tend to be impaired to an extent similar to that of glomerular filtration. Table 1.3 lists general factors that alter renal elimination.

### *Stereospecific Clearance*

A phenomenon that is worthy of note and has been described for some drugs is preferred stereospecific clearance of a particular enantiomer. That is, the *R* or *S* form might be cleared by the liver or kidneys at a greater rate. Since *R* and *S* isomers may differ in their activity, such preferential elimination might also have implications regarding drug activity.

Verapamil is a drug that displays stereoselectivity of both metabolism and effect as well as displaying first-pass hepatic metabolism. The calcium channel blocking properties of verapamil reside in the *S*-enantiomer while *R*-verapamil has slight local anesthetic properties that are probably of lit-

**Table 1.3**
**Factors that Alter Renal Elimination**

| | |
|---|---|
| Age | Drug interactions |
| Pregnancy | Dialysis |
| Renal disease | Protein binding |
| Urine pH | |
| Cardiac output | |

tle clinical significance. After oral administration, *S*-verapamil is more extensively metabolized by the liver on first-pass and thus relatively more *R*-verapamil and less *S*-verapamil enters the systemic circulation. With intravenous administration, both *R*-verapamil and *S*-verapamil enter the blood stream equally (10, 11). For this reason, at a given concentration of drug after oral administration there is relatively less *S*-verapamil and thus less effect on the atrioventricular (AV) node and its related arrhythmias than at the same drug level after intravenous administration.

## DOSING

### Initial Dose

Administration of the initial dose of a drug may be via one of three approaches. One may administer a small test dose to determine if there will be some sort of unexpected reaction, e.g., hypotension or bradycardia. This approach is commonly taken with β-blockers and angiotensin converting enzyme (ACE) inhibitors, among others. Second, one may administer a loading dose used to rapidly achieve a desired plasma level at the end of the first dosing interval. Third, one may administer the expected maintenance dose from the onset of therapy.

### Loading Dose

Loading doses are especially useful for drugs such as digoxin, amiodarone, and warfarin that normally take several days or weeks to reach a desired steady-state concentration (12). The loading dose is calculated on the basis of the following equation:

$$\mathrm{LD} = \frac{\mathrm{Cp} \times \mathrm{V_D}}{\mathrm{F}}$$

where Cp is the desired plasma concentration; $V_D$, the apparent volume of distribution; and F, the systemic availability (bioavailability). Thus, loading dose varies directly with the desired plasma concentration and the volume of distribution in which the drug must equilibrate (i.e., "fill") and inversely to bioavailability.

For example, in the case of procainamide administered to a 70-kg individual, the following is assumed (as per Table 14.3, Chapter 14):

Desired

$$Cp = 6 \text{ mg/L}$$

$$V_D = 2\text{L/kg}$$

$$\text{Weight} = 70 \text{ kg}$$

$$F = 0.9$$

Then

$$LD = \frac{(6)\ (2 \times 70)}{0.9} = 933 \text{ mg or approximately } 1 \text{ g}$$

## Maintenance Dosing and Drug Accumulation

Maintenance dosing can be accomplished by constant (intravenous) infusion of a drug or intermittent administration (oral or intravenous). One must decide the dosing rate and the dosing interval. The target average serum concentration for most drugs is in the middle of the therapeutic range, but for drugs for which this range is narrow, more precision in dosing is required. The therapeutic range may vary for an individual patient or an individual condition. For example, the serum levels of procainamide required to treat ventricular arrhythmias are generally higher than those for treating atrial arrhythmias.

An estimate of the elimination half-life (β half-life) is necessary to define the optimal dosing interval and to predict the time to reach a steady-state concentration. The elimination (β) half-life (β T 1/2) can be described by the following equation:

$$\beta\ T\ 1/2 = \frac{0.693\ V_D}{Cl}$$

where $V_D$ is the volume of distribution and Cl is total clearance. It is important to remember that half-life is influenced by both the volume of distribution and clearance. The half-life of a drug can change because of alterations in tissue or protein binding (volume of distribution changes) or because of changes in the function of organs that eliminate drugs, such as in renal or hepatic failure.

During each half-life, drug accumulates at 50% increments from the starting point to the new plateau:

| Half-life | Percent of Steady State |
|---|---|
| 1 | 50 |
| 2 | 75 |

| Half-life | Percent of Steady State |
|---|---|
| 3 | 88 |
| 4 | 94 |
| 5 | 97 |

Thus, close to steady-state serum concentration is achieved after about four half-lives of drug administration. Figure 1.4 shows drug accumulation for an intravenous drug with constant and with intermittent dosing. Oral drugs are, of course, given intermittently, though sustained-release products may be administered less frequently than every half-life because of their slow absorption during the dosing interval.

Once steady state is reached, the timing of the oral doses depends on the desired peak:trough ratio. Figure 1.5 and Table 1.4 show peak:trough ratios at various multiples of half-life. If the drug is given at intervals of every half-life, the peak:trough ratio will be 2:1. If it is given at two times half-life, this ratio is 4:1; at intervals of half of a half-life, 1.4:1.0. For drugs with narrow toxic:therapeutic ratios and a need for minimum effective levels to be maintained at all times (e.g., the antiarrhythmics), a narrow peak:trough ratio is generally desirable. In the case of antihypertensives in which levels can be

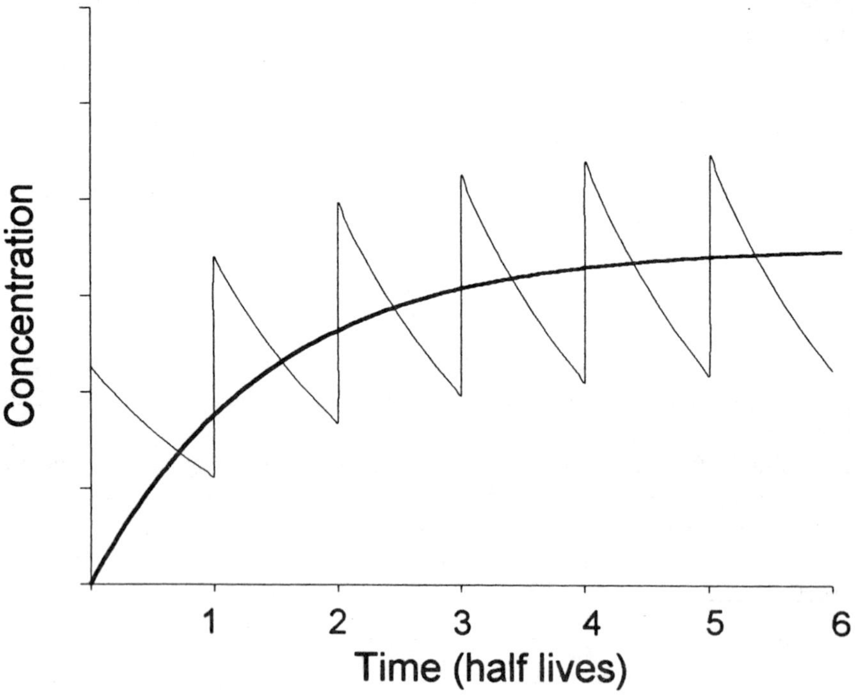


Figure 1.4. Variation in serum concentration with constant *(thick solid line)* and intermittent *(thin solid line)* dosing. See text for further discussion.

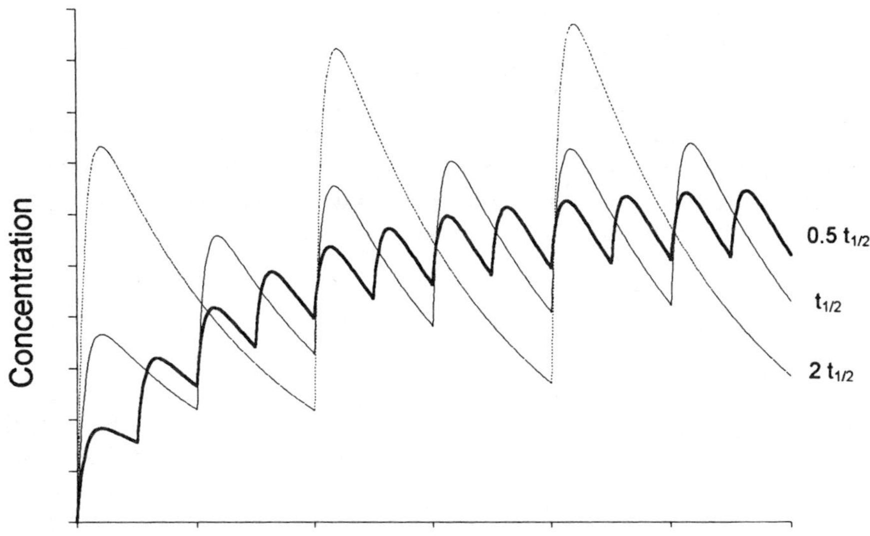


Figure 1.5. Serum concentration of drug administered with the same daily dose but at different dosing intervals. The *thick solid line* shows drug given at intervals of 0.5 of a β half-life, the *thin solid line* shows drug given at a full half-life, and the *dotted line* shows drug given at two times the half-life. Mean and peak trough levels vary with the dosing interval. (See also Table 1.4.)

**Table 1.4**
**Peak: Trough Ratios**

| Half-life ($T^1/_2$) Multiple | Peak: Trough |
|---|---|
| 0.5 $T^1/_2$ | 1.4:1.0 |
| 1.0 $T^1/_2$ | 2:1 |
| 2.0 $T^1/_2$ | 4:1 |
| 4.0 $T^1/_2$ | 16:1 |

somewhat more flexible, this situation may not apply. One should consider such circumstances in choosing a drug dose interval.

## PATHOPHYSIOLOGIC AND ENVIRONMENTAL FACTORS INFLUENCING DRUG RESPONSE

### Pathophysiologic Variables

Pathophysiologic changes in a variety of organ systems have important implications in the therapeutic management of patients. Age, obesity, genetics, and hepatic and renal function are important influences in this context (13).

#### *Age*

Physiologic changes known to occur with aging have numerous consequences for the pharmacologic management of elderly patients (14). Age-related decreases in drug absorption, distribution, metabolism, and elimination have been demonstrated. For example, cardiac output declines with age, resulting in a proportionate decrease in renal and hepatic blood flow (15), which influences the metabolism of several drugs. Digoxin, for one, exhibits age-related decreases in absorption rate, tissue distribution and renal elimination (16). Because the tissue distribution of digoxin can be influenced by renal function, both the initial dose and subsequent maintenance doses should be decreased appreciably to avoid toxicity in elderly patients.

Plasma concentration of albumin is often reduced in the elderly, which allows for greater unbound (free) drug and hence greater availability to tissues (17). These changes can cause aging patients to exhibit exaggerated sensitivity to highly protein-bound drugs such as propranolol, phenytoin, and warfarin.

The diminution in oxidative metabolism in elderly patients will not only slow the clearance of some drugs but, for drugs with first-pass metabolism, may also increase their bioavailability. The oral bioavailability of propranolol may be greater in elderly patients due to such a decrease in first-pass hepatic metabolism (18).

Aging also changes the physiologic responses to drugs. Elderly patients have decreased cardiac outputs, lower plasma volumes, decreased vasomotor tone, and decreased baroreceptor responses, all of which predisposes the elderly to hypotension from drugs that have the potential to lower blood pressure. Cellular loss and other physiologic changes in the central nervous system may contribute to an increase in acute confusional states observed in elderly patients exposed to certain cardiovascular drugs such as atropine, digitalis, and lidocaine. There are also examples of age-related alteration in the responses of other receptors. Warfarin sensitivity appears to be enhanced with increased age (19). Body composition changes with aging (see below), also influencing drug kinetics.

In summary, rational drug therapy in the elderly requires the incorporation of both pharmacokinetic and pharmacodynamic principles. Clinicians need to consider physiologic changes in absorption, distribution, and excretion as well as altered drug sensitivity when designing drug regimens in elderly patients.

### *Body Composition*

Body composition can be an important factor in the distribution and elimination of drugs. Again using the example of aging, the lean:fat ratio of body mass decreases as does total body water. Body fat may relatively increase by as much as 35%. These changes significantly reduce the tissue distribution of water-soluble drugs (such as digoxin) and relatively increase the tissue distribution of lipid-soluble drugs (such as propranolol) in the elderly.

Extreme obesity can influence the distribution of drugs in several ways (20). For example, an approximately twofold increase in the serum concentrations of α-1-acid glycoprotein has been observed in obese patients (21). Obese patients then may have a reduced pharmacologic response after administration of drugs that bind extensively to this protein (such as lidocaine). Increases in blood volume, cardiac size, cardiac output, and renal blood flow have also been observed consequent to obesity. These physiologic alterations can substantially alter the clearance of cardiovascular drugs such as procainamide (22).

### *Genetics*

Impressive variability in drug activity and kinetics can occur due to interindividual differences in genetic makeup (23). A noteworthy example is patients who have a hereditary resistance to the effects of warfarin (24) and thus exhibit suboptimal anticoagulation to the usual therapeutic doses of the drug.

Pharmacogenetic variability can also be displayed as altered capacities for drug metabolism. Phenotypic variations in the N-acetylation of some drugs will serve to alter their therapeutic efficacy as well as their side effects (25). Some alterations are also linked to the development of adverse effects. Genetically slow acetylators (observed in a high percentage of Italians and Greeks) are apparently predisposed to the development of systemic lupus erythematosus when treated with hydralazine or procainamide, since the parent compound and not the N-acetyl metabolite is involved with this untoward event (26). Genetic changes in oxidative metabolism have been associated with diminished first-pass drug metabolism (nifedipine), decreased elimination (metoprolol), increased elimination (flecainide), and decreased formation of active metabolites (propafenone).

Variations in response to drugs have also been observed among different racial groups. For example, black hypertensives have a reduced antihypertensive response to propranolol compared to white hypertensives (27). Conversely, Chinese men were found to have greater sensitivity than their white men counterparts to the heart rate and blood pressure effects of this particular drug (28).

*Renal Function*

Renal impairment influences pharmacology in many ways—directly via alteration in elimination or indirectly via impairment of many normal physiologic functions that occur in this state. There may be alteration in drug absorption via changes in gastric pH, gut motility, or edema (29) and in drug distribution via hypoalbuminemia, altered protein binding, or changes in body composition.

Regarding drug elimination, the clearance of a drug is determined by the sum of renal and nonrenal clearance. If only a small amount of drug is metabolized extrarenally, drug accumulation will occur as renal function worsens. Furthermore, active metabolites of drugs, such as N-acetylprocainamide, may also accumulate in renal insufficiency, contributing to excessive pharmacologic or toxic effects (30).

Drugs that are eliminated primarily by renal excretion are likely to need adjustments in dose or dosing interval as renal function declines. For many drugs, the changes in drug clearance vary along with changes in creatinine clearance, allowing some precision in the adjustment since creatinine clearance (CrCl) can be estimated by the Cockroft and Gault equation:

$$\text{CrCl} = \frac{(140 - \text{age})\ (\text{body weight in kg})}{72 \times \text{serum creatinine}}$$

In women, this result should be multiplied by 0.85.

Contrariwise, for an empiric approach to drug dosing in renal insufficiency, one may use published guidelines with consideration of individual physiologic characteristics. Use of drug assays to determine serum level, of course, enables more precise quantification of drug dosing in line with these changes in renal function.

Patients undergoing dialysis treatment fall into a special category. They require close attention to dose scheduling and the possible need for supplemental dosing for those drugs substantially cleared by dialysis (31).

*Hepatic Function*

Although hepatic dysfunction can influence the elimination of drugs handled by this organ, the kinetic changes are far less predictable than in the case of renal disease. The liver can affect both drug delivery to the body (first-pass effect) and elimination after a drug has entered the systemic circulation. Hepatic structural and functional abnormalities occur not only in common hepatocellular diseases such as hepatitis and cirrhosis but also in a variety of other pathophysiologic states, including congestive heart failure and metastatic and inflammatory diseases.

Hepatic disease states may alter hepatic blood flow, enterohepatic cycling, drug protein binding, and intrahepatic metabolic processes. The clearance of drugs can depend primarily on the rate of hepatic blood flow (in the case of the highly extracted "first-pass" drugs such as lidocaine and propranolol) or mainly on hepatic metabolism (for poorly extracted drugs such as diazepam, furosemide, and warfarin). In addition, a patient's sensitivity to hepatically cleared drugs depends not only on the severity of the hepatic disease but also on that patient's response to therapy in this condition.

For these reasons, the influence of hepatic disease on drug metabolism is often unpredictable in magnitude, exhibits large interpatient variations, and is not nearly as consistent as in those patients with renal impairment. Accordingly, there is no exact formula or specific dose adjustment that will precisely guide therapy in this state, and there is not an ideal liver function test capable of reflecting the severity of the underlying pathophysiologic problem (32). Tests that do indicate the potential for qualitative pharmacokinetics changes in drug metabolism include prothrombin time (absent vitamin K deficiency), serum albumin, and serum bilirubin. It has been suggested empirically that the dosage of highly extracted drugs should be reduced by at least 50% in patients with chronic liver disease such as cirrhosis (33).

### *Other Disease States*

A variety of other disease states can affect the behavior of drugs. Examples include cardiac failure, gastrointestinal disease, endocrine disorders, burn injury, and pulmonary disease. Congestive heart failure can affect the absorption as well as the clearance of drugs (34). As indicated earlier in the "Absorption and Distribution" section, this condition is especially pertinent to drugs with high hepatic extraction ratios (first-pass effect) in which drug metabolism and elimination are proportional to hepatic blood flow and thus cardiac output.

Gastrointestinal disease can either impair or enhance drug absorption (35). Achlorhydria (which is commonly found in elderly patients) may lead to increased (aspirin) or decreased (propranolol) absorption of drugs. Gastrectomy can produce malabsorption of drugs (such as digoxin and quinidine) as well as important nutrients (such as iron). Impaired absorption of digoxin can also occur in steatorrhea.

A reduction in gastric emptying and gastrointestinal blood flow as well as the presence of bowel edema in congestive heart failure can contribute to the impairment of drug absorption. With furosemide, for example, the extent of absorption is not affected by these abnormalities, but the rate of absorption is slowed, leading to a diminished clinical effect (3).

Common endocrine disorders, such as overactivity or underactivity of the thyroid gland, can alter the pharmacokinetics of certain drugs (36). For example, an increased dose of warfarin may be needed in patients with hypothyroidism and a decreased dose may be needed in hyperthyroidism, in both instances the result of an altered catabolism of the vitamin K-dependent clotting factors (37). Hyperthyroid patients are also relatively resistant to the effects of digoxin.

Severe burn injury, cancer, and acute myocardial infarction can affect drug pharmacokinetics by altering plasma protein binding (38). These disease states can be associated with increased concentrations of α-1-acid glycoprotein, a factor that may be especially important for drugs like propranolol and lidocaine. The rise in α-1-acid glycoprotein after acute myocardial infarction is associated with lidocaine accumulation, due to increased protein-bound but not free drug (39). Thus, the potential efficacy and toxicity of a given total plasma concentration of lidocaine may be misleading in this state.

Altered drug distribution has also been reported in pulmonary diseases. For example, the distribution of digoxin is diminished by approximately 50% in pulmonary disease. Moreover, quinidine exhibits higher protein binding in this patient population probably due to elevated α-1-acid glycoprotein.

Pregnancy can decrease both plasma albumin concentration and affinity to plasma proteins (40). These changes (as in aging, see above) increase sensitivity to drugs that are highly protein bound.

## Environmental Factors

Environmental factors are often overlooked when drug therapy is initiated, even though they play an important role in rational therapeutics. These factors include nutrition, drug-drug interaction, and noncompliance.

### *Dietary Factors*

The bioavailability of drugs can be increased, decreased, or not affected by food and nutritional status (41). Food-drug interactions can change both the rate and the extent of absorption (42). An extreme example of the enhanced effect of food on absorption has been observed with propafenone. The bioavailability of propafenone is increased more than 100% in the presence of food (43). Alternatively, food has been shown to reduce the bioavailability of captopril, atenolol, sotalol, and furosemide. The absorption of enalapril and isosorbide-5-mononitrate does not appear to be influenced by food.

For many drugs, food does not alter overall bioavailability but rather slows absorption and diminishes peak serum concentrations. These food-drug interactions may be utilized to improve patient compliance. In the case of nifedipine, an advantage of food-related slowing of absorption is that modifying peak serum levels also modifies adverse effects, such as hypotension and tachycardia. For quinidine and mexiletine, fewer undesirable side effects have been observed when they are administered with food. Food may also diminish the first-pass metabolism of certain drugs (See above "Absorption and Distribution" under "Applied Pharmacokinetics" ) but significant interindividual variation tends to occur. Conversely, starvation may lead to a dramatic rise in free fatty acids, which can displace highly protein bound drugs. This alteration will enhance the effect of highly bound drugs such as warfarin.

Specific dietary factors can also influence the metabolism and therapeutic effectiveness of drugs. It has been discovered that grapefruit juice can increase the bioavailability of nifedipine and felodipine (44). The bioflavonoids found in grapefruit juice appear to decrease first-pass metabolism. Ingestion of supplemental vitamin K contained in nutritional products or disproportionate ingestion of leafy vegetables are known to contribute to warfarin resistance (45).

### *Drug-Drug Interactions*

The literature is replete with information on possible drug-drug interactions, but only a small number have been studied carefully, and in some instances the ramifications have been overstated. Drug interactions can alter bioavailability, change the degree of protein binding, diminish the elimination of one or both drugs (pharmacokinetic interactions) or enhance or diminish a physiologic function (pharmacodynamic interactions). There are also several factors that can complicate both kinetic and dynamic drug interactions, such as disease state, dosage schedules, and genetic variability.

Not all drug-drug interactions are unwanted. Desirable interactions can be sought to increase therapeutic efficacy or to minimize toxicity, such as the combined use of low doses of thiazide diuretics and ACE inhibitors. Virtually all known adverse interactions are avoidable if the drugs are properly administered or if the mechanisms of the interaction are known. The drugs for which interactions are most important are those with significant therapeutic effects and low margins of safety, such as warfarin and digoxin.

### *Medication Compliance*

Possibly the most significant environmental factor in drug therapy is noncompliance with medication regimens (46). Despite documented improvements in patient awareness of cardiovascular health issues, estimates of medication compliance average about 50% for chronic diseases, and noncompliance to cardiovascular drugs brings about thousands of hospitalizations each year (47).

That even a minor alteration in compliance can have an influence is shown in Figure 1.6, which demonstrates that effects on serum level of missing just one dose of drug persist well past the time of reinitiation of therapy. On the other hand, an incorrect evaluation of compliance may lead to dosage increases, which may, in turn, result in unnecessary cost or

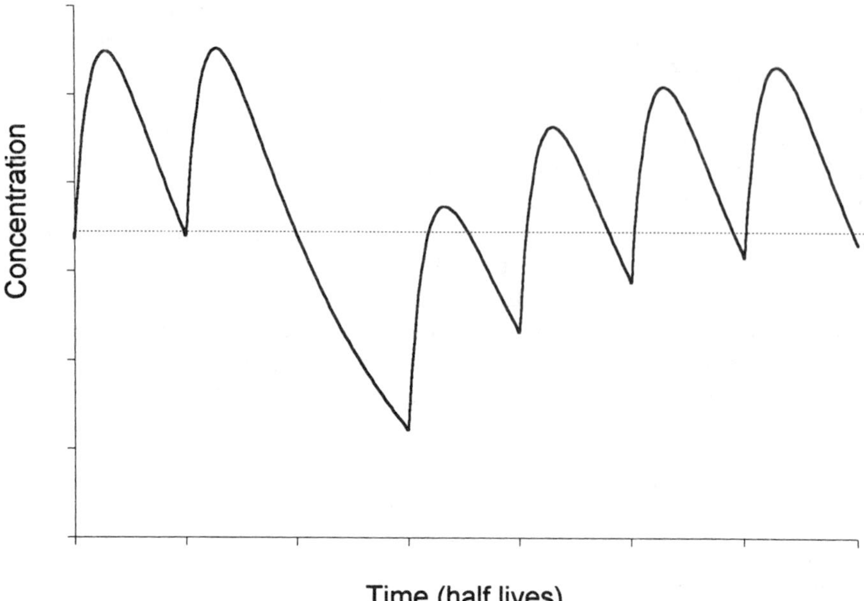


Figure 1.6. Drug levels *(solid line)* showing effects of one missed dose. The *dashed line* shows the minimum effective concentration for the drug. The first two serum peaks show steady-state during which the patient takes the drug every half-life interval and serum levels are always in the therapeutic range. The patient does not take the third dose, then resumes taking the medication for the fourth dose. Note the drug levels are below minimum effective concentration not only for the time of the missed dose but for a considerable time afterwards until steady-state is again achieved.

drug side effects. The clinical importance of noncompliance relates to the degree to which it interferes with achievement of the therapeutic goal. For example, medication noncompliance greatly contributes to the lack of control in hypertensive patients (48).

Compliance is reduced when the drug regimen is complicated, inconvenient, or of long duration as well as when there is no immediate relationship of medication discontinuance to symptoms (as in hypertensives). In patients with heart failure, medication errors have been shown to exceed 25% when two or three drugs are taken and to exceed 35% when five or more drugs are prescribed. In the case of the Lipid Research Clinic—Coronary Primary Prevention Trial of cholestyramine to lower serum cholesterol, the average compliance rate over the 7-year study was about 60% (49).

Although physicians are increasingly becoming aware that noncompliance is a significant health problem, they have considerable difficulty in predicting or assessing compliance in any individual patient (50). Methods to assess noncompliance tend to be unreliable, and moreover, individual patients rarely reveal their noncompliance. Checks on prescription filling or conducting pill counts are useful, but discrepancies between pill counts and physiologic measures used to determine consumption have been documented (51). Drug levels of pharmacologic markers are helpful, but their interpretation as a measure of compliance is complicated by pharmacokinetic differences among drugs as well as among patients (52).

One final and important note about compliance: time spent talking with patients and reviewing medication helps improve compliance considerably.

### *Chronotherapy*

Diurnal variation in physiology and disease has been the subject of considerable recent interest. The temporal association that exists between certain cardiovascular events and biorhythms may provide an interesting means for enhancing drug treatment strategies. The goal of chronotherapy is to optimize pharmacologic treatment via consideration of these temporal associations and thereby provide maximum effects at specific vulnerable risk periods (53).

Interesting observations in a number of clinical trials have highlighted the need for such consideration. For example, myocardial infarction has been observed to exhibit a circadian pattern with a higher frequency of occurrence in the morning hours and a second peak in the evening (54, 55). Patients who received β-adrenergic blockers in the morning were found not to have the morning cluster (56). Thus, it follows that long-acting β-blockers should be administered at night, whereas drugs with short half-lives should be given at appropriate intervals to be most effective in the morning and afternoon.

It is now established that aspirin can reduce the risk of myocardial infarction. The United States Physician's Health Study found that aspirin blunted the overall circadian variation of acute infarction, yielding a 60% reduction in its incidence during the morning hours compared with a 34% reduction for the remaining hours of the day (57). The protective effect of aspirin was particularly evident in the 3 hours immediately after rising from sleep.

Chronotherapy has potential for benefit in many cardiovascular diseases and more observations on this topic are sure to come forth.

### *Tolerance and Supersensitivity*

*Tolerance* can be defined as an initial favorable clinical response to therapy that abates during chronic therapy and cannot be restored with increasing doses. One of the most dramatic examples of drug tolerance in cardiovascular pharmacotherapy occurs with the use of organic nitrates. In the case of congestive heart failure, continuous delivery of organic nitrates for at least 24 hours will induce the onset of partial or complete vascular tolerance in approximately half of patients (58). A nitrate-free interval is needed to restore vascular responsiveness once a tolerant state is established. Factors that influence the development of tolerance to organic nitrates include dose, dosing frequency, duration of exposure, route of administration, and plasma level.

For catecholemines and adrenergic blockers, up and down regulation of receptors is important in the context of tolerance. With continued exposure to catecholamines, tolerance is ordinarily accompanied by a decrease in the number of adrenergic receptors. Conversely, treatment with adrenergic antagonists can lead to a supersensitivity of tissues to catecholamines due to an up-regulation of the adrenergic-receptor density (59). In some patients, when treatment with a β-blocker (e.g., propranolol), is abruptly discontinued, increased sensitivity to catecholamines becomes clinically evident, and unstable angina or myocardial infarction may occur (60). This rebound or withdrawal syndrome is apparently induced by the increase in the number of β-receptors. Supersensitivity and up-regulation have also been observed in patients with orthostatic hypotension.

## THERAPEUTIC DRUG MONITORING

Therapeutic drug monitoring (TDM), i.e., measuring and interpreting serum drug levels, is an aid in titrating an appropriate dosage for an individual patient. To be useful in therapeutic monitoring, a serum drug concentration should fulfill certain requirements (61), namely, the serum drug concentration must reflect the concentration at the receptor site, and the intensity and duration of the effect must temporally correlate with the receptor site concentration. In addition, there should be a therapeutic range (in steady state) in which there is a likelihood that the drug will be clinically effective and not toxic.

Although there is a clear therapeutic range for many drugs, it is often less than perfect and there is overlap both on the toxic end and the minimum effective therapeutic end (Fig. 1.7). For some drugs, e.g., antiarrhythmics, this range is relatively well defined. For others, however, e.g., digoxin, the overlap between ineffective, effective, and toxic concentrations can be considerable. Here, although serum level monitoring is still important, interpretation must be tailored to the individual patient. Another factor is that for some drugs effective concentrations may differ, depending on the particular condition treated. For example, as indicated above, it has generally been considered that the procainamide level required for ventricular tachycardia is greater than that for other arrhythmias.

For still other drugs, unfortunately there are no clear relationships between drug dose or concentration and drug effect. Furthermore, the effects of many drugs last much longer or bear no clear relationship to drug concentration. For example, the antihypertensive effect of several β-adrenergic blockers appears to last much longer than would be predicted by their elimination half-life.

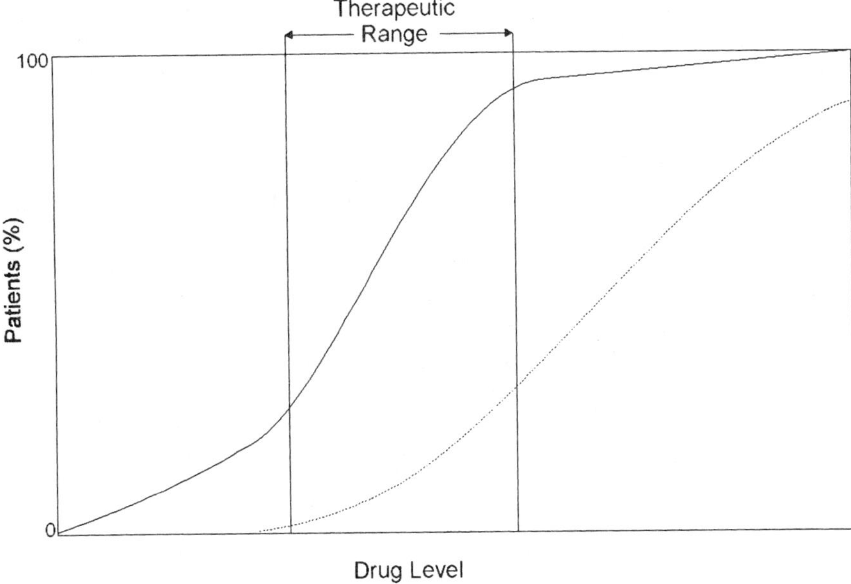


Figure 1.7. Schematic diagram of likely effectiveness *(solid line)* and toxicity *(dashed line)* of a drug in a population of patients. The vertical axis is percent of patients, the horizontal axis is drug level, and the central area shows the accepted therapeutic range. Although for most patients the therapeutic range is valid, for some toxicity occurs within this therapeutic range and for others effectiveness occurs below the range. The therapeutic range thus is an approximation.

## Optimal Sample Timing

Choosing an appropriate sampling time is crucial for the interpretation of serum drug concentrations. At a constant dosing rate, it will take four times the drug's half-life to attain more than 90% of the steady-state concentration (see above section on "Dosing"). After initiation of therapy with drugs with long half-lives and distribution phases, such as digoxin and warfarin, a considerable length of time will thus be required for steady state to be attained. The established therapeutic serum concentration ranges are based on samples collected after this phase, and therefore, sampling prior to attainment of the steady-state level may lead to premature and incorrect dosing adjustments (62).

A favorable time to obtain a serum level for oral drugs during steady state is just before the next dose. The "trough" level at this time is the minimum level that will occur and the most reproducible concentration during multiple dosing. If it is in the therapeutic range, then the patient will never have subtherapeutic concentrations (providing compliance is maintained). Peak or average steady-state concentrations correlate better with response or toxicity for some drugs. The time of peak concentrations, however, can vary depending on absorption rate, and many drugs are available in rapid and slow release formulations. The rapid forms usually peak in approximately 1 hour; however, slow release forms may take 2 to 4 hours to reach peak levels (Fig. 1.8).

## Active Metabolites

Many cardiovascular drugs are biotransformed into other compounds that are also pharmacologically active. When evaluating the therapeutic effects of these drugs, the clinician must take into account the relative contributions of all active compounds present in serum. Procainamide provides an illustration. Both procainamide and its major metabolite, N-acetylprocainamide (NAPA), have significant electrophysiologic and antiarrhythmic properties. The degree of metabolism of procainamide to NAPA is genetically determined and varies greatly among patients. Because NAPA is renally excreted, its concentration also varies greatly among individuals. The

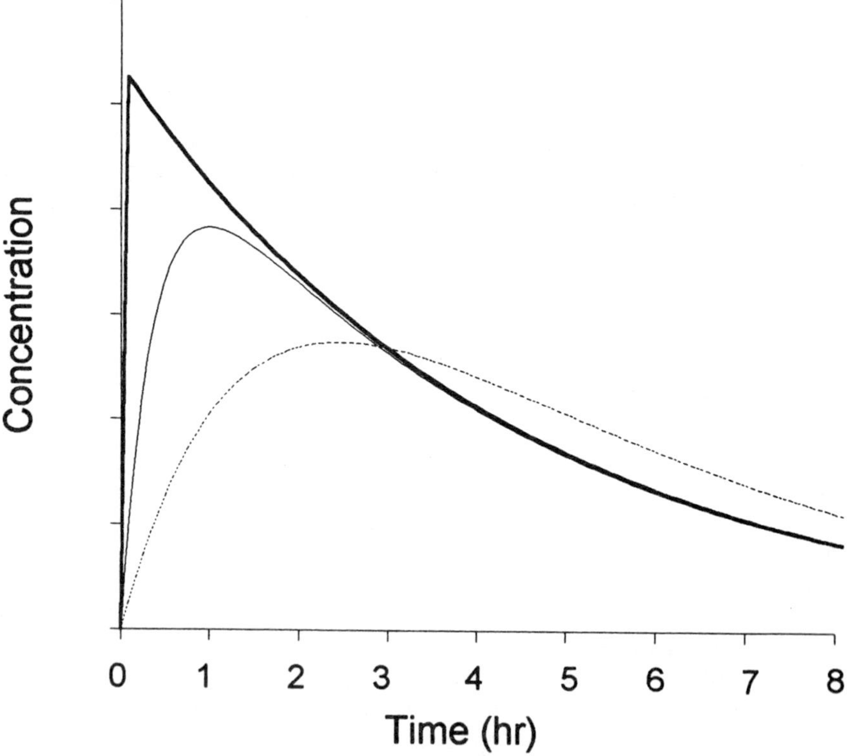


Figure 1.8. Comparison of serum levels after administration of a single rapid infusion of drug *(thick solid line)* and oral rapid *(thin solid line)* and oral sustained *(dashed line)* release. Elimination half-life is 3 hours, and absorption half-lives of fast and sustained release oral drug formulations are 7 and 70 minutes, respectively. Bioavailability of both oral drug formulations is 90%. Note delayed and blunted peak and more gradual decrease in serum level with sustained release oral agent.

failure to measure serum levels of NAPA may result in misleading conclusions concerning toxicity or efficacy. It has been suggested that the sum of both compounds be used to establish the therapeutic range, but this may not be accurate, as parent compound and metabolites have somewhat different pharmacodynamic properties (see Chapter 14).

### Protein Binding

The extent of binding of some drugs to plasma proteins may differ among patients. Although only free (unbound) drug can interact with receptors, free drug levels are not routinely monitored. Fortunately, for most drugs, the ratio of free to total serum concentration usually remains constant during a course of therapy. In some conditions, however, drug binding to serum protein may be substantially altered. For example, protein binding may be reduced in uremia and hypoalbuminemia or by another drug. Since the proportion of drug that is bound is inactive, these clinical states will lead to a downward movement of therapeutic windows and toxic ranges for the total serum drug levels.

The level of protein that the drug is bound to can also increase. As indicated earlier (see "Other Disease States" under "Pathophysiologic Variables"), α-1-acid glycoprotein is an acute phase reactant and rises in many conditions, such as myocardial infarction. It also binds many drugs, e.g., lidocaine and propranolol, and serum levels may be higher due to higher protein binding but with no change in free drug level and, therefore, effect.

### Summary of Therapeutic Drug Monitoring

In summary, obtaining a serum drug level is most useful but there is no guarantee that the information will be meaningful. The interpretation of drug concentrations can be influenced by factors that include sample timing, clinical status, pharmacokinetics, active metabolites, the analytic methodology used, and various peculiarities of the relationship of individual drug serum level to effect. This is not to minimize the value of serum levels in general but to maximize the chance of obtaining clinically meaningful and useful results when these factors are taken into account.

## METHODOLOGIES TO EVALUATE CONSEQUENCES OF DRUG THERAPY

This section will discuss various ways in which drug therapy is examined and its consequences evaluated. These ways include clinical trials, efficacy verses effectiveness considerations, pharmacoepidemiology, and pharmacoeconomics.

### Clinical Trials

The scientific standard for determining drug effect and toxicity is the randomized clinical trial, and our decision making on drug therapy should be guided by results of these trials. Clinical trials are the primary source of information about new drugs or new indications of older medications. It is gratifying for many clinical pharmacologists and others in both practice and academics that such thinking has finally taken hold among professionals and results of trials are carefully followed. Over the years, trial methodologies have constantly improved and become very precise.

A technique that has increased the usefulness of many clinical trials and has been used for evaluation of many treatments is metaanalysis (63). Although it is at times applied to observational studies, the most valuable use of this technique is in relation to randomized control trials. Metaanalysis is essentially a structured and systematic approach to combining and summing studies in literature review (as well as unpublished studies when appropriate) and thereby arriving at a larger overall database result to determine net effect (64). It is used when sample size of one study is too small and when there are qualitative differences in results among studies. When grouping studies, the technique takes into account the elemental design features of each study, including individual sample sizes and more subjective issues such as quality, extent of bias, and other aspects of study design.

Evaluating the effectiveness of intravenous fibrinolytic therapy to lower mortality in acute myocardial infarction illustrates the use and value of metaanalysis. Of the 24 randomized clinical trials included in an early metaanalysis (65), only 5 suggested any benefit from this therapeutic intervention in terms of mortality. Using metaanalysis, an overall reduction of mortality of approximately 22% was demonstrated. Large, multicenter, randomized trials later confirmed this finding. Other metaanalyses have covered a wide range of topics.

For a more complete discussion of clinical trials in general and metaanalysis specifically, various reviews are available (63, 66–70). As is seen in these reviews, considerable refinement of clinical trial technique is available, and yet despite the precision and value of techniques, including metaanalysis, it has recently become apparent that information derived solely from clinical trials may not be enough. Although such studies are still the foundation of drug therapy, more information is needed on therapeutic, epidemiologic, and economic aspects and consequences of drug therapy as it passes from trials into the population at large. We will now deal with some of these issues, which will become increasingly important in the future.

## Efficacy versus Effectiveness

Many trials of drug efficacy and safety fall somewhat short of providing the total information needed to make therapeutic decisions (71) for several reasons. First, the number of patients involved in the premarketing clinical trials may not be sufficient to detect the more unusual adverse effects, and the trials are often not long enough to detect delayed toxicity. Adverse effects of 1% or less are not reliably detected prior to marketing. Next, surrogate end points are often studied rather than the important clinical outcome. This problem was addressed in the Cardiac Arrhythmia Suppression Trial (CAST) (72), in which drugs that suppressed ventricular arrhythmias were surprisingly found also to increase rather than decrease sudden death and other mortality. Third, adverse effects of drugs on broad quality of life issues may be overlooked, even when they may be more important than the morbid events that are prevented. Fourth, in certain important patient groups, it may be difficult to predict the effects of new drugs, e.g, in the elderly, those with multiple illnesses, women, and minorities, as they have often been absent from clinical trials. Fifth, a statistically significant result, if small, does not necessarily mean that it is clinically significant. Sixth, over the course of time of a lengthy clinical trial, other information or approaches may come forth so as to make its results less relevant. Finally, compliance is often better in closely monitored trials than in the "real world."

An important distinction here may be the difference between a drug's *efficacy* and its *effectiveness*. Efficacy is determined in randomized trials and is essentially a measure of what a drug can do. Randomized clinical trials, however, have certain limitations, in that entry criteria tend to prevent inclusion of patients with comorbidity, low expected compliance, advanced age, and so forth. *Effectiveness* refers to what the drug does when it gets into the "real" (or postmarketing) world, i.e., when there is widespread use in a variety of situations that may have been incompletely evaluated in trials (often in patients with comorbidity, etc.). It is, therefore, a measure of what the drug will do. Effectiveness is more difficult to measure and thus far is assessed in observational studies, databases, and the like (73, 74). Recently, however, some clinical trials seem to have approached a determination of effectiveness. For example, utilization of broad entry criteria in the International Study of Infarct Survival (ISIS) (75) made it more of a pragmatic effectiveness trial (e.g., real world criteria for diagnosis of myocardial infarctions were used).

## Pharmacoepidemiology

The aforementioned considerations, the fact that information on dose options and non–Food and Drug Administration (FDA) approved use of drugs is often incomplete, and the need for rigorous postmarketing evaluation of the use and effects of drugs in large numbers of patients has led to the development of a new discipline in drug research known as *pharmacoepidemiology* (76). This approach utilizes epidemiological and like methods to study the effects and uses of drugs in the postmarketing phase and has made a number of contributions to more rational drug use.

Pharmacoepidemiology employs cohort, case-control, and like study designs to examine postmarketing drug use in large populations. These are observational and not controlled studies, but they are often derived from large automated databases that allow for efficient examinations of short-term and delayed drug effects in broad patient groups. For example, postmarketing surveillance of this type was used to quantitate the risk of first-dose syncope with prazosin. Local hospital and practice utilization review data may be helpful to provide preliminary information of this nature. Metaanalysis of observational data has also been used in these contexts.

Interest in pharmacoepidemiology is expanding and will continue to have an increasing impact on clinical medicine. For example, all hospitals are now required to document and evaluate adverse drug reactions that occur in their patients and to conduct ongoing drug utilization review programs. There is a need to expand the gathering of this type of information; however, there is also a need to develop appropriately rigorous methods to evaluate it as one moves from the bedrock of the randomized trial.

## Pharmacoeconomics

Because of the rising cost of medical care, economic analysis of drug and other treatments has become the subject of considerable interest. In this context the discipline of pharmacoeconomics has evolved. A pharmacoeconomic approach takes into account the entire direct economic impact of drugs on procedures, number of hospitalizations and length of stay, and when possible and appropriate, indirect costs such as lost work. For example, a drug for heart failure may be expensive but also reduce the number of hospitalizations, and delay the need for transplant. It may also ensure a more favorable work record. Such a drug would therefore have a very positive economic impact. Also taken into account are factors such as the type of reimbursement; e.g., a drug's total economic impact may be different in a managed care than in a fee-for-service environment (77–80).

In light of this economic interest, an important technique has also evolved to examine the value of pharmacotherapy and other treatment strategies: cost-effectiveness analysis. This technique examines the health outcomes of a treatment strategy compared to the resources that must be invested to adopt this strategy (74, 81, 82).

### *Cost-effectiveness Analysis*

Cost-effectiveness analysis combines clinical and economic information on clinical strategies into one formula. In this formula, the aggregate cost of an intervention is put in the numerator and divided by the effectiveness of the intervention in the denominator. Effectiveness may be expressed as number of lives saved or years of life prolonged (called *cost-effectiveness analysis*); it may be in years of life prolonged adjusted for quality of life (called *cost utility analysis*) or translated strictly into dollars (*cost benefit analysis*). [Note: the term *cost-effectiveness analysis* is often used as a rubric to encompass all three (74).] Results of analysis are most commonly expressed in cost per year of life saved (YLS) in cost-effectiveness analysis, costs/quality adjusted life year (QALY) in cost utility analysis, or net dollars in cost benefit analysis.

With the use of this technique, the value of various treatments, i.e., costs in relation to benefits, can all be considered on the same scale so that, for example, different pharmacologic treatments can be compared to each other as well as to interventional strategies. In addition, treatments of one disease, e.g., coronary artery disease, can be compared to those of another, e.g., Hodgkin's disease (74, 83–87).

**Methods of Conducting Cost-effectiveness Analysis.** In a cost-effectiveness analysis evaluating drug therapy, costs reflect total resources spent or saved. Here one adds the costs of the drug, hospitalization, and other costs associated with adverse effects, etc. From this expense, one subtracts savings resulting from drug-related prevention of events, e.g., fewer myocardial infarctions via lipid-lowering treatments or hospitalizations for congestive heart failure via ACE inhibitors. These net costs become the numerator of the cost-effectiveness formula. Costs of treatments not specifically related to therapy, e.g., cancer that may occur in the patients whose lives are prolonged by lipid-lowering therapy, have been variously included. In the denominator, one places effectiveness or the net benefit, which may be years of life saved, e.g., with β-blockers after myocardial infarction (88), ACE inhibition in congestive heart failure (89), or lipid-lowering therapy (90).

When performing cost-effectiveness analyses, one usually compares a given strategy to another and the results are then expressed as incremental or marginal cost-effectiveness. For example, one might compare lipid-lowering drug therapy with diet, as for bile acid sequestrants in the Lipid Research Clinic-Coronary Primary Prevention Trial (LRC-CPPT) (90). Here one determines the numerical difference in net costs of each intervention and divides by the difference in life expectancy. The difference is called the *incremental* or *marginal* cost-effectiveness. Thus, calculation of cost-effectiveness of lipid-lowering therapy (based on LRC-CPPT) (91) would be as follows:

$$\text{Cost Effectiveness} = \frac{\Delta C}{\Delta E}$$

$$\frac{\Delta C}{\Delta E} = \frac{\text{Cost}_{\text{Drug}} - \text{Cost}_{\text{Diet}}}{\text{LE}_{\text{Drug}} - \text{LE}_{\text{Diet}}} = \frac{\$}{\text{YLS}}$$

ΔC = Incremental cost
ΔE = Incremental effectiveness
Drug = Lipid-lowering therapy
Diet = Lipid-lowering preventive diet
LE = Life expectancy
YLS = Years of life saved

The results would be expressed in dollars/years of life saved.

In some instances, a strategy may be both cheaper and also more effective, i.e., it may save both dollars and lives. Such a strategy would be termed *dominant* (74). ACE inhibitor therapy for congestive heart failure falls in this category (89, 92).

In cost utility analysis, one takes quality of life into consideration. Generally, this is expressed as quality adjusted life years (QALYs), defined as the number of years of life experience multiplied by proportion representing the decrement due to less than perfect health (74, 84–86, 93, 94). For example, a year of life with severe angina may be worth only 0.7 years, one with with mild angina 0.9 years, etc. (95). Thus, if life expectancy is 3 years, with severe angina the corresponding QALY will be $3 \times 0.3 = 2.1$ years.

Other methodologic aspects in performing cost-effectiveness analysis include decision analysis, perspective targeting, discounting, and sensitivity analysis. Decision analysis is a fundamental technique used in cost-effectiveness analysis to quantify probabilities and outcomes. The Markov process, in which discrete time periods are considered to simulate the experience of a population as it moves through a disease process, is the decision analytic technique most commonly employed. For the lipid-lowering drug versus diet example above, the population is, of course, individuals with hyperlipidemia.

The perspective of a cost-effectiveness analysis refers to who stands to pay or reap a return from use of an intervention. For example, an analysis may look at costs from the point of view or perspective of society as a whole or from that of an HMO, hospital, insurance company, patient, and so forth. For analyses to be comparable to each other, they should take the broad societal perspective, but for specific purposes they may take the perspective of a specific entity or group such as an HMO. Perspective is discussed further in several references (74, 84, 86, 87).

Cost-effectiveness is not only a property of treatment; it also depends on the characteristics of the patient who receives the treatment. Directing cost-effectiveness analyses to specific patients (e.g., by age, sex, risk factors, etc.) is called *targeting.*

Discounting, a difficult concept for clinicians, is a method to devalue dollars spent in the future as well as future effectiveness to present value. Cost-effectiveness analysis usually considers time periods far into the future. Because of future uncertainties, there is time preference for current benefits and thus a reason to discount future costs and benefits. For example, there are many technological, medical, and economic uncertainties, e.g., technology may improve so as to make savings of lives by new means cheaper in the future, or other events may prevent a future death or, on the other hand, cause death to cancel the future benefit. Also, it is obvious that we would rather have a 1-year extension of life now than in the future. Discount rates of 3 to 5% are usually applied (more commonly 5%) to future costs and benefits (at times discounting is only applied to cost, but this is controversial).

Sensitivity analysis is part of virtually every cost-effectiveness analysis and is a method of overcoming uncertainty. Here changes and assumptions are varied and results computed. Sensitivity analysis addresses the question, what if? For example, what if the number of return visits after giving a drug for hyperlipidemia were five rather than two? How would this affect the overall cost-effectiveness? What if the expense of the drug were less than in the model? Sensitivity anaylsis is especially valuable in situations in which data are incomplete or inconclusive and expert opinion is relied on.

Table 1.5 is a list of cost-effectiveness values that have been derived for various drug therapies (81, 82). Such a list of cost-effectiveness comparisons is called a *league table.* It has been stated (in 1992) that a cost-effectiveness of $20,000 to $40,000/QALY is consistent with other funded programs such as hemodialysis and it may be considered "cost effective." Less than $20,000/QALY may be considered highly cost effective, $40,000 to $60,000/QALY borderline, $60,000 to $100,000/QALY expensive, and more than $100,000/QALY "unattractive" (96). As seen in Table 1.5, when interventions are subject to precise analysis, there are some surprises, e.g., preventive drug therapy can be expensive.

It is likely that in the future, cost-effectiveness analysis will be important in the evaluation of pharmacotherapy. It may be used to make policy and choose treatments (and here there are many ethical issues). It may also become an important consideration in drug pricing.

---

## GLOSSARY

***Active Metabolite:*** A product of drug metabolism that has pharmacologic activity (e.g., N-acetylprocainamide derived from procainamide).

***α-Half Life:*** The half-life decay representing the distributional phase, i.e. in a two-compartment model the α-half-life represents the half-life of distribution into the peripheral compartment. See also "β-half life."

***Area Under the Curve:*** The area under a serum concentration versus time profile (units are the product of concentration and time, i.e., μg/mL × hours).

***β-Half Life:*** The second half-life decay in a two-compartment model, representing the elimination phase. See also "α-half life."

***Bioavailability:*** The fraction of an administered dose that reaches the systemic circulation, defined as the area under the curve of oral administration divided by the area under the curve of intravenous administration.

***Central Compartment:*** A two-component model assumes two distinct areas of the body, a central compartment and a peripheral compartment. Drug initially and instantaneously distributes in the central compartment. This compartment includes blood and body tissues that are highly perfused and is also the compartment from which elimination occurs. See also "peripheral compartment."

***Clearance:*** A measure of the efficacy of drug elimination, defined as the volume of blood that is totally cleared of drug per unit of time. Systemic clearance is the sum of clearances by the individual eliminating organs.

**Table 1.5**
**Cost Effectiveness of Various Drug Treatments**

| Strategy | Condition | Patient Targeting | \$/YLS[a] \$/QALY*[a] |
|---|---|---|---|
| Lovastatin, 20 mg/day (97) | Hyperlipidemia[f] | 2°, chol ≥ 250 mg/dL♂, ages 45–54 | Dominant[b] |
| Enalapril (89) | CHF | EF ≤ 0.35 | Dominant[b] |
| β-Blocker (88) | Post MI | High risk | 3,800 |
| Anticoagulant (98) | Mitral stenosis | AF, ♀, age 35 | 4,400* |
| Lovastatin, 20 mg/day (97) | Hyperlipidemia[f] | 2°, chol ≥ 250 mg/dL♀, ages 45–54 | 4,900 |
| CABG surgery (99) | Chronic CAD | Severe angina<br>Left main disease[c] | 9,600* |
| Endocardial ICD (100) | VT/VF | | 15,500 |
| Propranolol (101) | Hypertension | | 17,700 |
| β-Blocker (88) | MI | Low risk | 20,450 |
| Lovastatin, 20 mg/day (97) | Hyperlipidemia[f] | 1°, chol ≥ 300 mg/dL, 3 RF, ♂, ages 55–64 | 21,200 |
| Hydrochlorothiazide (101) | Hypertension | | 26,600 |
| Streptokinase (102) | Acute MI | Age ≥ 75 | 28,300 |
| Captopril (103) | Post MI | EF ≤ 0.40 | 29,800*[d] |
| Oat bran (104) | Hyperlipidemia[f] | LRC-CPPT[e] extrapolated data | 33,100 |
| Epicardial ICD (100) | VT/VF | | 33,100 |
| CABG surgery (99) | Chronic CAD | Severe angina, 1 VD[c] | 76,400* |
| Lovastatin, 20 mg/day (97) | Hyperlipidemia[f] | 1°, chol ≥ 300 mg/dL<br>No RF, ♂, ages 55–64 | 82,000 |
| Captopril (88) | Hypertension | | 116,900[d] |
| Cholestyramine bulk drug (104) | Hyperlipidemia[f] | LRC-CPPT[e] | 121,000 |

**Table 1.5—*continued***
**Cost Effectiveness of Various Drug Treatments**

| Strategy | Condition | Patient Targeting | \$/YLS[a] \$/QALY*[a] |
|---|---|---|---|
| Anticoagulant (98) | Mitral Stenosis | NSR, ♀, age 35 | 182,400* |
| CABG surgery (99) | Chronic CAD | Mild angina, 1 VD[c] | 1,196,800* |
| Lovastatin, 20 mg/day (97) | Hyperlipidemia[f] | 1°, chol ≥ 300 mg/dL No RF, ♀, ages 35–44 | 2,121,400 |

[a]All values updated to 1994 dollars (105).
[b]Saves both money and lives.
[c]55-year-old man; EF ≥ 0.40.
[d]As patents on angiotensin converting enzyme inhibitors expire, the price of these drugs should decrease, leading to greater cost effectiveness.
[e]LRC-CPPT (Lipid Research Clinic-Coronary Primary Prevention Trial) patients were men, average age 48 years, 38% smokers, cholesterol ≥ 265 mg/dL, low-density lipoprotein ≥ 190 mg/dL.
[f]QALY; other values in column are YLS.
Abbreviations: 1° = Primary prevention; 2° = Secondary prevention; AF = atrial fibrillation; CABG = coronary artery bypass grafting; CAD = coronary artery disease; CHF = congestive heart failure; Chol = pretreatment cholesterol; ICD = implantable cardioverter defibrillator; Diast = diastolic blood pressure; EF = ejection fraction; MI = myocardial infarction; NSR = normal sinus rhythm; NYHA = New York Heart Association; QALY = quality adjusted life year; RF = other risk factors; VD = vessel disease; VF = ventricular fibrillation; VT = ventricular tachycardia; YLS = years of life saved.
Adapted with permission from Kupersmith J, Holmes-Rovner M, Hogan A, et al. Cost effectiveness analysis in heart disease. Part III: Ischemia, congestive heart failure and arrhythmias. Prog Cardiovasc Dis 1995; 37:307–346.

***Distribution Phase:*** The time in which drug diffuses or is transferred from intravascular to extravascular space (body tissue).

***Dose-Dependent Kinetics:*** See "zero order kinetics."

***Elimination Phase:*** The time to remove or transform drug in the systemic circulation.

***First Order Kinetics:*** A kinetic system in which the rate of drug metabolized or excreted is directly proportional to the concentration of that drug. Thus, the elimination half-life is constant and independent of dose or serum drug concentration.

***First-Pass Metabolism:*** The removal of a large fraction of drug dose by the liver before it reaches the systemic circulation.

***Half-Life:*** The time required for a concentration to be reduced to one-half of the original value.

***Hepatic Extraction:*** The fraction of drug in blood entering the liver that is removed by metabolism or biliary excretion.

***Loading Dose:*** A dose of drug given at the onset of therapy to rapidly provide a therapeutic level.

***Maintenance Dose:*** The dose of drug required to replace the amount of drug lost from the body so that a desired therapeutic effect can be maintained.

***Minimum Effective Concentration:*** The lowest drug concentration necessary to produce a desired pharmacologic effect; the lower limit of a therapeutic range.

***Peripheral Compartment:*** The sum of all body regions to which drug eventually distributes but is not in instantaneous equilibrium. See also "central compartment."

***Pharmacodynamics:*** The study of the biochemical and physiological effects of drugs and their mechanisms of action.

***Pharmacoeconomics:*** An approach that takes into account the entire economic impact of drug therapy.

***Pharmacokinetics:*** Study of the absorption, distribution, metabolism, and elimination of a drug and its metabolites in the body.

***Pharmacoepidemiology:*** The application of epidemiologic knowledge, methods, and reasoning to the study of the effects and uses of drugs in populations.

***Protein Binding:*** The reversible interaction between drug and protein in serum or tissue.

***Steady State:*** A condition of equilibrium achieved during chronic dosing when the rate of drug input equals the rate of drug elimination.

***Stereospecific Metabolism:*** The differential biotransformation or elimination of optical isomers (i.e., D or *S* or + or − form) of a drug.

***Tolerance:*** A state in which it is necessary to take progressively larger doses of drug to achieve the same degree of effect.

***Volume of Distribution:*** A hypothetical volume of body fluid that would be required to dissolve the total amount of drug at the same concentration as that found in the blood.

***Zero Order Kinetics:*** A kinetic system in which enzymes responsible for metabolism are saturable and kinetics are dose dependent. Thus, drug is metabolized at a constant rate independent of concentration, a true half-life does not exist, and there are steep increases in serum concentration once enzymes are saturated.

---

## REFERENCES

1. Williams RL. Dosage regimen design: pharmacodynamic considerations. J Clin Pharmacol 1992; 32:597–602.
2. Thompson GA. Dosage regimen design: a pharmacokinetics approach. J Clin Pharmacol 1992; 32:210–214.
3. Vasko MR, Brown-Cartwright D, Knochel JP, et al. Furosemide absorption altered in decompensated congestive heart failure. Ann Intern Med 1985; 102:314–318.
4. Nies AS, Shand DG. Clinical pharmacology of propranolol. Circulation 1975; 52:6–15.
5. Gibaldi M, Levy G. Pharmacokinetics in clinical practice: concepts. JAMA 1976; 235:1864–1868.
6. Greenblatt DJ, Koch-Weser J. Medical intelligence: drug therapy—clinical pharmacokinetics, Part I. N Engl J Med 1975; 14:702–705.
7. Greenblatt DJ, Koch-Weser J. Medical intelligence: drug therapy—clinical pharmacokinetics, Part II. N Engl J Med 1975; 19:964–969.
8. Stargel WW, Shand DG, Routledge PA, et al. Clinical comparison of rapid infusion and multiple injection methods for lidocaine loading. Am Heart J 1981; 102:872–876.
9. Riddell JG, McAllister CB, Wilkinson GR, et al. A new method for constant plasma drug concentrations: application to lidocaine. Ann Intern Med 1984; 100:25–28.
10. Eichelbaum B, Birkel P, Grube E, et al. Effects of verapamil on P-R intervals in relation to verapamil plasma levels following single i.v. and oral administration and during chronic treatment. Klin Wochenschr 1980; 58:919–925.
11. Echizen H, Vogelgesang B, Eichelbaum M. Effects of d,l-verapamil on atrioventricular conduction in relation to its stereoselective first-pass metabolism. Clin Pharmacol Ther 1985;38:71–76.
12. Gibaldi M, Levy G. Pharmacokinetics in clinical practice: applications. JAMA 1976; 235:1987–1992.
13. Koup JR. Disease states and drug pharmacokinetics. J Clin Pharmacol 1989; 29: 674–679.
14. Yuen GJ. Altered pharmacokinetics in the elderly. Clin Geriatr Med 1990; 6:257–267.
15. Wei JY. Age and the cardiovascular system. N Engl J Med 1992; 327:1735–1739.
16. Cusack B, Kelly JG, O'Malley K, et al. Digoxin in the elderly: pharmacokinetic consequences of old age. Clin Pharmacol Ther 1979; 25:772–776.
17. Greenblatt DJ. Reduced serum albumin in the elderly: a report from the Boston Collaborative Drug Surveillance Program. J Am Geriatr Soc 1979; 27:20–22.
18. Castleden CM, George CF. The effect of aging on the hepatic clearance of propranolol. Br J Clin Pharmacol 1979; 7:49–54.

19. Desforges JF. Management of drug therapy in the elderly. N Engl J Med 1989; 321: 303–309.
20. Blouin RA, Kolpek JH, Mann HJ. Influence of obesity on drug disposition. Clin Pharm 1987; 6:706–714.
21. Benedek IH, Fiske WD, Griffen WO, et al. Serum alpha 1-acid glycoprotein and the binding of drugs in obesity. Br J Clin Pharmacol 1983; 16:751–754.
22. Christoff PB, Conti DR, Naylor C, et al. Procainamide disposition in obesity. Drug Intell Clin Pharm 1983; 17:516–522.
23. Guttendorf RJ, Wedlund PJ. Genetic aspects of drug disposition and therapeutics. J Clin Pharmacol 1992; 32:107–117.
24. Alving BM, Strickler MP, Knight RD, et al. Hereditary warfarin resistance. Arch Intern Med 1985; 145:499–501.
25. May DG. Genetic differences in drug disposition. J Clin Pharmacol 1994; 34: 881–897.
26. Reidenberg MM, Levy M, Drayer DE, et al. Acetylator phenotype in idiopathic systemic lupus erythematosus. Arthritis Rheum 1980; 23:569–573.
27. Walle T, Byington RP, Furberg CD, et al. Biologic determinants of propranolol disposition: results from 1308 patients in the Beta-Blocker Heart Attack Trial. Clin Pharmacol Ther 1985; 38:509–518.
28. Zhou HH, Koshakji RP, Silberstein DJ, et al. Racial differences in drug response: altered sensitivity to and clearance of propranolol in men of Chinese descent as compared with American whites. N Engl J Med 1989; 320:565–570.
29. Talbert RL. Drug dosing in renal insufficiency. J Clin Pharmacol 1994; 34:99–110.
30. Gibson TP, Atkinson AJ, Mutusik E, et al. Kinetics of procainamide and N-acetylprocainamide in renal failure. Kidney Int 1977; 12:422–429.
31. Bennett WM. Guide to drug dosage in renal failure. Clin Pharmacokinet 1988; 15:326–354.
32. Chopra S, Griffin PH. Laboratory tests and diagnostic procedures in evaluation of liver disease. Am J Med 1985; 79:221–230.
33. Williams RL. Drug administration in hepatic disease. N Engl J Med 1983; 309: 1616–1622.
34. Shammas FV, Dickstein K. Clinical pharmacokinetics in heart failure: an updated review. Clin Pharmacokinet 1988; 15:94–113.
35. Parsons RL. Drug absorption in gastrointestinal disease with particular reference to malabsorption syndromes. Clin Pharmacokinet 1977; 2:45–60.
36. O'Connor P, Feely J. Clinical pharmacokinetics and endocrine disorders: therapeutic implications. Clin Pharmacokinet 1987; 13:345–364.
37. Shenfield GM. Influence of thyroid dysfunction on drug pharmacokinetics. Clin Pharmacokinet 1981; 6:275–297.
38. Bodenham A, Shelly MP, Park GR. The altered pharmacokinetics and pharmacodynamics of drugs commonly used in critically ill patients. Clin Pharmacokinet 1988; 14:347–373.
39. Routledge PA, Stargel WW, Wagner GS, et al. Increased alpha-1-acid glycoprotein and lidocaine disposition in myocardial infarction. Ann Intern Med 1980; 93:701–704.
40. Cumming AJ. A survey of pharmacokinetics data from pregnant women. Clin Pharmacokinet 1983; 8:344–354.
41. Anderson KE. Influences of diet and nutrition on clinical pharmacokinetics. Clin Pharmacokinet 1988; 14:325–346.
42. Neuvonem PJ, Kivisto KT. The clinical significance of food-drug interactions: a review. Med J Aust 1989; 150:36–40.
43. Axelson JE, Chan GL-Y, Kirsten ED, et al. Food increases the bioavailability of propanfenone. Br J Clin Pharmacol 1987; 23:735–741.
44. Bailey DG, Spence JD, Munoz C, et al. Interactions of citrus juices with felodipine and nifedipine. Lancet 1991; 337:268–269.
45. O'Reilly R, Rytand D. Resistance to warfarin due to unrecognized vitamin K supplementation. N Engl J Med 1980; 303:160–161.
46. Eraker SA, Kirscht JP, Becker MH. Understanding and improving patient compliance. Ann Intern Med 1984; 100:258–268.

47. Feldman JA, DeTullio PL. Medication noncompliance: an issue to consider in the drug selection process. Hosp Formul 1994; 29:204–211.
48. Sackett DL. Hypertension: V. Compliance with antihypertensive therapy. Can J Public Health 1980; 71:153–156.
49. Efrom B, Feldman D. Compliance as an explanatory variable in clinical trials. J Am Stat Assoc 1991; 86:9–26.
50. Roth HP, Caron HS. Accuracy of doctors' estimates and patients' statements on adherence to a drug regimen. Clin Pharmacol Ther 1978; 23:361–370.
51. Stephenson BJ, Rowe BH, Haynes RB, et al. Is this patient taking the treatment as prescribed? JAMA 1993; 269:2779–2781.
52. Levy G. A pharmacokinetics perspective on medication noncompliance. Clin Pharmacol Ther 1993; 54:242–244.
53. Manfredini R, Gallerani M, Salmi R, et al. Circadian rhythms and the heart: implications for chromotherapy of cardiovascular diseases. Clin Pharmacol Ther 1994; 56:244–247.
54. Peters RW, Mitchell LB, Brooks MM, et al. Circadian pattern of arrhythmia death in patients receiving flecainide or moricizine in the Cardiac Arrhythmia Suppression Trial (CAST). J Am Coll Cardiol 1994; 23:283–289.
55. Muller JE, Stone PH, Turi ZG, et al. Circadian variation in the frequency of onset of acute myocardial infarction. N Engl J Med 1985; 313:1315–1322.
56. Willich SN, Linderer T, Wegscheider K, et al. Increased morning incidence of myocardial infarction in the ISAM study: absence with prior β-adrenergic blockade. Circulation 1989; 80:853–858.
57. Ridker PM, Manson JE, Buring JE, et al. Circadian variation of acute myocardial infarction and the effect of low dose aspirin in a randomized trial of physicians. Circulation 1990; 82:897–902.
58. Elkayam U. Tolerance to organic nitrates: evidence, mechanisms, clinical relevance, and strategies for prevention. Ann Intern Med 1991; 114:667–677.
59. Motulsky HJ, Insel PA. Adrenergic receptors in man. N Engl J Med 1982; 307:18–29.
60. Shand DG, Wood AJJ. Propranolol withdrawal syndrome—why? Circulation 1978; 58:202–203.
61. Friedman H, Greenblatt DJ. Rational therapeutic drug monitoring. JAMA 1986; 256:2227–2233.
62. Spector R, Park GD, Johnson GF, et al. Therapeutic drug monitoring. Clin Pharmacol Ther 1988; 43:345–353.
63. Levine MAH. A guide for assessing pharmacoepidemiologic studies. Pharmacotherapy 1992; 12:232–237.
64. L'abbe KA, Detsky AS, O'Rourke K. Meta-analysis in clinical research. Ann Intern Med 1987; 107:224–233.
65. Yusuf S, Collins R, Peto R, et al. Intravenous and intracoronary fibrinolytic therapy in acute myocardial infarction: overview of results on mortality, reinfarction and side effects from 33 randomized controlled trials. Eur Heart J 1985; 6:556–585.
66. Pak C, Adams P. Techniques of patient-oriented research. New York: Raven Press, 1994.
67. Shapiro SH, Louis TA. Clinical trials: issues and approaches. New York: Marcel Dekker, 1983.
68. Iber FL. Conducting clinical trials. New York: Plenum, 1987.
69. Pocock SJ. Clinical trials: a practical approach. New York: John Wiley & Sons, 1983.
70. Spilker B. Guide to clinical trials. New York: Raven Press, 1991.
71. Ray WA, Griffin MR. Evaluating drugs after their approval for clinical use. N Engl J Med 1993; 329:2029–2032.
72. The Cardiac Arrhythmia Suppression Trial (CAST). Preliminary report: effect of encainide and flecainide on mortality in randomized trial of arrhythmia suppression after myocardial infarction. N Engl J Med 1989; 321:406–412.
73. Diamond GA, Denton TA: Alternative perspectives on the biased foundation of medical technology assessment. Ann Intern Med 1993; 118:455–464.
74. Kupersmith J, Holmes-Rovner M, Hogan A, et al. Cost effectiveness analysis in heart disease. I. General principles. Prog Cardiovasc Dis 1994; 27:161–184.

75. ISIS-2 (Second International Study of Infarct Survival) Collaborative Group. Randomized trial of intravenous streptokinase, oral aspirin, both or neither among 17,187 cases of suspected acute myocardial infarction: ISIS-2. Lancet 1988; 2: 349–360.
76. Strom BL. Pharmacoepidemiology: current status, prospects, and problems. Ann Intern Med 1990; 113:179–181.
77. McGhan WF, Lewis NJ. Guidelines for pharmacoeconomic studies. Clin Ther 1992; 14:486–494.
78. Jolicoeur LM, Jones-Grizzle AJ, Boyer JG. Guidelines for performing a pharmacoeconomic analysis. Am J Hosp Pharm 1992; 49:1741–1747.
79. Langley PC. The role of pharmacoeconomic guidelines for formulary approval: the Australian experience. Clin Ther 1993; 15:1154–1176.
80. Kozma CM, Reeder CE, Schulz RM. Economic, clinical, and humanistic outcomes: a planning model for pharmacoeconomic research. Clin Ther 1993; 15:1121–1132.
81. Kupersmith J, Holmes-Rovner M, Hogan A, et al. Cost effectiveness analysis in heart disease. II. Preventive therapies. Prog Cardiovasc Dis 1995; 37:243–271.
82. Kupersmith J, Holmes-Rovner M, Hogan A, et al. Cost effectiveness analysis in heart disease. III. Ischemic disease, congestive heart failure and arrhythmias. Prog Cardiovasc Dis 1995; 37:307–346.
83. Goldman L. Cost-effective strategies in cardiology. In: Braunwald E, ed. Heart disease. Philadelphia: WB Saunders, 1988;1680–1692.
84. Weinstein MC, Fineberg HV, Elstein AS, et al. Clinical decision analysis. Philadelphia: WB Saunders, 1980;228–265.
85. Weinstein MC, Stason WB. Foundations of cost-effectiveness analysis for health and medical practices. N Engl J Med 1977; 296:716–721.
86. Detsky AS, Naglie IG. A clinician's guide to cost-effectiveness analysis. Ann Intern Med 1990; 113:147–154.
87. Drummond MF, Stoddart GL, Torrance GW. Methods for the economic evaluation of health care programmes. Oxford, England: Oxford University Press, 1987.
88. Goldman L, Sia STB, Cook EF, et al. Costs and effectiveness of routine therapy with long-term beta-adrenergic antagonists after acute myocardial infarction. N Engl J Med 1988; 319:152–157.
89. Glick H, Cook J, Bourassa M, et al. for the SOLVD Investigators. Projections of the cost and benefits of enalapril treatment in patients with symptomatic heart failure (abst). J Am Coll Cardiol 1994; 1A:284A.
90. Oster G, Epstein AM. Primary prevention and coronary heart disease: the economic benefits of lowering serum cholesterol. Am J Public Health 1986; 76:647–656.
91. Lipid Research Clinics Program: The lipid research clinics coronary primary prevention trial results: I. Reduction in the incidence of coronary heart disease. JAMA 1984; 251:351–364.
92. Paul SD, Keaney KM, Eagle KA, et al. The costs and the effectiveness of angiotensin converting enzyme inhibition in patients with congestive heart failure (abst). Circulation 1992; (Suppl I): I-101.
93. Sox HC, Blatt MA, Higgins MC, et al. Medical decision making. Stoneham, MA: Butterworth , 1988.
94. Wright K. Should QALYs be programme-specific? J Health Econ 1988; 7:239–257.
95. Weinstein MC, Stason WB. Cost-effectiveness of coronary artery bypass surgery. Circulation 1982; (Suppl III): 56–66.
96. Goldman L, Gordon DJ, Rifkind BM, et al. Cost and health implications of cholesterol lowering. Circulation 1992; 85:1960–1968.
97. Goldman L, Weinstein MC, Goldman PA, et al. Cost-effectiveness of HMG-CoA reductase inhibition for primary and secondary prevention of coronary heart disease. JAMA 1991; 265:1145–1151.
98. Eckman MH, Levine HJ, Pauker SG. Decision analytic and cost-effectiveness issues concerning anticoagulant prophylaxis in heart disease. Chest 1992; 102:538S–549S.
99. Weinstein MC, Stason WB. Cost-effectiveness of coronary artery bypass surgery. Circulation 1982; 66 (Suppl III):56–66

100. Kupersmith J, Hogan A, Guerrero P, et al. Evaluating and improving the cost effectiveness of the implantable cardioverter defibrillator. Am Heart J 1995;130: 507–515.
101. Edelson JT, Weinstein MC, Toteson ANA, et al. Long-term cost-effectiveness of various initial monotherapies for mild to moderate hypertension. JAMA 1990; 263: 407–413.
102. Krumholz HM, Pasternak RC, Weinstein MC, et al. Cost effectiveness of thrombolytic therapy with streptokinase in elderly patients with suspected acute myocardial infarction. N Engl J Med 1992; 327:7–13.
103. Tsevat J, Duke D, Goldman L, et al. Cost-effectiveness of captopril therapy after myocardial infarction. Clin Res 1993; 41:180A (Abstract).
104. Kinosian BP, Eisenberg JM. Cutting into cholesterol. Cost-effective alternatives for treating hypercholesterolemia. JAMA 1988; 259:2249–2254.
105. Consumer Price Index, U.S. City Average. Washington, DC: U.S. Department of Labor, Bureau of Labor Statistics, 1994.
106. Scandinavian Simvastatin Survival Study Group. Randomized trial of cholesterol lowering in 4444 patients with coronary heart disease: the Scandinavian Sinvastatin Survival Study (4S). Lancet 1994;344:1383–1389.
107. Sheperd J, Cobbe SM, Ford I, et al. for the West of Scotland Coronary Prevention Study Group. Prevention of coronary heart disease with pravastatin in men with hypercholesterolemia. N Engl J Med 1995;333:1301–1307.

# PART II

# Lipid-Lowering Therapy: Risk Factor Reduction

CHAPTER 2

# Lipid-Lowering Drugs

William Virgil Brown, MD, Ngoc-Anh Le, PhD, and David Robertson, MD

This chapter will review the drugs that are currently used in reducing potentially harmful levels of cholesterol and triglyceride-carrying lipoproteins in plasma. The reduction of elevated concentrations of low-density lipoprotein (LDL)-cholesterol (c) has been the major indication in their prescription. Elevated levels of this lipoprotein are clearly related to coronary heart disease. LDL-c reduction is the major focus of the National Cholesterol Education Program in the United States (1). Drugs that are primarily useful in reducing LDL-c include the bile acid sequestrants, 3-hydroxy-3-methylglutaryl conzyme A (HMG-CoA) reductase inhibitors (statins), and niacin.

Marked elevations in plasma triglycerides involving very-low-density lipoprotein (VLDL) and chylomicrons are also considered to be conditions deserving drug therapy. Plasma triglyceride levels over 500 mg/dL (after diet changes and exercise programs have been adopted) are frequently treated with pharmacologic agents (2, 3). The major concern is the possibility of the "hyperchylomicronemic syndrome," which involves the development of severe hypertriglyceridemia with plasma concentrations over 1000 mg/dL and the potential for consequent pancreatitis (4). This syndrome is often manifest by eruptive xanthomata, hepatosplenomegaly, and dysfunction in other organs, including central nervous system and peripheral nerves, as well as the pancreas.

Triglyceride reduction may also be considered of value in patients with the syndrome of moderate hypertriglyceridemia (triglycerides 200–500 mg/dL) in the presence of moderately elevated LDL-c and low high-density lipoprotein (HDL)-cholesterol (c) (see Chapter 3). Agents that are already effective in reducing serum triglyceride values are niacin and the fibric acids.

This chapter will discuss the chemical structure, pharmacodynamics, mechanism of action, the efficacy in modifying lipoprotein levels, and the adverse effects of lipid-reducing drugs. In addition, it will provide a description of the current clinical use of lipid-reducing drugs, including most preparations available in this country and elsewhere in the world. The efficacy of these agents in primary and secondary prevention of arteriosclerotic cardiovascular disease is the subject of Chapter 3.

## THE BILE ACID SEQUESTRANTS

The current agents available include cholestyramine and colestipol (Fig. 2.1)

### History and Chemical Structure

Oral administration of the polymeric ion exchange resins cholestyramine or colestipol is used to bind bile acids in the intestinal tract, reducing their reabsorption in the distal bowel and increasing their excretion in the stool (5, 6). These agents were initially prescribed to reduce the bile acid accumulation in the skin and the associated pruritus seen in patients with partially obstructed biliary outflow tracts, as in biliary cirrhosis (7). The observed reduction in serum cholesterol led to their testing and subsequent approval for prescription for lowering cholesterol levels in the United States in 1972. Their demonstrated efficacy in lowering LDL cholesterol and in preventing heart disease in clinical trials, as well as their

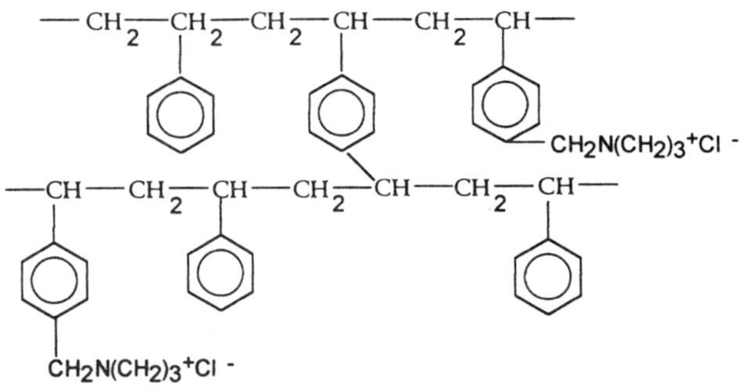

**Cholestyramine**

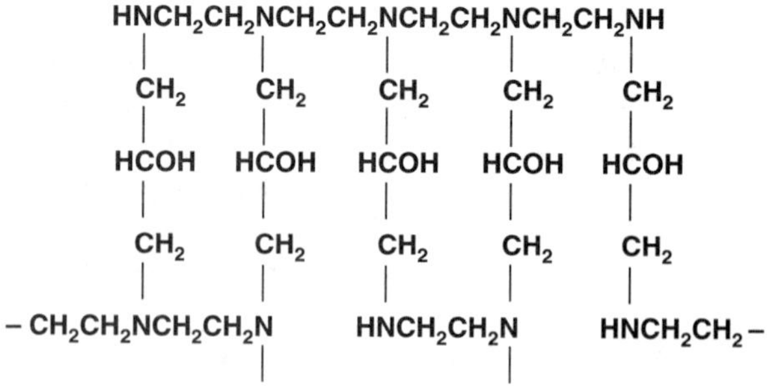

**Colestipol**

Figure 2.1 The chemical structure of cholestyramine resin and colestipol hydrochloride.

Education Program recommending these agents as first line treatment for hypercholesterolemia in patients without concurrent hypertriglyceridemia (1). Cholestyramine is a basic ion exchange resin synthesized as the copolymer of styrene and diphenylbenzene containing trimethylbenzammonium groups that provide a strong positive charge (8). It is prepared as the chloride salt in a fine granular powder of fractured irregular particles ranging in diameter from 45 to 225 μm. Colestipol is also the chloride salt of a basic ion exchange copolymer synthesized from diethylene triamine and 1 chloro 2,3-epoxy propane (8). It has multiple protonated amine groups providing positive charges that form ionic bonds with a variety of negative substances, including bile salts. Colestipol is supplied as a powder consisting of smooth, round beads, 50–400 μ in diameter.

## Pharmacology

When the bile acid sequestrants are consumed as suspensions of the powder in liquid or in capsular form at doses of 4–30 g per day, significant quantities of bile acids are adsorbed in the proximal small intestine, preventing their absorption into the body in the distal ileum (9, 10). In water, colestipol has been shown to bind up to 2 g of bile salts per gram of anhydrous resin (11). This very large capacity is dependent on the formation of micellar structures and is not due to a one-to-one ionic bonding. The actual capacity of these resins varies with the specific bile acid as well as with the pH of the medium and content of other salts or charged amphipathic molecules in the medium such as fatty acids and phospholipids. The observed increase in total daily fecal bile acid secretion is found to be less than 2 g with the usual maximum daily dosage of 24 g of cholestyramine (12). This is less than 5% of the demonstrated capacity in vitro (8). The observed maximal capacity for bile acid binding by colestipol in vitro is approximately one-fourth that of an equivalent weight of cholestyramine (8). In vivo, however, the two resins are only modestly different in their demonstrated ability to promote bile acid excretion in the stool. In this respect, a 5-g dose of colestipol is approximately equivalent to a 4-g dose of cholestyramine in accelerating bile acid loss from the intestine and in lowering cholesterol concentrations.

Bile acids excreted in the hepatic biliary tract consist of a complex mixture of compounds including conjugates of taurine and glycine. The last 100–200 cm of the ileum has the highest capacity to absorb and remove the bile acids from the intestinal contents, competing with the sequestrant beads. In theory, virtually all the bile acids would be removed from the resin and reabsorbed if the transit time were sufficiently slowed. The various bile acids are not treated equally by the sequestrants, with greater observed excretion of deoxy and chenodeoxycholic acids and their conjugated derivatives as compared to cholic acid (11). As a result, there is a relative rise in the concentration of cholic acid and its conjugates in gallbladder and intestinal bile during sequestrant therapy (13). The differential effects on bile acid excretion are not explained by the rate of binding of the various compounds in the intestinal tract but are predicted by the rate of dissociation of these bile acids from the complex with resin beads (8). The rates of dissociation from colestipol are more rapid than those from cholestyramine, and cholic acid is released more rapidly than the deoxycholic and chenodeoxycholic acids (11–13). These observations are consistent with the bile acid excretory patterns and the change in bile composition.

## Mechanism of Action

The hepatobiliary system and the gastrointestinal tract are responsible for excreting virtually all the cholesterol from the body. The sterols in the feces consist of cholesterol itself and its major metabolic products, the bile acids. In addition, bacteria in the colon generate a group of degradation products from these compounds. Some fecal cholesterol comes directly from the diet. The mean cholesterol intake in a Western individual varies from 200–600 mg/day, and approximately one-half of this is absorbed by the small intestine (14, 15). High doses of the bile acid sequestrants have been shown to moderately reduce cholesterol absorption during the first few days of treatment; however, there is little measurable effect on cholesterol absorption over the long-term.

In the normal adult man, 2–4 g of bile acids participate in a hepatobiliary-enteric cycle. After excretion in the duodenum, approximately 95% of the bile acids are reabsorbed in the distal ileum (14). While in the intestinal tract, these bile acids act as the body's detergent, solubilizing dietary triglycerides and cholesterol enabling enzymatic digestion and absorption. This "bile acid pool" is excreted and reabsorbed from five to ten times daily, with approximately 200–600 mg escaping into the colon under normal circumstances. Bile acid excretion may be increased from twofold to tenfold when the bile acid sequestrants are used in their customary clinical dosages. Interference with bile acid reabsorption causes a reduction in the concentration of bile acids returning to the liver. The consequent decline in hepatocyte concentration activates the genetic expression of the enzyme 7-α-hydroxylase, which controls the rate-limiting chemical modification of cholesterol in the synthetic pathway of bile acids (16). This enzyme catalyzes the formation of 7-α-hydroxycholesterol from cholesterol, initiating the synthesis of both cholic and chenodeoxycholic acids. As a result, there is a significant increase in the utilization of intracellular cholesterol for bile acid formation. The more rapid synthesis of bile acids quickly restores a total body pool of bile acids to near normal levels. The cholesterol content of liver cell membranes is reduced slightly, however, stimulating increased cholesterol synthesis by inducing the enzyme HMG Co-A reductase (17,18). Although increased hepatic cholesterol synthesis is stimulated, reduction in hepatic microsomal cholesterol also induces the synthesis of LDL receptors that are transported to the external aspect of the hepatic cell membrane where they are available to bind, remove, and degrade LDL (19). This increased uptake and degradation of LDL-c produces the clinically desirable effect of a fall in plasma LDL-c. A variety of studies using radiolabeled lipoproteins have demonstrated that the decline in LDL-c is a result of more rapid removal from the plasma space and a shortened residence time for these particles (20).

Within 3 to 4 weeks after the beginning of bile acid sequestrants, a new steady state is achieved with mean LDL-c reduction of 25–35% using the customary clinical dosage range of 12–30 g daily (5). Significant changes in the mean LDL-c are observed within 1 week of the beginning of therapy in groups of patients. There is both a decrease in particle number and a decrease in the cholesterol content of LDL. The decrease in particle number is reflected in the reduction in the number of apolipoprotein B-100 molecules present in the plasma, and this is consistent with the increased expression of LDL receptors that bind specifically to this protein as ligand (19,21). Strong evidence that this change is due specifically to the LDL receptor function and not to changes in other pathways of uptake has been provided by metabolic studies (22). As would be expected, patients who are genetically deficient in LDL receptor synthesis (homozygous familial hypercholesterolemia) show little or no responsiveness to bile acid sequestrant therapy (23).

Although LDL-c levels fall, an increase in the triglyceride-rich VLDL is frequently observed. VLDL is made in the liver as a vehicle for transport of triglyceride to peripheral tissues (see Figure 3.1, Chapter 3). When bile acid sequestrants are used, hepatic triglyceride synthesis has been found to increase (24). This may be due to the increased activity of the key regulatory enzyme, phosphatidic acid phosphatase, which is sensitive to the bile acid content of the liver cell (25). Reduction in chenodeoxycholic acid increases the activity, and feeding deoxycholic acid has been shown to produce a significant hypotriglyceridemic effect. In normal individuals with triglyceride levels less than 200 mg/dL, a rise in VLDL production rate of 10–50% is usually of little consequence. In patients with baseline triglyceride values of 500 mg/dL or greater, however, a marked increase in plasma triglycerides may be observed with the potential for clinical consequences (26). Fortunately, the development of pancreatitis or other severe sequelae has been rarely observed. In patients with the relatively uncommon disorder dysbetalipoproteinemia, there may be a marked increase in VLDL and chylomicron remnants during cholestyramine therapy (27). These individuals are known to have a genetic disorder in the processing of VLDL and chylomicrons, and the increased synthesis of triglyceride is more dramatically expressed as a rising plasma level with this metabolic impairment.

Another potentially beneficial effect of cholestyramine treatment may be a rise in HDL-c, usually from 2–6%. Bile acid sequestrant therapy has been associated with an increase in the number of larger and more lipid-rich HDL, referred to as $HDL_2$, with little or no change in the smaller and more dense $HDL_3$ (28). The major protein component of HDL, apolipoprotein A-I, also may show a significant rise as does a second constitutive protein, apolipoprotein A-II (29). It has been suggested that this change in the apolipoproteins is due to increased synthesis by the intestine.

### Clinical Use

Cholestyramine is available under the brand name Questran (Bristol-Myers Squibb, Princeton, New Jersey). The standard dose consists of 4 g of active resin and 5 g of additives, including sucrose. This preparation is provided as single dose, foil-wrapped packets or in cartons containing 378 g of powder. An enclosed scoop dispenses the standard dose of 9 g.

Cholestyramine is also formulated with aspartame as the sweetener (Questran-Light; Bristol-Myers Squibb, Princeton, New Jersey). With this preparation, approximately 5 g contains a 4-g dose of active resin. This is dispensed both in the individual packets as well as in 210-g containers.

Colestipol hydrochloride granules (Colestid; Upjohn, Kalamazoo, Michigan) is prepared without significant additives. The standard dose is 5 g, supplied in foil-wrapped packets or in bulk containers containing 300 or 500 g. Colestipol is also available as Flavored Colestid (the 7.5- g standard dose of which contains 5.0 g of active resin and 2.5 g of additional ingredients including aspartame) and Colestid tablets, each containing 1 g of active drug.

Elevated LDL cholesterol is the only lipoprotein abnormality for which clinical benefit has been demonstrated with the use of bile acid sequestrants (30,31). Elevation in LDL-c that is sustained after dietary and other lifestyle changes should be judged using the guidelines issued by the National Cholesterol Education Program (1). It is also important to document the triglyceride level and to avoid using these agents in patients who have significant hypertriglyceridemia. When triglyceride levels are persistently over 300 mg/dL, clinically significant increases may be observed. Therefore, the resins should be avoided until the triglyceride values are brought into a more desirable range.

Although a small rise in HDL cholesterol has been observed in group mean data, a 2–6% increase may be difficult to document with certainty in the individual patient (32). There is no documented benefit from raising HDL with these agents when LDL cholesterol levels are demonstrated to be within a desirable range.

The initial total daily dose of bile acid sequestrants should not exceed 10 g. This may be given as a single dose with a major meal of the day or divided as a twice daily regimen. Beginning with approximately one-third to one-half of the maximum dose reduces the gastrointestinal side effects and improves adherence. At this dose level, mean reductions in LDL cholesterol have been observed to be approximately 20% after 4–6 weeks (33). After reassessment of the lipoprotein levels and any adverse reactions, the dose may be doubled, given in equal quantities twice daily (34). The maximum dose of active resin has customarily been 24 g of cholestyramine or 30 g daily of colestipol hydrochloride. Mean reductions of LDL from 30–35% have been documented at these dose levels. Considerable variation in responsiveness among individuals has been noted, with some patients demonstrating a 50% reduction in LDL, whereas in others, the change is not significant. It is often difficult to determine whether lack of responsiveness is physiologic or due to problems with adherence to the regimen. Over the long term, a dosage range of 8–12 g is often the most effective regimen. Since compliance is more difficult and adverse effects are increased, higher dosages in many patients may produce diminishing returns. If additional reduction in LDL-c is desirable, prescribing a second drug with a different mechanism of action may prove to be more efficacious and less expensive (30, 35, 36). The addition of HMG Co-A reductase inhibitors or niacin provides very effective combinations with the bile acid sequestrants.

These agents are less convenient than simply taking a tablet, requiring the dispensing of a powder and its suspension in a liquid once or twice daily. The modern agents have no unpleasant odor or taste, and the resin beads can be made more palatable by being mixed with fruit juice or other carriers in the suspending liquid. Approximately 60% of patients report that the powder preparations are satisfactory when mixed in water as the only vehicle (37). Others, however, may find that the use of pureed foods (such as applesauce), frappes, carbonated beverages, and fruit juices provide useful alternatives if palatability problems occur. Such problems may also be effectively solved by simply changing the preparation, since there are different flavorings, additives, and textures available. It is often difficult to define the reason for preference of one preparation over another. Tablets of colestipol hydrochloride are available; however, each contains only 1 g of active resin, requiring 4 to 10 tablets be consumed at each dose. Tablets may prove to be a better choice for those who find the granularity of the suspended powder to be unpleasant (38).

Key elements in achieving compliance are (1) selecting the patient without contraindications, (2) informing the patient of the proven efficacy and safety of these agents, (3) explaining the adverse reactions and methods of avoiding them, and (4) beginning with a low dose, 4–10 g per day, and increasing only after 4–6 weeks.

## Adverse Reactions

The bile acid binding resins are not absorbed, and therefore, the adverse reactions are virtually confined to signs and symptoms of gastrointestinal tract dysfunction. Constipation, abdominal pain, eructation, "heart burn," and increased flatus have been among the common complaints. Diarrhea has occasionally been observed. Since these are all common problems, it is difficult in practice to know whether the drug is the causative agent in each case. Constipation has been the most easily documented problem, occurring in 30–50% of patients during the first 1–2 months of use (39). Monitoring of the 3800 patients who participated in the Lipid Research Clinic Coronary Primary Prevention Trial (LRC-CPPT) provided the largest, and perhaps the most objective, evaluation of adverse effects currently available (30). In this study, cholestyramine was used in a daily dose of 24 g (12 g twice a day). Adverse events were assessed at 2-month intervals. Half the patients had been assigned to take active drug and the other half placebo in a randomized and blinded fashion. The increase in specific complaints at the end of the first year and at the end of the seventh year of treatment compared with the placebo control group are presented in Table 2.1. A 39% incidence in complaints of constipation compared to 10% in the placebo group was noted during the initial year. However, there was no significant difference in the frequency of this complaint between the two groups after 7 years. Various remedies including fiber-rich dietary supplements and decreased compliance with the active medication may have helped resolve this issue.

The onset of constipation may relate to the reduced delivery of bile salts to the colon where they act as a normal stimulant. Starting with a dose of less than 10 g daily, increasing fluid intake, and altering the diet to contain more high fiber foods or adding fiber supplements usually reduces the problem. Increasing high fiber foods or using supplements with soluble fiber such as pectin, guar gum, or psyllium, is particularly attractive since they provide some additional cholesterol reduction (40, 41).

With higher doses, heartburn, nausea, and (rarely) vomiting may be observed. Taking the dosages immediately at mealtime or the use of antacids or simethicone preparations may relieve these symptoms during the early phases of treatment. Flatulence and belching have been attributed to air swallowing due to the frothing of the preparation with excessive stirring. Again, this disappears after the first few weeks of treatment in most patients.

The upper gastrointestinal tract complaints may be related to the release of cholecystokinin after bile acid sequestrant intake (42). This hormone causes increased gastrointestinal motility, relaxation of the lower esophageal sphincter, and contraction of the gallbladder. Diarrhea is a rare side effect without a well-documented etiology. The cholecystokinin release may be a contributing factor. Since certain dyes are present in some of the preparations, intestinal allergy may be another explanation. This can be treated by simply changing to another preparation.

Before beginning bile acid sequestrant treatment, it is important to record any history of bowel dysfunction. The existence of recurrent abdominal pain or colonic or anal-rectal disorders such as proctitis, hemorrhoids, recurrent constipation, or diarrhea may allow for effective prophylactic management or, in some cases, the decision to avoid these medications.

Bile acid sequestrants bind negatively charged compounds; therefore, other drugs may be adsorbed, reducing or delaying their transport through

**Table 2.1**
**Percent of Participants Reporting Moderate or Severe Side Effects with Cholestyramine[a]**

| | Pretreatment | | Year 1 | | Year 7 | |
|---|---|---|---|---|---|---|
| Side Effect | Placebo | Resin | Placebo | Resin | Placebo | Resin |
| Abdominal pain | 5 | 5 | 11 | 15 | 7 | 7 |
| Belching or bloating | 10 | 10 | 16 | 27 | 6 | 9 |
| Constipation | 3 | 4 | 10 | 39 | 4 | 8 |
| Diarrhea | 6 | 5 | 11 | 10 | 8 | 4 |
| Gas | 22 | 22 | 26 | 32 | 12 | 12 |
| Heartburn | 10 | 10 | 10 | 27 | 7 | 12 |
| Nausea | 4 | 3 | 8 | 16 | 4 | 3 |
| Vomiting | 2 | 2 | 5 | 6 | 3 | 2 |
| At least one gastrointestinal side effect | 34 | 34 | 43 | 68 | 26 | 29 |

[a]The adverse reactions reported during the Lipid Research Clinics Coronary Primary Prevention Trial (47) at the end of the first year and seventh year of treatment are given. The resin-treated patients received diet and cholestyramine, 12 g twice daily, for the entire period. The placebo-treated patients received an inactive powder to be taken in identical fashion. The treatment was randomized and double blind. Symptoms were treated according to protocol, including the use of fiber supplements and laxatives as necessary.

Data from The LRC-CPPT Study Group. The Lipid Research Clinics Coronary Primary Prevention Trial Results: (1) Reduction in incidence of coronary heart disease; (1) The relationship of reduction in incidence of CHD to cholesterol lowering. JAMA 1984; 251:351–374.

the intestinal epithelium. Clear evidence for such interference exists for β-adrenergic blocking agents, hydrochlorothiazide, furosemide, tetracycline, penicillin G, gemfibrozil, digoxin, and thyroxine (43). In general, it is best to assume that any drug may be adsorbed onto the resin beads and made less effective. All patients should be warned that other oral medications should be taken at least 1 hour before or 4–6 hours after cholestyramine or colestipol. The observed interference with exogenous thyroid hormone absorption caused concern about the enterohepatic circulation of exogenous thyroxine ($T_4$). Specific investigations of thyroid function have found no change in $T_4$ or thyroid-stimulating hormone (TSH) levels in patients over a 9-week period with colestipol administration up to 30 g per day (44).

A variety of chemical changes in the blood have been monitored. A small rise in alkaline phosphatase and an increased iron-binding capacity, both within the normal range, have been observed without any clinical symptoms or adverse effects over the 7 years of the LRC-CPPT noted (30). A drop in plasma β-carotene appeared to be consistent with this material being a normal component of the LDL molecule. There is no convincing evidence that body stores of any vitamin have been reduced by the use of these agents for 7–10 years.

Children with severe hypercholesterolemia such as those with familial hypercholesterolemia have been treated with good results and with no evidence of retardation of growth or development (45). Large doses given to young animals have also failed to alter normal gain in weight or growth (46). Hyperchloremic acidosis has been reported in metabolically compromised adults and very small children receiving large doses, but this appears to be a rare occurrence (47).

## HMG Co-A REDUCTASE INHIBITORS ("STATINS")

Currently available drugs include lovastatin, simvastatin, pravastatin, and fluvastatin. Atorvastatin is a fifth agent that is in the late stages of clinical development.

### History and Chemical Structure

The addition of a chemical isolated from the *Penicillium* mold was found to inhibit cholesterol synthesis in hepatic cells in culture. This initial compound mevastatin was shown to comparatively inhibit the rate-limiting enzyme in cholesterol synthesis HMG-CoA reductase. Lovastatin was the first of these drugs developed for clinical use and was approved for prescription in 1987. It is produced from cultures of *Aspergillus terreus*. The various chemical structures are shown in Figure 2.2. Simvastatin and pravastatin (not shown) are chemical modifications of lovastatin. Fluvastatin and atorvastatin are synthetic compounds designed to mimic the interaction of the naturally occurring drug with the HMG-CoA reductase enzyme (48,49). The drugs are administered either in the lactone ring (lovastatin or fluvastatin) or in the open acid form (pravastatin and fluvastatin). Structural features of all these compounds allow binding both at the active site and to a lipophilic region of the HMG-CoA reductase enzyme. The order of binding affinity among the currently available drugs is simvastatin>lovastatin>pravastatin>fluvastatin.

### Pharmacology

Absorption of the drugs is approximately 30% for lovastatin and pravastatin, 61–85% for simvastatin, and more than 90% for fluvastatin (50). Administration with food increases the plasma concentration after an oral dose of lovastatin. Food has the opposite effect on pravastatin and fluva-

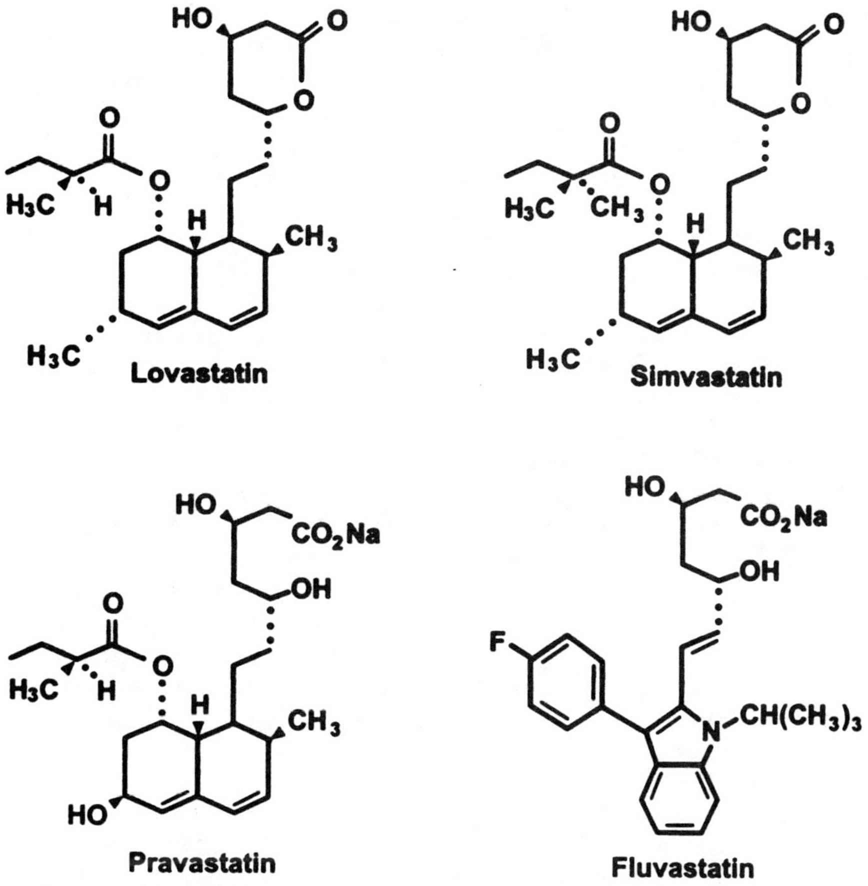

Lovastatin

Simvastatin

Pravastatin

Fluvastatin

Figure 2.2 Schematic depiction of the four drugs that inhibit 3-hydroxy—3-methylglutaryl coenzyme A ( HMG-CoA) reductase and are currently available for prescription use.

statin but no demonstrable effect on simvastatin. There is no significant effect on their efficacy in cholesterol reduction, however, by administration at meal time or during fasting. All statins have short plasma half-lives, ranging from 0.5–0.8 hours for fluvastatin to 3 hours for lovastatin and pravastatin. The liver is the major organ of uptake from plasma, with a major portion cleared on the first-pass through the liver. Studies in animals and tissue culture suggest that there may be a larger initial clearance by liver of lovastatin and fluvastatin. Other studies indicate that the open acid and more hydrophilic compound pravastatin is relatively excluded from nonhepatic tissues and is taken up by an active transport system in the liver similar, if not identical to, the bile acid transport system. It is not evident that these differences in metabolism have any meaningful clinical consequences. The primary route of excretion for the drugs other than pravastatin is biliary excretion. Pravastatin is excreted approximately equally in urine and stool, and small amounts are found in breast milk (50).

## Mechanism of Action and Clinical Use

HMG-CoA reductase is anchored in the membrane and lumen of the endoplasmic reticulum of all cells. The enzyme catalyzes the reduction of HMG-CoA to mevalonate, the first committed step in the pathway of cholesterol synthesis (51). In addition to cholesterol synthesis, this pathway is also responsible for the production of farnesyl phosphate, which serves as cell membrane anchor for several signal transduction proteins. The pathway also produces isopentenyl adenine, a precursor for transfer RNA (51). However, the clinical use of these drugs does not produce complete inhibition of mevalonate production, and cholesterol reduction can be achieved without adversely altering the other related synthetic pathways that include HMG-CoA reductase.

Evidence suggests that the HMG-CoA reductase inhibitors lower LDL-c through two mechanisms. First, the inhibition of HMG-CoA reductase activity decreases hepatic intracellular cholesterol levels, leading to compensatory increases in hepatocyte LDL receptors, resulting in increased LDL clearance from the plasma. Second, diminished synthesis of cholesterol in the liver reduces the rate of VLDL particle production and secretion, possibly through decreased availability of cholesterol to load apolipoprotein B-100 particles. The latter mechanism may be more important in patients with familial hypercholesterolemia (52).

The efficacy of these agents in lowering LDL cholesterol has been evaluated in a number of clinical trials. A recent review concludes that pravastatin has a potency similar to that of lovastatin, with only one-half of the dose of simvastatin required for equal effect. Approximately twice the milligram dose of fluvastatin is required to yield an LDL reduction equivalent to lovastatin or pravastatin. At maximal doses, the mean reduction in LDL by fluvastatin is 25–30%; by lovastatin and pravastatin, 30–35%; and by simvastatin, 35–40% (53) (Table 2.2). The initial reduction in LDL cholesterol, which has been demonstrated within 1 week of initiation of therapy (54), persists with long-term therapy (55). There is significant variation in the response among individuals with LDL-c reduction, varying from less than 5% to more than 50% for these drugs. More than 90% of patients will show more than a 15% decline in LDL-c. Since response is variable and adverse effects increase with dose, it is best to begin with a low dose and increase at 4- to 8-week intervals to achieve the targeted level of LDL-c.

## Adverse Events

The use of statins in clinical studies has been associated with a low rate of clinical and biochemical side effects as well as a high rate of patient compliance. Clinical side effects are generally short-term and self-limiting and

**Table 2.2**
**Low-Density Lipoprotein (LDL) Reduction by HMG CoA-Reductase Inhibitors**

| | Usual Daily Dose | Dosing Regimen | Percent LDL Reduction at Maximal Dose |
|---|---|---|---|
| Lovastatin | 10–80 mg | Up to 40 mg single daily dose at supper or bedtime; 80 mg dose as 40 mg b.i.d. | 30–35 |
| Simvastatin | 5–40 mg | Single dose at bedtime | 35–40 |
| Pravastatin | 10–40 mg | Single dose at bedtime | 30–35 |
| Fluvastatin | 20–40 mg | Single dose at bedtime | 25–30 |
| Atorvastatin | 10–80 mg | Single dose at bedtime | >50 |

b.i.d. = twice daily

include inconsistent changes in bowel habits, nausea, headaches, or malaise. Myalgias and muscle tenderness may occasionally occur but are not always associated with increases in the plasma concentrations of creatine kinase (53, 54). Overall, discontinuation rates in clinical trials are similar for the placebo and drug treatment groups (53). Persistent elevations of alanine aminotransferase (ALT) and aspartate aminotransferase (AST) occur in 2–3% of lovastatin-treated patients (55), 1.3% of fluvastatin-treated patients, and with an intermediate incidence for pravastatin and simvastatin treatment (50). The implications of these observed increases in ALT and AST levels are not fully understood. The secretion of these enzymes from liver cells in culture is enhanced with exposure to the statins. No permanent liver damage has been reported, and therefore, the transaminase rise may not reflect toxicity in the usual sense. However, a rise to three times the upper limit of normal is considered unacceptable, requiring a reduction in dosage or discontinuation of drug.

Muscle symptoms associated with an elevation of creatine kinase occur in 5% of patients treated with maximal doses of lovastatin, but only 0.2% have creatine kinase elevations that are more than 10 times the upper limits of normal (55). These adverse effects occur less frequently with lower doses (55). When muscle symptoms occur without creatine kinase elevation, or in the setting of mild elevation, continued therapy with more frequent monitoring or rechallenge after brief discontinuation of therapy is a reasonable strategy.

The production of steroid hormones from cholesterol in patients receiving long-term therapy with reductase inhibitors has been evaluated. In men and women treated with simvastatin for 12 months, there was no significant change in the cortisol response to corticotropin challenge, and no changes in sex steroid levels (56). In addition, both sperm quality and semen production remain intact (57). Despite in vitro data to suggest that inhibition of lymphocyte proliferation occurs with lovastatin, human studies have shown no clinically significant changes in any parameter of lymphocyte function in patients treated with lovastatin (58, 59). Theoretical considerations had suggested that the more hydrophilic reductase inhibitor pravastatin might have fewer central nervous system effects compared to the other more lipophilic reductase inhibitors. Studies, however, have shown that neither lovastatin nor pravastatin has significant effects on subjective or polysomnographic sleep measures (60, 61), and there were also no measurable effects of these drugs on cognitive function (60).

The most important drug interactions occur when the reductase inhibitors are combined with other lipid-lowering agents. Bile acid sequestrants have been shown to impair the absorption of pravastatin and fluvastatin; they should not be administered simultaneously with any of the reductase inhibitors (50). Concomitant administration of reductase inhibitors and fibric acid derivatives increase the risk of myopathy. There are reports, however, that patients who had myopathy while receiving the combination of lovastatin and gemfibrozil, and were subsequently treated with the combination of pravastatin and gemfibrozil, did not have recurrence of muscle symptoms (62). Therefore, it is reasonable to add a reductase inhibitor to a fibric acid treatment regimen in patients with significant elevations of both LDL-c and triglycerides. Symptoms and the activity of ALT and AST should be monitored 6–8 weeks after a dosage change. Combined treatment of lovastatin and nicotinic acid has been said to have a risk of myopathy of approximately 3% (50). Myopathy was not reported in a small number of patients treated with a combination of fluvastatin and niacin (63).

The macrolide antibiotics also increase the risk of myopathy in patients receiving reductase inhibitor therapy. If treatment with erythromycin, clarithromycin, or azithromycin is strongly indicated in patients receiving reductase inhibitors, then the lipid-lowering agent should be discontinued temporarily until antibiotic therapy is completed. Immunosuppressants, particularly cyclosporin, also increase the risk of myopathy in patients treated with reductase inhibitors. Although the incidence has been estimated at 30% in patients receiving lovastatin (50), packaging information allows for the coadministration of pravastatin and cyclosporin. Therefore, this becomes the agent of choice in patients with solid organ transplants receiving cyclosporin.

Propranolol has been shown to reduce the systemic bioavailability but not the clinical efficacy of pravastatin and lovastatin. The β-blocker may increase first-pass hepatic extraction of the reductase inhibitors (50). Because the desired effects of reductase inhibitors occur mainly in the liver, this may not be of significance. This effect has not been seen with fluvastatin or simvastatin.

Simvastatin may increase the prothrombin time in patients treated with warfarin, and dose adjustments may need to be made when reductase inhibitors are started in patients previously stabilized on warfarin. Digoxin levels increase slightly in patients receiving simvastatin, but this effect was not seen with fluvastatin (50).

The magnitude of the cholesterol-lowering effect of lovastatin has been compared in patients on several classes of antihypertensives: calcium channel antagonists, β-blockers, diuretics, and angiotension-converting enzyme (ACE) inhibitors (64). No class of antihypertensives impaired the lipid-lowering action of lovastatin, but calcium channel antagonists increased the potency of lovastatin by approximately 5% (with borderline significance). Antihypertensive therapy did not increase the rate of adverse reactions associated with reductase inhibitor therapy. Despite the analysis of 1475 patients on antihypertensive agents, this study should be interpreted cautiously, since analysis was ad hoc and the numbers of patients in drug treatment groups were not balanced (64).

## NIACIN

### Current Available Drugs

Crystalline nicotinic acid is supplied as tablet or capsule in 50–500- mg doses. It is distributed both as over-the-counter and prescription products by many suppliers. Delayed release forms of niacin are also available in a variety of preparations, including Slo-niacin (Upsher-Smith Laboratories, Minneapolis, Minnesota) and Enduracin (Endurance Products Company, Portland, Oregon).

### History and Pharmacology

Nicotinic acid or its amide derivative, nicotinamide (vitamin $B_3$), are essential nutrients in mammalian metabolism (65). Niacin is converted to nicotinamide in the mammalian liver, which is the substrate for nicotinamide adenine dinucleotide (NAD). This compound, along with its phosphate derivative, NADP, act as hydrogen-transferring coenzymes for a series of physiologically important dehydrogenases. Less than 20 mg/day provides the recommended dietary allowance for this purpose When used in doses of 1 or more g/day, niacin, but not nicotinamide, has pharmacologic effects resulting in the reduction of serum cholesterol and triglycerides (66). Niacin has a broad range of effects, reducing VLDL and chylomicrons in patients with severe hypertriglyceridemia, VLDL and chylomicron remnants in dysbetalipoproteinemia, and LDL in hypercholesterolemia. It also increases HDL-cholesterol in patients with various lipoprotein disorders. It has been used alone or in combination with other lipid-lowering drugs in a series of studies that have demonstrated reduction in vascular disease incidence. However, the common occurrence of both annoying and serious adverse reactions have limited the use of this drug in the clinic. Its optimal use requires appropriate patient education and monitoring.

When crystalline niacin is taken orally in large doses, it is rapidly absorbed and rapidly excreted in the urine as a series of metabolites (Fig. 2.3). The peak blood levels are reached within 30–60 minutes (67). The half-life in the plasma is approximately 1 hour. Ninety percent of the oral dose is recovered in the urine primarily as nicotinuric acid (68). With doses of 3–6 g/day, up to 20% of the total excreted mass may be the unaltered compound. At usual dietary intakes, niacin is predominantly converted to nicotinamide, which is then further metabolized and excreted as N-methyl nicotinamide or in N-methyl-2 pyridone carboxamide (69). Thus, the pattern of urinary excretion varies greatly with the dose administered.

Sustained plasma levels of 0.5–2.0 μg/mL of free nicotinic acid appear to produce the maximum pharmacological effects on lipid levels (70). Although a 1-g dose of crystalline niacin produces a peak plasma level of 10–40 μg/mL, the rapid excretion results in levels below those needed for maximal pharmacological effects within a few hours. As a consequence, the drug must be administered in divided doses during the day, or a method for its delayed release into the plasma space must be used. Capsules containing niacin trapped in a wax matrix or packaged in plastic casings of minimal porosity are among the techniques that have been devised to delay release into the intestinal contents and, thereby, delay absorption of the drug into the bloodstream (66). The delayed release of niacin after absorption from the bowel has been achieved by esterifying the drug to polyhydric alcohols, such as tetranicotinol fructose, pentaerythritol tetranicotinate, *meso*inositol tetranicotinate, and sorbitol hexanicotinate. These compounds are absorbed primarily intact. They are then subjected to the slow action of esterases in liver and in other tissues, allowing the release of the nicotinic acid over prolonged periods. These agents are currently not available in the United States.

## Mechanism of Action

Niacin therapy reduces VLDL synthesis (71). Since VLDL is converted to intermediate-density lipoprotein (IDL) and ultimately to LDL (see Figure 3.1, Chapter 3), the reduction of the latter two lipoproteins is a natural consequence of niacin treatment. There is also evidence that VLDL particles are cleared more rapidly before they can be fully processed to LDL (71). With current techniques, it is difficult to differentiate between reduction in synthesis of VLDL particles and more rapid removal of large VLDL particles early in the chain of events involving lipolysis of the triglyceride. On the other hand, endogenous labeling techniques have allowed more accurate measurement of triglyceride synthesis and secretion

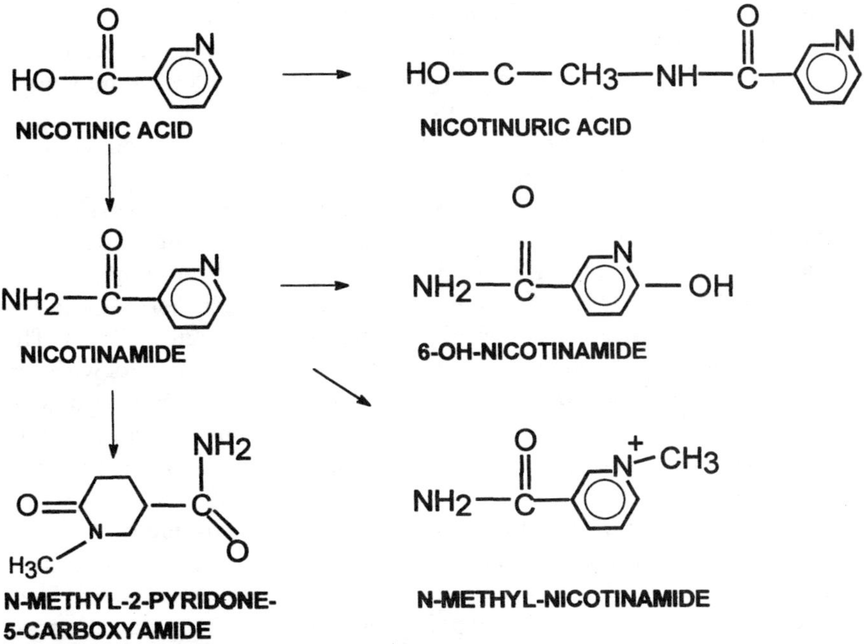

NICOTINIC ACID

NICOTINURIC ACID

NICOTINAMIDE

6-OH-NICOTINAMIDE

N-METHYL-2-PYRIDONE-5-CARBOXYAMIDE

N-METHYL-NICOTINAMIDE

Figure 2.3 Nicotinic acid is converted rapidly to nicotinamide and subsequently to nicotinamide adenine dinucleotide (not shown). It may also be metabolized to 6-hydroxy-nicotinamide, N-methyl-nicotinamide, or N-methyl-2-pyridone-5-carboxyamide. When high doses are given, nicotinuric acid may become one of the major metabolites, and it is excreted rapidly into the urine.

into the plasma space, and studies using these techniques indicate a reduced triglyceride production rate with modest increases in VLDL triglyceride clearance.

Most studies indicate that the clearance of LDL is not significantly altered (71,72). Reduced triglyceride synthesis was initially thought to be a result of suppressing free fatty acid mobilization from adipose tissue stores (73). Free fatty acids supply the major substrate for hepatic triglyceride production, and it was shown early that large doses of niacin could suppress the release of substrate from adipocytes. More detailed studies, however, found that this was a very transient effect, lasting for only approximately1 hour, and that during prolonged treatment, the mean free fatty acid level in plasma was actually elevated (74). Current evidence, therefore, is most consistent with the liver being the primary target of this drug, suppressing triglyceride synthesis by mechanisms yet to be explained. An alteration in the lipoprotein particle structure leading to enhanced clearance of VLDL and VLDL remnants after initial action by lipoprotein lipase has also been considered as a possible niacin effect. A reduction in a series of apolipoproteins known to reside on the VLDL particle has been found during treatment of hypolipoproteinemic subjects with niacin (70). These changes are in approximate proportion to the decrease in the number of VLDL particles circulating; therefore, it is unknown whether these changes may play a causative role or simply are a consequence of reduced VLDL secretion from the liver.

Because VLDLs compete with chylomicrons for the lipase enzymes in peripheral tissues and perhaps for the clearance of remnant particles in the liver, prolonged chylomicron life span in the plasma is often associated with high VLDL levels. The reduction of VLDL in this setting leads to a simultaneous reduction in chylomicrons and chylomicron remnants.

A rise in HDL-c of 10–40% has been observed in both normal and hyperlipoproteinemic persons when niacin treatment is begun (75,76). The most dramatic increase in HDL-c is usually observed in patients with hypertriglyceridemia. Such patients often have increased clearance rates for HDL particles and the reduction in triglycerides returns this rapid catabolism toward normal with a longer residence time for HDL in the blood stream (76, 77).

Lipoprotein (Lp) (a) is a lipoprotein generated by the modification of LDL through the attachment of a second protein to apolipoprotein B-100. This particle is not metabolized by the normal LDL receptor and has been associated in case control studies with increased vascular disease risk. Lp(a) has been reduced by approximately one-third by niacin therapy in several studies (69, 78), although not all investigators have found plasma concentration of Lp(a) to be reduced (79). The mechanism by which this reduction occurs or the clinical benefit to the patient is not known.

## Clinical Use

Niacin has been used in doses up to 12 g per day; however, the usual dose range is 2–4 g/day of crystalline niacin and up to 2 g/day of the delayed release form. With higher doses one usually finds only a modest increase in effectiveness with regard to lipoprotein levels, but adverse reactions continue to occur with significantly higher frequency. In this dosage range, a reduction in triglycerides of 20–60% and a reduction in total plasma cholesterol of 15–30% can be expected in most patients (80, 81). There is considerable individual variability in response. This may be related in part to the underlying disorder of lipoprotein metabolism. Increased HDL may be quite significant at lower doses. At 1 g/day of niacin, a rise in HDL may continue over many months, achieving 25–30% increases in concentration (75). The clinical benefit in terms of cardiovascular disease endpoints has not been assessed in clinical trials using such low doses.

The largest percentage reductions in LDL cholesterol (20–30%) usually occur in individuals with normal triglyceride levels (less than 200 mg/dL) and with LDL values above 160 mg/dL. These patients may also demonstrate a 15–20% reduction in VLDL triglyceride. In persons with fasting plasma triglycerides that are over 500 mg/dL, 50–70% reductions are common (82). In such patients, LDL reduction may be minimal. Dysbetalipoproteinemia is a specific genetic disorder due to abnormal processing of VLDL to LDL with a considerable rise in VLDL remnants. This results in a marked increase in the mass of triglyceride and cholesterol in small VLDL and in the IDL fraction. The plasma of patients often shows a dramatic reduction in both cholesterol and triglyceride levels with niacin therapy (83).

Niacin has been used in combination with the bile acid sequestrants producing a reduction in LDL of 40–50% (84, 85). This combination may be particularly useful in patients with familial combined hyperlipidemia who have both increased VLDL and LDL levels. In combination with the HMG CoA reductase inhibitors, the effect of niacin may be additive in reducing LDL cholesterol (86). The adverse effects seen occasionally with the statins, including liver dysfunction and myopathy, may occur more frequently and require monitoring for elevations in levels of ALT and AST (87).

Crystalline niacin therapy should begin with a low dose given with meals three or four times daily. The major initial adverse effect is cutaneous flushing. This can be attenuated by gradually increasing the dose over a few weeks, by administering the drug with food, and by strict compliance to the regimen. Since the flushing reaction is due to the release of a prostaglandin, inhibiting cyclooxygenase with aspirin therapy (one or two 325-mg tablets daily) has been found to reduce this reaction (88). The initial niacin regimen might include the use of 50- or 100-mg tablets administered four times daily. The dose may be doubled at intervals of 3–7 days if the flushing episodes have abated. At the appropriate time, 500-mg tablets may be used after reaching a total daily dose of 1.5–2.0 g. After this dose has been taken for 4–6 weeks, lipoprotein values should be assessed. In addition, uric acid, fasting plasma glucose, ALT, and AST activity should be measured in the plasma. If there has not been an adequate reduction of cholesterol or triglyceride and no laboratory abnormalities are detected that suggest liver dysfunction, hyperuricemia, or hyperglycemia, the dose may be increased to 3 g/day. Further increases are possible, but it is usually unwise to exceed a total dose of 4.5 g/day. Some patients will be able to tolerate 8–12 g/day, but this is usually not necessary. Greater efficacy and safety can be achieved by adding other drugs with different mechanisms of action.

Delayed release niacin offers the advantage of administration once or twice daily. The usual regimen is 0.5 –1.0 g twice a day. LDL reduction appears to be somewhat greater with delayed release niacin, so that the 2-g dose is roughly equivalent to 4 g of crystalline niacin (81). However, triglyceride reduction is equivalent at a given dose, and the HDL-c elevation is greater with crystalline niacin at any dose level. Although the adverse effects of cutaneous flushing may be less with the delayed release form, they are still observed in some patients.

The low cost of niacin is a distinct advantage; high quality preparations can be obtained, providing a dose of 3 g/day for under $10/month. Other preparations, however, may exceed this price by twentyfold. The frequency of adverse reactions and the efficacy in lipid lowering may vary among preparations. It is best to purchase this agent from a well-documented supplier. This does not necessarily require the use of a prescription formulation since high quality niacin is available as an over-the-counter drug.

## Adverse Reactions

The frequency of adverse reactions with niacin therapy requires systematic and careful monitoring of patients. Most of these are only annoying (cutaneous flushing, abdominal discomfort) and usually can be ameliorated with treatment. Other side effects are more serious (hyperuricemia, hyperglycemia) or potentially fatal (hepatic failure). Table 2.3 lists the adverse reactions observed with niacin therapy and gives an estimate of their frequency when crystalline niacin is used at a dose of 3–6 g daily. It should be noted that the delayed release forms may produce less cutaneous flushing; however, hepatic dysfunction and gastrointestinal side effects may be more frequent (81, 89, 90).

Approximately 90% of patients will experience cutaneous flushing during the early phases of therapy. This consists of a sensation of sudden unexplained warmth, usually developing within 1 hour after the dose but potentially occurring at any time during the day. The skin may appear reddened over the face and upper body, and occasionally over the entire body. This has been attributed to the release of a prostaglandin $D_2$ ($PgD_2$) from the endothelium causing marked vasodilatation in the skin (91). Rarely, this may be accompanied by a drop in blood pressure with dizziness. Preparation of the patient by administering aspirin or other cyclooxygenase inhibitors at low dose may markedly ameliorate this effect. A tachyphylaxis will occur over time; however, it is important to avoid missing more than one or two doses, since the capacity to release the prostaglandin will increase in the interval. It is also useful to avoid hot liquids immediately after taking niacin, since this appears to accentuate the rate of absorption. Other cutaneous reactions may include chronic persistent pruritus and, less commonly, hyperpigmentation of skin folds about the neck and the axillae or groin, typical of acanthosis nigricans. The latter usually requires several months of therapy at high dose.

Direct gastric irritation may occur, causing abdominal discomfort and nausea. This is often ameliorated by food and antacids but made worse by hot liquids. Inflammatory diseases of the intestinal tract, including peptic ulcer, regional ileitis, ulcerative colitis, and others, may be exacerbated by niacin. One should explore the medical history for evidence of such disorders prior to using this drug.

The rise in AST and ALT levels above the upper limits of normal is seen in 5 % or more of patients taking 3 g of crystalline niacin daily. The patient

**Table 2.3**
**Adverse Reactions Observed with Niacin Therapy**

| Adverse Reaction | Estimated Frequency[a] | % |
|---|---|---|
| Skin | | |
| Cutaneous flushing | Very common | (≥ 90) |
| Pruritus | Common | (10–50) |
| Rash | Common | (5–30) |
| Dry skin | Less common | (5–10) |
| Acanthosis nigricans | Less common | (<5) |
| Gastrointestinal tract | | |
| Abdominal pain | Common | (10–20) |
| Nausea | Common | (5–10) |
| Vomiting | Less common | (1–5) |
| Anorexia | Less common | (1–5) |
| Diarrhea | Less common | (1–5) |
| Liver | | |
| Elevated AST and ALT | Common | (5–10) |
| Elevated alkaline phosphatase | Less common | (1–3) |
| Elevated bilirubin | Rare | (<1) |
| Heart | | |
| Cardiac arrhythmias | Less common | (1–5) |
| Muscle | | |
| Myopathic changes | Rare | (<1) |
| Eye | | |
| Cystic maculopathy | Rare | (<1) |
| Metabolic | | |
| Elevated uric acid | Common | (5–10) |
| Abnormal GTT | Common | (5–10) |
| Elevated fasting glucose | Common | (5–10) |
| Weight loss | Less common | (1–5) |

[a]The frequency estimates refer to patients taking crystalline niacin in the dose range of 3–6 g/day for several months or longer. Gastrointestinal side effects may be two or three times more common with delayed release forms.
ALT = Alanine aminotransferase; AST = Aspartate aminotransferase; GTT = Glucose Tolerance Test.

usually experiences no specific symptoms but may have noted loss of appetite, mild nausea, and lethargy. Occasionally, severe hepatic dysfunction has occurred with jaundice and hepatic failure (90, 92). Reports of hepatic failure have been associated with a change of dosage form, particularly the use of high dose ( more than 2 g/day) delayed release form, even after demonstrated tolerance of crystalline niacin at the same daily dosage (90, 92). An unexplained further fall in VLDL and LDL levels or a fall in HDL level may be signs of significant hepatic dysfunction. When mild liver dysfunction is present, a reduction in dose by 50% may be followed by return to normal liver tests, and continued treatment with this agent may be possible. If there is evidence of severe liver dysfunction, the drug should be discontinued immediately.

A myopathic syndrome marked by myalgias and increased AST and creatine phosphokinase (CPK) levels has been described in several case reports (90). This appears to be quite a rare problem, as indicated by the lack of a single such occurrence among 750 patients who were given nicotinic acid at a dose of 3 g/day for 5 years as part of the Coronary Drug Project (93). This syndrome may be triggered by the concomitant use of other drugs, such as ethanol, gemfibrozil, or HMG Co-A reductase inhibitors.

A disorder of the retina referred to as *cystic maculopathy* may occur after prolonged use of niacin. This is thought to be secondary to the accumulation of fluid within the retinal tissue, producing swelling and cystic lesions located in a sunburst distribution around the macula. Patients may complain of a donut-shaped blurring in their visual field. Fortunately, this is an uncommon adverse effect occurring in less than 1% of patients (94). Patients' visual symptoms appear to be a sensitive indicator of this problem, since an ophthalmological survey of a large number of patients using niacin failed to find a single asymptomatic patient (95). To date, this disorder has completely disappeared on discontinuation of niacin.

Cardiovascular side effects may include palpitation and tachycardia associated with the cutaneous flushing episodes. However, severe cardiac arrhythmias have been noted with niacin therapy. Atrial fibrillation and other arrhythmias were described with greater frequency in the niacin-treated group when compared to placebo-treated patients in the Coronary Drug Project (93). Although few patients will have cardiac signs or symptoms that might be attributed to niacin therapy, the existing rhythm disturbances should be a relative contraindication to the use of this drug.

The worsening of hyperuricemia is predictable in patients who have preexisting elevated uric acid levels, and gouty attacks have been precipitated by niacin treatment (93). Some individuals with normal uric acid levels also seem to have a significant increase. Uric acid levels should be monitored during the first few months and annually thereafter. Patients with gouty arthritis or significant hyperuricemia should not be treated with this agent.

An increase in fasting plasma glucose level and the appearance of significant glucose intolerance has been observed in 5–10% of patients (81, 93). This may be due to the worsening of an underlying insulin-resistance syndrome and the exacerbation of subclinical non–insulin-dependent diabetes mellitus. Moderate increases in fasting plasma glucose level or known glucose intolerance are relative contraindications. This is particularly true when a strong family history of non–insulin-dependent diabetes mellitus is detected. Patients with frank diabetes have been treated, but approximately 50% require discontinuation of the drug due to the worsening glycemic control (81). The success rate may be higher in insulin-dependent patients.

## FIBRIC ACID DERIVATIVES

Currently available fibric acid derivatives are clofibrate, gemfibrozil, bezafibrate, fenofibrate, ciprofibrate, and etofibrate (Fig. 2.4).

### History and Chemical Structure

Clofibrate (*p*-chlorophenoxyisobutyric acid) was introduced as a hypolipidemic drug in the United Kingdom in 1962 and in the United States in 1967. A series of similar compounds have become available for prescription use over the past 25 years. The phenoxyisobutyric acid structure is common to all of these agents and this has given the generic name "fibric acid" to this class of lipid-lowering drugs. Clofibrate and then gemfibrozil were the most commonly used lipid-lowering drugs in the United States during the 1970s and early 1980s. Fenofibrate became the dominant lipid-lowering drug in Europe during the same period. The marked reduction in triglycerides and the moderate reduction in cholesterol seen in many patients, combined with a relatively low incidence of adverse reactions and ease of use, made them a popular choice for management of hyperlipidemia. Their long-term efficacy in lipid modification and in changing the incidence of cardiovascular disease has been studied in large randomized trials with clofibrate (93, 96) and gemfibrozil (97) (these are discussed in Chapter 3). These trials have provided useful information about prolonged changes in lipoprotein levels as well as frequency of adverse effects.

In all agents other than gemfibrozil, a chlorine atom or a chlorinated ring structure is located in the para position relative to the oxygen atom of the phenoxy ring (Fig. 2.4). In gemfibrozil, the ring structure contains methyl groups at the ortho and meta positions. This compound also differs in that the isobutyric acid derivative is connected through an ethylene bridge. Clofibrate and fenofibrate are esterified with ethanol and isopropanol, respectively, whereas the remainder of the group are formulated in the free-acid form. All of these agents can produce profound reductions in triglyceride levels in hypertriglyceridemic patients (98, 99). This effect is roughly equivalent among the various members of the group when used at maximum dosage levels (100). They also raise HDL cholesterol by 5–20%. LDL is reduced by 5–20%. Bezafibrate, fenofibrate, and ciprofibrate may be somewhat more effective in LDL reduction, although few studies have provided direct comparisons between members of this group. The LDL reduction is most dramatic in patients with triglyceride levels below 200 mg/dL. In hypertriglyceridemia, with LDL levels in the normal range,

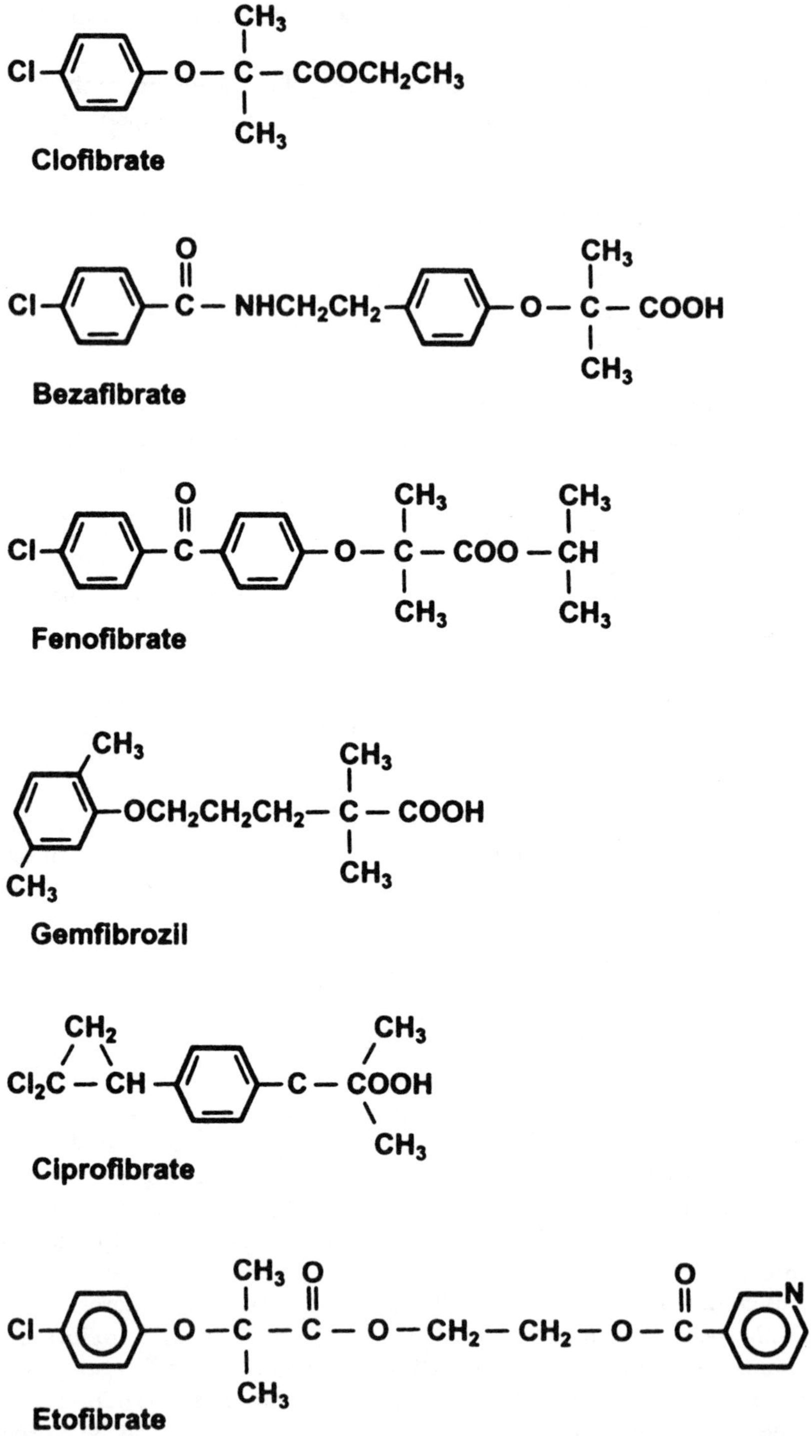

Clofibrate

Bezafibrate

Fenofibrate

Gemfibrozil

Ciprofibrate

Etofibrate

Figure 2.4 Chemical structure of fibric acid derivatives used worldwide. In the United States, only clofibrate and gemfibrozil are currently available for prescription use.

these drugs may produce no effect or paradoxically, an increase in LDL-c (99–101).

### Pharmacology and Mechanism of Action

After oral administration, more than 90% of the dose is absorbed and peak levels are usually reached within 2 to 4 hours (98, 102, 103). The ester bonds of clofibrate and fenofibrate are hydrolyzed in plasma or tissues into the active acid forms. All these drugs are bound avidly to albumin and other plasma proteins. The clearance rates from plasma vary widely, with half-lives of approximately 1.5–2.0 hours for gemfibrozil and bezafibrate (103) and up to 25 hours for clofibrate and fenofibrate (102). The major route of excretion is in the urine, after glucuronide conjugation in the liver. In normal humans, 60–90% of clofibrate, gemfibrozil, fenofibrate, and bezafibrate are excreted in the urine; the remainder appears in the stool after biliary excretion. The quantities of these drugs that undergo enterohepatic cycling are probably sizable. As a result, renal impairment markedly prolongs the half-life of these agents and requires a dose reduction. This prolonged clearance is a particularly significant problem with fenofibrate. The half-life of this agent has been found to be increased by as much as sevenfold in patients with renal failure (104). Fenofibrate is therefore contraindicated in patients with renal disease. The doses of other fibric acid derivatives should be reduced significantly with renal or hepatic dysfunction.

Plasma triglyceride reduction of 20–70% is the dominant effect of fibric acid therapy, and the various agents are approximately equivalent in their triglyceride-reducing effect at maximum dosage levels. The plasma concentrations of both VLDL and chylomicrons are reduced. IDL and LDL levels also decline in most patients. A rise in HDL-c is a common finding.

This series of changes in the lipoproteins has been related to a complex of metabolic and biochemical changes observed in hepatic and plasma lipoprotein metabolism. The synthesis of triglyceride in the liver and the transport of VLDL into the plasma space are reduced in animal and human studies (98, 105). This has been attributed to a reduction in the flow of free fatty acids from the adipose tissue (106, 107) and to increased oxidation of fatty acids in the liver (105). Several studies, using radioactive tracers, have strongly indicated that the major reason for VLDL triglyceride reduction is increased plasma clearance (108–110). The dominant enzyme activity responsible for removing triglyceride from VLDL and chylomicrons, lipoprotein lipase, is increased in postheparin plasma and in muscle tissue following fibrate treatment (98, 105, 111). However, this change is often quite small and does not correlate well with the triglyceride reduction observed in groups of patients. Recently, a more consistent theory has been proposed involving structural changes in VLDL and chylomicrons with reduced apolipoprotein C-III content (112, 113). This apolipoprotein is a known inhibitor of lipoprotein lipase and when increased quantities are present on the surface of triglyceride rich lipoproteins, there is inhibited interaction of the particle with receptors in the liver that are responsible for the uptake and degradation of the VLDL and chylomicron remnants. Apolipoprotein C-III is an important component of VLDL and chylomicrons that regulates the clearance of these lipoproteins. The plasma content of this protein has been shown to be reduced after fibric acid treatment (114). Recently, in animal and tissue culture studies, the hepatic synthesis of apolipoprotein C-III has been shown to be reduced by fibric acid treatment (112, 113). This was attributed specifically to suppression of the apolipoprotein C-III gene transcription through the suppression of hepatic nuclear factor IV (113). These observations and other studies have suggested that overproduction of apolipoprotein C-III may be one etiologic mechanism in those hypertriglyceridemic syndromes that are responsive to fibric acid treatment.

Alterations in LDL metabolism are quite complex when these drugs are used. In patients with elevated LDL levels but without hypertriglyceridemia, a reduction in LDL levels is believed to result from an increase in the number of LDL receptors in the liver and other tissues (115). The increase in LDL receptors may be the result of a reduction in cholesterol in the hepatocyte due to increased cholesterol secretion in the bile (116) and a reduction in cholesterol synthesis, as observed in animal studies (117). A fall in intrahepatic cholesterol content is known to result in a stimulation of the transcription of the gene for the LDL receptor protein, thus increasing the receptor numbers.

In patients with hypertriglyceridemia, the reduction in LDL-c is often blunted, and an increase in the concentration of this lipoprotein may occur. This apparent paradoxical effect has several potential explanations. First, the patients who have very high levels of VLDL and chylomicrons have abnormally high LDL clearance through pathways other than the LDL receptor (118). The fibric acid derivatives appear to reduce the role of these non-LDL receptor pathways. Secondly, the LDL particle in patients with hypertriglyceridemia is usually smaller, containing less cholesterol and somewhat more triglyceride. These smaller particles may be more rapidly cleared. Their lower cholesterol content belies the number of LDL particles in the plasma. The reduced cholesterol in LDL is in part a result of the transfer of cholesterol ester to the large number of triglyceride-rich particles through the action of cholesterol ester transfer protein present in the plasma. This protein exchanges cholesterol ester for triglyceride, enriching the LDL with triglyceride which can be removed by plasma lipase enzymes. The result is a much smaller, cholesterol-poor particle in these patients with hypertriglyceridemia. When the triglyceride pool in VLDL and chylomicrons is reduced, the cholesterol ester content of LDL then increases, as does the particle size (119–121). This often occurs without a significant change in the apolipoprotein B concentration, indicating that the number of LDL particles has remained relatively unchanged. The final LDL cholesterol concentration will reflect the balance of these competing factors.

In hypertriglyceridemic patients, the HDL is also smaller and cholesterol poor with increased triglyceride content (119–121). Cholesterol ester transfer protein exchanges cholesterol ester for triglyceride with these particles in a manner similar to that of LDL (see also Chapter 3). Fibrate treatment reduces the available triglyceride for this exchange process, resulting in a more normal cholesterol content in the HDL particles. A second reason for rising HDL-c may be due to effects on clearance of HDL particles. Small, dense HDL particles have been observed to have a shorter life span in plasma than larger, more cholesterol-rich particles. The apolipoprotein content of HDL may change with an increase in apolipoprotein A-I and apolipoprotein A-II (122) (and thus an increase in size). Often, the increase in apolipoprotein A-II is more dramatic, for reasons that are not explained.

Lp(a) is present in the plasma in increased quantities in some patients with coronary heart disease. This lipoprotein is a modification of LDL produced by the covalent attachment of a second protein synthesized in the liver. The quantity of this material is strongly determined by genetic factors. Attempts to reduce elevated levels of Lp(a) with the fibric acid derivatives have generally been unsuccessful (123).

## Clinical Use

Fibric acid derivatives are used primarily in the context of hypertriglyceridemia. These drugs may be an effective treatment in patients with triglyceride levels persistently higher than 500 mg/dL after maximum efforts with diet modification, exercise, and weight loss. When LDL cholesterol is elevated in those with triglyceride levels between 300 and 500 mg/dL, a fibrate may be considered an appropriate first-line drug. The alternative is niacin (discussed earlier), which is usually less expensive. The significant list of contraindications will, however, eliminate niacin from consideration in many patients, leaving the fibric acid group as the best choice for triglyceride control.

After 4–6 weeks, a reevaluation of lipoprotein levels will often reveal that the triglyceride value is less than 300 mg/dL and that HDL has risen 5–20%. The LDL cholesterol may have changed little. If LDL is in the target range, no further drug therapy may be needed. If the LDL remains above the desired level, addition of a second drug may be necessary. Bile acid sequestrants or HMG CoA reductase inhibitors are possible choices for further LDL reduction. The sequestrants should be used only if the triglyceride level has fallen below 300 mg/dL. If plasma triglyceride levels remain elevated, the reductase inhibitors are appropriate because they often lower triglyceride levels by approximately 20%.

In severe hypertriglyceridemia, persistence of triglyceride levels of more than 500 mg/dL may justify the combination of niacin and a fibric acid derivative.

Patients taking fibrates with other lipid-lowering drugs that act within the liver (niacin or reductase inhibitors) should be more frequently and rigorously monitored for liver or muscle dysfunction. Measuring ALT and AST and accessing symptoms of myopathy are indicated at intervals of 4–8 weeks while the dose is adjusted and at 3-month intervals after a stable dosage has been achieved.

The recommended doses of the various fibrates are given in Table 2.4. Reduction of the dose, usually by half or more, is indicated if there is mild renal or hepatic disease. Severe liver disease or renal failure is usually a contraindication for this class of drugs.

## Adverse Reactions

Several large scale double-blind, randomized, placebo-controlled clinical trials have provided detailed and objective information regarding the rate of adverse events with clofibrate (94, 96) and gemfibrozil (97). Data on other drugs in this class come from smaller studies and studies lasting for shorter periods of time. There are no studies giving significant data on the adverse reactions in a direct comparative sense. The larger studies have included only middle-aged men; therefore, adverse events in women and the elderly are less well studied. The major adverse drug effects are reported in Table 2.5.

### *Gastrointestinal Reactions*

Five to ten percent of patients complain of mild to moderate abdominal pain. This may be due to direct gastric or upper intestinal exposure to the

**Table 2.4**
**Recommended Doses of Fibrate Derivatives**

| Fibrate Derivative | Daily Dosing Schedule | Total Daily Dose |
|---|---|---|
| Bezafibrate | Twice | 600 mg |
| Ciprofibrate | Once | 100 mg |
| Clofibrate | Twice | 2000 mg |
| Etofibrate | Once or twice[a] | 1000 mg |
| Fenofibrate | Once[a] | 300 mg |
| Gemfibrozil | Twice | 1200 mg |

[a]Most studies conducted with two or three times daily dosing, but once daily appears to be equally efficacious.

**Table 2.5**
**Reported Adverse Drug Effects with Fibric Acid Derivatives**

| | |
|---|---|
| Gastrointestinal | Nausea eructation, flatulence, diarrhea, abdominal pain |
| Integumental | Rash, urticaria, hair loss, increased sweating |
| Musculoskeletal | Myalgias, elevated CPK and SGOT |
| Hepatic | Lithogenic bile, gallstones[a], elevated SGPT and SGOT |
| Psychoneurologic | Dizziness, fatigue, headache, insomnia, impotence |
| Cardiovascular | Atrial and ventricular arrhythmias[a] |
| Hematologic | Leukopenia, anemia |
| Drug interactions | Potentiates coumarins; increases incidence of myositis with reductase inhibitors |

[a]Documented only for clofibrate in the Coronary Drug Project and the World Health Organization Study.
CPK = creatine phosphokinase; SGOT = serum glutamic oxaloacetic transaminase; SGPT = serum glutamic pyruvic transaminase.

drug, either as a chemical irritant or through the release of hormones that increase intestinal motility, such as cholecystokinin. In the Coronary Drug Project (93) and World Health Organization (96) studies with clofibrate, abdominal discomfort led to increased diagnosis of cholecystitis and more cholecystectomies were performed. Several studies of bile composition have found increased cholesterol content relative to other components, such as bile acids and phospholipids (124). As a result, the bile is more prone to form cholesterol gallstones with all fibric acid derivatives. Clofibrate is the only member of this group that has been documented to increase gallbladder disease. This is probably due in part to the larger number of patients followed for prolonged periods in clinical trials with this drug.

### *Musculoskeletal Reactions*

Several cases of lethargy, weakness, and muscle tenderness have been associated with increased creatinine phosphokinase (CPK) levels in patients during clofibrate treatment (125). This syndrome has been seen with gemfibrozil and other fibric acid derivatives, particularly when combinations of drugs were used. It is a rare side effect when normal liver and renal function exist and in the absence of other drugs. This side effect was not observed in the 1900 patients treated in the Helsinki Heart Study with gemfibrozil for 5 years (97).

### *Hepatic Reactions*

Approximately, 1–2% of patients have shown a rise in the plasma activity of enzymes characteristic of hepatocellular disease (93, 97). These values return to normal when the drug is discontinued or the dose level is reduced. No convincing evidence of permanent liver damage has been presented.

### *Cardiovascular Reactions*

Rare cardiac arrhythmias have been described with clofibrate and correlated with blood concentrations of this drug in one study (93, 126).

### *Hematologic Reactions*

Leukopenia, decreased hemoglobin, and decreased hematocrit are uncommon observations that may be attributable to this group of drugs. Decreased platelet aggregation has been observed in a series of studies, and fibrinogen level may be reduced in some patients, but no adverse events have been related to these observations (127).

### *Integumental Reactions*

An allergic rash has been observed as well as urticaria and pruritus. Reported hair loss and increased sweating are less well documented adverse effects.

### *Other chemical changes*

Urea and creatinine levels have been noted to rise, but this is rare and of unclear significance. A small decrease in glucose and uric acid levels have been observed in a few patients. Fenofibrate is an exception in that it has well documented uricosuric effects, and uric acid level commonly falls in patients treated with this drug (127).

### *Cancer*

The World Health Organization Study involving 5000 patients showed a trend toward higher cancer rates in clofibrate-treated patients (96). The actual increase in cancer over this period of time was not statistically significant and no specific type of cancer was noted to increase in frequency. When these patients were followed for an additional 5-year period, there was no difference in the cancer rates for those who were treated with active drug or placebo. Trials with other fibric acid derivatives have not shown a significant change in cancer rate, and it is possible that the observations in the World Health Organization Study were spurious. A similar observational follow-up of participants in the Helsinki Heart Study showed no difference in cancer rates during the 5 years after the Study ended.

*Drug interaction*

Fibric acid derivatives are well documented to potentiate the anticoagulant effects of warfarin derivatives. These anticoagulants have been used successfully in reduced dosage and with appropriate monitoring during treatment with the fibrates. The myopathy noted above has been reported to be more frequent when these agents are combined with lovastatin and other HMG CoA reductase inhibitors.

## INDICATIONS FOR DRUG THERAPY

In addition to the discussion in this chapter, see also Chapter 3.

### Treatment of Elevated LDL-c

National guidelines call for reduction of LDL-c in an effort to reduce risk of coronary heart disease (1). These guidelines recommend dietary and lifestyle changes prior to the institution of drug treatment. Since many risk factors contribute to the incidence of coronary heart disease (Table 2.6) and since LDL-c appears to be a continuous risk factor, patients with higher total risk (predicted by all risk factor measures) should be treated most aggressively. The guidelines offer "threshold values" for beginning drug treatment and specific target values of LDL-c categorized by the risk

**Table 2.6**
**Major Risk Factor for Coronary Heart Disease Suggested for Use in Setting Goals for Therapy of Elevated LDL-c**

| Risk factor |
|---|
| Age<br>Man 45 years of age or older<br>Woman 55 years of age or older; over 45 if premature menopause and no estrogen replacement therapy |
| Family History<br>Definite coronary artery disease in first degree relatives: men under 55 years or women relatives under 65 years of age |
| Current cigarette smoking<br>Ten cigarettes or more per day |
| High blood pressure<br>Blood pressure greater than 140/90 or use of antihypertensive medication. |
| Low HDL-c<br>HDL-c less than 35 mg/dL |
| Diabetes mellitus<br>IDDM or NIDDM by American Diabetes Association criteria |

IDDM = insulin dependent diabetes mellitus; NIDDM = Non–insulin-dependent diabetes mellitus.

status of the individual patient (Table 2.7). Highest risk patients are those who have already manifested arteriosclerotic vascular disease in the coronary, carotid, or peripheral vessels. These individuals should seek drug therapy if the LDL-c remains above 130 mg/dL after several weeks of diet. The target LDL cholesterol in such patients is less than 100 mg/dL. In those with more than two other risk factors, drug therapy should begin at LDL-c levels of 160 mg/dL or higher with a target of reducing LDL to less than 130 mg/dL. For middle-aged individuals with LDL levels over 190 but with only one or no other risk factors, drug therapy should be used to reduce this value to less than 160. In very low risk individuals who are young (women less than 45 and men less than 35) without other major risk factors, LDL-c may not require drug therapy at values up to 220 mg/dL. If there is a strong family history of early coronary disease or other risk factors in such young individuals, good clinical judgement may call for drug therapy at lower LDL-c values. Currently, there are no specific recommendations suggesting that we avoid therapy in the elderly. It should be noted that we do not have extensive data on the value of treating individuals over 70 years. In those patients, however, whose life expectancy is 5 or more years and whose quality of life and attitudes suggest a preventive approach in the cardiovascular area, drug therapy may be as strongly indicated as in younger patients. There is no evidence that treating such patients will be less beneficial than treating those in their 50s or 60s.

**Table 2.7**
**LDL-c Concentrations Suggested for Clinical Decision Making Regarding Drug Therapy After Diet Treatment[a]**

| Risk Status | Consider Drug | Target Level |
|---|---|---|
| Arteriosclerosis clinically diagnosed-definite CAD, CVD, or PVD | >130 mg/dL | <100 mg/dL |
| No CVD known but two or more major risk factors for CVD (Table 2.5) | >160 mg/dL | <130 mg/dL |
| No CVD known and one or no major risk factor for CVD | >190 mg/dL | <160 mg/dL |
| No CVD known and no major risk factors in men <30 or women <40 years | >220 mg/dL | <160 mg/dL |

[a]All patients should be given counseling regarding a low cholesterol, low saturated fat diet, weight loss, and exercise. All other risk factors should be given appropriate treatment. If LDL-c does not fall below the values given above, drug therapy is recommended. Family history of early vascular disease should be given careful attention, particularly in concentration regimen for a young person. Some believe that diabetes mellitus is the equivalent of two major risk factors. An HDL-c concentration over 60 mg/dL might be considered a "negative risk factor," allowing less aggressive treatment in a person with only two other risk factors.
CAD = coronary artery disease; CVD = cardiovascular disease; PVD = peripheral vascular disease.

In the selection of the initial drug, many factors should be considered, including safety, patient characteristics, specific contraindications for a given drug, as well as the magnitude of change necessary to achieve the target value. When the triglyceride value is less than 200 mg/dL, bile acid sequestrants should be considered as first line drug therapy because of their long record of safety and efficacy. In patients who have very high LDL-c, sequestrants may provide a 20–30% reduction, which should be additive to the reduction that may be achieved by combining with other medications. The statins are also an attractive choice since they offer high efficacy in achieving major reduction in LDL-c in most patients, with an excellent safety record over the past 7 to 10 years. The combination of a sequestrant and a statin in low doses has many advantages. The additive effects may produce LDL-c levels that are reduced by 50–60% below baseline. Since lower doses of these two medications may be adequate, this combination has proven to be very cost effective in several studies (35, 36, 128). When this combination is used, the bile acid sequestrant is often given before dinner as a single dose and the reductase inhibitor at bedtime, 4–6 hours later. The two drugs should not be given simultaneously because of the potential adsorption and reduced absorption of the reductase inhibitor. The use of niacin in combination with bile acid sequestrants provides for a very low cost combination; however, there are more side effects observed, as noted earlier. In patients whom cost is a major consideration and in whom there are no contraindications for niacin therapy, it is recommended that this combination be considered.

Cost effectiveness in preventing coronary disease has been calculated in several studies, often using the index of dollars per year of life saved. Generally very attractive cost effectiveness estimates are calculated for the treatment of patients who already have manifest vascular disease (36–38).

## Indications for Drug Therapy in Hypertriglyceridemia

High triglyceride values often indicate lack of control of other metabolic abnormalities, including diabetes, hypothyroidism or nephrotic syndrome. When these disorders are brought under optimal control, the triglyceride value often falls considerably and occasionally to within the normal range (less than 200 mg/dL). Weight loss is often the most effective treatment that can be applied. If, however, after maximum dietary therapy has been achieved, triglycerides remain above 400 mg/dL, it is appropriate to consider drug therapy. Only two current drugs produce a significant triglyceride reduction. These are niacin and fibric acid derivatives. In general, if there are no contraindications to the use of niacin, it should be considered first line therapy. Niacin offers quite impressive triglyceride reduction, as well as LDL reduction, and very significant HDL elevation. However, in many patients, contraindications such as hyperuricemia, elevated blood glucose level, various inflammatory conditions, or gastrointestinal abnormalities prevent the use of niacin therapy. There is also evidence that many patients will not tolerate the cutaneous flushing reactions that are so frequent with this drug treatment. In such patients, the fibric acid derivatives are a very valuable option. After the maximum triglyceride reduction has been achieved with these agents, the LDL may be outside the guidelines calling for additional drug therapy. The elevated LDL-c may then be controlled by the addition of a bile acid sequestrant. These agents are preferable since they provide no additional systemic toxic effects. If this is not adequate or not acceptable to the patient, the combination of a statin with either niacin or a fibric acid derivative can be used. It should be remembered that liver dysfunction and myopathic changes appear somewhat more frequently when statins are combined with either niacin or a fibrate.

---

## REFERENCES


1. Grundy SM, Bilheimer D, Chait A, et al. Summary of the Second Report of the National Cholesterol Education Program (NCEP) Expert Panel on Detection, Evaluation, and Treatment of High Blood Cholesterol in Adults (Adult Treatment Panel II). JAMA 1993; 269:3015.
2. Consensus Conference. Treatment of hypertriglyceridemia. JAMA 1984; 251:1196–1200.
3. Consensus Conference. The hypertriglyceridemias: risk and management. Am J Med 1991; 68:1A–42A.
4. Greenberg BH, Blackwelder WC, Levy RI. Primary type V hyperlipoproteinemia. A descriptive study of 32 families. Arch Intern Med 1977; 87:526.
5. Hunninghake DB. Bile acid sequestrants. In: Rifkind BM, ed. Drug treatment of hyperlipidemia. New York: Marcel Dekker, 1991; 89–102.
6. Ast M, Frishman WH. Bile acid sequestrants. J Clin Pharmacol 1990;30:99–106.
7. Van Itallie TB, Hashim SA, Crampton RS, et al. Treatment of puritus and hypercholesterolemia of primary biliary cirrhosis with cholestyramine. N Engl J Med 1961; 265:469–474.
8. Benson GM, Haynes C, Blanchard S, et al. In vitro studies to investigate the reasons for the low potency of cholestyramine and colestipol. J Pharm Sci 1993: 82:80.
9. Packard C J, Shepherd J. The hepatobiliary axis and lipoprotein metabolism: effects of bile acid sequestrants and ileal bypass surgery. J Lipid Res 1982; 23:1081.
10. Shepherd J. Mechanism of action of bile acid sequestrants and other lipid lowering drugs. Cardiology 1989; 76(Suppl 1):65.
11. Konechnik TJ, Kos R, White JL. In vitro adsorption of bile salts by colestipol hydrochloride. Pharm Res 1989; 6:619.
12. Miettinen TA. Effects of hypolidemic drugs on bile acid metabolism in man. Adv Lipid Res 1981;18:65.
13. Garbutt JT, Kenney TJ. Effect of cholestyramine on bile acid metabolism in normal man. J Clin Invest 1972; 51:2781.
14. Dietschy JM, Wilson JD. Regulation of cholesterol metabolism. N Engl J Med 1970; 282:1128–1138, 1179, 1193.
15. Grundy S M. Dietary and drug regulation of cholesterol metabolism in man. In: Paoletti R, Glueck CJ, eds. Lipid pharmacology, vol 2. New York: Academic Press, 1976: 127–161.
16. Myant NB, Mitropoulos KA. Cholesterol-7-a-hydroxylase. J Lipid Res 1977; 18:135.
17. Kim DN, Rogers DH, Li JR, et al. Effects of cholestyramine on cholesterol balance parameters and hepatic HMG CoA reductase and cholesterol-7-a-hydrolase activities. Exp Mol Pathol 1977;26:434.
18. Mitropoulos KA, Knight BL, Reeves BE. 3-Hydroxy-3-methylglutaryl coenzyme A reductase. Biochem J 1980; 185:435.

19. Brown MS, Goldstein JL. A receptor-mediated pathway for cholesterol homeostasis. Science 1986; 232:234.
20. Levy RI, Langer T. Hypolipidemic drugs and lipoprotein metabolism. Adv Exp Med Biol 1972; 26:155.
21. Witztum JL, Schonfeld G, Weidman SW, et al. Bile acid sequestrant therapy alters the composition of LDL and HDL. Metabolism 1995.
22. Shepherd J, Bicker S, Lorimer AR, et al. Receptor-mediated LDL catabolism in man. J Lipid Res 1979; 20:999.
23. Breslow JL, Spaulding DR, Lux SE, et al. Homozygous familial hypercholesterolemia. New Engl J Med 1975; 293:900.
24. Angelin B, Einarsson K, Hellstrom K, et al. Effects of cholestyramine and chenodeoxycholic acid on the metabolism of endogenous triglyceride in hyperlipoproteinemia. J Lipid Res 1978; 19:1017.
25. Angelin B, Bjorkhem I, Einarsson K. Influence of bile acids on the soluble phosphatidic acid phosphatase in rat liver. Biochem Biophys Res Commun 1981; 100:606.
26. Crouse J R. Hypertriglyceridemia: a contraindication for use of bile acid resins. Am J Med 1987;83:243.
27. Hoogwerf BJ, Peters RJ, Frantz ID Jr, et al. Effect of clofibrate and colestipol singly and in combination of plasma lipids and lipoproteins in type III hyperlipoproteinemia. Metabolism 1985;34:978.
28. Shepherd J, Packard CJ. Effects of drugs on HDL metabolism. In:. Gotto VAM, Smith LC, Allen B, eds. Atherosclerosis. New York: Springer Verlag, 1980; 591.
29. Shepherd J, Packard CJ, Morgan J, et al. The effects of cholestyramine on HDL metabolism. Atherosclerosis 1979; 33:433.
30. The LRC-CPPT Study Group. The Lipid Research Clinics Coronary Primary Prevention Trial Results: (I) Reduction in incidence of coronary heart disease; (II) The relationship of reduction in incidence of CHD to cholesterol lowering. JAMA 1984; 251:351–374.
31. Watts GF, Lewis B, Brunt JNH, et al. Effects on CAD of lipid-lowering diet, or diet plus cholestyramine, in the St Thomas Atherosclerosis Regression Study (STARS). Lancet 1992; 339:563–569.
32. Gordon DJ, Knoke J, Probstfield JL, et al. HDL-cholesterol and coronary heart disease in hypercholesterolemic men: the Lipid Research Clinics Coronary Primary Prevention Trial. Circulation 1979; 74:1217.
33. Superko HR, Greenland P, Manchester RA, et al. Effectiveness of low-dose colestipol therapy in patients with moderate hypercholesterolemia. Am J Cardiol 1992; 70:135.
34. Hunninghake DB, Peterson F, Swenson M, et al. Efficacy of once vs twice-a-day dosage of cholesterylamine in type IIa hyperlipoproteinemia. Pharmacology 1979; 21:176 (Abstract).
35. Tonstad S, Ose L, Gorbitz, Harrison EM, et al. Effectiveness of low-dose lovastatin combined with low-dose colestipol in moderate and severe hypercholesterolemia. Scand J Clin Lab Invest 1993; 53:457–463.
36. Heudebert GR, van Ruiswyk J, Hiatt J, et al. Combination drug therapy for hypercholesterolemia. The trade-off between cost and simplicity. Arch Intern Med 1993; 153:1828–1837.
37. Jungnickel PW, Shaefer MS, Maloley PA, et al. Blind comparison of patient preference for flavored colestid granules and questran light. Ann Pharmacol 1993; 27: 700–703.
38. Hunninghake DB, Stein EA, Bremner WF, et al. Dose-response study of colestipol tablets in patients with moderate hypercholesterolemia. Am J Therap 1995;2: 180–189.
39. Insull W, Davidson MH, Demke AM, et al. The effects of colestipol tablets compared with colestipol granules on plasma cholesterol and other lipids in moderately hypercholesterolemic patients. Atherosclerosis 1995;112:223–235.
40. Spence JD, Huff MW, Heidenheim P, et al. Combination therapy with colestipol and psyllium mucilloid in patients with hyperlipidemia. Arch Intern Med 1995;123:493–499.
41. Bell LP, Hectorne K, Reynolds H, et al. Cholesterol lowering effects of psyllium hydrophilic mucilloid. JAMA 1989; 261:3419.

42. Palasciano G, Chiloiro M, Belfiore A, et al. Cholestyramine alters feedback mechanism of bile acids and cholecystokinin in the regulation of gallbladder motility in humans. Hepatology 1989; 10:603 (Abstract).
43. Hunninghake DB. Resin therapy. Adverse effects and management. In: Fears J, Barcelona JR, eds. Pharmacological control of hyperlipidemia. Prous Science Publishers, SA, 1986; 67–89.
44. Witztum JL, Laurence SJ, Schonfeld G. Thyroid hormone and thyrotropin levels in patients placed on colestipol hydrochloride. J Clin Endocrinol Metab 1978;46:838.
45. Stein EA. Treatment of familial hypercholesterolemia with drugs in children. Arterioscler Thromb 9(Suppl I):I-145–I-151.
46. Schneider DL, Gallo DG, Sarett HP. Effect of cholestyramine on cholesterol metabolism in young adult swine. *P. S. E. B. M.* 1966;121:1244.
47. Scheel PJ, Whelton A, Rossiter K, et al. Cholesterylamine-induced hyperchloremic metabolic acidosis. J Clin Pharmacol 1992; 32:536.
48. Grundy, SM. HMG CoA reductase inhibitors: clinical applications and therapeutic potential. In: Rifkind BM, ed. Drug treatment of hyperlipidemia. New York: Marcel Dekker, 1991;139–167.
49. Schonfeld G. HMG CoA reductase inhibitors. In: LaRosa JC, ed. Practical management of lipid disorders. Fort Lee, NJ: Healthcare Communications, 1992; 75–90.
50. Blum CB. Comparison of properties of four inhibitors of HMG CoA reductase. Am J Cardiol 1994; 73:3D–11D.
51. Goldstein JL, Brown MS. Regulation of the mevalonate pathway. Nature 1990; 343:425–430.
52. Grundy SM, Vega GL. Influence of mevinolin on metabolism of LDL in primary moderate hypercholesterolemia. J Lipid Res 1985; 26:1466–1475.
53. Illingworth DR, Tobert JA. A review of clinical trials comparing HMG CoA reductase inhibitors. Clin Ther 1994;16:366–385.
54. Illingworth DR. Therapeutic use of lovastatin in the treatment of hypercholesterolemia. Clin Ther 1994; 16:2–26.
55. Bradford RH, Shear CL, Chremos AN, et al. Expanded Clinical Evaluation of Lovastatin (EXCEL) study results: two-year efficacy and safety follow-up. Am J Cardiol 1995;74:667–673.
56. Azzarito C, Boiardi L, Zini M, et al. Long-term therapy with high-dose simvastatin does not affect adrenocortical and gonadal hormones in hypercholesterolemic patients. Metabolism 1992;41:148–153.
57. Purvis K, Tollefsrud A, Rui H, et al. Short-term effects of treatment with simvastatin on testicular function in patients with heterozygous familial hypercholesterolemia. Eur J Clin Pharmacol 1992; 42:61–64.
58. Cutts JL, Bankhurst AD. Reversal of lovastatin-mediated inhibition of natural killer cell cytotoxicity by interleukin 2. Cell Physiol 1990;145:244–252.
59. Kobashigawa JA., Katznelson S, Laks H, et al. Effect of pravastatin on outcomes after cardiac transplantation. N Engl J Med 1995;333:621–627.
60. Kostis JB, Rosen RC, Wilson AC. Central nervous system effects of HMG CoA reductase inhibitors: lovastatin and pravastatin on sleep and cognitive performance in patients with hypercholesterolemia. J Clin Pharmacol 1994;34:989–996.
61. Partinen M, Pihl S, Strandberg T, et al. Comparison of effect on sleep of lovastatin and pravastatin in hypercholesterolemia. Am J Cardiol 1994;73:876–880.
62. Rosenson RS, Frauenheim WA. Safety of combined pravastatin-gemfibrozil therapy. Am J Cardiol 1994; 74:499–500.
63. Jacobson TA, Amorosa LF. Combination therapy with fluvastatin and niacin in hypercholesterolemia. Am J Cardiol 1994; 73:25D–29D.
64. Pool JL, Shear CL, Downton M, et al. Lovastatin and coadministered antihypertensive/cardiovascular agents. Hypertension 1992;19:242–248.
65. Darby WJ, McNutt KW, Tod-Hunter EN. Niacin. Nutr Rev 1975;33:289–297.
66. Brown WV, Howard WJ, Field L. Nicotinic acid and its derivatives. In: Rifkind BM, ed. Drug treatment of hyperlipidemia. New York: Marcel Dekker, 1990; 189–213.
67. Carlson LA, Oro L, Ostman J.. Effect of a single dose of nicotinic acid on plasma lipids in patients with hyperlipoproteinemia. Acta Med Scand 1968;183:457–465.

68. Mrochek JE, Jolley RI, Young DS.. Metabolic response on humans to ingestion of nicotinic acid and nicotinamide. Clin Chem 1976;22:1821–1827.
69. Carlson LA, Hamsten A, Asplund A. Pronounced lowering of serum levels of lipoprotein Lp(a) in hyperlipidemic subjects treated with nicotinic acid. J Intern Med 1989;226:271–276.
70. Wahlberg G, Holmquist L, Walldins G, et al. Effects of nicotinic acid on concentrations of serum apolipoproteins: B, C-I, C-II, C-III and E in the hyperlipidemic patients. Acta Med Scand 1988;224:319–327.
71. Grundy SM, Mok HYI, Zech L, et al. Influence of nicotinic acid on metabolism of cholesterol and triglyceride in man. J Lipid Res 1989;22:24–36.
72. Froberg SO, Boberg J, Carlson LA, et al. Metabolic effects of nicotinic acid and its derivatives. In : Hans Huber Publishers, 1971;167–181.
73. Carlson LA, Oro L. The effect of nicotinic acid on the plasma free fatty acids. Acta Med Scand 1962; 172:641–645.
74. Carlson LA, Olsson AG. Effect of nicotinic acid on serum lipids and lipoproteins. In: Olsson AG, ed. Treatment of hyperlipoproteinemia. New York:Raven Press, 1984; 115–119.
75. Alderman JD. Effect of a modified, well tolerated niacin regimen on serum total cholesterol, HDL-c and the cholesterol to HDL ratio. Am J Cardiol 1989;64:725–729.
76. Blum CE, Levy RI, Eisenberg S, et al. HDL metabolism in man. J Clin Invest 1977;60:795–807.
77. Shepherd J, Packard CJ, Patsch JR, et al. Effects of nicotinic acid therapy on plasma HDL subfraction and composition and on apoA metabolism. J Clin Invest 1979;63: 858–867.
78. Guvakav A, Hoeg JM, Kostner G, et al. Levels of lipoprotein Lp(a) decline with neomycin and niacin treatment. Atherosclerosis 1985;57:293–301.
79. Kostner G, Klein G, Krempler F. Can serum Lp(a) concentration be lowered by drugs and or diet? In: Carlson LA, Olsson AG, ed. Treatment of hyperlipoproteinemia. New York: Raven Press,1984; 154–156.
80. Figge HL, Figge J, Souney PF, et al. Nicotinic acid: a review of its clinical use in the treatment of lipid disorders. Pharmacotherapy 1988;8:287–294.
81. Gray DR, Morgan T, Chretien S, et al. Efficacy and safety of controlled-release niacin in dyslipoproteinemic veterans. Ann Intern Med 1994;121:252–258.
82. Carlson LA, Olsson AG, Ballantyne D. On the rise in LDL and HDL in response to the treatment of hypertriglyceridemia in type IV and type V hyperlipoproteinemia. Atherosclerosis 1977;26:603–609.
83. Carlson LA, Olsson AG. Effects of hypolipidemic drugs on serum lipoproteins. In: Eisenberg S, ed. Progress in biochemical pharmacology. New York: S Karger, 1990;238–257.
84. Kane JP, Malloy JJ, Tun P. Normalization of LDL levels in heterozygous familial hypercholesterolemia with combined drug regimen. N Engl J Med 1981;304:2541–2548.
85. Hotz W. Nicotinic acid and its derivatives. A short survey. Adv Lipid Res 1983;20: 195–217.
86. Malloy MJ, Kane JP, Kunitake ST, et al. Complimentary of colestipol, niacin and lovastatin in the treatment of severe familial hypercholesterolemia. Arch Intern Med 1987;107:616–623.
87. Reaven P, Witztum JL. Lovastatin, nicotinic acid and rhabdomyolysis. Arch Intern Med 1988;109:595–597.
88. Jay RH, Dickson AC, Betterridge DJ. Effects of aspirin upon the flushing reaction induced by niceritrol. Br J Clin Pharm 1990;29:120–122.
89. Knopp RH, Ginsberg J, Albers JJ, et al. Contrasting effects of unmodified and time-release forms of niacin or lipoproteins in hyperlipidemic subjects: clues to mechanism of action of niacin. Metabolism 1985;34:642–650.
90. Brown WV. Niacin for lipid disorders. Postgrad Medicine 1995;98:185–196.
91. Morrow JD, Parsons WG, Roberts LJ. Release of markedly increased quantities of prostaglandin $D_2$ in vivo in humans following the administration of nicotinic acid. Prostaglandins 1989;38:263–274.

92. Christiansen NA, Achor RWP, Berge KG, et al. Nicotinic acid treatment of hypercholesterolemia: comparison of plain and sustained action preparations and report of two cases of jaundice. JAMA 1961;177:546–550.
93. The Coronary Drug Project Research Group. Clofibrate and niacin in coronary heart disease. JAMA 1975;231:360–381.
94. Gass JDM. Nicotinic acid maculopathy. Am J Opthalmol 1973;76:500–510.
95. Millay RH, Klein ML, Illingworth DR. Niacin maculopathy. Ophthalmology 1988; 95:930–936.
96. WHO Investigators. WHO Cooperative Trial on primary prevention of ischaemic heart disease with clofibrate to lower serum cholesterol: final mortality follow-up. Lancet 1984;2:600–604.
97. Frick MH, Elo O, Haapa K, et al. Helsinki Heart Study: primary prevention trial with gemfibrozil in middle-aged men with dyslipidemia. N Engl J Med 1987;317: 1237–1245.
98. Todd PA, Ward A. Gemfibrozil: a review of its pharmacodynamic and pharmacokinetic properties and therapeutic use in dyslipidemia. Drugs 1988;36:314–339.
99. Goldberg AC, Schonfeld G, Feldman EB, et al. Fenofibrate for the treatment of type IV and V hyperlipoproteinemias: a double-blind, placebo-controlled, multicenter US study. Clin Therapy 1989;11:69–83.
100. Hunninghake DB, Peters J. Effects of fibric acid derivatives on blood lipid and lipoprotein levels. Am J Med 1987;83(Suppl 5B):44–49.
101. Wilson DE, Lees RS. Metabolic relationships among the lipoproteins: reciprocal changes in the concentrations of VLDL and LDL in man. J Clin Invest 1972; 251:1052–1062.
102. Balfour JA, McTavish D, Heel RC. Fenofibrate: a review of its pharmacodynamic and pharmacokinetic properties and therapeutic use in dyslipidemia. Drugs 1990; 40:260–290.
103. Monk JP, Todd PA. Bezafibrate: a review of its pharmacodynamic and pharmacokinetic properties and therapeutic use in hyperlipidemia. Drugs 1987;3:539–576.
104. Desager JP, Costermans J, Verberckmoes R, et al. Effect of human dialysis on plasma kinetics of fenofibrate in chronic renal failure. Nephron 1982;31:51–54.
105. Kloer HU. Structure and biochemical effects of fenofibrate. Am J Med 1987;83 (Suppl 5B):328.
106. Kissebah AH, Adams BW, Harrigan P, et al. The mechanism of clofibrate and tetranicotile fructose on the kinetics of plasma free fatty acids and triglyceride transport in type IV and in type V hypertriglyceridemia. Eur J Clin Invest 1974;4:163–174.
107. Rifkind BM. Effect of CPIB ester on plasma free fatty acid levels in man. Metabolism 1966;15:673–675.
108. Grundy SM, Vega GL. Fibric acids: effects on lipids and lipoprotein metabolism. Am J Med 1987;83(Suppl 5B):9–20.
109. Shepherd J, Packard CJ, Stewart JM. Apolipoprotein A and B metabolism during bezafibrate therapy in hypertriglyceridemic subjects. J Clin Invest 1984;74:2164–2177.
110. Packard CJ, Clegg RJ, Dominiczak MH, et al. Effects of bezafibrate on apoB metabolism in type III hyperlipoproteinemic subjects. J Lipid Res 1986;27:930–938.
111. Boberg J, Boberg M, Gross R, et al. The effect of treatment with clofibrate on hepatic triglyceride and lipoprotein lipase activities of post-heparin plasma in male patients with hyperlipoproteinemia. Atherosclerosis 1977;267:499–503.
112. Staels B, Vu-Dac N, Kosykh VA, et al. Fibrates downregulate apoC-III expression independent of induction of peroxisomal acyl CoA oxidase. J Clin Invest 1995;95: 705–712.
113. Hertz R, Bishara-Shieban J, Bar-Tana J. Mode of action of peroxisome proliferators as hypolipidemic drugs. J Biol Chem 1995;270:13470–13475.
114. Fruchart JC, Davignon J, Bard JM, et al. Effect of fenofibrate on type III hyperlipoproteinemia. Am J Med 1987;83(Suppl 5B):71–74.
115. Stewart JM, Packard CJ, Lorimer AR, et al. Effects of bezafibrate on receptor-mediated and receptor-independent LDL catabolism in type II hyperlipoproteinemia. Atherosclerosis 1984;44:355–364.

116. Kesaniemi YA, Grundy SM. Influence of gemfibrozil and clofibrate on metabolism of cholesterol and plasma triglyceride in man. JAMA 1984;251:2241–2246.
117. Bernt J, Gaumert R, Still J. Mode of action of the lipid-lowering agents clofibrate and BM-15,075 on cholesterol biosynthesis in rat liver. Atherosclerosis 1978;30: 147–152.
118. Shepherd J, Caslake MJ, Lorimer MR, et al. Fenofibrate reduces LDL catabolism in hypertriglyceridemic subjects. Arteriosclerosis 1985;5:162–168.
119. Eisenberg S, Gavish D, Oschry Y, et al. Abnormalities in VLDL, LDL and HDL in hypertriglyceridemia: reversal toward normal with bezafibrate treatment. J Clin Invest 1984;74:470–482.
120. Goldberg AC, Schonfeld G, Anderson C, et al. Fenofibrate affects the composition of lipoproteins. Am J Med 1987;83(Suppl 5B):60–65.
121. Knopp RH, Walden CE, Warnick R, et al. Effect of fenofibrate treatment on plasma lipoprotein lipids, HDL cholesterol subfractions and apolipoprotein B, A-I, A-II, E. Am J Med 1987;83(Suppl 5B):75–84.
122. Saku K, Gartside DS, Hind BA, et al. Mechanism of action of gemfibrozil on lipoprotein metabolism. J Clin Invest 1985;75:1702–1712.
123. Albers JJ, Cabana VG, Warnick GR, et al. Lp(a) lipoprotein: relationship to sinking prebetalipoprotein, hyperlipoproteinemia and apoB. Metabolism 1975;24: 1047–1054.
124. Palmer RH. Effects of fibric acid derivatives on biliary lipid composition. Am J Med 1987;83(Suppl 5B):37–43.
125. Langer T, Levy RI. Acute muscular syndrome associated with administration of clofibrate. N Engl J Med 1968;279:856–858.
126. LaRosa JC, Brown WV, Frommer P, et al. Clofibrate-induced ventricular arrhythmia. Am J Cardiol 1969:23:266–269.
127. Brown WV. Fenofibrate, a third-generation fibric acid derivative. Proceedings of a symposium. Am J Med 1987:83(Suppl 5B):1–89.
128. Schrott HG, Stein EA, Dujovne CA, et al. Enhanced LDL cholesterol reduction and cost-effectiveness by low-dose colestipol plus lovastatin combination therapy. Am J Cardiol 1995;75:34–39.

CHAPTER 3

# Primary and Secondary Prevention of Coronary Heart Disease

John A. Farmer, MD, and Antonio M. Gotto, Jr, MD, DPhil

During the past several decades, a large body of evidence has accumulated in support of the lipid hypothesis, which postulates that elevated serum cholesterol increases risk for coronary heart disease (CHD) and that cholesterol lowering reduces the risk. Support derives from observational epidemiological, genetic, experimental, and clinical studies. The interventional studies indicate that normalization of the lipid profile by dietary, pharmacologic, or surgical (partial ileal bypass) intervention decreases the risk for atherosclerotic events and may slow progression and induce regression of atherosclerotic lesions. This chapter reviews the rationale for pharmacologic intervention against hyperlipidemia, including evidence from clinical trials of the effect of pharmacologic lipid lowering on CHD lesions and events and guidelines for evaluation and treatment.

## RATIONALE FOR LIPID LOWERING

### Lipoprotein Metabolism

Lipids are transported in the circulation in multimolecular, spherical particles termed *lipoproteins,* which are composed of a core of cholesteryl ester and triglyceride surrounded by a surface monolayer of phospholipid, cholesterol, and apolipoproteins (Fig. 3.1). The lipoproteins are distinguished by composition, density, size, and electrophoretic mobility (Table 3.1).

#### *Triglyceride-Rich Lipoproteins*

Chylomicrons and very-low-density lipoprotein (VLDL) are the initial particles of exogenous and endogenous lipid transport, respectively. The major lipid in these lipoproteins is triglyceride, derived from dietary fats or synthesized by the liver. The apolipoprotein (apo) B-48 on the surface of chylomicrons reflects their intestinal origin; the apo B-100 of VLDL, which is secreted by the liver, is characteristic of lipoproteins throughout the endogenous cascade. At the capillary endothelium, triglyceride in these triglyceride-rich lipoproteins is hydrolyzed through the action of lipoprotein lipase, which is activated by apo C-II on the lipoprotein surface. Hydrolysis of chylomicron and VLDL triglyceride frees fatty acids to be used

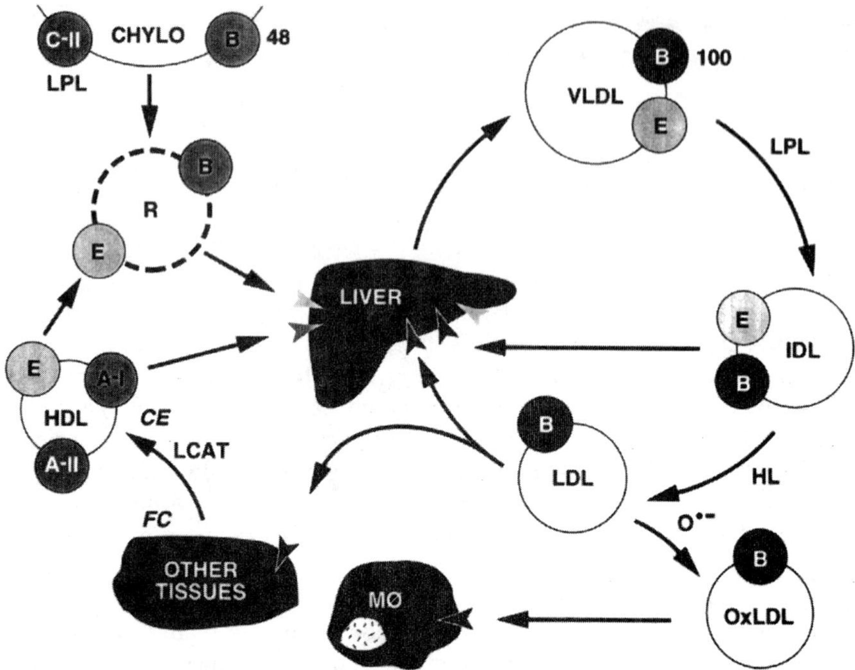


Figure 3.1. The exogenous and endogenous plasma lipid pathways. *CE* = cholesteryl ester; CHYLO = chylomicron; *FC* = free (unesterified) cholesterol; HDL = high-density lipoprotein; HL = hepatic lipase; IDL = intermediate-density lipoprotein; LCAT = lecithin:cholesterol acyltransferase; LDL = low-density lipoprotein; LPL = lipoprotein lipase; Mì = macrophage; O·− = oxygen free radical; OxLDL = oxidized LDL; R= chylomicron remnant; VLDL = very-low-density lipoprotein. Lipoproteins are shown with their major apolipoproteins (A-I, A-II, B-48, B-100, C-II, E). Reprinted with permission from International Lipid Information Bureau. The ILIB lipid handbook for clinical practice: blood lipids and coronary heart disease. Houston: ILIB, 1995.

as energy by muscle tissue or to become stored energy in adipose tissue. The C and A apolipoproteins released on hydrolysis transfer to high-density lipoprotein (HDL), as do other surface components made redundant by the shrinking chylomicron and VLDL cores.

### *Receptor-Mediated Clearance of Apolipoprotein B–Containing Lipoproteins*

Chylomicron remnants are quickly removed from the circulation, apparently through receptor-mediated recognition and binding of apo E by the liver. Some intermediate-density lipoprotein (IDL) particles, which remain after the hydrolysis of VLDL, are cleared by apo E–mediated uptake by the B/E receptor in the liver; others remain in the circulation, where, through the action of hepatic lipase, they are further hydrolyzed to form low-density lipoprotein (LDL). The sole major apolipoprotein remaining in

**Table 3.1**
**Classification and Properties of Plasma Lipoproteins**

| Lipoprotein Class | Major Lipids | Apolipoproteins | Density (g/mL) | Diameter (Å) | Electro-phoretic Mobility |
|---|---|---|---|---|---|
| Chylomicrons | Dietary triglyceride, cholesteryl ester | A-I, A-II, A-IV, B-48, C-I, C-II, C-III, E | <0.95 | 800–5000 | Origin |
| Chylomicron remnants | Dietary cholesteryl ester | B-48, E | <1.006 | >300 | Origin |
| VLDL | Endogenous triglyceride | B-100, C-I, C-II, C-III, E | <1.006 | 300–800 | Pre-β |
| IDL | Cholesteryl ester, triglyceride | B-100, E | 1.006–1.019 | 250–350 | Broad-β |
| LDL | Cholesteryl ester | B-100 | 1.019–1.063 | 180–280 | β |
| $HDL_2$ | Cholesteryl ester | A-I, A-II, C-I, C-II, C-III, E | 1.063–1.125 | 90–120 | α |
| $HDL_3$ | Cholesteryl ester | A-I, A-II, C-I, C-II, C-III, E | 1.125–1.210 | 50–90 | α |

LDL is apo B-100, by which LDL is bound by the B/E receptor (LDL receptor) and removed from the circulation.

Approximately 70% of circulating cholesterol is carried in LDL particles, which deliver cholesterol to peripheral cells for use in forming cell membranes and steroid hormones. LDL cholesterol level has been directly correlated with risk for CHD and is the primary target of intervention in the treatment guidelines of the second Adult Treatment Panel (ATP II) of the US National Cholesterol Education Program (1). LDL not removed by the B/E receptor is removed through alternative pathways, including scavenger receptors on macrophages. Oxidation or other chemical modification is thought to be necessary for LDL to be recognized by the scavenger receptor. Unlike the B/E receptor, the activity of which is down-regulated as intracellular cholesterol content increases, the scavenger receptor continues to accumulate lipid, and the macrophage can become a foam cell. Foam cells are the chief constituents of the fatty streak, the initial lesion in atherogenesis.

In individuals with hypertriglyceridemia, triglyceride from VLDL can be transferred to LDL in exchange for cholesteryl ester through the action of cholesteryl ester transfer protein. The triglyceride is then hydrolyzed, resulting in small, dense LDL. Because these LDL particles contain proportionately less cholesterol than normal, buoyant LDL, the number of LDL particles may be elevated although the LDL cholesterol level is normal. Individuals with a predominance of small, dense LDL, termed *LDL subclass pattern B,* have been reported to have a threefold increased risk for myocardial infarction (MI) compared with individuals with a predominance of normal, buoyant LDL, termed LDL subclass pattern A (2). Some evidence suggests that LDL subclass pattern is genetically influenced, although it is generally not expressed before adulthood in men or before menopause in women (3). Some studies suggest that triglyceride lowering—for example, by fibric acid derivative therapy—can change LDL subclass pattern B to pattern A (4).

### *HDL and Reverse Cholesterol Transport*

HDL is considered cardioprotective and may be the vehicle of the putative process of reverse cholesterol transport. Through this process, HDL is thought to return cholesterol from peripheral tissues to the liver for excretion. Nascent HDL is believed to be secreted as discoidal precursor particles; these particles acquire phospholipid and cholesterol from the surfaces of chylomicrons and VLDL during lipolysis and from cell membranes. Lecithin–cholesterol acyltransferase (LCAT) acts upon these discoidal particles to transform them into mature, spherical HDL with a core rich in cholesteryl ester. Through continued acquisition of phospholipid and cholesterol, and through continued esterification by LCAT, the smaller $HDL_3$ is transformed into the larger $HDL_2$, thus increasing the cholesterol-carrying capacity of HDL and enhancing the efficiency of reverse cholesterol transport.

Cholesteryl ester from HDL may be exchanged for triglyceride from the triglyceride-rich lipoproteins through the action of cholesteryl ester transfer protein. The cholesteryl ester then continues in the exogenous and endogenous lipolytic cascades and is ultimately removed from the circulation with chylomicron remnants, IDL, and LDL (Fig. 3.1). The triglyceride transferred to HDL is hydrolyzed by hepatic lipase, and $HDL_2$ reverts to $HDL_3$, decreasing its cholesterol content and reducing the volume of reverse cholesterol transport.

The cardioprotection of HDL may instead be indirect. High levels of HDL may be the result of efficient metabolism of triglyceride-rich lipoproteins, which are cleared from the circulation before cholestryl ester transfer proteins transfer their triglyceride to HDL for subsequent lipolysis (5). Potential direct protective mechanisms ascribed to HDL are stimulation of endothelial repair (6), prostacyclin stabilization (7), and prevention of lipid oxidation (8).

## Observational Epidemiological Studies

Numerous epidemiological studies conducted in different countries and among different ethnic groups have established a strong positive relation between serum cholesterol level and risk for CHD (9, 10). In populations that consume diets high in saturated fat and cholesterol, serum cholesterol level is increased, and coronary and peripheral atherosclerosis develops at an accelerated rate. Conversely, circulating cholesterol level is decreased and prevalence of atherosclerosis is reduced in populations that consume diets low in saturated fat and cholesterol.

The possibility that genetic differences accounted for geographic or ethnic differences in rates of atherosclerotic disease was clearly refuted by comparison of men of Japanese descent living in Japan with those living in the United States. In the Ni-Hon-San Study, Japanese men in Japan consumed less fat and cholesterol (fat 15% of total calories, cholesterol 457 mg/day) than Japanese emigrants and their sons in Hawaii (fat 33% of total calories, cholesterol 545 mg/day) and California (fat 38% of total calories, cholesterol 536 mg/day) (11). Elevated serum cholesterol levels (260 mg/dL or greater) were more common in Hawaii than in Japan and more common in California than in Hawaii; mean serum cholesterol levels were progressively higher in Hawaii and California than in Japan (12). Accordingly, the age-adjusted incidence of MI and CHD death in Japan was 50% lower than that in Hawaii, which was 50% lower than that in California (13).

Among the 356,222 men screened for the Multiple Risk Factor Intervention Trial (MRFIT), the relation between total cholesterol level and CHD mortality was found to be curvilinear (14). With each successive decile of serum cholesterol, 6-year CHD mortality increased. Mortality in the highest decile (total cholesterol 264 mg/dL or more) was four times higher than that in the lowest decile (total cholesterol 167 mg/dL or less).

In the Framingham Heart Study, total cholesterol level was directly related to cardiovascular mortality and total mortality in men and women aged less than 50 years (15). For each 10 mg/dL increase in cholesterol, cardiovascular mortality increased 9% and total mortality increased 5%.

### Genetic Evidence

The relation between cholesterol level and the development of CHD has also been established in studies of genetic disorders characterized by elevated cholesterol. In patients with these disorders, CHD can develop without any other risk factors present.

In familial hypercholesterolemia, LDL accumulates in the blood because of a lack of competent B/E receptors to remove these particles from the circulation (16). In the heterozygous form of this disorder, individuals have half the normal number of competent LDL receptors, and LDL cholesterol levels are typically twice as high as in normal individuals. In these patients, symptomatic CHD generally occurs by age 40–50 in men and by age 50–60 in women. In homozygous familial hypercholesterolemia, competent LDL receptors are absent, and LDL cholesterol levels reach 500–1000 mg/dL. Homozygotes typically develop symptomatic CHD before age 20.

Among other genetic disorders associated with increased LDL cholesterol levels and increased CHD risk are familial defective apo B-100, in which a defect in the apo B-100 molecule prevents its recognition and binding by the B/E receptor, and familial combined hypercholesterolemia, characterized by elevations in cholesterol and triglyceride levels within a family, although both levels may not be elevated within an individual.

## Experimental Studies

Studies in a variety of animal species have demonstrated that atherosclerosis can be induced by diets rich in saturated fat and cholesterol (17, 18) and reversed by converting to a low-fat, low-cholesterol diet (19). The Watanabe heritable hyperlipidemic rabbit provides a model for familial hypercholesterolemia, because this species lacks the B/E receptor and is susceptible to the development of severe atherosclerosis.

## Clinical Trial Evidence

Studies in which cholesterol lowering was accomplished by diet, drugs, surgery (partial ileal bypass), or some combination of these treatments have demonstrated a reduction in CHD risk, in support of the lipid hypothesis. In general, these studies indicate a 2–3% decrease in CHD incidence with each 1% decrease in total cholesterol level. Angiographically monitored studies have shown that the progression of atherosclerotic lesions can be decreased with aggressive lipid lowering. In addition, data from clinical trials are now available to demonstrate a reduction in all-cause mortality. Representative major studies are described.

### *Primary Prevention*

Trials in subjects without clinical evidence of CHD have used single-agent lipid-lowering drug therapy to supplement diet in efforts to decrease rates of CHD events. Decreases in CHD incidence have been clear—for example, significant mean decreases of 19%, 20%, 34%, and 31% in nonfatal MI and CHD death were seen in the Lipid Research Clinics Coronary Primary Prevention Trial (LRC-CPPT), the World Health Organization (WHO) Cooperative Trial, the Helsinki Heart Study, and the West of Scotland Coronary Prevention Study (WOSCOPS), respectively, described. However, primary prevention trials are hampered by the need for large numbers of subjects and lengthy duration to demonstrate a benefit in coronary mortality or total mortality. Metaanalysis of the LRC-CPPT, the WHO Cooperative Trial, the Helsinki Heart Study, and the Wadsworth–Veterans Administration trial (20) (a diet trial that did not exclude individuals with existing CHD), indicated that risk for fatal MI decreased a mean 14% with treatment, but that difference did not reach statistical significance (21). Risk for nonfatal MI decreased 26% and risk for combined fatal and nonfatal MI decreased 23% with treatment in these trials; both of these decreases were significant. These four published trials were not of sufficient statistical power to determine total mortality.

**Lipid Research Clinics Coronary Primary Prevention Trial.** The LRC-CPPT is considered a landmark study because it was the first trial to demonstrate unequivocally that reduction of cholesterol level by pharmacologic means results in a statistically significant decrease in CHD events. The trial randomized 3806 men, aged 35–59 years, without known CHD but at increased risk because of hypercholesterolemia (total cholesterol level 265 mg/dL or more, LDL cholesterol level 190 mg/dL or more, triglyceride level 300 mg/dL or less) to receive the bile-acid sequestrant cholestyramine, 24 g/day, or placebo; average time on trial was 7.4 years (22). A moderate cholesterol-lowering diet (cholesterol 400 mg/day, polyunsaturated:saturated fat ratio 0.8) was prescribed for all subjects. The trial design had predicted a 28% decrease in total cholesterol level in subjects adhering to the cholestyramine treatment regimen, but the actual reduction was less than anticipated because of poor patient compliance. Many patients had trouble taking the drug, predominantly because of gastrointestinal side effects; average dose taken was only about 14 g/day.

Diet alone decreased total cholesterol a mean 5% and LDL cholesterol a mean 8% in the placebo group. In the group also treated with cholestyramine, total cholesterol decreased 13% and LDL cholesterol decreased 20% from baseline. Although the lipid lowering achieved in the drug-treated group was less than anticipated, incidence of fatal and nonfatal MI was significantly reduced 19% in this group. The impact on CHD mortality was directly related to the degree of cholesterol lowering. The other cardiovascular endpoints evaluated in the trial were also beneficially affected by cholestyramine treatment: development of angina pectoris was reduced 20%, new positive exercise test results were reduced 25%, and incidence of coronary bypass surgery was reduced 21%. There was no reduction in total mortality, however, because of an increase in noncardiovascular deaths, primarily due to accidents and violence, in the drug-treated group. There was no difference in cancer deaths between the treatment groups.

The LRC-CPPT substantiated the lipid hypothesis and gave rise to the rule of thumb that a 1% decrease in total cholesterol is associated with a 2% reduction in CHD events. In the subgroup of subjects whose cholesterol level decreased 25% or more, CHD risk was reduced 64% (23).

**World Health Organization Cooperative Trial.** The WHO Cooperative Trial, begun in 1965, studied the impact of the fibric acid derivative clofibrate in dyslipidemic men, aged 30–59 years, whose lipid profile placed them in the upper tertile of total cholesterol distribution (24). More than 10,000 subjects were randomized to receive clofibrate, 1.6 g/d, or placebo; mean time on trial was 5.3 years.

Clofibrate lowered total cholesterol level 9% from baseline and reduced the incidence of nonfatal MI 25%. CHD incidence decreased a significant

20%. The CHD mortality rate was not successfully lowered, however, and there was a statistically significant increase in total mortality in the group receiving clofibrate. Further analysis almost 8 years after the trial's completion revealed that the excess mortality with clofibrate treatment decreased from 47% during the trial to 11% during the entire 13-year follow-up period and was no longer significant (25). Additional large studies, designed specifically to examine effects on total and noncardiovascular mortality and using later generation agents capable of achieving substantial cholesterol reductions, are necessary to answer the mortality question in primary prevention.

**Helsinki Heart Study.** The Helsinki Heart Study was conducted in 4081 men, aged 40–55 years, with no known CHD but considered at increased risk because of non-HDL cholesterol levels higher than 200 mg/dL (26). All subjects received dietary counseling before being randomized to the fibric acid derivative gemfibrozil, 1200 mg/day, or placebo for 5 years. Unlike the LRC-CPPT, which was limited to subjects with elevated LDL levels, the Helsinki Heart Study also included subjects with elevated VLDL levels and subjects with elevations in both LDL and VLDL levels.

In the group receiving gemfibrozil, total cholesterol level decreased 10%, LDL cholesterol level decreased 11%, HDL cholesterol level increased 11%, and triglyceride level decreased 35% compared with the group receiving placebo. In drug-treated subjects with best compliance (at least 1100 mg/day), LDL cholesterol level decreased 15%, HDL cholesterol level increased 14%, and triglyceride level decreased 45%.

Incidence of fatal and nonfatal MI and cardiac death was reduced 34% in the group treated with gemfibrozil. Further analysis indicated that CHD risk was reduced 71% in a subgroup characterized by an LDL cholesterol:HDL cholesterol ratio greater than 5 and a triglyceride level greater than 200 mg/dL; this subgroup at high risk for CHD events accounted for about 10% of the study population (27).

**West of Scotland Coronary Prevention Study.** WOSCOPS randomized 6595 men aged 45–64 years with no history of MI to receive pravastatin, 40 mg/day, or placebo (28). Subjects with stable angina who had not been hospitalized within the previous year were not excluded. Mean LDL cholesterol level at baseline (after 2 months of lipid-lowering dietary therapy) was 192 mg/dL; entry lipid criteria included an LDL cholesterol level of at least 155 mg/dL on two assessments despite dietary therapy, at least 174 mg/dL on at least one assessment, and no more than 232 mg/dL on one assessment. Mean follow-up was 4.9 years.

Although data were analyzed by intent to treat as well as by treatment received, specific lipid changes have been published only for the latter analysis at the time of this writing. In subjects who actually received pravastatin, total plasma cholesterol decreased 20%, LDL cholesterol decreased 26%, triglyceride decreased 12%, and HDL cholesterol increased 5%.

For the combined primary endpoint of either definite nonfatal MI or CHD death as a first event, the relative risk in the group randomized to pravastatin was significantly decreased 31% compared with the group randomized to placebo. There was no significant difference in death from noncardiovascular causes between treatment groups. The pravastatin group had a 22% reduction in death from any cause compared with the placebo group ($P = 0.051$).

*Secondary Prevention*

A number of major clinical trials using clinical or angiographic endpoints have studied the efficacy of single-agent or combination-agent pharmacologic therapy plus diet in patients with CHD. In angiographically monitored trials, the reduction in clinical events has often been disproportionate to the small decrease in the size of atherosclerotic lesions, and it has been suggested that lipid lowering stabilizes lesions, thereby reducing their susceptibility to rupturing (29). The relative anatomic benefit in mild, moderate, and severe lesions varies among these trials.

**Coronary Drug Project.** The Coronary Drug Project was a large trial of pharmacologic monotherapy with various agents in 8341 men, aged 30–64 years, who had a history of documented MI (30). Three treatment arms were discontinued before the completion of the 5-year trial because of adverse effects: the group randomized to conjugated estrogens, 5 mg/day, experienced an excess of nonfatal MI and insufficient efficacy; the group randomized to dextrothyroxine, 6 mg/day, had excess mortality; and the group randomized to conjugated estrogens, 2.5 mg/day, had an excess incidence of thromboembolism and excess cancer mortality as well as a small increase in total mortality.

In the 1103 subjects randomized to receive clofibrate, 1.8 g/day, total cholesterol level decreased 6% and triglyceride level decreased 22%. These alterations in the lipid profile were accompanied by a decrease in fatal and nonfatal MI, although this difference was not statistically significant. Total mortality was not affected by clofibrate treatment.

In the 1119 subjects randomized to receive nicotinic acid, 3 g/day, total cholesterol level decreased 10% and triglyceride level decreased 26%. At the end of the trial, incidence of nonfatal MI was significantly reduced 27% compared with the placebo group, but there was no difference in total mortality or CHD death. At 15-year follow-up, however, the group that received nicotinic acid demonstrated 11% lower all-cause mortality than the group randomized to placebo, which was a significant improvement (31). Suggested mechanisms for this difference were reduced progression of atherosclerotic lesions during the trial and early prevention of nonfatal MI.

**National Heart, Lung, and Blood Institute Type II Coronary Intervention Study.** The National Heart, Lung, and Blood Institute (NHLBI) Type II Coronary Intervention Study randomized 143 men and women to receive diet plus cholestyramine at a projected dose of 24 g/day or diet plus placebo for 5 years (32). Subjects were aged 21–55 years and had angiographic evidence of CHD and an LDL cholesterol level above the 90th percentile for the general population that remained after diet.

In the cholestyramine group, total cholesterol level decreased 17% and LDL cholesterol level decreased 26% from baseline, compared with decreases of 1% and 5% in the placebo group. HDL cholesterol level increased 8% in the drug-treated group and 2% in the placebo group; triglyceride level increased 28% and 26%, respectively.

The primary endpoint was change in the severity of CHD as determined by visual comparison of angiograms obtained at baseline and at 5-year follow-up. Definite or probable regression of coronary atherosclerotic lesions was seen in approximately 7% of subjects in each group. Definite or probable progression without regression was seen in significantly fewer cholestyramine-treated subjects (32%) than placebo-treated subjects (49%). Among lesions causing 50% or greater stenosis at baseline, progression was seen in 12% of cholestyramine-treated subjects compared with 33% of placebo-treated subjects, which was a significant difference. The risk of progression, death, or nonfatal MI was reduced 40% in the drug-treated group, but this difference was not significant.

**St Thomas' Atherosclerosis Regression Study.** The St Thomas' Atherosclerosis Regression Study (STARS) compared the effects of diet plus cholestyramine, diet alone, and usual care in 90 men, aged less than 66 years, with CHD (33). Mean total cholesterol was 280 mg/dL. The STARS diet reduced total fat intake to 27% of total calories, saturated fat intake to 8–10% of total calories, and dietary cholesterol to 100 mg/1000 kcal; ω-6 and ω-3 polyunsaturated fatty acid intake was increased to 8% of total calories, and intake of plant-derived soluble fiber was increased to an equivalent of 3.6 g polygalacturonate/1000 kcal.

Total cholesterol level decreased 25% in the group receiving diet plus cholestyramine and 14% in the group receiving diet alone; LDL cholesterol level decreased 36% and 16% in the two respective groups. These levels decreased only 2% and 3%, respectively, in the group receiving usual care.

After an average of 39 months, change in the mean absolute width of coronary artery segments was evaluated by quantitative coronary angiography and was found to be correlated with the LDL cholesterol level and with the LDL cholesterol:HDL cholesterol ratio. In the group receiving diet plus cholestyramine, mean absolute width of coronary artery segments increased 0.103 mm, and in the group receiving diet alone, mean absolute width increased 0.003 mm, compared with a decrease of 0.201 mm in the group receiving usual care.

A cardiovascular event or events, defined as CHD death, MI, coronary surgery, angioplasty, or stroke, occurred in 1 subject receiving diet plus cholestyramine, 3 subjects receiving diet alone, and 10 subjects receiving usual care. Both active-treatment groups showed significant benefit compared with the control group.

**Monitored Atherosclerosis Regression Study.** In the Monitored Atherosclerosis Regression Study (MARS), 270 men and women (91% men), aged 37–67 years, with angiographically defined CHD and total cholesterol of 190–295 mg/dL were randomized to receive the 3-hydroxy-3-methylglutaryl coenzyme A (HMG-CoA) reductase inhibitor lovastatin at a high dose (80 mg/day) or placebo for 2 years (34). Of these subjects, 64% had total cholesterol less than 240 mg/dL, 60% had previous MI, and 41% had angina. Baseline and follow-up angiograms were evaluated visually and by quantitative coronary angiography.

In the lovastatin-treated group, the mean total cholesterol level decreased 32% and the LDL cholesterol level decreased 45%, compared with decreases of 2% and 3% in the placebo group. HDL cholesterol increased 8% and triglyceride decreased 22% in lovastatin-treated subjects, compared with increases of 2% and 4% in placebo-treated subjects.

The primary endpoint was mean per-patient change in percent diameter stenosis as assessed by quantitative coronary angiography. The mean change was a 1.6% increase in the lovastatin-treated group and a 2.2% increase in the placebo group; that is, progression occurred in both groups, and the amount of progression was higher in the placebo-treated group (a nonsignificant difference). Significant improvement with lovastatin treatment was reported in lesions causing at least 50% stenosis at baseline; in these lesions, the 5-year change was a 4.1% decrease in the lovastatin-treated group (indicating regression) compared with a 0.9% increase in the placebo-treated group.

Among secondary endpoints, mean per-patient minimum lumen diameter for all lesions decreased less in the lovastatin-treated group than in the placebo-treated group, indicating less progression with lovastatin treatment, but this difference was not significant. In lesions causing at least 50% stenosis at baseline, mean minimum lumen diameter increased 0.13 mm in the lovastatin group, compared with a decrease of 0.04 mm in the placebo group; this improvement with lovastatin treatment was statistically significant.

Anatomic change was also measured by a global change score determined by visual assessment of baseline and follow-up angiograms. The mean global change score in lovastatin subjects (+0.41) was significantly lower than in placebo subjects (+0.88), indicating less progression with lovastatin treatment. In subgroup analysis by total cholesterol level, improvement was seen in subjects with cholesterol less than 240 mg/dL as well as in subjects with cholesterol of 240 mg/dL or greater.

By quantitative assessment, significantly fewer lovastatin subjects demonstrated progression only (29% compared with 41% of placebo subjects) and significantly more demonstrated regression only (23% compared with 12% of placebo subjects). By visual determination (global change score), significantly fewer lovastatin subjects demonstrated progression (47% compared with 65% of placebo subjects) and significantly more demonstrated regression (23% compared with 11% of placebo subjects).

The lovastatin group had fewer clinical coronary events, defined as MI, angioplasty, coronary artery bypass surgery, coronary death, and hospitalization for unstable angina, but this trend did not reach significance. Events totaled 22 in the lovastatin group and 31 in the placebo group.

**Canadian Coronary Atherosclerosis Intervention Trial.** The Canadian Coronary Atherosclerosis Intervention Trial (CCAIT) randomized 331 men and women, aged 21–70 years, with angiographically demonstrated diffuse CHD and total cholesterol level of 220–300 mg/dL to receive lovastatin or placebo for 2 years (35). The dose of lovastatin was titrated to reduce LDL cholesterol level to 90–130 mg/dL; mean dose was 36 mg/day. All subjects received dietary counseling. The primary endpoint was the mean per-patient change in minimum lumen diameter for all lesions measured, as determined by quantitative coronary angiography.

Total cholesterol decreased 21% and LDL cholesterol decreased 29% from baseline in the lovastatin-treated group, compared with decreases of less than 2% in the placebo-treated group. HDL cholesterol level increased 7.3% and triglyceride level decreased 8% with lovastatin, compared with increases of 3% and 4%, respectively, with placebo.

Primary-endpoint analysis showed coronary lesion progression in both groups, but progression was less severe in the group receiving lovastatin: a decrease of 0.05 mm in mean minimum lumen diameter compared with a decrease of 0.09 mm in the group receiving placebo. Evaluated by percent diameter stenosis, lesions in lovastatin subjects progressed less (1.7%) than lesions in placebo subjects (2.9%). Both of these results were significantly different between treatment groups.

Progression only was reported in 33% of lovastatin subjects compared with 50% of placebo subjects, which was a significant difference. Per-lesion progression was also significantly improved with lovastatin : 7% of lesions in lovastatin subjects progressed compared with 9% of lesions in placebo subjects. New lesions developed in 16% of lovastatin subjects compared with 32% of placebo subjects, which was a significant difference.

Regression was seen in 19% of lovastatin subjects, compared with 13% of placebo subjects, and regression without progression was seen in 10% and 7%, respectively. These differences between treatment groups were not significant.

Among lesions causing less than 50% diameter stenosis at baseline, which accounted for most lesions in the study, significantly fewer progressed in the lovastatin group (7%) than in the placebo group (11%). Of lesions causing at least 50% diameter stenosis at baseline, only six lesions in the lovastatin group and eight lesions in the placebo group progressed.

Clinical coronary events, defined as cardiac death, MI, and unstable angina, were less frequent in the lovastatin group (15 events in 14 subjects) than in the placebo group (20 events in 18 subjects), but this difference was not significant.

**Pravastatin Limitation of Atherosclerosis in the Coronary Arteries.** The Pravastatin Limitation of Atherosclerosis in the Coronary Arteries (PLAC I) study was a randomized, placebo-controlled, multicenter trial that examined the impact of lipid lowering with the HMG-CoA reductase inhibitor pravastatin in 408 men and women with at least one coronary lesion causing at least 50% stenosis and LDL cholesterol level of 130–190 mg/dL after diet (36). After 3 years of treatment, mean diameter of coronary artery segments able to be evaluated by quantitative coronary angiography decreased 0.02 mm/year in the prevastatin group and 0.04 mm/year in the placebo group, but the difference between groups was not statistically significant. Minimal diameter decreased 0.03 mm/year in the pravastatin group and 0.05 mm/year in the placebo group, which was a statistically significant difference.

Total cholesterol decreased 19%, LDL cholesterol decreased 28%, and HDL cholesterol increased 7% in subjects receiving pravastatin. This group also experienced significantly fewer fatal and nonfatal MIs (8) than the placebo group (17).

**Multicentre Anti-Atheroma Study.** The Multicentre Anti-Atheroma Study (MAAS) was conducted in 381 men and women, aged 30–67 years, with atherosclerosis in at least two coronary artery segments, total cholesterol of 210–310 mg/dL, and triglyceride less than 350 mg/dL (37). Approximately half had had previous MI. All subjects received dietary instruction according to the usual practice of each participating center and were randomized to receive the HMG-CoA reductase inhibitor simvastatin, 20 mg/day, or placebo for 4 years. Quantitative coronary angiography was used to measure diffuse coronary atherosclerosis, defined as the per-patient average of mean lumen diameter of all coronary segments, and focal coronary atherosclerosis, defined as the per-patient average of minimum lumen diameter of all atheromatous segments, whether diseased at baseline, follow-up, or both.

In the simvastatin group, total cholesterol decreased 23%, LDL cholesterol decreased 31%, HDL cholesterol increased 9%, and triglyceride decreased 18%, compared with the placebo group.

In the simvastatin subjects, mean lumen diameter decreased 0.02 mm compared with a decrease of 0.08 mm in placebo subjects, and minimum lumen diameter decreased 0.04 mm compared with a decrease of 0.13 mm in placebo subjects. Both differences were significant. Diameter stenosis increased 1.0% in the simvastatin group and 3.6% in the placebo group.

In mildly and moderately diseased segments, defined as those with less than 50% stenosis at baseline, mean lumen diameter decreased 0.02 mm with simvastatin and 0.07 mm with placebo. Minimum lumen diameter for these lesions decreased 0.01 mm with simvastatin and 0.06 mm with placebo. However, simvastatin exerted a greater treatment effect in severely diseased segments, defined as those with 50% or more stenosis at baseline. In these segments, mean lumen diameter decreased 0.07 mm with simvastatin and 0.24 mm with placebo, and minimum lumen diameter increased 0.19 mm with simvastatin and decreased 0.01 mm with placebo.

Progression only was reported in 23% of simvastatin subjects and 32% of placebo subjects. Both progression and regression were seen in 5% of simvastatin subjects and 13% of placebo subjects, and lesion stabilization was seen in 53% of simvastatin subjects and 43% of placebo subjects. Regression only was reported in 19% of simvastatin subjects compared with 12% of placebo subjects.

Cardiac death was reported in 4 subjects of each group. MI occurred in 11 simvastatin subjects, compared with 7 placebo subjects, but the difference was not significant. Percutaneous transluminal coronary angioplasty or coronary artery bypass surgery was performed in 23 simvastatin subjects, compared with 34 placebo subjects, but this benefit with treatment was not significant.

**Scandinavian Simvastatin Survival Study.** The Scandinavian Simvastatin Survival Study (4S) was the first cholesterol-lowering trial of sufficient size and duration designed to evaluate total mortality. In this multicenter trial, 4444 men and women, aged 35–70 years, were randomized to receive simvastatin or placebo; median time on trial was 5.4 years (38). Entry criteria were total cholesterol level of 210–310 mg/dL, triglyceride level of no more than 220 mg/dL after diet, and a history of acute MI or angina pectoris. Most subjects had had previous MI; only 21% of the study population had angina alone. The dose of simvastatin was titrated to reduce total cholesterol level to 115–200 mg/dL, and the initial dose of 20 mg/day was increased to 40 mg/day in 37% of the simvastatin subjects and decreased to 10 mg/day in 2 subjects. The study was designed to have 95% power to detect a 30% reduction in total mortality, the sole primary endpoint. Analysis was intent to treat.

In the simvastatin-treated group, total cholesterol decreased 25%, LDL cholesterol decreased 35%, HDL cholesterol increased 8%, and triglyceride decreased 10%. Respective changes in the placebo group were increases of 1%, 1%, 1%, and 8%.

Subjects randomized to receive pharmacologic therapy demonstrated a highly significant 30% decrease in total mortality. CHD mortality was also improved with simvastatin treatment; this 42% reduction accounted for the major improvement in overall survival, because there was no difference in noncardiovascular deaths between treatment groups. Deaths caused by trauma, suicide, and cancer, which had been implicated as possible complications of lipid lowering in the LRC-CPPT, WHO, and Helsinki trials, were not increased in 4S.

The secondary endpoint was major coronary events (coronary death, nonfatal MI, and resuscitated cardiac arrest). The risk of suffering one of these coronary events was 34% lower in the simvastatin group; this difference was highly significant.

Subset analyses included in the trial's design evaluated mortality and major coronary events in women and in subjects aged 60 years or more. The death rate in women was quite low and similar between the two groups: 7% in the simvastatin group and 6% in the placebo group. However, incidence of major coronary events was significantly decreased 35% in women in the simvastatin group. In older subjects, relative risk reductions for mortality and for major coronary events with simvastatin treatment was less than in the overall study population, but these endpoints were still significantly improved.

**Cholesterol Lowering Atherosclerosis Study.** Combination-drug therapy was evaluated in the Cholesterol Lowering Atherosclerosis Study (CLAS), conducted in 162 nonsmoking men, aged 40–59 years, with previous coronary bypass surgery, progressive atherosclerosis, and total cholesterol level of 185–350 mg/dL (39). Subjects were randomized to receive either a cholesterol-lowering diet (cholesterol less than 125 mg/day, fat 22% of total calories, polyunsaturated fat 10% of total calories, saturated fat 4% of total calories) and a combination of the bile acid sequestrant colestipol, 30 g/d, and nicotinic acid, 3–12 g/d, or a somewhat less restrictive cholesterol-lowering diet (cholesterol less than 250 mg/day, fat 26% of total calories, polyunsaturated fat 10% of total calories, saturated fat 5% of total calories) and placebo. During a 6-week pretrial period, all subjects received both study drugs to determine compliance and to ensure a response in total cholesterol of at least 15%. Angiograms made at baseline and after 2 years of treatment were assessed visually to derive a coronary global change score, which was the primary endpoint of the study.

In the drug-treated group, total cholesterol decreased 27% and LDL cholesterol decreased 43%, compared with decreases of 4% and 5% in the placebo group. Combination-drug therapy decreased triglyceride 22% compared with 5% in the placebo group, and increased HDL cholesterol 37% compared with 2% in the placebo group.

The average global change score was smaller in the drug-treated group (+0.3) than in the placebo group (+0.8), indicating less progression with aggressive treatment. Among drug-treated subjects, progression was reported in 39%, lesion stabilization was reported in 45%, and regression was reported in 16%. Among placebo-treated subjects, progression was reported in 60%, lesion stabilization was reported in 36%, and regression was reported in 4%.

In the native coronary arteries, the number of lesions that progressed per subject and the percentage of subjects with new lesions were significantly reduced in the group receiving combination-drug therapy. In the saphenous vein bypass grafts, the percentage of subjects with any adverse change and the percentage of subjects with new lesions were significantly reduced in the drug-treated group. There was no difference in new closures in either of these vessels between treatment groups.

Cardiovascular event rates were not significantly different between the two treatment groups.

Risk factor analyses were conducted in each treatment group to determine predictors of disease progression (40). On univariate analysis, apo C-III was found to have a significant effect on progression in both treatment groups, and diastolic blood pressure and plasma levels of total cholesterol, LDL cholesterol, apo B, non-HDL cholesterol, and triglyceride were all significant predictors of progression in the placebo group. Multivariate analysis identified the content of apo C-III in HDL as an independent risk factor predictive of progression in drug-treated subjects; in placebo-treated subjects, the best predictor of progression was non-HDL cholesterol. These findings suggest that triglyceride-rich lipoproteins are involved in disease progression. Sequestration into HDL of apo C-III, which inhibits lipoprotein lipase activity, is thought to facilitate catabolism of chylomicrons and VLDL and to increase removal of their potentially atherogenic remnants from the circulation.

CLAS was extended an additional 2 years in 103 subjects (41). Lipid changes in drug-treated subjects were maintained during the second 2-year period. At 4-year follow-up, progression was seen in 48% of drug-treated subjects, compared with 85% of placebo-treated subjects, and regression was seen in 18% of drug-treated subjects, compared with 6% of placebo-treated subjects. Both nonprogression and regression were significantly more frequent in the drug-treated group. This group also had significantly fewer subjects with new lesions in the native coronary arteries (14% compared with 40% in the placebo-treated group) and in the saphenous vein bypass grafts (16% compared with 36% in the placebo-treated group).

**Familial Atherosclerosis Treatment Study.** The Familial Atherosclerosis Treatment Study (FATS) was conducted in 120 men, aged 62 years or less, with elevated plasma apo B level (more than 125 mg/dL), at least one coronary lesion causing at least 50% stenosis or three coronary lesions causing at least 30% stenosis, and family history of CHD (42). Subjects received dietary therapy and were randomized to receive a combination of lovastatin, 40–80 mg/day, and colestipol, 30 g/d; a combination of nicotinic acid, 4–6 g/d, and colestipol, 30 g/d; or conventional therapy for 2.5 years. Subjects randomized to conventional therapy whose baseline LDL cholesterol level was greater than the 90th percentile for age received colestipol, 30 g/d, instead of placebo; 43% of subjects in this treatment group received colestipol. The primary endpoint was mean change in percent stenosis for the worst lesion in each of nine proximal segments, as assessed by quantitative coronary angiography.

In the group receiving lovastatin plus colestipol, total cholesterol decreased 34%, LDL cholesterol decreased 46%, HDL cholesterol increased 15%, and triglyceride decreased 9%. In the group receiving nicotinic acid plus colestipol, total cholesterol decreased 23%, LDL cholesterol decreased 32%, HDL cholesterol increased 43%, and triglyceride decreased 30%. Corresponding changes in the group receiving conventional therapy were decreases of 3%, 7%, and 5%, and an increase of 15%.

Mean percent stenosis for the nine worst proximal lesions decreased 0.7 percentage points in the group treated with lovastatin plus colestipol and 0.9 percentage points in the group treated with nicotinic acid plus colestipol (indicating regression), compared with an increase of 2.1 percentage points in the group receiving conventional therapy (indicating progression). Proximal lesions causing at least 50% stenosis at baseline decreased 3.9 percentage points and 6.5 percentage points, respectively, in the active-treatment groups compared with an increase of 1.2 percentage points in the conventional-therapy group. Mean percent stenosis in proximal lesions causing less than 50% stenosis at baseline increased 0.2 percentage points in both active-treatment groups compared with an increase of 2.4 percentage points in the conventional-therapy group. Minimum lumen diameter for the nine worst proximal lesions increased 0.012 mm in the group receiving lovastatin plus colestipol and 0.035 mm in the group receiving nicotinic acid plus colestipol, but decreased 0.050 mm in the group receiving conventional therapy.

Progression as the only lesion change was seen in 21% of subjects receiving lovastatin plus colestipol, 25% of subjects receiving nicotinic acid plus colestipol, and 46% of subjects receiving conventional therapy. Regression only was seen in 32%, 39%, and 11% of the respective groups.

Cardiovascular events, defined as death, MI, and need for peripheral or coronary bypass or angioplasty, were reduced 73% in the active-treatment groups. Events were reported in 3 subjects randomized to lovastatin plus colestipol, 2 subjects randomized to nicotinic acid plus colestipol, and 10 subjects randomized to conventional therapy.

**University of California, San Francisco, Arteriosclerosis Specialized Center of Research Intervention Trial.** The University of California, San Francisco, Arteriosclerosis Specialized Center of Research (UCSF-SCOR) Intervention Trial evaluated the effects of colestipol, 15–30 g/day; nicotinic acid up to 7.5 g/day; and lovastatin, 40–60 mg/day in various binary and ternary combinations in 72 men and women with heterozygous familial hypercholesterolemia (43). When the LRC-CPPT results were published, UCSF-SCOR subjects randomized to placebo were also offered colestipol, 15 mg/day, which 44% chose to receive. All subjects received dietary instruction. During the 26-month trial, 90% of drug-treated subjects received nicotinic acid, 80% received colestipol, and 40% received lovastatin.

The total cholesterol level decreased 31% and the LDL cholesterol level decreased 39% in the drug-treated group, compared with decreases of 9% and 12% in the control group. The HDL cholesterol level increased 25% and 1% in the respective groups, and triglyceride decreased 21% in drug-treated subjects and increased 4% in control subjects.

The primary endpoint of mean within-patient change in percent area stenosis as evaluated by quantitative coronary angiography decreased 1.53 percentage points in drug-treated subjects, indicating regression, and increased 0.80 percentage points in control subjects, indicating progression. This change was significantly different between treatment groups. In a separate analysis of women in the study, the primary endpoint was significantly different between treatment groups; the difference was not significant in separate analysis of men in the study.

Progression was seen in 20% of drug-treated subjects compared with 41% of control subjects. Regression was seen in 32.5% of drug-treated subjects compared with 12.5% of control subjects. There was a strong trend toward regression and away from progression with drug treatment, but this trend did not reach significance.

## GUIDELINES FOR TREATMENT

On the basis of the established relation between serum cholesterol and CHD incidence, the National Cholesterol Education Program includes both a population approach and an individual approach to lipid lowering as a means of preventing CHD. The population strategy is intended to decrease blood cholesterol levels in the population as a whole, through changes in diet and increased physical activity (44). The individual approach of the ATP II targets the detection and treatment of people at high risk for CHD because of elevated blood cholesterol. The ATP II guidelines are stratified according to presence or absence of CHD or other atherosclerotic disease, although the distinction between primary prevention and secondary prevention may be largely semantic in patients with subclinical atherosclerosis.

### Risk Factors Other Than Hypercholesterolemia

CHD risk is influenced by both lipid and nonlipid factors. Among lipid risk factors, the ATP II guidelines focus on reduction of LDL cholesterol, because of the overwhelming evidence linking elevated LDL cholesterol and CHD incidence. Emphasis is also placed on altering other modifiable risk factors. In addition, the overall risk profile, reflecting both modifiable and nonmodifiable risk factors, is used in deciding upon treatment of dyslipidemia.

#### *Low HDL Cholesterol*

Numerous epidemiologic studies have shown a strong, inverse relation between low HDL cholesterol level and risk for CHD. In the Framingham Heart Study, CHD incidence was eight times higher in men and women with an HDL cholesterol level of 35 mg/dL or less than in men and women with an HDL cholesterol level of 65 mg/dL or greater (45). An analysis of four prospective studies (Framingham [45], Lipid Research Clinics Prevalence Mortality Follow-up Study [46], LRC-CPPT [22, 23], and MRFIT [47]) indicates that each increase in HDL cholesterol of 1 mg/dL decreased CHD risk 2% in men and 3% in women (48). Clinical trials are under way to evaluate specifically the hypothesis that increasing HDL cholesterol will decrease CHD morbidity and mortality.

### *Cigarette Smoking*

The use of tobacco products has been shown to increase risk for CHD and other atherosclerotic diseases (49) as well as for diseases such as chronic obstructive pulmonary disease and various malignancies. Cessation of cigarette smoking is an effective and risk-free means of decreasing CHD and all-cause morbidity and mortality. Risk decreases more than 50% within the first year of smoking cessation and, within 2–3 years, decreases to that of individuals who have never smoked (50). Smoking cessation is estimated to reduce risk for MI 50–70% (51).

Smoking increases risk for CHD by a number of mechanisms, including increased coronary spasm, clotting abnormalities, and lowering of the HDL cholesterol level. Substitution of low-tar products does not appear to reduce CHD risk appreciably. Instead, intensive efforts should be made to eliminate the consumption of tobacco products. The physician should give patients who smoke explicit advice to quit and should provide appropriate follow-up to encourage compliance.

### *Hypertension*

In observational studies, the association between blood pressure and CHD events is positive and continuous (52). The increased risks associated with hypertension for congestive heart failure, renal failure, malignant hypertension, dissecting aneurysm, and stroke have been shown to be reduced effectively with blood pressure lowering; however, results with CHD incidence have been disappointing. Although the effect of lowering blood pressure on CHD risk has been less impressive in individual trials, in a metaanalysis of 14 trials together enrolling 37,000 subjects, blood pressure was lowered 6 mm Hg in treated subjects, compared with control subjects, and CHD events were reduced 14% (53). This decrease in mortality was less than expected on the basis of observational epidemiology correlating hypertension and CHD; the discrepancy may have been due to adverse effects of antihypertensive medication on the lipid profile. In a metaanalysis that evaluated CHD incidence (CHD death and nonfatal MI) in approximately 420,000 men and women in nine prospective observational studies, a prolonged difference of 6 mm Hg in diastolic blood pressure was associated with a 23% decrease in CHD incidence (54).

### *Obesity*

In the Framingham Heart Study, relative weight was found to be predictive of CHD incidence in both men and women (55). Among subjects aged less than 50 years, CHD incidence was two times as high in men in the most obese tertile as in the leanest tertile, and almost two and one-half times as high in women in the most obese tertile as in the leanest tertile.

The increased risk for CHD conferred by obesity appears to be associated with other CHD risk factors, namely hypercholesterolemia (56), low HDL cholesterol (57), hypertension (58), and diabetes mellitus (59). Although the independent risk for CHD imparted by obesity is not clear, weight reduction in overweight patients is an essential part of both primary and secondary prevention because of the effect of obesity on these other risk factors.

### *Physical Inactivity*

In observational epidemiological studies, regular moderate physical activity has been shown to decrease CHD risk. For example, in a study in 10,269 men aged 45–84 years, CHD mortality was 36% higher in sedentary subjects than in active subjects, although this difference was not significant, at least in part because of the small number of CHD deaths during the 8-year study (60). Initiating moderately vigorous physical activity during the trial decreased risk for CHD death 41%, which was a significant reduction. In 10.5-year follow-up of 12,138 men in MRFIT, CHD mortality was reduced 27% in subjects (intervention and control groups combined) who engaged in moderate physical activity compared with less active subjects (61).

The cardioprotective effect of regular physical activity may be attributable to direct effects on the heart (62). In addition, physical activity may contribute indirectly by improving HDL cholesterol level (63), blood pressure (64), body weight (65), and insulin resistance (66). Increased physical activity is an integral part of primary and secondary prevention of CHD.

### *Diabetes Mellitus*

Abnormal glucose tolerance and overt diabetes are associated with an increased risk for CHD (67). Risk for CHD death is almost two times as high in diabetic men and more than three times as high in diabetic women, compared with nondiabetics (68). It is estimated that 75–80% of adults with diabetes die of CHD, cerebrovascular disease, or peripheral vascular disease (69). In patients with diabetes mellitus, atherosclerosis occurs more often and at an earlier age, and women with diabetes do not share the relative premenopausal cardioprotection of women without diabetes. The lipid profile of patients with diabetes is characterized by increased serum triglyceride level and decreased HDL cholesterol level. Although patients with diabetes typically have several CHD risk factors, associated risk factors do not account for all of the risk conferred by diabetes (70).

Although the necessary level of control of diabetes has been a controversial issue for several decades, in the recently completed Diabetes Control and Complications Trial, conducted in 1441 patients with insulin-dependent diabetes mellitus, aged 13–39 years, the group randomized to tight glucose control with intensive insulin therapy had a 41% reduction in all major cardiovascular and peripheral vascular events combined, although this difference was not significant (71). No such data are available for patients with non–insulin-dependent diabetes mellitus.

### *Age*

Chronological age is a major nonmodifiable risk factor. Of individuals who die of MI, approximately four-fifths are aged 65 years or older (72). In the Framingham Heart Study, the development of CHD increased with age in both men and women (73). Because middle-aged and elderly patients are at much higher short-term risk for CHD events than younger patients with the same LDL cholesterol level, intervention is more likely to reduce event rates in a short time period in older patients. Although relative risk for CHD by total cholesterol level decreases with age, the attributable risk (amount of CHD attributed to a risk factor) increases. For example, in the observational, primary prevention Kaiser Permanente Coronary Heart Disease in the Elderly Study of 2746 men aged 60–79 years, excess CHD mortality associated with elevations in total cholesterol increased more than five times with age (74). The ATP II does not exclude elderly patients from lipid-lowering therapy on the basis of age.

The same risk factors operative in the general population have been shown to apply to elderly patients (75, 76). Although more studies specific to risk in the elderly are needed, findings to date suggest that risk factor intervention reduces risk for cardiovascular events in the elderly. In subgroup analysis of 4S subjects aged 60–70 years, incidence of major coronary events was reduced 29% with cholesterol-lowering therapy (39). In the Systolic Hypertension in the Elderly Program (SHEP), conducted in men and women aged 60 years or older (mean 71.6 years), major cardiovascular events were reduced 32% in subjects who received antihypertensive medication (77).

Because clinical benefit from lipid lowering is typically not seen in clinical trials until after approximately 2 years of therapy, the patient's life expectancy should be taken into account when considering aggressive intervention. Assessment of overall health status and competing illnesses should inform treatment decisions. Special care must be taken when considering pharmacologic therapy in the elderly, because of increased susceptibility to adverse drug effects in this population.

### *Gender*

In 26-year follow-up of Framingham subjects aged 35–84 years, 60% of all coronary events occurred in men and 40% occurred in women (78).

Among Framingham women of all ages, CHD morbidity rate was only half that of Framingham men, and not until age 75 did CHD morbidity or CHD mortality of women approach that of men. The CHD mortality rate in women was about 10 years behind that in men, and CHD morbidity in women in the oldest age group (75–84 years) was 40 times that of women in the youngest age group (35–44 years). Because of the relatively low CHD risk in premenopausal women, the ATP II recommends delaying drug therapy in this group unless the patient is otherwise at high risk because of severely elevated LDL cholesterol or other risk.

With menopause, CHD incidence increases rapidly in women. In postmenopausal women, LDL cholesterol increases and HDL cholesterol may decrease (79). These lipid changes are thought to be estrogen mediated. Estrogen-replacement therapy (described below) may provide an alternative to drug therapy in some postmenopausal women.

### *Family History of Premature Atherosclerotic Disease*

Another nonmodifiable CHD risk factor is a positive family history of premature atherosclerosis. In observational epidemiological studies, family history of CHD has been shown to be an independent CHD risk factor, even after adjusting for other risk factors (80). The family history should evaluate not only the presence of CHD but also the presence and age of onset of CHD risk factors—including hypercholesterolemia—in all first-degree relatives. Patients with a positive family history of atherosclerotic disease and dyslipidemia may have a genetic dyslipidemia, and for these patients, it may be helpful to include second-degree relatives in the family history.

### *Coronary Heart Disease*

Patients with established CHD or other atherosclerotic disease are at the highest risk for MI or CHD death. Reinfarction occurs in 16% of men and 20% of women within 4 years after an MI, and risk for sudden death is four to six times higher in patients with previous MI than in the general population (72). As shown above, a number of large clinical trials in patients with CHD have demonstrated that the progression of atherosclerosis can be decreased and the incidence of cardiovascular events reduced with aggressive cholesterol lowering. In addition, results of the 4S trial (38) show a significant reduction in all-cause mortality rate in this population. The ATP II recommends that the presence of CHD be determined by definite clinical and laboratory evidence of MI or of clinically significant myocardial ischemia, or by a history of coronary artery surgery or of coronary angioplasty. Angiography can be useful in documenting CHD in symptomatic patients but is not recommended solely to identify the presence of CHD.

Large-vessel peripheral arterial disease has been reported to increase risk for CHD morbidity and CHD mortality 2.4 times in men and 3.6 times in women (81). The ATP II recommends that the determination of peripheral arterial disease be based on the finding of abdominal aortic aneurysm or on clinical signs and symptoms of ischemia to the extremities, accompanied by angiographic evidence of substantial atherosclerosis or abnormalities of segment-to-arm pressure ratios or flow velocities.

Carotid disease has also been reported to increase risk for CHD events. In a longitudinal study conducted in 1288 men, the presence of small carotid plaques was associated with a fourfold increased risk for MI; the presence of large carotid plaques was associated with a greater than sixfold increased risk for MI compared with men with no ultrasound evidence of carotid atherosclerosis at baseline (82).

Early results from the Atherosclerosis Risk in Communities (ARIC) Study, a prospective observational study of 15,800 middle-aged men and women in the United States, show mean carotid intimal–medial artery wall thickness as determined by ultrasound to be predictive of CHD events (definite or probable MI and definite CHD death) at a mean 2.2 years' follow-up (Chambless LE, Barnes R, Folsom AR, Heiss G, Hutchinson R, Patsch W, Sharrett R, Szklo M, Wu K, Rosamond W. Carotid artery wall thickness is associated with incident coronary heart disease: early results of the ARIC Study [abstract]. In: Unpublished abstracts book of the Third International Conference on Preventive Cardiology, Oslo, Norway, 27 June–1 July 1993). The race-adjusted and age-adjusted CHD relative risk (95% confidence interval) for 1 standard deviation (0.16 mm) in intimal–medial thickness was 1.24 (1.07–1.43) for men and 1.44 (1.16–1.80) for women. Adjusted also for diastolic blood pressure, pack-years of smoking, and total cholesterol level, the relative risk was 1.17 (1.00–1.36) for men and 1.32 (1.04–1.66) for women.

The ATP II recommends that the presence of carotid disease be determined by the concurrence of cerebral symptoms (transient ischemic attacks or stroke) and angiographic or ultrasound evidence of significant atherosclerosis.

## Evaluation of Lipid Levels

The ATP II recommends that total cholesterol be measured at least every 5 years in all adults aged 20 years or older. HDL cholesterol should also be measured if accuracy can be assured. Nonfasting samples may be used for these determinations. The need for determining other lipid levels is based on the presence or absence of CHD, total cholesterol and HDL cholesterol levels, and the degree of CHD risk, although the physician may choose a full fasting lipoprotein profile as the initial assessment.

### *Primary Prevention*

In primary prevention, risk status is estimated by the sum of positive and negative risk factors, with clinical judgment used to evaluate the severity of risk.

Positive risk factors are as follows:

- Age (45 years or older in men; 55 years or older, or premature menopause without estrogen-replacement therapy, in women)
- Family history of premature CHD (MI or sudden death before the age of 55 in father or other male first-degree relative, or before the age of 65 in mother or other female first-degree relative)
- Current cigarette smoking
- Hypertension (140/90 mm Hg or higher, or on antihypertensive medication)
- Low HDL cholesterol (less than 35 mg/dL)
- Diabetes mellitus

Negative risk factor (if present, subtract 1 risk factor) is as follows:

- High HDL cholesterol (60 mg/dL or greater)

In the ATP II's algorithm, a net of two or more risk factors in primary prevention indicates high risk, and patients with this risk profile require more vigorous intervention than patients with less than two risk factors. Although obesity is not included in the algorithm because it is usually found in conjunction with risk factors that are listed (i.e., hypertension, hyperlipidemia, low HDL cholesterol, and diabetes mellitus), it should be a target for intervention, as should physical inactivity.

In patients not known to have atherosclerotic disease, if both total cholesterol and HDL cholesterol are at desirable levels (less than 200 mg/dL and 35 mg/dL or more, respectively), general education should be provided on diet, physical activity, and risk factor reduction. Testing should be repeated within 5 years. If total cholesterol is borderline high (200–239 mg/dL) but otherwise the patient is at low risk (HDL cholesterol 35 mg/dL or more and fewer than two other risk factors present), information should be provided on dietary modification, physical activity, and risk factor reduction. Testing and dietary information should be repeated in 1–2 years.

In patients at higher risk, a full fasting lipoprotein analysis should be performed. In primary prevention, that includes patients with low HDL cholesterol (less than 35 mg/dL) regardless of the total cholesterol level, patients with borderline-high total cholesterol and two or more other risk factors, and patients with high total cholesterol (240 mg/dL or more).

### *Secondary Prevention*

In individuals with established CHD or other atherosclerotic disease, full fasting lipoprotein analysis should be the initial test. Because LDL cholesterol levels in patients recovering from an acute coronary event may be lower than baseline for several weeks after the event, values obtained during this time should be evaluated accordingly.

### *Lipoprotein Analysis*

Full fasting lipoprotein analysis includes measurement of total cholesterol, HDL cholesterol, and serum triglyceride levels and calculation of LDL cholesterol level by the Friedewald formula (all values mg/dL):

$$\text{LDL cholesterol} = \text{total cholesterol} - \text{HDL cholesterol} - (\text{triglyceride} \div 5)$$

This formula is not accurate if the triglyceride level is greater than 400 mg/dL or if the patient has type III hyperlipidemia or apo $E_{2/2}$ phenotype. Triglyceride must be measured after a 12-hour fast to allow clearance of chylomicrons.

Although levels of other lipoprotein variables, including individual apolipoproteins, lipoprotein subclasses, and lipoprotein(a) [Lp(a)], have been evaluated as CHD risk predictors, the ATP II does not recommend their routine assessment because of limited availability of reliable measurements and questions about the clinical impact of their modification. At present, these measurements remain research procedures.

### *Classification of Risk by LDL Cholesterol Level*

In primary prevention (Table 3.2), an LDL cholesterol level less than 130 mg/dL is considered desirable, and patients in this category should have their total cholesterol and HDL cholesterol levels measured again within 5 years and be provided with general education on diet, physical activity, and risk factor reduction. An LDL cholesterol level of 130–159 mg/dL is considered borderline high in primary prevention. Patients in this category are further classified according to risk profile. Patients with borderline-high LDL cholesterol and fewer than two other risk factors should be provided with information on dietary therapy and physical activity; they should be reevaluated annually with repeat lipoprotein analysis, reinforcement of dietary education, and risk factor reduction.

**Table 3.2**
**Low-Density Lipoprotein (LDL) Cholesterol Classification in Adults**

| Patient Status | Classification | LDL Cholesterol Level (mg/dL) |
|---|---|---|
| Primary prevention | Desirable | <130 |
| | Borderline high risk | 130–159 |
| | High risk | ≥160 |
| Secondary prevention | Optimal | ≤100 |
| | Higher than optimal | >100 |

Reprinted from National Cholesterol Education Program. Second report of the Expert Panel on Detection, Evaluation, and Treatment of High Blood Cholesterol in Adults (Adult Treatment Panel II). Circulation 1994; 89: 1329–1445.

Patients with borderline-high LDL cholesterol and at least two other risk factors and patients with high LDL cholesterol (160 mg/dL or more) should undergo clinical evaluation, including history, physical examination, and laboratory tests, to better characterize risk status and to determine any cause of secondary dyslipidemia or, if possible, any familial disorder. The physical examination should include examining for manifestations of dyslipidemia (which include corneal arcus, xanthelasmas or xanthomas) and hepatosplenomegaly and for evidence of atherosclerosis (which can be detected by peripheral pulses and vascular bruits). The genetic lipid disorders most commonly encountered are familial combined hyperlipidemia, polygenic hypercholesterolemia, familial hypercholesterolemia, and type III hyperlipidemia. Possible causes of secondary dyslipidemia include diabetes mellitus, hypothyroidism, nephrotic syndrome, obstructive liver disease, and certain drugs. Any cause of secondary dyslipidemia should be treated and LDL cholesterol should be reevaluated. If LDL cholesterol level remains elevated, dietary therapy should be initiated (Table 3.3). All treatment decisions should be based on the average of two or more LDL cholesterol determinations; if two values differ by more than 30 mg/dL, a third assessment should be made and the three averaged.

In secondary prevention, a more aggressive approach is warranted to decrease the high probability of MI or CHD death. An LDL cholesterol level of 100 mg/dL or less is considered optimal (Table 3.2); patients in this category should receive individualized instruction on diet and physical activity and should repeat the fasting lipoprotein analysis annually. Patients with an LDL cholesterol level higher than 100 mg/dL should undergo full clinical evaluation, including treatment of any causes of secondary dyslipidemia, as discussed above. These patients should then proceed with dietary therapy. As in primary prevention, treatment decisions should be based on the average of two or more LDL cholesterol determinations.

**Table 3.3**
**Dietary Therapy Treatment Levels in Adults**

| | LDL Cholesterol Level (mg/dL) | |
|---|---|---|
| Risk | Initiation Level | Goal |
| Without CHD, <2 other risk factors | ≥160 | <160 |
| Without CHD, ≥2 other risk factors | ≥130 | <130 |
| With CHD or other atherosclerotic disease | >100 | ≤100 |

CHD = coronary heart disease; LDL = low density lipoprotein.
Reproduced from National Cholesterol Education Program. Second report of the Expert Panel on Detection, Evaluation, and Treatment of High Blood Cholesterol in Adults (Adult Treatment Panel II). Circulation 1994; 89:1329–1445.

## Dietary Therapy

Lifestyle intervention should include not only modification of eating habits but also increased physical activity as appropriate, weight control, and risk factor reduction. The ATP II provides a stepped approach to dietary intervention (Table 3.4), beginning with the Step I Diet, which is recommended for the general population aged at least 2 years and is the initial therapy in primary prevention. Patients whose LDL cholesterol level remains elevated after 3 months' adherence to a Step I Diet should proceed to the Step II Diet. In secondary prevention and in patients already adhering to a Step I Diet at the time of assessment, the Step II Diet is the initial therapy. Particularly for the Step II Diet, a dietitian may be helpful in individualizing the diet, ensuring adequate nutrition, and promoting adherence.

The Step I Diet may be expected to reduce total cholesterol 5–7% in individuals previously consuming a typical American diet; advancing to the Step II Diet may be expected to reduce total cholesterol level an additional 5–13% (83). Weight reduction typically enhances the cholesterol-lowering response.

## Drug Therapy

If target LDL cholesterol levels are not reached despite adherence to maximal dietary therapy, lipid-lowering drug therapy may be considered in addition to diet in patients whose LDL cholesterol level remains at or above the initial level for drug therapy (Table 3.5). An adequate trial of diet

**Table 3.4**
**Dietary Therapy for High Blood Cholesterol**

| Nutrient | Step I Diet[a] | Step II Diet |
|---|---|---|
| Total fat | ≤30% of total calories | |
| Saturated fat | 8–10% of total calories | <7% of total calories |
| Polyunsaturated fat | ≤10% of total calories | |
| Monounsaturated fat | ≤15% of total calories | |
| Carbohydrates | ≥55% of total calories | |
| Protein | ~15% of total calories | |
| Cholesterol | <300 mg/day | <200 mg/day |
| Total calories | Sufficient to achieve and maintain desirable weight | |

[a]Recommended eating pattern for all healthy individuals in the United States age 2 years or older.
Reproduced from National Cholesterol Education Program. Second report of the Expert Panel on Detection, Evaluation, and Treatment of High Blood Cholesterol in Adults (Adult Treatment Panel II). Circulation 1994;89:1329–1445.

**Table 3.5**
**Drug Therapy Treatment Levels in Adults**

| Risk | LDL Cholesterol Level (mg/dL) | |
|---|---|---|
| | Consideration Level | Goal |
| Without CHD, <2 other risk factors | ≥190[a] | <160 |
| Without CHD, ≥2 other risk factors | ≥160 | <130 |
| With CHD or other atherosclerotic disease | ≥130[b] | ≤100 |

[a]In younger patients (men aged less than 35 years and premenopausal women) with LDL cholesterol 190–220 mg/dL, drug therapy may be delayed if other risk is absent.
[b]In patients with CHD and LDL cholesterol 100–130 mg/dL, the physician should exercise clinical judgment in deciding whether to initiate drug therapy.
CHD = coronary heart disease; LDL = low-density lipoprotein.
Reproduced from National Cholesterol Education Program. Second report of the Expert Panel on Detection, Evaluation, and Treatment of High Blood Cholesterol in Adults (Adult Treatment Panel II). Circulation 1994;89:1329–1445.

is usually 6 months, but may be shorter in patients with marked hypercholesterolemia that would not be expected to be reduced adequately by diet alone and in patients with CHD. Drug therapy always supplements but does not replace dietary therapy. In patients recovering from an acute coronary event, the LDL cholesterol level will generally rise in subsequent weeks; intensive dietary therapy and risk factor reduction should be implemented prior to discharge and follow-up lipid measurements scheduled for 6–8 weeks later.

Great care needs to be taken in determining whether to initiate lipid-lowering drug therapy, which will likely be lifelong. The potential benefit must be weighed against potential adverse effects and costs of long-term therapy. Drug therapy is not appropriate in patients for whom sufficient benefit is not expected, such as those with short life expectancy, poor cardiac prognosis, or other severe medical conditions.

The ATP II recommendation of delaying drug therapy in primary prevention in men aged less than 35 years and in premenopausal women, unless LDL cholesterol level is 220 mg/dL or more or the patient has additional risk, requires clinical judgment as to the patient's overall risk. In secondary prevention in patients whose LDL cholesterol level is 100–129 mg/dL despite maximal dietary therapy, clinical judgment should be employed in the decision about whether to initiate drug therapy.

The lipid-lowering agents approved in the United States are bile acid sequestrants (cholestyramine and colestipol), nicotinic acid, HMG-CoA reductase inhibitors ("statins" —fluvastatin, lovastatin, pravastatin, and simvastatin), fibric acid derivatives (clofibrate, which is little used, fenofibrate, which is not yet available, and gemfibrozil), and probucol (see also

Chapter 2 for drug characterisitcs). Alternatively, estrogen-replacement therapy is considered by some clinicians for lipid lowering in postmenopausal women, although it does not have US Food and Drug Administration approval for this indication or for reducing CHD risk.

Patients receiving drug therapy should be monitored at 6–8 weeks after initiation of therapy (or 4–6 weeks after nicotinic acid dosage has been stabilized) and again 6 weeks later. At least two fasting lipoprotein analyses and careful evaluation of adherence are required to assess efficacy of a given dosage. If single-drug therapy does not produce adequate lipid lowering after 3 months, the addition of a second agent may be considered (Table 3.6). The potential benefit of additional lipid lowering must be weighed against the potential for additional side effects and possible drug interactions. Combination therapy, however, may decrease side effects, decrease cost, and increase compliance, since utilization of agents with synergistic mechanisms of action may allow lower doses of each drug. Combination therapy is especially useful in patients with established CHD, to reduce LDL cholesterol level to less than 100 mg/dL, and in patients with severe genetic conditions, who would not be expected to respond to maximum dosage of an individual hypolipidemic agent. In secondary prevention in patients whose LDL cholesterol level is 100–129 mg/dL with single-drug therapy, clinical judgment should be used in the decision about whether to introduce a second drug.

When the LDL cholesterol goal has been attained, patients should be followed up every 8–12 weeks for the first year and every 4–6 months thereafter. Patients should be monitored for potential drug side effects as

**Table 3.6**
**Drug Selection in Adults:**
**National Cholesterol Education Program Recommendations**

| Hyperlipidemia | Single drug | Combination drug |
|---|---|---|
| Elevated LDL cholesterol and triglyceride <200 mg/dL | Bile acid sequestrant<br>HMG-CoA reductase inhibitor<br>Nicotinic acid | Bile acid sequestrant + HMG-CoA reductase inhibitor<br>Bile acid sequestrant + nicotinic acid<br>HMG-CoA reductase inhibitor + nicotinic acid[a] |
| Elevated LDL cholesterol and triglyceride 200–400 mg/dL | Nicotinic acid<br>HMG-CoA reductase inhibitor<br>Gemfibrozil | Nicotinic acid + HMG-CoA reductase inhibitor[a]<br>HMG-CoA reductase inhibitor + gemfibrozil[b]<br>Nicotinic acid + bile acid sequenstrant<br>Nicotinic acid + gemfibrozil |

[a]Possible increased risk for myopathy or liver dysfunction.
[b]Increased risk for myopathy; must be used with caution.
HMG-CoA = 3-hydroxy-3-methylglutaryl coenzyme A; LDL = low density lipoprotein.
Reproduced from National Cholesterol Education Program. Second report of the Expert Panel on Detection, Evaluation, and Treatment of High Blood Cholesterol in Adults (Adult Treatment Panel II). Circulation 1994;89:1329–1445.

well as drug efficacy. A fasting lipoprotein analysis is required annually. Patients need to be advised to continue their medication after the LDL cholesterol goal has been met, since upon discontinuation of drug therapy, LDL cholesterol will return to pretreatment levels.

## Estrogen-Replacement Therapy

Estrogen-replacement therapy may be used instead of drug therapy in postmenopausal women with elevated LDL cholesterol. The increase in CHD risk that occurs with menopause has been shown by prospective observational studies to be reduced in women taking estrogen (84, 85); confirmation by large clinical trials is still needed. Although estrogen favorably affects LDL cholesterol and HDL cholesterol levels, triglyceride may be increased, particularly in patients with hypertriglyceridemia. Triglyceride should be monitored during the initial months of estrogen-replacement therapy; if triglyceride is markedly increased, estrogen should be discontinued. Because of an increased risk for endometrial hyperplasia and endometrial cancer with unopposed estrogen use, progestin is administered concomitantly in women with a uterus, although progestin use decreases the beneficial effect of estrogen on lipid levels. However, in the randomized Postmenopausal Estrogen/Progestin Interventions (PEPI) trial, conducted in 875 healthy postmenopausal women aged 45–64 years, the estrogen-mediated increase in HDL cholesterol was not eliminated by progestin coadministration though it was somewhat blunted (86). Additional benefits of estrogen-replacement therapy include decreased risk for osteoporosis.

Although estrogen-replacement therapy provides an alternative to lipid-lowering drug therapy, the potential risks of long-term estrogen use, which may include increased risk for breast cancer, must be considered. Patients receiving estrogen should be monitored for early signs of uterine cancer and screened for breast cancer as generally recommended. Estrogen does not, at the time of this writing, have an FDA indication for lipid lowering or for reducing CHD risk.

## Treatment of Hypertriglyceridemia

The role of serum triglyceride in CHD risk is less well defined than that of LDL cholesterol. Although univariate analyses of data from prospective studies have found a direct association between serum triglyceride level and CHD incidence, the association tends to weaken on multivariate analysis controlling for other variables and, perhaps in part because of the metabolic interrelation between HDL and the triglyceride-rich lipoproteins, may disappear altogether in analyses controlling for HDL cholesterol (87). Further, fasting triglyceride measurements can vary considerably within an individual, which can lead to misclassification of subjects in epidemiological and clinical trials, (88) and between individuals, which may account for the disappearance of the association of serum triglyceride with CHD risk on multivariate analysis controlling for more accurately measured lipids such as HDL cholesterol (89). Postprandial lipemia has not usually been considered in risk assessment; however, it may be that measurement of triglyceride-rich particles postprandially would more accurately describe their risk associations, because of the potential cytotoxicity of remnant particles (90) as well as the possibility that these partially catabolized, triglyceride-rich particles deliver cholesterol to the vessel wall (91). In recent studies, markers of postprandial metabolism of triglyceride-rich lipoproteins have been shown to be at least as accurate as HDL cholesterol in distinguishing CHD cases from controls (92, 93). The evaluation of serum triglyceride as a risk factor is complicated as well by the heterogeneity of the triglyceride-rich particles and their remnants. Chylomicrons and VLDL are not thought to be directly atherogenic, but their remnants may be.

The ATP II classifies serum triglyceride as normal (less than 200 mg/dL), borderline high (200–400 mg/dL), high (400–1000 mg/dL), and very high (more than 1000 mg/dL). Hypertriglyceridemia in the presence of existing CHD, familial combined hyperlipidemia, or diabetes or a positive family history of early atherosclerosis suggests that intervention is warranted. The primary therapy for hypertriglyceridemia is lifestyle modification: control of body weight, consumption of a diet low in saturated fat and cholesterol, institution of a regular exercise program, stopping smoking, and in some patients, restricting alcohol intake. Patients with hypertriglyceridemia frequently are physically inactive, obese, and glucose intolerant.

In patients with primary borderline-high triglyceride, the ATP II notes that drug therapy (see Table 3.6) may be considered in the presence of CHD, a family history of premature CHD, a combination of high total cholesterol (more than 240 mg/dL) and low HDL cholesterol (less than 35 mg/dL), or a genetic hypertriglyceridemia associated with increased CHD risk (e.g., type III hyperlipidemia, familial combined hyperlipidemia). The therapy selected should decrease LDL cholesterol, increase HDL cholesterol, and decrease the number of VLDL particles and their remnants. Although some triglyceride-lowering agents may increase LDL cholesterol levels in some patients, the clinical significance of a minor increase in LDL cholesterol in such cases is unclear. This increase reflects primarily the higher content of cholesteryl ester in the larger, lipid-rich LDL particles.

Although high triglyceride levels (400–1000 mg/dL) are not sufficiently elevated to cause pancreatitis, they may easily increase to very high levels in some patients and, especially in patients with a history of acute pancreatitis, may require treatment with a triglyceride-lowering drug. In general, treatment should be as for borderline-high triglyceride, with particular emphasis placed on controlling causes of secondary hypertriglyceridemia. In most patients, triglyceride elevation is the result of both primary and secondary factors; the most common secondary factor is obesity.

Very high triglyceride also is usually caused by a combination of primary and secondary factors. Because of the increased risk for pancreatitis, vigorous immediate intervention is warranted to lower triglyceride in these patients. Treatment strategies include discontinuing triglyceride-raising drugs, controlling diabetes mellitus, restricting alcohol intake, and limiting dietary fat to 10–20% of total calories. If nonpharmacologic measures do not decrease triglyceride levels to below 1000 mg/dL, drug therapy may be instituted. Because very high triglyceride can seldom be reduced to normal levels, a reasonable goal of therapy is a triglyceride level less than 500 mg/dL. No effective drug therapy is available for chylomicronemia.

The combination of elevated triglyceride and low HDL cholesterol is the typical dyslipidemia of patients with diabetes. The American Diabetes Association Consensus Development Panel on the Detection and Management of Lipid Disorders in Diabetes recommends that hypertriglyceridemia and hypercholesterolemia in adult patients with diabetes be treated primarily by diet, exercise, and glucose control (69). In patients with diabetes who do not have evidence of macrovascular disease, vigorous treatment is recommended for a triglyceride level of 200 mg/dL or more or an LDL cholesterol level of 130 mg/dL or greater. If triglyceride remains 400 mg/dL or greater or if LDL cholesterol remains 160 mg/dL or more after 6 months of treatment, pharmacologic therapy should be considered. The goal of pharmacologic therapy is to decrease triglyceride to less than 200 mg/dL and to decrease LDL cholesterol to less than 130 mg/dL. In diabetic patients without macrovascular disease who smoke or who have an HDL cholesterol level of 35 mg/dL or less, hypertension, or a family history of premature CHD, pharmacologic therapy should be considered if triglyceride remains 200 mg/dL or greater or LDL cholesterol remains 130 mg/dL or greater. In diabetic patients with evidence of macrovascular disease, the goal of lipid-lowering therapy is a triglyceride level of 150 mg/dL or less and an LDL cholesterol level of 100 mg/dL or less. Patients with diabetes whose triglyceride level is 1000 mg/dL or more require immediate attention because of the risk for pancreatitis and other complications of chylomicronemia.

## Treatment of Low HDL Cholesterol

Because of the increased risk for CHD associated with low HDL cholesterol, increasing HDL cholesterol should be incorporated in overall management of blood lipids. Lifestyle changes are the primary therapy and should include dietary modification, weight reduction in overweight patients, smoking cessation in smokers, and increased exercise in sedentary patients. Elimination of drugs that lower HDL cholesterol levels should also be considered but may not be feasible, for example, in the treatment of some patients with β-blockers.

In primary prevention in patients with low HDL cholesterol and other CHD risk factors, particularly those with a family history of CHD, lifestyle changes should be employed to reduce modifiable risk factors. Hypertension and diabetes should be treated as appropriate. If drug therapy is indicated for a concomitant elevation in LDL cholesterol, the drug selected ideally should be one that also increases HDL cholesterol. In primary prevention in patients with low HDL cholesterol but otherwise low CHD risk (acceptable LDL cholesterol and negative family history of premature CHD), drugs are not generally recommended to increase HDL cholesterol.

In secondary prevention, lifestyle changes remain the primary therapy. In addition, hypertension and diabetes should be treated as is appropriate. In patients with CHD, including those with high normal triglyceride, if drug therapy is required to decrease LDL cholesterol to 100 mg/dL or less, an agent that also increases HDL cholesterol is a good choice. In patients whose LDL cholesterol is initially less than 100 mg/dL, nicotinic acid may be considered to increase low HDL cholesterol.

## SUMMARY

Intensive lipid lowering in clinical trials has proved the lipid hypothesis by successfully preventing coronary events in subjects at high risk for these events whether because of dyslipidemia or known CHD. In metaanalysis of major primary prevention trials, a 10% decrease in total cholesterol led to reductions of 25% in nonfatal MI, 12% in fatal MI, and 22% in all MIs; respective decreases in major nonangiographic secondary prevention trials were 19%, 12%, and 15% (94). A metaanalysis of angiographically monitored secondary prevention trials (NHLBI Type II, STARS, CLAS, FATS, and UCSF-SCOR) indicated that pharmacologic lipid lowering reduced risk for CHD events 58% (21). Angiographic trials have also demonstrated that the progression of atherosclerotic lesions can be retarded and even reversed with aggressive lipid-lowering therapy, providing direct evidence that the natural course of CHD is modifiable with treatment. In addition, with the publication of the 4S and WOSCOPS results, pharmacologic lipid lowering has been shown to reduce total mortality.

Trials are under way to determine the effect on CHD risk of altering lipid levels other than LDL cholesterol. For example, the HDL Intervention Trial is evaluating the effect of increasing HDL cholesterol by pharmacologic means in secondary prevention.

Evaluation and treatment guidelines established by the ATP II are stratified according to the gradient of risk for CHD events in patients with or without established CHD. Although patients who already have CHD are at the highest risk for subsequent CHD events, risk in patients without CHD is increased by the presence of other known risk factors, some of which can be modified to reduce the likelihood that CHD will develop. Pharmacologic therapy provides a safe and effective means of magnifying the effects of dietary therapy to achieve the degree of lipid lowering necessary to decrease CHD risk.

## REFERENCES


1. National Cholesterol Education Program. Second report of the Expert Panel on Detection, Evaluation, and Treatment of High Blood Cholesterol in Adults (Adult Treatment Panel II). Circulation 1994; 89:1329–1445.
2. Austin MA, Breslow JL, Hennekens CH, et al. Low-density lipoprotein subclass patterns and risk of myocardial infarction. JAMA 1988; 260:1917–1921.
3. Austin MA, King M-C, Vranizan KM, et al. Inheritance of low-density lipoprotein subclass patterns: results of complex segregation analysis. Am J Hum Genet 1988; 43:838–846.
4. Eisenberg S, Gavish D, Oschry Y, et al. Abnormalities in very low, low, and high density lipoproteins in hypertriglyceridemia: reversal toward normal with bezafibrate treatment. J Clin Invest 1984; 74:470–482.
5. Patsch JR. Triglyceride-rich lipoproteins and atherosclerosis. Atherosclerosis 1994; 110:S23–S26.
6. Kuhn FE, Mohler ER, Satler LF, et al. Effects of high density lipoprotein on acetylcholine induced coronary vasoreactivity. Am J Cardiol 1991; 68:1425–1430.
7. Aoyama T, Yui Y, Morishita H, et al. Prostacyclin stabilization by high density lipoprotein is decreased in acute myocardial infarction and unstable angina pectoris. Circulation 1990; 81:1784–1791.
8. Klimov AN, Gurevich VS, Nikiforova AA, et al. Antioxidative activity of high density lipoproteins in vivo. Atherosclerosis 1993; 100:13–18.
9. Keys A, ed. Coronary heart disease in seven countries [American Heart Association Monograph 29]. Circulation 1970; 41(Suppl 1):1–211.
10. Gotto AM Jr, LaRosa JC, Hunninghake D, et al. The cholesterol facts: a summary of the evidence relating dietary fats, serum cholesterol, and coronary heart disease: a joint statement by the American Heart Association and the National Heart, Lung, and Blood Institute. Circulation 1990; 81:1721–1733.
11. Kagan A, Harris BR, Winkelstein W Jr, et al. Epidemiologic studies of coronary heart disease and stroke in Japanese men living in Japan, Hawaii and California: demographic, physical, dietary and biochemical characteristics. J Chronic Dis 1974; 27:345–364.
12. Marmot MG, Syme SL, Kagan A, et al. Epidemiologic studies of coronary heart disease and stroke in Japanese men living in Japan, Hawaii and California: prevalence of coronary and hypertensive heart disease and associated risk factors. Am J Epidemiol 1975; 102:514–525.
13. Robertson TL, Kato H, Rhoads GG, et al. Epidemiologic studies of coronary heart disease and stroke in Japanese men living in Japan, Hawaii and California: incidence of myocardial infarction and death from coronary heart disease. Am J Cardiol 1977; 39:239–243.
14. Stamler J, Wentworth D, Neaton JD, for the MRFIT Research Group. Is relationship between serum cholesterol and risk of premature death from coronary heart disease continuous and graded? Findings in 356 222 primary screenees of the Multiple Risk Factor Intervention Trial (MRFIT). JAMA 1986; 256:2823–2828.
15. Anderson KM, Castelli WP, Levy D. Cholesterol and mortality: 30 years of follow-up from the Framingham Study. JAMA 1987; 257:2176–2180.
16. Brown MS, Goldstein JL. A receptor-mediated pathway for cholesterol homeostasis. Science 1986; 232:34–47.
17. Reiser R, Sorrels MF, Williams MC. Influence of high levels of dietary fats and cholesterol on atherosclerosis and lipid distribution in swine. Circ Res 1959; 7:833–846.
18. Radcliffe JD, St Martin M, Alexander K. The effect of dietary cholesterol level on serum cholesterol and development of atherosclerosis in Japanese quail. Nutr Rep Int 1985; 31:1357–1361.
19. Armstrong ML, Warner ED, Connor WE. Regression of coronary atheromatosis in rhesus monkeys. Circ Res 1970; 27:59–67.
20. Dayton S, Pearce ML, Hashimoto S, et al. A controlled clinical trial of a diet high in unsaturated fat in preventing complications of atherosclerosis. Circulation 1969; 40(Suppl 2):II-1–II-63.

21. Rossouw JE. The effects of lowering serum cholesterol on coronary heart disease risk. Med Clin North Am 1994; 78:181–195.
22. Lipid Research Clinics Program. The Lipid Research Clinics Coronary Primary Prevention Trial results. I. Reduction in incidence of coronary heart disease. JAMA 1984; 251:351–364.
23. Lipid Research Clinics Program. The Lipid Research Clinics Coronary Primary Prevention Trial results. II. The relationship of reduction in incidence of coronary heart disease to cholesterol lowering. JAMA 1984; 251:365–374.
24. Committee of Principal Investigators. A co-operative trial in the primary prevention of ischaemic heart disease using clofibrate. Br Heart J 1978; 40:1069–1118.
25. Committee of Principal Investigators. WHO cooperative trial on primary prevention of ischaemic heart disease with clofibrate to lower serum cholesterol: final mortality follow-up. Lancet 1984; 2:600–604.
26. Huttunen JK, Manninen V, Mänttäri M, et al. The Helsinki Heart Study: central findings and clinical implications. Ann Med 1991; 23:155–159.
27. Manninen V, Tenkanen L, Koskinen P, et al. Joint effects of serum triglyceride and LDL cholesterol and HDL cholesterol concentrations on coronary heart disease risk in the Helsinki Heart Study: implications for treatment. Circulation 1992; 85:37–45.
28. Shepherd J, Cobbe SM, Ford I, et al. for the West of Scotland Coronary Prevention Study Group. Prevention of coronary heart disease with pravastatin in men with hypercholesterolemia. N Engl J Med 1995; 333:1301–1307.
29. Brown BG, Zhao X-Q, Sacco DE, et al. Lipid lowering and plaque regression: new insights into prevention of plaque disruption and clinical events in coronary disease. Circulation 1993; 87:1781–1791.
30. Coronary Drug Project Research Group. Clofibrate and niacin in coronary heart disease. JAMA 1975; 231:360–381.
31. Canner PL, Berge KG, Wenger NK, et al, for the Coronary Drug Project Research Group. Fifteen year mortality in Coronary Drug Project patients: long-term benefit with niacin. J Am Coll Cardiol 1986; 8:1245–1255.
32. Brensike JF, Levy RI, Kelsey SF, et al. Effects of therapy with cholestyramine on progression of coronary arteriosclerosis: results of the NHLBI Type II Coronary Intervention Study. Circulation 1984; 69:313–324.
33. Watts GF, Lewis B, Brunt JNH, et al. Effects on coronary artery disease of lipid-lowering diet, or diet plus cholestyramine, in the St Thomas' Atherosclerosis Regression Study (STARS). Lancet 1992; 339:563–569.
34. Blankenhorn DH, Azen SP, Kramsch DM, et al. Coronary angiographic changes with lovastatin therapy: the Monitored Atherosclerosis Regression Study (MARS). Ann Intern Med 1993; 119:969–976.
35. Waters D, Higginson L, Gladstone P, et al. Effects of monotherapy with an HMG-CoA reductase inhibitor on the progression of coronary atherosclerosis as assessed by serial quantitative arteriography: the Canadian Coronary Atherosclerosis Intervention Trial. Circulation 1994; 89:959–968.
36. Pitt B, Mancini GBJ, Ellis SG, et al., for the PLAC I Investigators. Pravastatin Limitation of Atherosclerosis in the Coronary Arteries (PLAC I); reduction in atherosclerosis progression and clinical events. J Am Coll Cardiol 1995; 26:1133–1139.
37. MAAS Investigators. Effect of simvastatin on coronary atheroma: the Multicentre Anti-Atheroma Study (MAAS). Lancet 1994; 344:633–638.
38. Scandinavian Simvastatin Survival Study Group. Randomised trial of cholesterol lowering in 4444 patients with coronary heart disease: the Scandinavian Simvastatin Survival Study (4S). Lancet 1994; 344:1383–1389.
39. Blankenhorn DH, Nessim SA, Johnson RL, et al. Beneficial effects of combined colestipol-niacin therapy on coronary atherosclerosis and coronary venous bypass grafts. JAMA 1987; 257:3233–3240.
40. Blankenhorn DH, Alaupovic P, Wickham E, et al. Prediction of angiographic change in native human coronary arteries and aortocoronary bypass grafts: lipid and non-lipid factors. Circulation 1990; 81:470–476.
41. Cashin-Hemphill L, Mack WJ, Pogoda JM, et al. Beneficial effects of colestipol-niacin on coronary atherosclerosis: a 4-year follow-up. JAMA 1990; 264:3013–3017.

42. Brown G, Albers JJ, Fisher LD, et al. Regression of coronary artery disease as a result of intensive lipid-lowering therapy in men with high levels of apolipoprotein B. N Engl J Med 1990; 323:1289–1298.
43. Kane JP, Malloy MJ, Ports TA, et al. Regression of coronary atherosclerosis during treatment of familial hypercholesterolemia with combined drug regimens. JAMA 1990; 264:3007–3012.
44. National Cholesterol Education Program. Report of the Expert Panel on Population Strategies for Blood Cholesterol Reduction. Circulation 1991; 83:2154–2232.
45. Gordon T, Castelli WP, Hjortland MC, et al. High density lipoprotein as a protective factor against coronary heart disease. The Framingham Study. Am J Med 1977; 62:707–714.
46. Jacobs DR Jr, Mebane IL, Bangdiwala SI, et al, for the Lipid Research Clinics Program. High density lipoprotein cholesterol as a predictor of cardiovascular disease mortality in men and women: the follow-up study of the Lipid Research Clinics Prevalence Study. Am J Epidemiol 1990; 131:32–47.
47. Multiple Risk Factor Intervention Trial Research Group. Multiple Risk Factor Intervention Trial: risk factor changes and mortality results. JAMA 1982; 248:1465–1477.
48. Gordon DJ, Probstfield JL, Garrison RJ, et al. High-density lipoprotein cholesterol and cardiovascular disease: four prospective American studies. Circulation 1989; 79:8–15.
49. Jonas MA, Oates JA, Ockene JK, et al. Statement on smoking and cardiovascular disease for health care professionals. Circulation 1992; 86:1664–1669.
50. US Surgeon General. The health benefits of smoking cessation: a report of the Surgeon General, 1990. (DHHS publication no. (CDC) 90-8416.) Rockville, MD: US Department of Health and Human Services, Public Health Service, Office on Smoking and Health, 1990.
51. Manson JE, Tosteson H, Ridker PM, et al. The primary prevention of myocardial infarction. N Engl J Med 1992; 326:1406–1416.
52. MacMahon S, Peto R, Cutler J, et al. Blood pressure, stroke, and coronary heart disease. Part 1, prolonged differences in blood pressure: prospective observational studies corrected for the regression dilution bias. Lancet 1990; 335:765–774.
53. Collins R, Peto R, MacMahon S, et al. Blood pressure, stroke, and coronary heart disease. Part 2, short-term reductions in blood pressure: overview of randomised drug trials in their epidemiological context. Lancet 1990; 335:827–838.
54. MacMahon S, Cutler JA, Stamler J. Antihypertensive drug treatment: potential, expected, and observed effects on stroke and on coronary heart disease. Hypertension 1989; 13(Suppl I):I-45–I-50.
55. Hubert HB, Feinleib M, McNamara PM, et al. Obesity as an independent risk factor for cardiovascular disease: a 26-year follow-up of participants in the Framingham Heart Study. Circulation 1983; 67:968–977.
56. Denke MA, Sempos CT, Grundy SM. Excess body weight: an underrecognized contributor to high blood cholesterol levels in white American men. Arch Intern Med 1993; 153:1093–1103.
57. Garrison RJ, Wilson PW, Castelli WP, et al. Obesity and lipoprotein cholesterol in the Framingham offspring study. Metabolism 1980; 29:1053–1060.
58. Berchtold P, Jorgens V, Finke C, et al. Epidemiology of obesity and hypertension. Int J Obes 1981; 5(Suppl 1):1–7.
59. Hartz AJ, Rupley DC, Kalkhoff RD, et al. Relationship of obesity to diabetes: influence of obesity level and body fat distribution. Prev Med 1983; 12:351–357.
60. Paffenbarger RS Jr, Hyde RT, Wing AL, et al. The association of changes in physical-activity level and other lifestyle characteristics with mortality among men. N Engl J Med 1993; 328:538–545.
61. Leon AS, Connett J, for the MRFIT Research Group. Physical activity and 10.5 year mortality in the Multiple Risk Factor Intervention Trial (MRFIT). Int J Epidemiol 1991; 20:690–697.
62. Fletcher GF, Blair SN, Blumenthal J, et al. Statement on exercise: benefits and recommendations for physical activity programs for all Americans: a statement for health professionals by the Committee on Exercise and Cardiac Rehabilitation of the Council on Clinical Cardiology, American Heart Association. Circulation 1992; 86:340–344.

63. Blair SN, Cooper KH, Gibbons LW, et al. Changes in coronary heart disease risk factors associated with increased treadmill time in 753 men. Am J Epidemiol 1983; 118:352–359.
64. Jennings G, Nelson L, Nestel P, et al. The effects of changes in physical activity on major cardiovascular risk factors, hemodynamics, sympathetic function, and glucose utilization in man: a controlled study of four levels of activity. Circulation 1986; 73:30–40.
65. Després J-P, Pouliot M-C, Moorjani S, et al. Loss of abdominal fat and metabolic response to exercise training in obese women. Am J Physiol 1991; 261:E159–E167.
66. Helmrich SP, Ragland DR, Leung RW, et al. Physical activity and reduced occurrence of non-insulin-dependent diabetes mellitus. N Engl J Med 1991; 325:147–152.
67. Butler WJ, Ostrander LD, Carman WJ, et al. Mortality from coronary heart disease in the Tecumseh Study: long-term effect of diabetes mellitus, glucose tolerance and other risk factors. Am J Epidemiol 1985; 121:541–547.
68. Barrett-Connor EL, Cohn BA, Wingard DL, et al. Why is diabetes mellitus a stronger risk factor for fatal ischemic heart disease in women than in men? The Rancho Bernardo Study. JAMA 1991; 265:627–631.
69. American Diabetes Association Consensus Development Conference on the Detection and Management of Lipid Disorders in Diabetes. Detection and management of lipid disorders in diabetes. Diabetes Care 1993; 16(Suppl 2):106–112.
70. Pyörälä K, Laakso M, Uusitupa M. Diabetes and atherosclerosis: an epidemiologic view. Diabetes Metab Rev 1987; 3:463–524.
71. Diabetes Control and Complications Trial Research Group. The effect of intensive treatment of diabetes on the development and progression of long-term complications in insulin-dependent diabetes mellitus. N Engl J Med 1993; 329:977–986.
72. American Heart Association. Heart and stroke facts: 1995 statistical supplement. Dallas: American Heart Association, 1994.
73. Castelli WP. Epidemiology of coronary heart disease: the Framingham Study. Am J Med 1984; 76(2A):4–12.
74. Rubin SM, Sidney S, Black DM, et al. High blood cholesterol in elderly men and the excess risk for coronary heart disease. Ann Intern Med 1990; 113:916–920.
75. Castelli WP, Wilson PWF, Levy D, et al. Cardiovascular risk factors in the elderly. Am J Cardiol 1989; 63:12H–19H.
76. Barrett-Connor E, Suarez L, Khaw K, et al. Ischemic heart disease risk factors after age 50. J Chronic Dis 1984; 37:903–908.
77. SHEP Cooperative Research Group. Prevention of stroke by antihypertensive drug treatment in older persons with isolated systolic hypertension. Final results of the Systolic Hypertension in the Elderly Program (SHEP). JAMA 1991; 265:3255–3264.
78. Lerner DJ, Kannel WB. Patterns of coronary heart disease morbidity and mortality in the sexes: a 26-year follow-up of the Framingham population. Am Heart J 1986; 111:383–390.
79. Matthews KA, Meilahn E, Kuller LH, et al. Menopause and risk factors for coronary heart disease. N Engl J Med 1989; 321:641–646.
80. Shea S, Ottman R, Gabrieli C, et al. Family history as an independent risk factor for coronary artery disease. J Am Coll Cardiol 1984; 4:793–801.
81. Criqui MH, Langer RD, Fronek A, et al. Mortality over a period of 10 years in patients with peripheral arterial disease. N Engl J Med 1992; 326:381–386.
82. Salonen JT, Salonen R. Ultrasonographically assessed carotid morphology and the risk of coronary heart disease. Arterioscler Thromb 1991; 11:1245–1249.
83. Kris-Etherton PM, Krummel D, Russell ME, et al. The effect of diet on plasma lipids, lipoproteins, and coronary heart disease. J Am Diet Assoc 1988; 88:1373–1400.
84. Stampfer JM, Colditz GA, Willett WC, et al. Postmenopausal estrogen therapy and cardiovascular disease: ten-year follow-up from the Nurses' Health Study. N Engl J Med 1991; 325:756–762.
85. Bush TL, Barrett-Connor E, Cowan LD, et al. Cardiovascular mortality and noncontraceptive use of estrogen in women: results from the Lipid Research Clinics Program Follow-up Study. Circulation 1987; 75:1102–1109.
86. Writing Group for the PEPI Trial. Effects of estrogen or estrogen/progestin regimens

on heart disease risk factors in postmenopausal women: the Postmenopausal Estrogen/Progestin Interventions (PEPI) trial. JAMA 1995; 273:199–208.
87. Austin MA. Plasma triglyceride and coronary heart disease. Arterioscler Thromb 1991; 11:2–14.
88. Austin MA. Plasma triglyceride as a risk factor for coronary heart disease: the epidemiologic evidence and beyond. Am J Epidemiol 1989; 129:249–259.
89. Criqui MH, Heiss G, Cohn R, et al. Plasma triglyceride level and mortality from coronary heart disease. N Engl J Med 1993; 328:1220–1225.
90. Chung BH, Segrest JP, Smith K, et al. Lipolytic surface remnants of triglyceride-rich lipoproteins are cytotoxic to macrophages but not in the presence of high density lipoprotein: a possible mechanism of atherogenesis? J Clin Invest 1989; 83:1363–1374.
91. Zilversmit DB. Atherogenesis: a postprandial phenomenon. Circulation 1979; 60: 473–485.
92. Groot PH, van Stiphout WA, Krauss XH, et al. Postprandial lipoprotein metabolism in normolipidemic men with and without coronary artery disease. Arterioscler Thromb 1991; 11:653–662.
93. Patsch JR, Miesenbock G, Hopferwieser T, et al. Relation of triglyceride metabolism and coronary artery disease. Arterioscler Thromb 1992; 12:1336–1345.
94. Rossouw JE, Lewis B, Rifkind BM. The value of lowering cholesterol after myocardial infarction. N Engl J Med 1990; 323:1112–1119.

# PART III

# Therapy of Ischemic Heart Disease

# CHAPTER 4

## Principles of Therapy in Ischemic Heart Disease and Use of Antiischemic Drugs

Prakash C. Deedwania, MD, and
William W. Parmley, MD

Coronary artery disease (CAD) is a leading cause of death and disability in the United States and most other industrialized countries. The prevalence of CAD increases with age, and some recent studies have demonstrated that CAD is the leading cause of death in the elderly (more than 65 years old) (1). Even in women who are relatively protected from CAD in the premenopausal period, after 65 years of age CAD becomes the leading cause of death. With improved survival, increased life expectancy, and the large number of elderly Americans in the population, the number of patients with CAD is likely to increase. The exact prevalence of CAD is not known, but it is estimated that more than 6 million Americans have clinically significant CAD. The economic consequences of CAD in the United States are also quite significant. Some estimates suggest an enormous cost of approximately $100 billion for conditions associated with CAD (2).

Almost every practicing clinician, especially the internist and the primary care physician, encounters patients with CAD on a regular basis. In recent years, most primary care physicians have become accustomed to referring their patients with CAD to the cardiologist for workup and management. However, with the rapidly changing environment in the health care arena, it is likely that the primary care physician will be responsible for the care of most patients with stable CAD. In this chapter, we will review the essential aspects of the pathophysiology of myocardial ischemia and the rational use of antianginal drugs in patients with stable CAD.

### ANGINA VERSUS MYOCARDIAL ISCHEMIA

In general, most patients with CAD present to the clinician because of chest discomfort or other anginal equivalent symptoms (e.g., shortness of breath). Traditionally, management of patients with angina has consisted of therapy prescribed for control of symptoms; however, several recent studies have demonstrated that, although control of anginal symptoms is of obvious importance to relieve patients' discomfort, the presence of ischemia determines the prognosis of patients with stable CAD (3–5).

Myocardial ischemia is the most common expression of stable CAD. Although many patients with ischemia have associated anginal symptoms, recent studies suggest that angina is a relatively insensitive and nonspecific predictor of significant CAD (3). The lack of anginal symptoms does not imply absence of severe and potentially lethal coronary stenosis (3). Even in patients with significant CAD, lack of anginal symptoms does not predict benign prognosis. The severity of anginal symptoms also does not correlate well with the extent of CAD and long-term prognosis (3). Holter monitoring in patients with angina pectoris and stable CAD has demonstrated that most patients with CAD have frequent episodes of silent ischemia during daily life (3–6). Silent ischemia during Holter monitoring is defined as the presence of ST-segment depression without associated chest pain. The presence of myocardial perfusion abnormalities during episodes of ST-segment depression recorded on Holter monitoring provides strong evidence regarding the ischemic nature of the ST-segment changes (3).

Several recent studies have shown that silent ischemia occurs frequently despite control of symptoms, and the presence of such residual silent ischemia is associated with an adverse clinical outcome and increased risk of death. Advanced obstructive CAD may exist with minimal or no symptoms and can progress rapidly, leading to a lethal outcome with little warning, and, in some cases, sudden death may be the initial manifestation of CAD (3). It has been estimated that 18% of coronary attacks occur with sudden death as the first event. Detection of ischemic ST-segment depression during exercise testing in asymptomatic individuals has been shown to predict higher risk of subsequent coronary events and death. Recent data suggest that symptom-guided therapy does not abolish all ischemic events and more than 40% of patients with stable angina treated with one or more antianginal drugs have silent ischemic events during daily life (3, 4).

The mechanism or mechanisms responsible for the presence of angina during some episodes of myocardial ischemia and the absence of symptoms during many other ischemic episodes is not known. Several possible explanations have been proposed, including increased pain threshold, lesser magnitude and shorter duration of ischemia, and presence of a defective anginal warning system. Whatever the mechanism might be, it is reasonably well established that most patients with CAD have far more frequent episodes of silent ischemia than anginal symptoms. It has also been proven beyond doubt that it is the presence of ischemia (regardless of the associated symptoms) that determines the eventual prognosis in patients with CAD. It is therefore critical for the clinician prescribing therapy for patients with ischemic heart disease to aim not only for the control of symptoms but also for the suppression of myocardial ischemia.

## PATHOPHYSIOLOGIC BASIS OF MYOCARDIAL ISCHEMIA

Myocardial ischemia occurs whenever there is an imbalance between myocardial oxygen demand and myocardial oxygen supply (Fig. 4.1). In general, the most common reason for myocardial ischemia is the presence

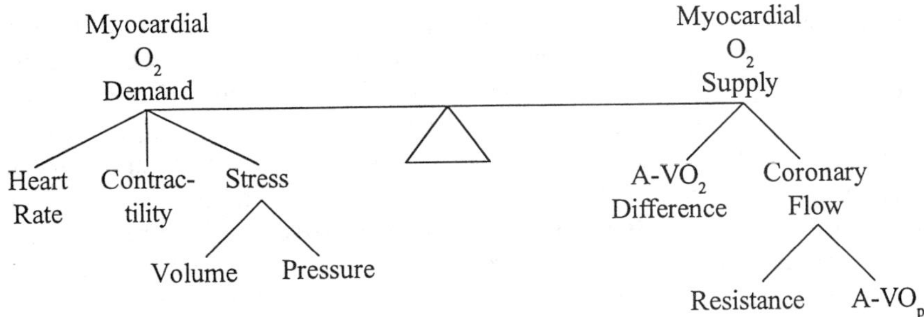


Figure 4.1. The balance of myocardial oxygen demand and myocardial oxygen supply is schematically depicted. Myocardial oxygen demand is largely determined by the heart rate, myocardial contractility, and left ventricular (LV) stress, which is related to LV volume and systolic blood pressure. Myocardial oxygen supply depends on coronary blood supply and the oxygen carrying capacity of blood. A-V=arterial-venous.

of obstructive CAD secondary to coronary atherosclerosis. The three major determinants of myocardial oxygen demand are heart rate, myocardial contractility, and ventricular wall tension. Left ventricular wall tension is largely related to ventricular volume and systolic blood pressure. Any conditions associated with an increase in one or more of these determinants of myocardial oxygen demand can result in myocardial ischemia if there is insufficient coronary reserve secondary to CAD (7).

The atherosclerotic process begins with the development of distinct subintimal thickening that eventually leads to development of plaque formation (8). Further progression of the atherosclerotic process in the plaques leads to localized luminal stenosis of varying severity in the coronary artery. Myocardial ischemia occurs whenever there is an imbalance between myocardial oxygen demand and coronary blood flow. The onset of ischemia triggers several events, including profound metabolic abnormalities and development of diastolic and systolic dysfunction of the myocardium.

## Coronary Vasospasm and Endothelial Dysfunction

Although coronary obstructive disease has been considered absolutely essential for the occurrence of angina at times of increased demands, it does not explain angina not associated with increased oxygen demands, or the presence of angina in patients who show normal coronary arteries. Many investigators have confirmed the role of coronary vasospasm in patients with anginal syndromes by demonstrating angiographic evidence of severe vasospasm of one or more coronary arteries during spontaneous anginal attacks, along with prominent ST-segment elevation and massive reversible transmural perfusion defect on thallium-201 scintigraphy. It is therefore essential to discuss the available evidence to support the role of coronary flow abnormalities in patients with ischemic heart disease. When myocardial ischemia and angina in patients with stable CAD are not easily predictable, a dynamic variability in coronary vasomotor tone is usually present that further decreases the cross-sectional lumen of the coronary artery already reduced as the result of an atherosclerotic lesion. The alteration of coronary vasomotor tone occurs due to a varying degree of endothelial dysfunction at the site of the stenosis (9). Although the atherosclerotic lesion is fairly stable, the perfusion of a particular area of the myocardium can be reduced due to dynamic changes in the luminal diameter associated with abnormal intimal activity overlying the stenosis. During the atherosclerotic process there are structural changes in the endothelium that lead to eventual endothelial dysfunction. Vasoconstriction of the vessel can occur through loss of normal dilator responses and development of abnormal (paradoxical) constrictor response to exercise, acetylcholine, and other vasodilating substances (9–12). Some studies have also demonstrated a deterioration of endothelial-mediated vasodilator response during exposure to noxious stimuli, including increased plasma cholesterol levels, increased plasma low-density lipoprotein (LDL) cholesterol, elevated glucose levels, and during persistent and significant elevation of blood pressure (12, 13). Long-term observation of healthy subjects in the Framingham heart study has identified these noxious stimuli as risk factors for development of coronary artery disease (14). Based on results of several recent studies, it has been suggested that effective risk factor modification such as lowering plasma cholesterol may result in improved endothelial function and a reduction in the risk of coronary events as well as anginal symptoms with only a modest regression in the severity of atherosclerotic lesions.

Another potential mechanism for reduction in myocardial blood flow could involve an increased resistance to blood flow in the coronary arterioles; constriction of distal coronary arteries or collateral vessels, or both; and a decrease in subendocardial flow due to increased intracavitary pressures (e.g., heart failure) (15). Although more work is needed to establish the clinical significance of endothelial dysfunction, it is evident that abnormalities of endothelial function, abnormalities of the distal coronary artery tone, as well as abnormal hemodynamic status can affect blood supply to the myocardium, resulting in the development of ischemia in patients with stable CAD (9–15).

## The Role of Increased Oxygen Demand

In the vast majority of patients with obstructive CAD, the predominant cause of myocardial ischemia appears to be an increase in myocardial oxygen demand in presence of a fixed coronary reserve. The increase in myocardial oxygen demand occurs largely due to increases in heart rate, blood pressure, or myocardial contractility. In most patients this is manifested by development of ischemia during periods of physical or mental stress. Treadmill exercise testing usually performed in patients with CAD induces ischemia by increasing myocardial oxygen demand. However, several recent studies have suggested that most ischemic episodes during daily life occur with minimal or no physical activity (3–5). These findings have led some to question the role of increased oxygen demand in the pathogenesis of myocardial ischemia. Recently, the evaluation of heart rate and blood pressure monitoring on a continuous basis in ambulatory patients with stable CAD revealed that most ischemic episodes were preceded by an increase in the heart rate and systolic blood pressure (16). The increased myocardial oxygen demand preceding episodes of spontaneous ischemia seen in patients during routine daily activities is also responsible for the surge of ischemia in the early morning hours when patients initiate physical activities (3,16). Approximately 20–30% of ischemic episodes are not preceded by an increase in myocardial oxygen demand, and it is likely that these ischemic events are triggered by abnormalities of coronary blood flow.

A clear understanding of the pathophysiology of myocardial ischemia has obvious clinical relevance in the approach to a patient with stable CAD. In each patient, intervention aimed at reducing symptoms or suppressing myocardial ischemia may be best selected based on the underlying pathophysiologic processes responsible for myocardial ischemia. A thorough and detailed clinical history should provide the clinician with important clues regarding the predominant mechanism responsible for anginal and ischemic episodes. For example, when angina occurs predominantly during periods of increased catecholamine activity and enhanced sympathetic tone, the most likely mechanism would appear to be increased demand; whereas when the anginal threshold shows variability and angina occurs at rest, during sleep, or with mild exertion, a coronary vasomotion abnormality might be playing a dominant role.

## CLASSIFICATION OF PATIENTS WITH ANGINA

Based on a good understanding of the pathophysiologic process, the selection of appropriate therapy varies depending upon the clinical picture of the patient with angina. In order to better define the pathophysiologic process involved, it is useful to classify patients into various categories before developing a treatment plan. Such classification helps the clinician choose the appropriate drug for a given patient. Most patients fit into the first category of chronic exertional angina, which usually occurs whenever the patient reaches a fixed threshold beyond which there occurs an imbalance because of increased myocardial oxygen demand and reduced coronary blood flow secondary to fixed atherosclerotic obstructive CAD. This condition is also classified as *fixed threshold angina*. On the other hand, there are some patients who have no limitation of their activity and are able to perform vigorous exercise without any angina, but they develop angina while at rest (rest angina). Myocardial ischemia and angina usually occur in these patients secondary to dynamic obstruction (vasospastic angina) of the coronary artery. It had been previously suggested that vasospasm occurs in these patients because of an imbalance between α-receptor (vasoconstrictory) and β-receptor (vasodilatory) activity. Recent data, however, tend to suggest that the endothelial dysfunction seen in early stages of atherosclerosis is responsible for vasospasm. Although in general most patients with vasospastic angina do not have significant fixed obstructive disease, careful review of angiographic data suggests that many may have irregularities in their coronary arteries indicating early stages of the atherosclerotic process that leads to endothelial dysfunction.

Prinzmetal's angina (variable threshold angina) usually occurs in patients with fixed atherosclerotic CAD who also demonstrate evidence of dynamic narrowing (vasospasm), usually in areas with mild obstructive lesions. These patients can have variable anginal threshold levels so that on some occasions they can develop rest angina due to vasospasm, whereas on other occasions they will develop ischemia and angina only with vigorous physical exercise or mental stress. Although it is not clear why these patients develop coronary vasospasm on some occasions and not on others, it has been shown that certain situations, such as exposure to cold, anger, mental stress, and excessive alcohol abuse, tend to bring on their vasospastic attack. In contrast, the usual factors responsible for increased myocardial oxygen demand (e.g., physical activity) would lead to the exertional component of angina. Based on these discussions, it should be fairly evident that the appropriate choice of therapy varies a great deal based on the precise pathophysiologic mechanism responsible for myocardial ischemia and angina.

## THERAPEUTIC CONSIDERATIONS IN PATIENTS WITH ISCHEMIC HEART DISEASE

The goals of therapy in patients with CAD primarily consist of providing freedom from symptoms, enhancing quality of life, and improving the adverse clinical outcome associated with the disease (Table 4.1). To achieve these goals, a multifaceted approach is needed in the management of patients with stable CAD. The main goals of this approach should be not only to treat angina but also to reduce or suppress myocardial ischemia. This approach must take into consideration changes in lifestyle to help the patient avoid situations that trigger episodes of angina such as emotional distress, large meals, cold environment, and sudden exertion to which the patient is not accustomed. In addition, smoking cessation should be encouraged in all patients with angina because nicotine is one of the most potent vasoconstrictors and it also increases catecholamine level, thereby affecting both supply and demand sides of the balance. Modification of risk factors for CAD should be strongly emphasized, because the presence of risk factors is of pivotal importance not only in the development, but also

**Table 4.1**
**Goals of Therapy in Patients with Angina Pectoris**

| |
|---|
| Relieve symptoms |
| Improve functional capacity |
| Improve quality of life |
| Suppress myocardial ischemia |
| Prevent progression of coronary artery disease |
| Reduce risk of coronary events |
| Improve survival |

in the progression, of CAD. Risk factor modification is often neglected by most clinicians, but recent knowledge gained in this area now makes it mandatory to institute such therapy in most patients with CAD.

## Modification of Risk Factors for Coronary Artery Disease

Recently, sufficient new information has become available to suggest that modification of risk factors can and does result in a reduced risk of acute myocardial infarction and cardiac death. Although this topic is discussed in detail in Chapter 3, it will be described briefly here because of its relevance in patients with angina. Several studies in patients with angiographically proven CAD have evaluated the effects of diet and lipid-lowering drugs on clinical outcome and demonstrated that, compared to placebo, there was a greater degree of nonprogression and regression of CAD in patients receiving lipid-lowering treatment (17–23). Total adverse events (including death, nonfatal infarction, and worsening angina requiring coronary revascularization) were significantly reduced in patients receiving active therapy (20–24). It has also been demonstrated that in angina patients with angiographic CAD who are treated with a regular physical exercise program and a low-fat, low-cholesterol diet, there is slower progression of CAD (22). A recent study has demonstrated that with intense risk factor modification (including regular exercise, vegetarian diet, and weight reduction), patients with angina showed evidence not only of modest regression of coronary stenosis but also of decreased size and severity of perfusion abnormalities on resting dipyridamole position emission tomography (PET) after 5-year follow-up (23).

Despite these encouraging results, overall risk factor modification appears to achieve rather modest beneficial results in patients with documented CAD. This may be partly because implementation of such interventions requires extremely demanding changes in lifestyle that are associated with compliance problems and less than optimal duration of intervention as well as a limited follow-up for a relatively short period of time (24). The risk factors that are most amenable to modification are cigarette smoking, systemic hypertension, obesity, physical inactivity, and elevated serum cholesterol levels.

## Antiischemic Drug Therapy for Angina Pectoris and Ischemia

Antianginal drugs are used primarily to restore the balance by reducing myocardial oxygen demand or enhancing coronary blood flow. Several classes of antianginal drugs (nitrates, calcium channel blockers, and β-blockers) are available, and they produce a wide range of cardiovascular effects (Table 4.2). The efficacy of these drugs has been evaluated by their effects on relief of angina pectoris as well as their ability to reduce the degree of ischemia detected during exercise testing in patients with stable CAD. Traditionally, this has been a good objective, since episodes of angina, time to onset of angina during exercise, and time to occurrence of electrocardiographic evidence of ischemia can be readily measured. Recent evidence, however, from several studies in patients with CAD indicate that evaluation of angina may be not enough, and even the evaluation of ischemia during exercise stress testing may be inadequate in the evaluation of total ischemic burden in patients with CAD. This is largely because a great amount (70% or more) of ischemia is asymptomatic and can be detected only during Holter monitoring. As a result of the new information regarding findings of ischemia during Holter monitoring in patients with CAD, therapy with conventional antianginal drugs recently has been evaluated more objectively for its antiischemic effects outside the exercise laboratory. Most of the antianginal drugs seem effective in reducing the frequency and severity of anginal attacks and improving the functional capacity during exercise testing. Several studies, however, in patients with stable angina have revealed that drug therapy aimed at control of symptoms does not eliminate or adequately suppress episodes of silent ischemia detected during Holter monitoring. These findings may have important future clinical implications because ischemia determines prognosis in patients with stable CAD.

**Table 4.2**
**Antiischemic Actions of Antianginal Drugs**

| | Nitrates | β-Blockers | $Ca^{++}$ Blockers |
|---|---|---|---|
| Myocardial oxygen demand | | | |
| Heart rate | ↑ | ↓↓ | ↑↓ |
| Contractility | ↔↑ | ↓↓ | ↑↔↓ |
| Systolic pressure | ↓ | ↓↓ | ↓↓ |
| LV volume | ↓↓ | ↑↔ | ↑↓ |
| Mycardial oxygen supply | | | |
| Coronary vasodilation | ↑ | ↓↔ | ↑↑ |
| Epicardial blood flow | ↑ | ↓ | ↑↑ |
| Collateral blood flow | ↑ | ↔↓ | ↑ |
| Dilation at site of atheroma | ↑↑ | ↔ | ↑ |

$Ca^{++}$ = calcium channel; LV = left ventricular; ↓ = decreased; ↑ = increased; ↔ = no predominant effect.

The specific actions of various antianginal drugs on myocardial oxygen demand and coronary blood flow will now be discussed in detail. Emphasis will be placed on their unique properties and pharmacologic actions, and clinical guidelines will be provided for achieving maximum success with the given drug in patients with stable CAD and angina.

### *Nitrates*

Nitrates have been used for their antianginal effects for more than a century. They are the only agents that immediately alleviate an attack of angina regardless of the underlying mechanism triggering the attack. Nitrates seem to exert their antianginal and antiischemic effect through a combination of peripheral venodilation (reduced preload), arterial vasodilation (reduced afterload) at higher doses, and dilation of the coronary vessels (Table 4.2) (25–27). At the doses used in clinical practice to treat patients with angina and CAD, nitrates exert their antiischemic effect primarily by reducing preload through pooling of blood in the peripheral and splanchnic venous beds, resulting in reduced venous return. This in turn produces a reduced ventricular volume and lower intracavitary pressure. All of these effects result in a decrease in ventricular wall stress (28). At relatively small doses, nitrates can produce dilatation at the site of the coronary stenosis (especially in eccentric lesions) and seem capable of increasing collateral flow with improved subendocardial perfusion in areas of ischemic myocardium (29).

Treatment with nitrates can also relieve spontaneous coronary vasospasm and the exercise-induced spasm at the site of epicardial coronary atheroma (30). Nitrates appear to be direct vasodilators that will exert their effect in the absence of endothelial-derived relaxant factor (EDRF) and other vasodilator substances (for example, denuded endothelium). After entering the vessel wall nitrates seem to be metabolized to nitric oxide (a direct endothelial relaxant agent), which also has antiplatelet properties (27, 31). Nitric oxide stimulates production of cyclic guanosine monophosphate (cGMP) that in turn causes inhibition of calcium influx into the cell or enhances exit of calcium from the cell, or both. These effects on calcium transport result in vessel wall relaxation and dilatation. The mechanism through which cGMP promotes vascular smooth muscle relaxation is not fully known. Table 4.3 summarizes the important pharmacologic differences between various nitrate preparations. The details of pharmacologic properties of various nitrates are described in Chapter 7. This chapter will concentrate on the important issues regarding the practical problem of nitrate tolerance, which has been identified as the major limitation of nitrate usage.

**Development of Tolerance to Nitrates.** Although nitrates are highly effective for treatment of an anginal attack and can be used to prevent an attack if taken before an activity that is known to precipitate angina, their long-term use can be associated with a relatively fast devel-

**Table 4.3**
**Comparative Pharmacology of Different Nitrate Preparations**

| | Dose (mg) | Onset of Action (min) | Peak Action (min) | Duration (min) |
|---|---|---|---|---|
| Sl NTG | .3–.8 | 2–5 | 4–8 | 10–30 |
| SL ISDN | 2.5–10 | 5–20 | 15–60 | 45–120 |
| Oral NTG | 6.5–19.5 | 20–45 | 45–120 | 120–360 |
| Oral ISDN (b.i.d., t.i.d.)[a] | 10–60 | 15–45 | 45–120 | 120–360 |
| Buccal NTG | 1–3 | 2–5 | 4–10 | 30–300 |
| NTG 2% Oint. | 0.5–2 in. | 15–60 | 30–120 | 180–480 |
| NTG patch (12 h-on, 12 h-off) | 5–10 | 30–60 | 60–180 | 18–24 h |
| Oral ISMN | 20–40 | 60 | 60–240 | 300 |

[a]Eccentric dosing with 12–14-hour nitrate-free interval to avoid nitrate tolerance.
h = hour; ISDN = isosorbide dinitrate; ISMN = isosorbide mononitrate; mg = milligrams; min = minutes; NTG = nitroglycerin; SL = sublingual.

opment of tolerance. Nitrate tolerance has been described as the reduced effect of a particular dose of nitrate and the need for a higher dose to sustain efficacy (32, 33). Some factors that have been described as playing an important role in the development of nitrate tolerance include the amount and frequency of dosing, the duration of treatment, nitrate blood levels, and the particular pharmacokinetic profile of the nitrate being used (32). The problem of rapid tolerance to long-term administration of nitrates limits their efficacy as antianginal and antiischemic agents. Several reports from studies using various types of nitrates (oral, transdermal preparations) indicate that partial to complete development of tolerance will occur rapidly, depending on the amount and frequency of administration (32–37). The available evidence from these reports suggests that tolerance develops quickly during long-term administration of nitrates, particularly with preparations such as transdermal patches that deliver the drug at a constant rate and provide constant plasma concentrations (37). Nitrate tolerance seems to be less prominent during treatment with preparations and dosing schedules that provide abrupt or quick rises and falls in plasma concentrations during the dosing interval (37, 38). Therefore it seems unlikely that a continuous prophylactic antianginal effect can be achieved with the currently available nitrate preparations. Tolerance seems to be partial rather than absolute and it can disappear quickly after a period of abstinence from nitrate use (37).

*Mechanism of Nitrate Tolerance.* The precise mechanism responsible for nitrate tolerance is not known. Tolerance to the vascular effects of nitrates might be related to oxidation or depletion of sulfhydryl groups, which can result in reduced production of cGMP with no further effect on calcium transport across the cell and consequent loss of ability to relax the vessel wall (39). Other potential mechanisms have been postulated, including reflex activation of neurohumoral factors with enhanced vasoconstriction or sodium retention (or both) associated with probable expansion of the plasma volume (40, 41). Although none of these theories has been fully studied, it is possible that a combination of these mechanisms might play a role in development of nitrate tolerance (37, 42).

*How to Avoid Nitrate Tolerance.* The most effective way to prevent nitrate tolerance is to provide dosage schedules that will result in peaks and valleys of plasma nitrate levels. This can be achieved by providing nitrates for only some portion of the 24-hour schedule and having nitrate-free intervals in between the dosing intervals (37–42). It has been suggested that a nitrate-free period of at least 8 hours or more is required to maintain responsiveness to nitrates (43). Use of sulfhydryl donor *N*-acetylcysteine in large doses has been found to reverse nitrate tolerance (44). This approach, however, does not appear to be a practical one in the management of nitrate tolerance. The use of angiotensin-converting enzyme inhibitors (captopril, a sulfur-containing compound, and enalapril) also has been proposed to avoid nitrate tolerance; however, the initial studies have shown mixed results, and this treatment needs further evaluation (41, 45).

A potential problem that has been associated with the intermittent administration of nitrates is the risk for rebound or breakthrough phenomenon during which a patient might experience increased frequency of angina, particularly at night, during the prolonged nitrate-free interval (26, 32). This does not seem to present a significant clinical problem, however, partly because only a few patients receive nitrates as their sole antianginal therapy. Most patients receive other longer-acting antianginal drugs in addition to nitrates. Although the rebound phenomena has not been fully studied and its clinical significance is not fully established, it should be considered a potential explanation in a patient on nitrates who complains of recurrence of angina during nitrate-free periods (46).

Because steady use of nitrates is associated with rapid development of tolerance, these drugs can be provided only for some hours every day. It is, therefore, essential to customize therapy with these agents according to the individual patient's needs. Sublingual nitroglycerin is clearly effective in relieving acute anginal attacks and is suitable when angina occurs on an infrequent basis. For prophylactic use of nitrates during a longer period, the patient could be instructed to take isosorbide dinitrate, 20 to 30 mg, two or three times daily using an "eccentric" dosing schedule according to need. Isosorbide dinitrate can be prescribed at 8 am and 12 noon, or at 8 am, 12 noon, and at 5 pm. Alternatively, the patient could use transdermal nitroglycerin patches during the day and remove them before going to bed (with an emphasis on leaving at least a 12-hour patch-free interval at night to help restore vascular responsiveness). For patients who experience angina in the early morning hours, it is necessary to consider using agents with longer antianginal activity such as β-blockers or one of the calcium channel antagonists.

In general, nitrates are safe drugs at the recommended therapeutic doses. The most common side effect is the development of headache that on occasion can be severe. Although, in most cases, the headache disappears over time, when needed over-the-counter analgesic agents can be useful in relieving headaches. Another potentially serious side effect is the rare occurrence of hypotension and inappropriate bradycardia (usually with sublingual nitrates) with resultant presyncope or syncope. These reactions can be reversed by assumption of the supine position and elevation of the legs. Atropine can also reverse this reaction, which seems to be triggered by excessive parasympathomimetic (vagal) activity.

### β-*Adrenergic Blockers*

β-Blockers have established an important role in the management of patients with CAD. β-Blockers exert their antianginal effect primarily by decreasing myocardial oxygen demand (Table 4.2). The antiischemic actions include reduction in heart rate at rest, attenuation of the degree of heart rate increment during exercise, decreased blood pressure, and reduced force of contraction. Other effects, such as prolongation of the diastolic phase of the cardiac cycle, might also help improve myocardial oxygen supply by improving coronary flow to the ischemic regions. β-Blockers work largely by binding to specific receptors in cardiac muscle (particularly $\beta_1$ receptors); in doing so they competitively inhibit the binding of catecholamines with resultant attenuated cardiac response to sympathetic stimulation. Through their negative inotropic effect, β-blockers may increase left ventricular (LV) volume, LV end-diastolic pressure, and increased pulmonary capillary pressure. This may cause the patient to experience dyspnea and limit functional capacity. In patients with evidence of LV dysfunction there is a risk that these agents may precipitate LV decompensation, leading to development of congestive heart failure (CHF). Some recent data, however, indicate that even in patients with CHF and ischemic heart disease, β-blockers are beneficial and improve LV performance (see also Chapters 11 and 13).

In patients with stable CAD, β-blockers have proved to be important therapeutic agents as monotherapy as well as adjunctive therapy to nitrates (47). These β-blockers are particularly useful in the treatment of exertional angina. Because of their negative inotropic and chronotropic actions, β-blockers attenuate the increase in myocardial oxygen demand secondary to increased catecholamine levels associated with physical exertion or emotional stress. β-Blockers are the drugs of choice for patients with chronic exertional angina.

**Cardioselective Versus Nonselective β-Blockers.** Cardioselective β-blockers ($\beta_1$ receptor blockers) are preferred over agents that are nonselective and that possess $\beta_2$ receptor blocking activity. Because stimulation of $\beta_2$ receptors is associated with arterial vasodilation, blockade of $\beta_2$ receptors might be associated with risk of developing generalized and especially focal coronary vasoconstriction due to unopposed α vasoconstrictor activity in the areas of coronary atheroma (48). There is some clinical evidence to indicate that this is a relatively frequent problem during treatment with noncardioselective β-blockers. The addition of a nitrate or a calcium channel blocker can counteract the vasoconstrictive influence of nonselective β-blockade (49). Stimulation of $\beta_2$ receptors is also associated with relaxation of bronchial smooth muscle and when $\beta_2$ receptors are blocked by nonselective β-blockers, there is a risk of triggering bronchoconstriction and wheezing. This is especially a problem in patients with bronchial asthma or chronic obstructive pulmonary disease, and in such patients use of cardioselective β-blockers is preferred. It should, however, be noted that at progressively higher doses the cardioselective β-blockers also begin to loose $\beta_1$ selective action because of a greater degree of binding to $\beta_2$ receptors.

**Contraindications for β-Blocker Use.** β-Blockers have several side effects that limit their clinical usefulness. The clinician should be cautious when using β-blockers in patients with persistent bradyarrhythmias, atrioventricular conduction abnormalities, or clinical congestive heart failure, although they are not absolutely contraindicated in these conditions. Other relative contraindications to the use of β-blockers include the presence of reactive airway disease, peripheral arterial insufficiency, and brittle diabetes mellitus (patients who have had hypoglycemic episodes).

**Other Practical Considerations when Using β-Blockers.** β-Blockers have different properties such as water or lipid solubility and mild intrinsic ability to stimulate the β-receptors (partial intrinsic sympathomimetic activity) (Table 4.4). The water soluble β-blockers such as nadolol and atenolol appear to be less prone to cross the blood-brain barrier. This translates into a lower incidence of central nervous system side effects such as depression and generalized fatigue. These are fairly uncommon side effects and should be noted, especially in elderly patients using β-blockers. β-Blockers with α-adrenergic blocking activity may be useful in CAD patients with angina who suffer from claudication in the extremities, hypertension, or both.

**Table 4.4**
**Comparative Doses and Actions of Commonly Used β-Blockers**

| | Dose/Day (mg) | Cardioselectivity | ISA | Lipidsoluble | Plasma half-life (h) | Elimination Route | CNS Effects | I.V. Route | Safety in Diabetes | Safety in PVD |
|---|---|---|---|---|---|---|---|---|---|---|
| Propranolol | 160–480 | – | – | ++++ | 3–6 | hepatic | +++ | + | poor | poor |
| Metoprolol | 100–200 | + | – | ++ | 3–4 | hepatic | + | + | good | good |
| Atenolol | 50–200 | + | – | + | 6–9 | renal | +, – | – | good | good |
| Nadolol | 40–320 | – | – | + | 12–24 | renal | –, + | – | poor | poor |
| Timolol | 20–40 | – | –, + | +, ++ | 3–5 | hepatic | ++ | – | poor | poor |
| Pindolol | 20–40 | – | +++ | ++ | 8 | renal | ++ | – | poor | poor |
| Labetalol | 200–800 | –, also $\alpha_1$ | + | + | 6–8 | hepatic | –, + | – | poor | poor |
| Betaxolol | 10–20 | + | – | + | 14–22 | renal | + | – | good | good |

$\alpha_1$ = alpha-adrenergic receptor blocker; CNS = central nervous system; h = hours; ISA = intrinsic sympathomimetic activity; I.V. = intravenous; mg = milligrams; PVD = peripheral vascular disease; – = not present; + = present.

After the decision has been made to initiate treatment with a β-blocker, the choice of specific agent will depend on factors such as other medical conditions coexistent in a particular patient, the potential side effects, the duration of action of the drug, and the need for cardioselectivity. It is prudent to initiate treatment with a low dose and progressively increase the dose while monitoring for adverse reactions. The maintenance dose of β-blocker should be titrated to achieve the desired therapeutic effects. Evaluation for adequacy of dosage can be made by assessment during exercise stress testing by monitoring the heart rate and blood pressure responses. After treatment with a β-blocker has been initiated, ideal therapeutic goals should include a reduction in frequency or suppression of anginal attacks, a relative attenuation of heart rate response during exercise (to less than a 50% increment above the resting heart rate), resting heart rate of 50 to 60 beats/minute, attenuation of blood pressure response during exercise, and absence of serious intolerable adverse reactions.

**β-Blocker Withdrawal Phenomenon.** A significant potential problem in patients with CAD who are receiving treatment with a β-blocker is the risk of developing withdrawal symptoms after abrupt discontinuation of the drug. During treatment with β-blockers there is an upward regulation in β-receptors associated with an increase in the density, affinity, and sensitivity of β-receptors. Whenever β-blocker therapy is stopped, β-receptors are down-regulated; however, this process takes a lot longer than up-regulation. Because down-regulation is slower, if β-blocker therapy is abruptly withdrawn, the β-receptors have a heightened response to stimulation by catecholamines, resulting in excessive increases in heart rate and blood pressure (50). Some of the manifestations of acute β-blocker withdrawal in patients with CAD include exacerbation of angina, frequent ventricular ectopy, and risk of developing acute myocardial infarction and sudden death (51, 52). Any condition associated with increased sympathetic activity can potentiate the occurrence of β-blocker withdrawal. Some of the common reasons for β-blocker withdrawal are patient noncompliance, running out of medication, and often preoperative and postoperative status.

### *Calcium Channel Blockers*

Calcium channel blockers are a heterogeneous group of drugs that produce a relative restriction of calcium influx into the cell through calcium channels. The depletion of intracellular calcium leads to a variety of hemodynamic and electrophysiologic effects in the cardiovascular system (Table 4.2). Each drug binds to specific chemical subunit or receptors at different locations in the interior of the calcium channel (53). It has been suggested that because various calcium channel blockers bind to different sites or types of calcium channel, synergistic action could occur when two or more different calcium channel blockers are used in the same patient.

Calcium channel blockers produce significant vasodilation at the level of coronary and systemic arterial beds, decrease myocardial contractility, and depress the automaticity and conduction of the sinoatrial and atrioventricular nodes. Their net actions are, however, influenced by the reflex activation of sympathetic activity (Table 4.5). This is especially true for the dihydropyridine class of calcium channel blockers, such as nifedipine. Nifedipine exerts a very potent vasodilator action in the systemic circulation that triggers a pronounced baroreceptor stimulation and also results in reflex increases in catecholamine levels. This heightened sympathetic activity causes an increase in heart rate and enhanced conduction through the atrioventricular node. The ultimate effect on the heart depends on the complex interaction between the direct effects and the indirect effects through reflex sympathetic stimulation. The mode of administration could also affect the hemodynamic effects of each drug on the heart. For example, intravenous administration of verapamil will produce more pronounced hypotension or cardiac failure than oral administration. On the other hand, the pronounced positive chronotropic effect of nifedipine secondary to reflex stimulation by catecholamines could increase myocardial oxygen demand and may trigger an episode of myocardial ischemia.

Calcium channel blockers decrease myocardial oxygen demand by afterload reduction and a decrease in myocardial contractility. They seem to be the most potent coronary vasodilators currently available for clinical use. Calcium channel blockers are highly effective in attenuating coronary spasm at the site of coronary atheroma (54). These drugs also improve collateral blood flow and have the potential for increasing or redistributing blood flow to the ischemic myocardium (55, 56). These properties make the agents quite useful in the treatment of patients with stable CAD, particularly patients with Prinzmetal's angina. All calcium channel blockers seem to have a negative inotropic action that could be of clinical concern in the treatment of patients with depressed LV function. In the animal model only verapamil has been found to diminish the inotropic response that occurs during exercise. Conversely, recent studies have shown that certain calcium channel blockers (e.g., amlodipine or felodipine) have the potential for improving LV function in patients with CHF (57). In addition, calcium channel blockers can improve diastolic dysfunction, which is often present in patients with advanced CAD, particularly the elderly (58).

Recently, significant concern has been expressed about the use of short-acting calcium channel blockers in patients with hypertension and ischemic heart disease (59, 60). This is largely due to the finding of increased risk of myocardial infarction in patients treated with short-acting drugs such as nifedipine (59). It should, however, be noted that this risk has not at this time been demonstrated with use of newer long-acting calcium channel blockers (e.g., amlodipine or felodipine).

In summary, calcium channel blockers are highly effective antianginal

**Table 4.5**
**Comparison of Cardiovascular Actions of Calcium Channel Blockers**

| | Nifedipine | Diltiazem | Verapamil | Amlodipine | Nifedipine GITS | Diltiazem CD |
|---|---|---|---|---|---|---|
| Heart rate | ↑↑ | ↓,↔ | ↔, ↓ | ↔ | ↔, ↑ | ↓ |
| Systemic resistance | ↑↑↑↑ | ↑↑ | ↓↓↓ | ↓ | ↓ | ↓ |
| Coronary resistance | ↓↓↓↓ | ↓↓ | ↓↓ | ↓↓ | ↓↓↓ | ↓ |
| Cardiac preload | ↓ | ↓, ↔ | ↓, ↔ | ↓ | ↓ | ↓,↔ |
| Cardiac output | ↑↑ | ↑ or ↔ | ↑ or ↓ | ↑ | ↑ | ↔ |
| AV nodal conduction | ↔ | ↓ | ↓↓ | ↔ | ↔ | ↓ |
| Onset of action (min) | 20 | 15 | 30 | 60–360 | 20–60 | 120 |
| Plasma half-life (h) | 1.5–5 | 2–6 | 3–7 | 30–50 | 2 | 5–8 |
| Elimination route | renal | hepatic | renal | hepatic | renal | hepatic |
| Dose/day (mg) | 30–120 | 120–480 | 240–480 | 5–10 | 30–90 | 120–360 |

AV = atrioventricular; CD = controlled delivery; GITS = gastrointestinal therapeutic system; h = hour; mg = milligram; min = minutes; ↑ = increased; ↓ = decreased; ↔ = no predominant effect.

drugs that can be used safely in patients with reactive airways, peripheral arterial insufficiency, and diabetes mellitus. If a patient does not respond to one calcium channel blocker, there may be adequate response to another calcium channel blocker that blocks a different calcium channel.

*Combination Therapy*

Many patients with severe CAD do not respond to therapy with a single antianginal drug. In some, the highest possible dose of a given agent may not be well tolerated (e.g., β-blocker). The use of two or more antianginal drugs in combination can allow for management with lower doses of each agent, which will help reduce adverse effects and improve compliance. Also, because of the synergistic effect, combination therapy could be more effective in suppressing anginal episodes than either agent given alone. The superiority of combination therapy results from differing hemodynamic actions and synergistic effects on coronary blood flow of the different antianginal drugs to be combined to achieve a more effective control of symptoms (61). An appropriate combination should cancel the undesirable actions and prevent any increase in myocardial oxygen demand. A typical combination would be use of a nitrate preparation with a nitrate-free period of 10–12 hours and a long-acting β-blocker. Another possibility would be a calcium channel blocker such as diltiazem or verapamil and a nitrate, or a β-blocker and a calcium channel blocker such as nifedipine. When making a decision to use combination therapy for treatment of angina, the physician should ideally evaluate the cardiac actions of each agent being considered and establish that the effects of the drugs to be used will complement each other. Also, in the evaluation of combination therapy for a particular patient, other associated medical conditions should be considered. A large number of studies have evaluated a variety of combination treatments and indicate that combination therapy is more effective than any monotherapy. However, because of the added expenditure of drugs and increased risk of adverse experiences with combination therapy, such treatment strategy should be utilized only when treatment with a single agent is not effective in controlling anginal symptoms or ischemic manifestations.

## Efficacy of Antianginal Therapy for Reducing Total Ischemic Burden

Recent evidence from several studies in patients with stable angina and CAD indicate that, despite control of symptoms, most patients continue to manifest evidence of myocardial ischemia during daily life. Furthermore, findings from these studies indicate that clinical outcome in patients with CAD seems to be linked primarily to the presence of transient myocardial ischemia and, to a lesser degree, to the frequency and severity of angina. These results have encouraged clinicians to consider more aggressive anti-ischemic therapy that is effective in controlling total ischemic burden (i.e., angina as well as silent ischemia). Although it seems prudent, little hard evidence is available to support such a therapeutic approach.

Several recent studies have evaluated the antiischemic effects of antianginal drugs given as monotherapy or as combination therapy during prolonged ambulatory Holter monitoring in patients with stable CAD (61–63). Most of these studies have reported positive results characterized by significant reductions in the frequency and duration of transient myocardial ischemia during active treatment phases, especially with β-blocker therapy. Despite control of angina, however, none of these studies achieved complete suppression of ischemia. In each of these studies there were patients who continued to have ischemic episodes during the monitoring period while receiving active treatment. Before such an approach and enthusiasm for total suppression of ischemia can be supported, it would be important to demonstrate that total suppression of ischemia is essential for improving the adverse prognosis associated with presence of silent ischemia. Based on the available data, it appears reasonable to suggest that Holter monitoring for ischemia would be most useful to identify the high-risk subset of patients with established CAD, especially when they are to be treated medically. Holter monitoring does not appear to be needed for ischemia in patients who fail to demonstrate inducible ischemia during a treadmill exercise test.

## SELECTION OF ANTIANGINAL DRUGS BASED ON CLINICAL PICTURE AND ASSOCIATED CONDITIONS

The selection of the best treatment for patients with angina pectoris varies depending on the clinical picture. In general, most patients with stable angina can be successfully treated initially with medical therapy. The goals of therapy (Table 4.1) are not only relief of symptoms and, as such, the selection of appropriate antianginal drugs should also take into account the goal of reducing the risk of coronary events and improving survival. Because many patients with angina pectoris also have other concomitant cardiac conditions, the selection of antianginal drugs also varies accordingly. Table 4.6 summarizes our recommendations for selection of antianginal drugs in a variety of common clinical settings.

### Chronic Exertional Angina

For patients with chronic exertional angina, nitrates are still considered the initial therapy of choice. Most patients with stable angina respond to treatment with various forms of nitrates. As mentioned, nitrates are available in sublingual, oral, buccal, ointment, and sustained-release forms (Table 4.3). Most of these forms have been found to relieve symptoms and increase exercise endurance in patients with chronic exertional angina. Nitrates are usually well tolerated and are comparatively inexpensive. In pa-

**Table 4.6**
**Suggested Antianginal Drug Choices in Patients with Stable Angina and Comorbid Conditions**

| | Initial Drug | Second Drug | Third Drug |
|---|---|---|---|
| Chronic exertional or effort angina (infrequent) | Nitrate | β-blocker | $Ca^{++}$ blocker |
| Chronic exertional or effort angina (frequent) | β-blocker | Nitrate | $CA^{++}$ blocker |
| Angina at rest or nocturnal | $Ca^{++}$ blocker | Nitrate | β-blocker (cardioselective) |
| History of prior MI | β-blocker | Nitrate | $Ca^{++}$ blocker |
| Bradyarrhythmias or AV blocks | Nitrate | $Ca^{++}$ blocker (N, A) | |
| Supraventricular tachyarrhythmias | β-blocker | $Ca^{++}$ blocker (D, V) | Nitrate |
| Congestive heart failure | Nitrate | $Ca^{++}$ blocker (A) | β-blocker (cardioselective) |
| Hypertrophic cardiomyopathy (IHSS) | β-blocker | $Ca^{++}$ blocker (D, V) | |
| Peripheral vascular disease | $Ca^{++}$ blocker | Nitrate | β-blocker (cardioselective) |
| Chronic renal failure | Nitrate | $Ca^{++}$ blocker (D)[a] | β-blocker[a] (cardioselective) |
| IDDM | Nitrate | $Ca^{++}$ blocker | β-blocker (cardioselective)[b] |
| COPD | Nitrate | $Ca^{++}$ blocker | β-blocker (cardioselective)[b] |

[a]Hepatic metabolism.
[b]In small doses.
A = amlodipine; AV = atrioventricular; $Ca^{++}$ = calcium channel; COPD = chronic obstructive pulmonary disease; D = diltiazem; IDDM = insulin dependent diabetes mellitus; IHSS = idiopathic hypertrophic subaortic stenosis; ISA = intrinsic sympathomimetic activity; MI = myocardial infarction; N = nifedipine; V = verapamil.

tients with mixed angina, calcium blockers are a suitable initial choice, since coronary vasospasm may play an important role in their disease.

If a nitrate given in the maximum tolerated dose is not sufficient to achieve the therapeutic goal, the clinician should add another antianginal drug. A β-blocker is a good addition to a nitrate, as discussed in the section on combination therapy. If β-blockers are not tolerated or are contraindicated, a calcium blocker can be added to the treatment regimen. Most patients with chronic stable angina respond to treatment with an appropriately selected combination of drugs.

Except for patients with left main coronary artery disease or three-vessel disease with LV dysfunction, coronary artery bypass grafting should be considered only when medical therapy with the appropriate combination given in the maximum tolerated dose has failed. Percutaneous transluminal coronary angioplasty may be suitable for patients with ideal anatomic lesions and severe symptoms.

## Vasospastic and Prinzmetal's Angina

Many patients have a history that clearly indicates coronary vasospasm to be the predominant mechanism responsible for their anginal symptoms. As shown in Table 4.2, calcium blockers are by far the most potent coronary vasodilatory agents and should be considered first-line therapy in these patients. Several studies have shown the clinical efficacy of these agents in such patients, even when nitrates and β-blockers failed to control symptoms. All calcium blockers are effective in treatment of such patients, and selection of a specific compound should be based on the patient's clinical features. For example, verapamil is contraindicated in patients with bradycardia, atrioventricular block, or heart failure, whereas nifedipine has been found to be safe in these patients.

If a calcium blocker cannot be used, a nitrate is a suitable alternative. Large doses of nitrates are usually needed, however, and some patients still may not respond. A cardioselective β-blocker should be used only when symptoms continue despite treatment with a calcium blocker and a nitrate or exercise-induced symptoms are present. Coronary artery revascularization usually does not provide therapeutic benefit to patients with vasospasm who do not have a significant fixed lesion.

## Treatment of Angina with Associated Illness

### *Congestive Heart Failure*

β-Blockers and the calcium blocker verapamil are contraindicated in patients with congestive heart failure. However, if the patient is already taking a β-blocker, it should not be abruptly discontinued, to avoid precipitating unstable angina or acute myocardial infarction. Instead, the dosage of the β-blocker should be gradually tapered under close monitoring to avoid β-blocker withdrawal phenomenon. It is likely that with the introduction of new β-blockers (e.g., carvedilol and bucindolol, which are currently investigational) that are safe and even beneficial in patients with CHF, the clinician will have a selection of β-blockers that can be used in patients with heart failure.

Nitrates are usually considered the most suitable first-line agents, since they also help in treatment of CHF. Nitrates reduce venous return to the heart and decrease LV volume and end-diastolic pressure. The calcium blockers amlodipine and felodipine appear to be safe and suitable alternatives, since they are vasoselective and have been shown to improve LV function also. Unlike verapamil, amlodipine and felodipine have no negative inotropic effects clinically.

### *Systemic Hypertension*

β-Blockers and calcium blockers appear to be effective for patients with systemic hypertension and angina. Control of hypertension improves anginal discomfort considerably. A cardioselective β-blocker should be considered when a vasospastic component is suspected. If the patient is elderly, a water-soluble β-blocker, such as nadolol or atenolol, produces fewer central nervous system side effects and is therefore better tolerated. A calcium blocker might be an even more appropriate choice because these agents are better tolerated by elderly patients than are β-blockers.

### *Recent Acute Myocardial Infarction*

The incidence of sudden death after acute myocardial infarction has been shown to be reduced with use of either selective or nonselective β-blockers. Thus, treatment with a β-blocker is most suitable for patients with a history of recent myocardial infarction. However, if LV dysfunction is present in such patients, β-blockers can cause further decompensation and decrease cardiac output, although some recent studies suggest that β-blockers might be safe and even effective in patients with CHF. The addition of a nitrate or calcium blocker (with heart rate reducing effect) may be beneficial in some patients; however, calcium channel blockers are also contraindicated in patients with left ventricular dysfunction.

### *Hypertrophic Obstructive Cardiomyopathy*

β-Blockers and calcium blockers are effective in decreasing the subvalvular gradient present in this clinical condition. Both classes of agents achieve this hemodynamic effect through negative inotropic action. Nitrates and strenuous physical activity, on the other hand, might worsen the subvalvular obstructive gradient and lead to aggravation of anginal symptoms.

### *Bradyarrhythmia and Atrioventricular Block*

Patients with high-grade atrioventricular conduction abnormalities or sick sinus syndrome should be treated initially with a nitrate or dihydropyridine calcium blocker (nifedipine, amlodipine, or nicardipine) since these agents have negligible adverse electrophysiologic effects on sinoatrial automaticity or atrioventricular conduction velocity. β-Blockers and the calcium blockers verapamil and diltiazem are relatively contraindicated.

### *Supraventricular Tachyarrhythmia*

If no congestive heart failure or other underlying pathologic condition that might cause supraventricular tachyarrhythmia is present, a trial of a β-blocker or either of the calcium blockers verapamil or diltiazem is appropriate. These agents adequately control ventricular rate and might even terminate tachyarrhythmia, which if left uncontrolled, can compromise coronary perfusion and worsen myocardial ischemia. Control of ventricular response decreases myocardial oxygen demand and helps relieve symptoms.

### *Chronic Obstructive Pulmonary Disease*

A nitrate or calcium blocker is an appropriate choice in a patient with chronic obstructive pulmonary disease. Calcium blockers might even have a salutary effect in these patients because of their bronchodilating action and because they promote a reduction in pulmonary vascular resistance. In general, use of nonselective β-blockers is considered hazardous in patients with chronic obstructive pulmonary disease, because these compounds might trigger bronchospastic episodes that may lead to worsening of ventilatory insufficiency. When used in high doses, even the cardioselective β-blockers may induce bronchoconstriction in patients with chronic airway disorders.

### *Diabetes Mellitus*

In insulin-dependent diabetic patients, β-blockers may mask symptoms of hypoglycemia and allow prolonged hypoglycemic episodes by inhibiting glycogenolysis. These problems might not be clinically important in the patient whose diabetes is controlled with dietary measures alone. Neither nitrates nor calcium blockers interfere with hypoglycemic symptoms, and they do not cause any alteration in glucose tolerance. Therefore, these are more appropriate options in treatment of anginal symptoms in insulin-dependent patients. If a β-blocker must be used, a low-dose cardioselective agent is preferable, and the patient should be educated and followed carefully and frequently for evidence of hypoglycemic episodes.

### *Renal Failure*

Since nitrates are primarily metabolized by the liver, they are fairly safe in patients with renal failure. The calcium channel blocker diltiazem is metabolized predominantly by the liver and would be safer than nifedipine or verapamil in patients with impaired renal function. Also, as shown in Table 4.4, metoprolol is preferred over atenolol because metoprolol is primarily elminated by the hepatic route.

## SUMMARY

The most appropriate treatment for a patient with angina pectoris depends on the underlying pathophysiologic process and whether other associated illness is present. Each patient's clinical history must be carefully reviewed so that the hemodynamic process responsible for the clinical picture can be ascertained before therapy is prescribed. If symptoms are produced mostly by an increase in myocardial oxygen demand, efforts should be directed toward reducing the demand or improving coronary blood flow to meet the demand, or both. If symptoms appear to occur secondary to vasospasm, treatment should be directed toward relief of spasm with potent vasodilating agents, such as calcium channel blockers. Most patients have a clinical picture consistent with mixed angina and may require combination therapy. Treatment of associated illnesses and the safety of pharmacologic agents used in their presence should also be carefully considered. Finally, it should be noted that if the prescribed treatment is to be successful in reducing the incidence of serious cardiac events and prolonging life, the therapy should be effective in not just relieving anginal symptoms but also reducing the total ischemic burden on the heart.

---

## REFERENCES

1. Gillum R. Trends in acute myocardial infarction and coronary artery disease death in the United States. J Am Coll Cardiol 1993;23:1273–1277.
2. Healthy people 2000: National health promotion and disease prevention objectives. (DHHS publication no. (PHS) 91-50212.) Washington, DC: US Department of Health and Human Services, 1991.
3. Deedwania P, Carbajal E. Silent myocardial ischemia. A clinical perspective. Arch Intern Med 1991;151:2373–2382.
4. Deedwania P, Carbajal E. Prevalence and patterns of silent myocardial ischemia during daily life in stable angina patients receiving conventional antianginal drug therapy. Am J Cardiol 1990;65:1090–1096.
5. Deedwania P, Carbajal E. Silent ischemia during daily life is an independent predictor of mortality in stable angina. Circulation 1990;81:748–756.
6. Yeung A, Barry J, Orav J, et al. Effects of asymptomatic ischemia on long term prognosis in chronic stable coronary disease. Circulation 1991;83:1598–1604.
7. Cohn, P. Silent myocardial ischemia in patients with a defective anginal warning system. Am J. Cardiol 1980;45:697–702.
8. Selwyn A, Yeung A, Ryan T, et al. Pathophysiology of ischemia in patients with coronary artery disease. Prog Cardiovasc Dis 1992;35:27–39.
9. Nabel E, Ganz P, Gordon J, et al. Dilation of normal and constriction of atherosclerotic coronary arteries caused by the cold pressor test. Circulation 1988;77:43–52.
10. Nabel E, Selwyn A, Ganz P. Large coronary arteries in humans are responsive to changing blood flow: an endothelium-dependent mechanism that fails in patients with atherosclerosis. J Am Coll Cardiol 1990;16:349–356.
11. Zeiher A, Drexler H, Wollschlaeger H, et al. Progressive endothelial dysfunction with different early stages of coronary atherosclerosis. Circulation 1991;83:391–401.
12. Heistad D, Armstrong M, Marcus M, et al. Augmented responses to vasoconstrictor stimuli in hypercholesterolemic and atherosclerotic monkeys. Circ Res 1984; 54: 711–718.
13. Vita J. Treasure C, Nabel E, et al. The coronary vasomotor response to acetylcholine relates to risk factors for coronary artery disease. Circulation 1990;81:491–497.
14. Gordon T, Kannel W. Premature mortality from coronary heart disease: the Framingham study. JAMA 1971;215:1617–1625.
15. Pupita G, Maseri A, Kaski J, et al. Myocardial ischemia caused by distal coronary artery constriction in stable angina pectoris. N Engl J Med 1990;323:514–520.

16. Deedwania P, Nelson J. Pathophysiology of silent myocardial ischemia during daily life. Circulation 1990;82:1296–1304.
17. Roussouw JE. The effects of lowering serum cholesterol on coronary heart disease risk. Med Clin North Am 1994;78:181–195.
18. Scandinavian Simvastatin Survival Study Group. Randomized trial of cholesterol lowering in 4444 patients with coronary heart disease: The Scandinavian Simvastatin Survival Study (4S). Lancet 1994;344:1383–1389.
19. Brown G, Albers J, Fisher L, et al. Regression of coronary artery disease as a result of intensive lipid lowering therapy in men with high levels of apolipoprotein B. N Engl J Med 1990;323:1289–1298.
20. Kane J, Malloy M, Ports T, et al. Regression of coronary atherosclerosis during treatment of familial hypercholesterolemia with combined drug regimens. JAMA 1990; 264:3007–3012.
21. Cashin-Hemphill L, Mack W, Pogoda J, et al. Beneficial effects of colestipol-niacin on coronary atherosclerosis. a 4 year follow-up. JAMA 1990;264:3013–3017.
22. Schuler G, Hambrech R, Schlierf G, et al. Regular physical exercise and low-fat diet. Effects on progression of coronary artery disease. Circulation 1992;86:1–11.
23. Gould KL, Ornish D, Scherwitz L, et al. Changes in myocardial perfusion abnormalities by positron emission tomography after long-term, intense risk factor modification. JAMA 1995;274:894–901.
24. Vos J, Feyter P, Simoons M, et al. Retardation and arrest of progression or regression of coronary artery disease. Prog Cardiovasc Dis 1993;35:435–454.
25. Abrams J. New insights into the management of myocardial ischemia. Overview. Am Heart J 1990;120:719–721.
26. Thadani U. Role of nitrates in angina pectoris. Am J Cardiol 1992;70:43B–53B.
27. Mangione N, Glasser S. Phenomenon of nitrate tolerance. Am Heart J 1994;128: 137–145.
28. Goldstein R, Bennet E, Leech G. Effects of glyceryl trinitrate on echocardiographic left ventricular dimensions during exercise in the upright position. Br Heart J 1979;42:245–254.
29. Bassenge E, Stewart K. Effects of nitrates on various vascular sections and regions. Z Kardiol 1986;75(Suppl 3):1–7.
30. Gage J, Jess D, Murakami T, et al. Vasoconstriction of stenotic coronary arteries during dynamic exercise in patients with classic angina pectoris: reversibility by nitroglycerin. Circulation 1986;73:865–871.
31. Diodati J, Theroux P, Latour J, et al. Effects of nitroglycerin at therapeutic doses on platelet aggregation in unstable angina pectoris and acute myocardial infarction. Am J Cardiol 1990;66:683–688.
32. Amsterdam E. Rationale for intermittent nitrate therapy. Am J Cardiol 1992;70: 55G–60G.
33. Thadani U, Fung H, Darke A, et al. Oral isosorbide dinitrate in angina pectoris: comparison of duration of action and dose-response relation during acute and sustained therapy. Am J Cardiol 1982;49:411–416.
34. Crean P, Ribeiro P, Crea F, et al. Failure of transdermal nitroglycerin to improve chronic stable angina: a randomized placebo-controlled, double-blind, double crossover trial. Am Heart J 1984;108:1494–1500.
35. Parker J. Nitrate therapy in stable angina pectoris. N Engl J Med 1987;316: 1635–1642.
36. Flaherty J. Nitrate tolerance. A review of the evidence. Drugs 1989;37:523–550.
37. Elkayam U. Tolerance to organic nitrates: evidence, mechanisms, clinical relevance, and strategies for prevention. Ann Intern Med 1991;114:667–677.
38. Thadani U, Whitsett T, Hamilton S. Nitrate therapy for myocardial ischemic syndrome: current perspectives including tolerance. Curr Probl Cardiol 1988; 13: 731–784.
39. Needleman P, Johnson E. Mechanism of tolerance development to organic nitrates. J Pharmacol Exp Ther 1973;184:709–715.
40. Parker JD, Farrell B, Fenton T, et al. Counter-regulatory responses to continuous and intermittent therapy with nitroglycerin. Circulation 1991;84:2336–2345.
41. Parker JD, Parker JO. Effect of therapy with an angiotensin converting enzyme in-

hibitor on hemodynamic and counterregulatory responses during continuous therapy with nitroglycerin. J Am Coll Cardiol 1993;21:1445–1453.
42. Parker JO, Farrel B, Lahey KA, et al. Effect of intervals between doses on the development of tolerance to isosorbide dinitrate. N Engl J Med 1987;316:1440–1444.
43. Gumbrielle T, Freedman S, Fogarty L, et al. Efficacy, safety and duration of nitrate-free interval to prevent tolerance to transdermal nitroglycerin in effort angina. Eur Heart J 1992;13:671–678.
44. Torresi J, Horowitz J, Dusting G. Prevention and reversal of tolerance to nitroglycerin with N-acetylcysteine. J Cardiovasc Pharmacol 1985;7:777–783.
45. Dakak N, Makhoul N, Flugelman M, et al. Failure of captopril to prevent nitrate tolerance in congestive heart failure secondary to coronary artery disease. Am J Cardiol 1990;66:608–613.
46. DeMots H, Glasser S. Intermittent transdermal nitroglycerin therapy in the treatment of chronic stable angina. J Am Coll Cardiol 1989;13:786–795.
47. Prichard B. Beta-adrenoreceptor blocking drugs in angina pectoris. In: Avery GX, ed. Cardiovascular drugs. Vol 2: Beta-adrenoreceptor blocking drugs. Baltimore: University Park Press, 1978: 85–118.
48. Kern J, Ganz P, Horowitz J, et al. Potentiation of coronary vasoconstriction by beta-adrenergic blockade in patients with coronary artery disease. Circulation 1983;67: 1178–1185.
49. Prida X, Feldman R, Hill J, et al. Comparison of selective (beta 1) and nonselective (beta 1 and beta 2) beta-adrenergic blockade on systemic and coronary hemodynamic findings in angina pectoris. Am J Cardiol 1987;60:244–248.
50. Nattel S, Rangno R, Loon G. Mechanism of propranolol withdrawal phenomena. Circulation 1979;599:1158–1164.
51. Alderman E, Coltart K, Wettach G, et al. Coronary artery syndromes after sudden propranolol withdrawal. Ann Intern Med 1974;81:625–627.
52. Miller R, Olson H, Amsterdam E, et al. Propranolol withdrawal rebound phenomenon: exacerbation of coronary events after abrupt cessation of antianginal therapy. N Engl J Med 1975;293:416–418.
53. Glossmann H, Ferry D, Goll A, et al. Molecular pharmacology of the calcium channel: evidence for subtypes, multiple drug-receptor sites, and channel subunits. J Cardiovasc Pharmacol 1984;6(Suppl 4):S608–S621.
54. Hossack K, Brown B, Stewart K, et al. Diltiazem induced blockade of sympathetically mediated constriction of normal and diseased coronary arteries: lack of epicardial coronary dilatory effect in humans. Circulation 1984;70:465–471.
55. Matsuzaki M, Gallagher K, Patritti J, et al. Effects of calcium entry blocker (diltiazem) on regional myocardial flow and function during exercise in conscious dogs. Circulation 1984;69:801–814.
56. Backe R, Tockman B. Effect of nitroglycerin and nifedipine on subendocardial perfusion in the presence of a flow limiting coronary stenosis in the awake dog. Circ Res 1982;50:678–687.
57. Reicher-Reiss H, Barasch E. Calcium antagonists in patients with heart failure. A review. Drugs 1991;42:343–364.
58. Bonow R. Effects of calcium channel blocking agents on left ventricular diastolic function in hypertrophic cardiomyopathy and in coronary artery disease. Am J Cardiol 1985;55:172B–178B.
59. Psaty BM, Heckbert SR, Koepsell TD, et al. The risk of myocardial infarction associated with antihypertensive drug therapies. JAMA 1995;274:620–625.
60. Yusuf S. Calcium antagonists in coronary artery disease and hypertension. Time for reevaluation? Circulation 1995;92:1079–1082.
61. Glasser S, Friedman R, Talibi T, et al. Safety and compatibility of betaxolol hydrochloride combined with diltiazem or nifedipine therapy in stable angina pectoris. Am J Cardiol 1994;73:213–218.
62. Hassan E, Davies G. Optimal control of myocardial ischemia: the benefit of a fixed combination of atenolol and nifedipine in patients with chronic stable angina. Br Heart J 1992;68:291–295.
63. Deanfield J, Detry J, Lichtlen P, et al. Amlodipine reduces transient myocardial ischemia in patients with coronary artery disease: double blind circadian anti-ischemia program in Europe (CAPE trial). J Am Coll Cardiol 1994;24:1460–1467.

CHAPTER 5

# Management of Patients with Stable Coronary Disease

Roxana Mehran, MD, and Richard Gorlin, MD

Coronary artery disease is a major cause of morbidity and mortality in the United States as well as in other industrialized countries. In the United States alone it is estimated that atherosclerosis is responsible for more than half of all adult deaths. Coronary artery disease presents clinically in several syndromes ranging from the acute coronary syndromes of myocardial infarction (MI) and unstable angina to chronic stable angina and silent ischemia.

This chapter focuses on pharmacologic treatment of chronic ischemic coronary disease. A brief overview of the pathophysiology of this disease, including the molecular aspects, sets the stage for constructing rational therapeutic regimens. We shall discuss patient management with special attention to the various pharmacologic options but with reference to the role of direct revascularization as well.

Although the picture of angina today may match the original description made by Heberden 200 years ago (1), the past decade has revealed much about this disease. Current research on the pathogenesis of atherosclerosis at the molecular level has brought us closer to understanding this disease.

## PATHOPHYSIOLOGY

### Atherogenesis

Most chronic stable angina results from obstructive atherosclerosis, although clearly, angina can occur in most forms of valvular heart disease, hypertension, some congenital heart disease, and occasionally without clear-cut etiology.

Atheromas have both acute and chronic forms. One of the most puzzling dilemmas in atherogenesis is the conversion of a chronic atheroma to an acute one. Clearly, acute inflammation, cytokines, and a variety of other moieties acting on intimal tissue reach a point at which the physical and biochemical balance in the plaque engenders fissuring, rupture, hemorrhage, and thrombosis. It is most likely in the healing process (with or without transient coronary occlusion or myocardial infarction) that luminal narrowing occurs as a byproduct of reendothelialization over a residual thromboatheroma (Fig. 5.1). Frequent fissuring and healing can even

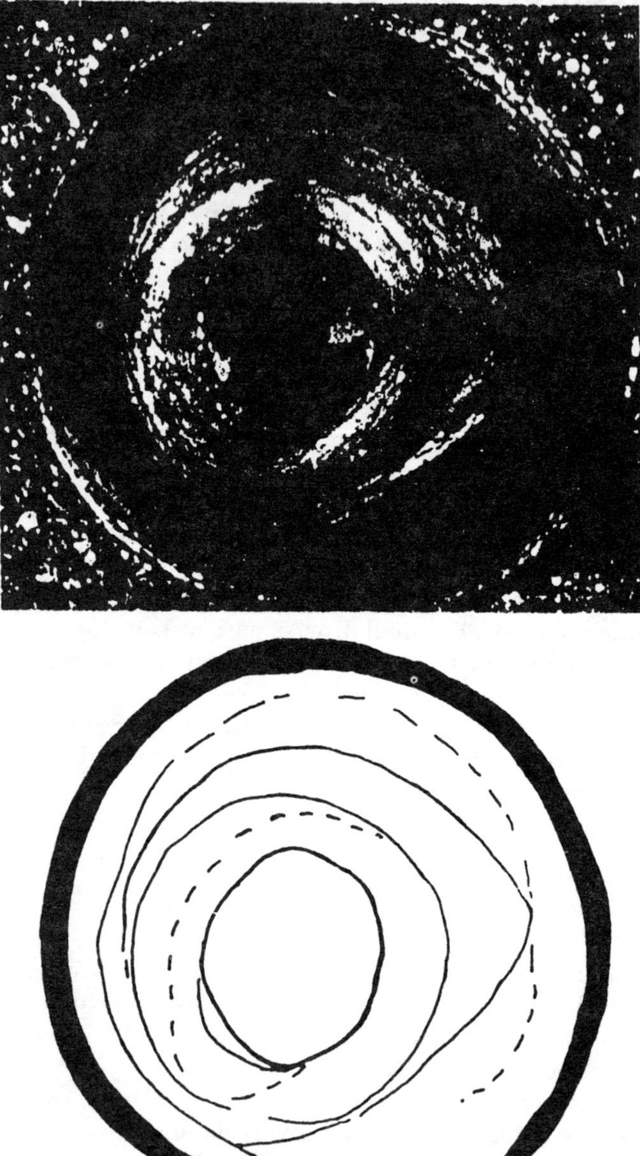

Figure 5.1. Thrombotic occlusion of a coronary artery. *Top,* Micrograph. *Bottom,* Diagram of component layers of lesion. Reproduced with permission from Fulton WFM. The coronary arteries: arteriography, microanatomy and pathogenesis of obliterative coronary artery disease. Springfield, IL: Charles C. Thomas, 1965;242.

give an "onion ring" appearance to the artery, and the resulting coronary stenosis may ultimately be flow limiting.

A stable lesion usually contains fewer macrophages or monocytes, and platelets are not activated in comparison with what is seen with an acute unstable plaque, which does have an inflammatory component.

## Physiology of Myocardial Blood Flow and Metabolism

In order to understand the management of myocardial ischemia and angina pectoris, one must pay special attention to the physiology of myocardial blood flow. Imbalance of myocardial supply and demand has long been recognized as explaining ischemia (Fig. 5.2). Any cardiac demand that outstrips the available oxygen supply leads to ischemia and, potentially, angina, whereas absolute reduction in flow can also deprive even resting myocardium of its energy supply.

### *Increased Energy Demand*

On the demand side of the equation, several factors come into play. These include the major determinants of myocardial work load: blood pressure, heart rate, contractility, and left ventricular cavity size. Control of these factors is well understood as forming a major cornerstone of pharmacotherapy.

### *Inadequate Myocardial Blood Flow*

By contrast, augmentation or even maintenance of blood flow in a diseased heart is less well understood, is critically dependent on appreciation of new knowledge, and forms the other cornerstone of therapy.

### *The Endothelium and Vascular Smooth Muscle*

The myocardium is oxygen dependent and, therefore, eventually flow dependent. Caliber and flow in the coronary vessels are controlled by vas-

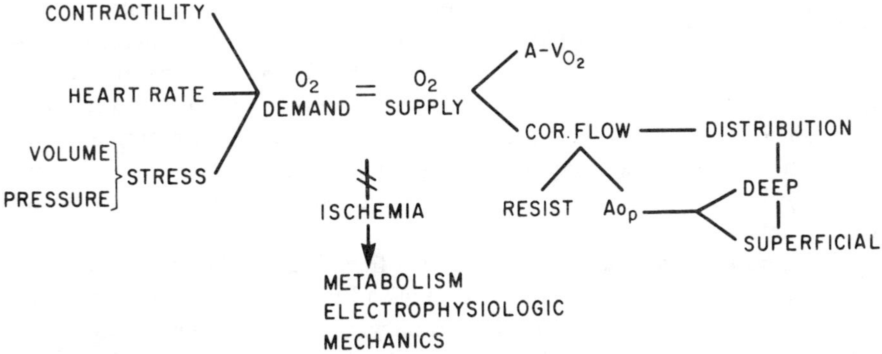

Figure 5.2. Cardiac energy demand-supply system. $Ao_P$ = Aortic pressure. Reproduced with permission from Gorlin R. Physiology of myocardial blood flow and metabolism. In: Gorlin R. Coronary artery disease. Philadelphia: W.B. Saunders, 1976;71.

cular smooth muscle tone. Vascular smooth muscle may be affected by mediators that act directly on vascular smooth muscle in any size vessel and by those that act on the endothelium itself. The endothelium is remarkably active, both in maintaining a nonthrombogenic surface and in elaborating a variety of substances that directly affect vascular smooth muscle. Because a number of stimuli work through the endothelium, they are considered to be endothelium-dependent modulators of coronary flow. An understanding of the actions of these vasoactive substances is crucial in the selection of therapy for patients with atherosclerotic coronary disease. The intact vascular endothelium secretes endothelium-derived relaxing factor, primarily nitric oxide, which is a vasodilator (2). Certain other vasorelaxants also work through the endothelium, such as prostacyclin and serotonin (3). Serotonin acts as a vasodilator through the endothelium (4) but as a vasoconstrictor when acting directly upon vascular smooth muscle (5–7). Endothelin, a novel polypeptide, is a major vasoconstrictor (8).

The endothelium may be dysfunctional, and this may be one of the early stages of atherogenesis. Nabel and coworkers (9) showed that angiographically normal segments of mildly atherosclerotic coronary arteries fail to dilate when exposed to papaverine-induced increased blood flow. Although these vessels were angiographically normal, the patients had atherosclerotic disease, supporting the hypothesis that endothelial dysfunction occurs early in atherosclerosis.

Four major risk factors for atherosclerosis appear to be associated with endothelial dysfunction. These are hypertension (10), diabetes mellitus (11), smoking (12), and hypercholesterolemia (13). Thus, therapy directed at increasing myocardial blood flow capacity must consider control of these risk factors as well as how to offset inappropriate endothelium-dependent control of vascular smooth muscle by pharmacologic means.

## The Obstructed Coronary Artery

Coronary arteries with atherosclerotic obstruction are unable to meet the increased demand for blood flow placed on the heart by increased hemodynamic activity. Resting blood flow is not affected until the luminal diameter is reduced by 90%. During hyperemia in response to demand, however, coronary flow is affected much earlier, at luminal diameters of about 50%. The ratio of peak hyperemic to resting blood flow, or coronary flow reserve, is, in fact, used to characterize coronary stenoses both clinically and experimentally.

The coronary vascular system is a low-flow, high-resistance circulation at rest but during vasodilation it becomes a high-flow, low-resistance one.

Gould (14) has proposed that the coronary circulation is dependent on two resistances: stenosis resistance and vascular bed resistance (Fig. 5.3). Once the stenosis is sufficient to impose the same resistance as the distal vascular bed at full dilatation, further changes in coronary blood flow are determined

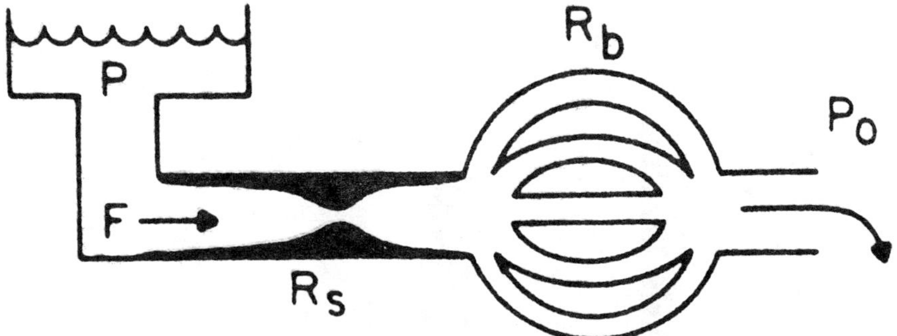


Figure 5.3. Diagrammatic representation of coronary flow as two resistances (R). Coronary flow is determined primarily by $R_b$ if $R_b$ is large compared to $R_s$. $R_s$ has a greater effect on flow as it approaches or exceeds $R_b$. $R_b$ = narrowed tube resistance; $R_s$ = distal vascular bed resistance. Adapted with permission from Gould KL. Quantification of coronary artery stenosis in vivo. Circ Res 1985;57:341–353.

by changes in the caliber of the stenosis. This is why it is important to use therapeutic agents that dilate the large coronary arteries, particularly when there are critical coronary stenoses. Once the demand for increased flow is placed on the system, lesser stenoses of about 60% become physiologically significant because the vasodilator reserve has been exhausted. Pharmacologic dilation of the large vessels is crucial prior to any stimulus for increased flow demand. A "steal" phenomenon results when the small resistance vessels beyond the obstruction are fully dilated because of marginal hypoperfusion. Any stimulus that produces vasodilation elsewhere in the coronary bed may shunt blood away from the potentially ischemic segment (15).

Left ventricular hypertrophy as it occurs in patients with hypertension, aortic stenosis or regurgitation, and hypertrophic cardiomyopathy is another determinant of myocardial oxygen supply and demand. The process of left ventricular hypertrophy elongates the pathway from epicardium to endocardium as well as increases the muscle mass to be perfused by the preexisting capillary network (16; 17).

In chronic stable angina, ischemia involves modulation of coronary blood flow by both the anatomic and functional aspects of the coronary stenosis, the fixed reserve capacity for vascular dilation, and the regulation of microvascular tone.

Contrary to expectations, coronary stenoses exhibit dynamic behavior in patients with chronic angina pectoris. This was first found by Brown and colleagues (18), who demonstrated the effects of sublingual nitroglycerin on moderate and severe coronary stenoses as well as on normal segments (Fig. 5.4). They showed that coronary stenoses thought to be fixed were able to dilate. They later showed that sublingual nitroglycerin produced coronary vasodilation that was most pronounced in the smaller arteries (19). Furthermore, severe stenoses responded more dramatically than lesser ones.

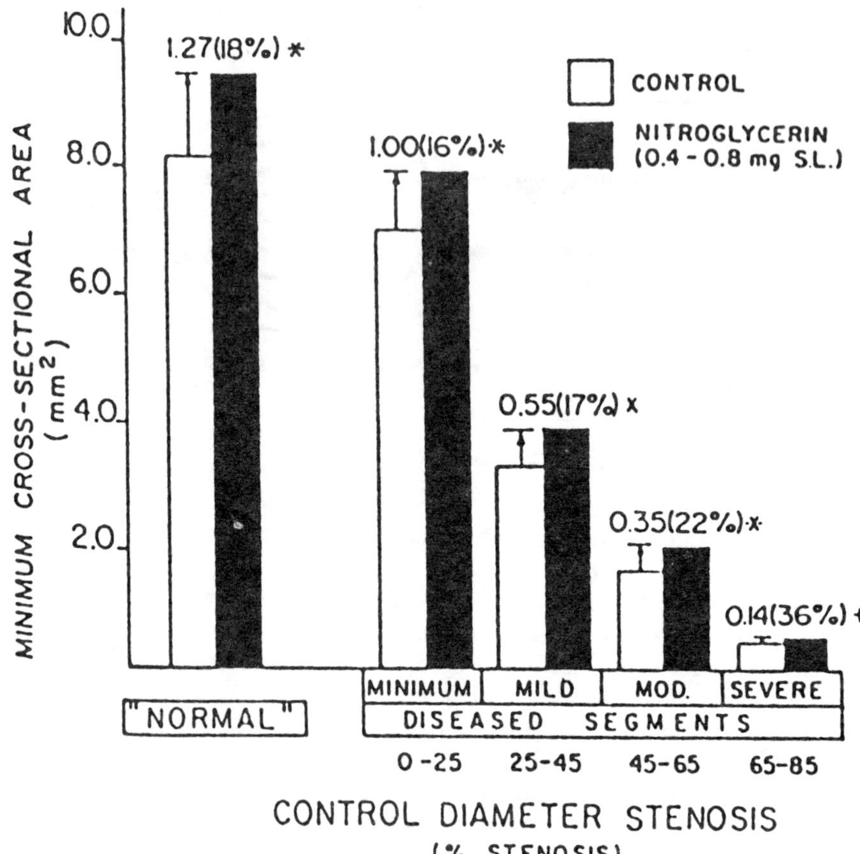


Figure 5.4. The effect of sublingual (S.L.) nitroglycerin on normal and diseased epicardial coronary arteries. Each bar represents the average value of all luminal areas in each of the five groups, either before or after nitroglycerin. Mod = moderate. x = $P < 0.05$; * = $P < 0.01$; + = $P < 0.005$. Reproduced with permission from Brown BG, Bolson E, Peterson RB, et al. The mechanism of nitroglycerine action: stenosis vasodilation as major component of drug response. Circulation 1981;64:1089–1097.

### *Collateral Vessels*

When a fixed coronary obstruction produces a pressure difference between segments of a coronary artery, collateral vessels are recruited from coronary arteries with normal (or at least higher) perfusion pressure. The amount of collateral flow varies from patient to patient according to the number and size of the vessels and seems to be augmented by nitrates (20) and by protracted exercise training (21).

## Extracoronary hemodynamic functions

Myocardial blood flow occurs during left ventricular diastole. When diastole begins, flow accelerates along the course of the epicardial artery. An obstruction in an epicardial artery is hydraulically significant in diastole because rapid inflow to the myocardium occurs during this phase (22).

The left ventricular pressure also influences myocardial blood flow. When left ventricular diastolic pressure is elevated, as in acute left ventricular failure, the diastolic intramyocardial pressures increase and thereby limit myocardial blood flow by narrowing the perforator arteries and by diminishing the trans-myocardial perfusion gradient (Fig. 5.5).

Intramyocardial blood flow is regulated by hydraulic conditions, by the small resistance vessels at the arteriolar level, and, in the presence of disease, by the coronary collateral system. Net coronary perfusion pressure may be compromised in three ways resulting in ischemia: first, through loss of pressure across the coronary stenosis; second, by elevated left ventricular diastolic pressure; and third, through severe impairment of the perfusion pressure time integral including slow diastolic relaxation (Fig.5.5). Thus, many hemodynamic factors can either aid or impair coronary perfusion (22).

In addition, many physiologic mediators may contribute to ischemia in patients with coronary artery disease, including activity of the sympathetic nervous system and vasoactive amines, such as norepinephrine and

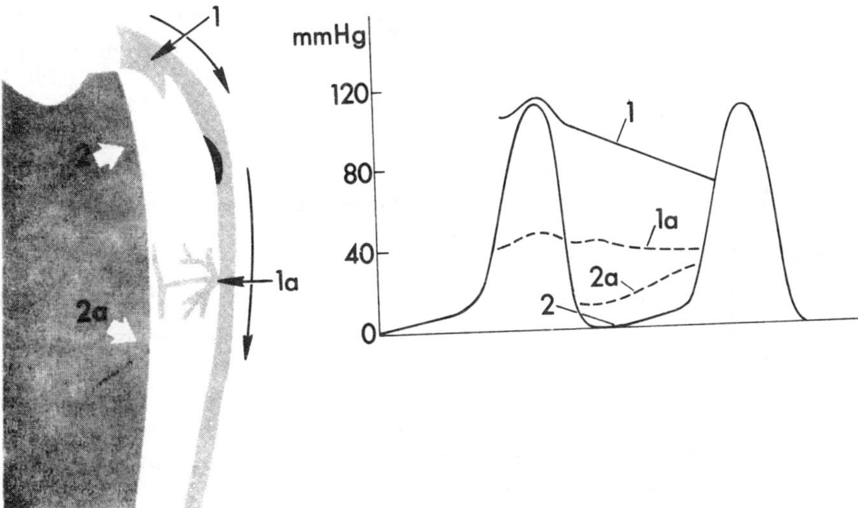


Figure 5.5. Hemodynamic factors influencing perfusion of subendocardial layers of left ventricle. *Left,* Cross-section of left ventricular myocardium with an epicardial coronary artery exhibiting severe proximal obstruction. Branches to the subendocardial region are depicted. 1 = normal coronary artery perfusion pressure. 2 = normal intracavitary diastolic pressure. The difference between 1 and 2 is the net diastolic perfusion pressure under normal conditions. When there is an obstruction beyond point 1, perfusion pressure at 1a is reduced. If, in addition, there is left ventricular failure, then intracavitary pressure (and therefore intramyocardial pressure) during diastole will be correspondingly elevated (2a). Thus, net perfusion pressure will be reduced to the difference between 1a and 2a. Reproduced with permission from Gorlin R. Physiology of myocardial blood flow and metabolism. In: Gorlin R. Coronary artery disease. Philadelphia: W.B. Saunders, 1976.

other catecholamines, serotonin, thromboxane, and endothelin. Finally, anemia, hypoxia, or carbon monoxide retention can adversely affect myocardial oxygenation by reducing oxygen transport per unit of blood flow. This places an additional burden on the coronary flow system by depleting the available vasodilator reserve.

## THERAPY

Both new invasive and pharmacotherapeutic approaches of the past decades have provided increased choices in the decision tree. Evaluation of the patient, as always, is the critical preliminary step in determining selection of therapy. In addition to the coronary disease itself, considerations must include the patient's lifestyle, diet, exercise level, stress, and other comorbid conditions. Thus, a thorough history and physical examination are of utmost importance.

Therapy for chronic stable angina begins with identification of factors, including obesity, smoking, hypertension, diabetes, hypercholesterolemia, anemia, and thyrotoxicosis, that may precipitate or exacerbate myocardial ischemia, either through increasing energy demand or compromising supply. The physician is then faced with the choice of noninvasive and invasive tests, or both, first to make the diagnosis, then to determine if there is any demonstrable ischemia, and finally, to identify patients who would benefit from early revascularization. Additional workup, possibly including imaging to identify stress-induced abnormalities of perfusion or contraction and coronary angiography, or both, allows delineation of the special subset of patients with three-vessel disease and impaired left ventricular function, who require direct revascularization (see below).

### Pharmacotherapy

Once the decision is made to treat the patient medically, the physician must choose the agent or agents with the most therapeutic benefit, fewest side effects, and greatest cost-effectiveness.

The currently available antianginal agents work to modulate either demand or supply, or both (Table 5.1). The ideal agent would, obviously, decrease demand and increase myocardial blood supply without side effects and at a low cost to the patient.

The cornerstone of medical therapy in chronic stable angina is the appropriate use of the three major classes of antianginal drugs: nitrates, β-receptor blockers, and calcium channel antagonists.

#### *Nitrates*

Nitrates have long been the mainstay of therapy for angina pectoris.

**Mechanism of Action.** Nitrates are potent dilators of veins and arteries by releasing nitric oxide during catabolism, but nitrates differ in how they generate nitric oxide. For example, nitroglycerin seems to require a re-

**Table 5.1**
**Physiologic Effects of Medical Therapy for Chronic Stable Angina Pectoris**

| | | Nitrates | β-blockers | Calcium Blockers |
|---|---|---|---|---|
| Oxygen and Coronary Flow Demand | Arterial pressure | ↓ | ↓ | ↓ |
| | Ventricular volume | ↓ | ± | ↓ |
| | Heart rate | ↑ | ↓↓ | ↓ (or ↑) |
| | Inotropy | ± | ↓↓ | ↓ or ± |
| Oxygen and Coronary Flow Supply | Increase coronary diameter/dilate stenosis | ↑↑ | ± | ↑ |
| | Increase collateral flow | ↑ | ± | ? |
| | Prevent/relieve vasoconstriction | ↑↑ | ± | ↑ |
| | Improve transmyocardial gradient | ↑↑ | ↑ | ± or ↓ |

↓ = decreased; ↓↓ = greatly decreased; ↑ = increased; ↑↑ = greatly increased.

duced sulfhydryl group to release nitric oxide (23) whereas nitroprusside does not. Nitrates enter vascular smooth muscle cells and are activated at the plasma membrane. Nitric oxide, or endothelium-derived relaxing factor, through the denitration process, stimulates guanylate cyclase. Guanylate cyclase enhances conversion of guanylate trisphosphate to cyclic guanosine monophosphate (cGMP), which is the key mediator of vascular smooth muscle relaxation (24). cGMP, in turn, precipitates activation of protein kinase, protein phosphorylation, and smooth muscle relaxation.

Nitrates favorably modify both the supply and demand sides of the equation to relieve ischemia. They operate differently in the venous and arterial beds (24). Venodilation causes pooling in the periphery and the splanchnic bed and decreases preload by decreasing ventricular volume and pressure. This, in turn, decreases myocardial mechanical load and oxygen demand. Nitrates also reduce afterload impedance by dilating or relaxing the arterial tree, including the aorta. Both diseased and normal segments of the large epicardial coronary arteries dilate. Dilation of the large arteries, however, increases coronary blood flow only if there are critical stenoses to be dilated. Nitrovasodilators affect the coronary microcirculation to a lesser degree, and only at very high doses.

The effects of nitrates on different sizes of diseased and normal coronary arteries are well demonstrated (18, 25). Gage and colleagues (26) demonstrated consistent dilation in all epicardial coronary arteries, with or without stenosis, with the use of nitrates (Fig. 5.6). During exercise, normal vessels remain essentially unchanged in caliber (and may even dilate), while the diseased vessels constrict. Once nitrates are given, this effect is eliminated, and even the stenotic vessel dilates.

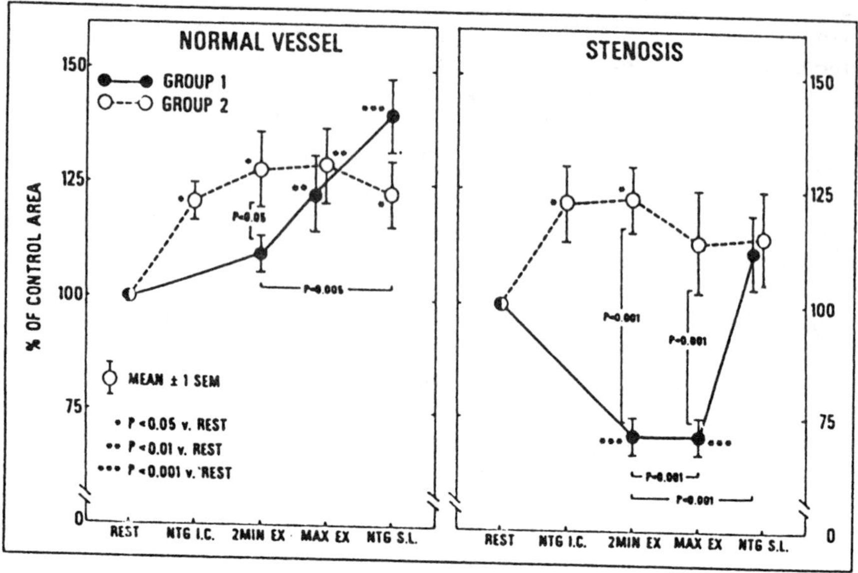


• **Patients exercised to angina, then given NTG SL.**
o **Patients pretreated with NTG IC, then exercised.**

Figure 5.6. Responses to dynamic exercise in patients without (group 1) and with (group 2) pretreatment with intracoronary nitroglycerin, expressed as percentage of resting luminal area. Normal vessels dilated during exercise to 123% of control values, and were further dilated by sublingual nitroglycerin (140%). Intracoronary nitroglycerin induced dilation of normal vessels to 121% of resting values, and dilation persisted at the same level during subsequent exercise (129%). In stenotic vessels, exercise induced a narrowing of stenoses to 71% of control, which dilated to 112% of resting values after sublingual nitroglycerin was given at the end of exercise. Intracoronary nitroglycerin administered to group 2 patients produced dilation of stenosis (122%) that persisted during exercise (114%), thereby preventing the exercise-induced narrowing of stenosis seen in group 1. NTG = nitroglycerin; I.C.= intracoronary; S.L.= sublingual; 2 MIN EX = 2 minutes of supine bicycle exercise; MAX EX = the end of symptom-limited exercise. Reproduced with permission from Gage JE, Hess OM, Muradami T, et al. Vasoconstriction of stenotic coronary arteries during dynamic exercise in patients with classic angina pectoris: reversibility by nitroglycerine. Circulation 1986;73:865–876.

Other emerging concepts in nitrate efficacy include enhanced endothelial function, possible antiplatelet activity, and prevention or reversal of distal coronary bed or collateral constriction (27).

**Nitrovasodilator Agents.** Nitrates may be divided into the short-acting and long-acting preparations (Table 5.2). Sublingual nitroglycerin remains the drug of choice for acute anginal attacks, but its short half-life precludes use for long-term prophylaxis. Many patients benefit from using sublingual nitroglycerin prior to engaging in activities that precipitate chest pain, and this prophylactic use must be emphasized to the patient.

Transdermal patches are useful in some patients, although variable absorption at different skin sites and development of tolerance with contin-

**Table 5.2**
**Nitrate Therapy for Chronic Stable Angina Pectoris**

| | Route | Dosage | Duration of Action |
|---|---|---|---|
| Nitroglycerin | S.I. tablets<br><br>Transmucosal tablets<br>2% ointment<br>Transdermal patch | 0.3–0.6 mg p.r.n.<br>up to 3 tablets<br>1–3 mg q 5 h t.i.d.<br>1–2 mg q 4 h 12–14 h/d<br>One patch 12–14 h/d | Short half-life, peak effect 2–3 min lasting ≤ 1 h<br>4–5 h<br>Inadequate data<br>Effective within 1–2 h, prescribed; duration of effect 8–12 h[a] |
| Isosorbide dinitrate | SL tablet<br><br>Oral<br><br>Extended release tablets | 2.5–10.00 mg q 2–3 h<br><br>30–60 mg b.i.d. or<br>10–30 mg t.i.d.<br>40–80 mg q.d to t.i.d. | Effective within 5 min; lasts ≤ 1 h<br>Effective 2–8 h after single dose†[b]<br>Effective 8–12 h |
| Isosorbide-5-mononitrate | Immediate release<br><br>Extended release | 20 mg AM & PM<br>7 h apart<br>60–120 mg q.d | Effective 6–10 h<br><br>Effective ≤ 9 h |

[a]Tolerance when used for 24 h.
[b]Q.i.d. dose produces tolerance.
b.i.d. = twice a day; d = day; h = hour; p.r.n. = as required; q = every; S.L. = sublingual; t.i.d. = three times a day.
Adapted with permission from Drugs for stable angina pectoris. Medical Letter 1994;36:111–114; and Thadani U. Medical therapy of stable angina pectoris. Cardiol Clin 1991:9:73–87.

uous use have limited their employment. Intermittent treatment with the patches prevents tolerance but may cause rebound nocturnal angina and decrease early morning exercise capacity (28; 29).

Nitroglycerin ointment has a duration of action from 3–8 hours. To be effective, it should be spread over a skin surface of 5–6 square inches.

The widely used oral isosorbide dinitrate is excreted through the liver and kidneys. The first-pass hepatic extraction may result in a mean bioavailability of 19–25% (30).

Isosorbide mononitrate, which bypasses the liver metabolism, has a duration of action from 6–10 hours. This preparation is nearly 100% bioavailable without any active metabolites. The usual dose of 20 mg at 7 AM and 2 PM does not produce tolerance or rebound nocturnal angina (31).

A sustained-release product, Imdur (Key Pharmaceuticals, Kenilworth, New Jersey), can be given once daily in a dose of 60–120 mg and still permit about an 8- to 10-hour nitrate-free interval.

**Efficacy of Dosing.** The clinical hallmark of absorption is production of headache, flushing, and occasionally, dizziness. Should two or three nitroglycerin tablets (0.3–0.4 mg) fail to relieve the anginal pain, unstable angina, acute MI, or incorrect diagnosis should be suspected, and a physician should be contacted. Patients should be instructed in the proper use of their nitroglycerin tablets and should store them in dark glass vials to be discarded after 4 months.

**Nitrate Tolerance.** The exact mechanism of nitrate tolerance is not known. Several mechanisms have been proposed. The vasodilatory effects are related to cGMP production. This compound attenuates calcium release from sarcoplasmic reticulum and thereby reduces permeability to extracellular calcium (32). A reduced sulfhydryl group is essential for nitric oxide production and release. Nitric oxide interacts with a sulfhydryl group to form S-nitrosothiol compound, which stimulates cGMP. Tolerance has been associated with depletion of cGMP, with decreased intracellular stores of reduced sulfhydryl groups.

Pharmacokinetic changes have also been proposed as a possible cause of nitrate tolerance. Over time, absorption, distribution, and elimination of the nitrates may change and thereby alter levels of nitrates and their metabolites.

Rebound vasoconstrictive forces offsetting vasodilation have also been suggested as a mechanism for nitrate tolerance. One study showed increased heart rate and elevated plasma renin activity accompanied by hemodynamic tolerance in patients with congestive heart failure (33).

Tolerance, the major drawback to nitrate therapy, may be avoided by planning a nitrate-free interval of at least 8 hours, whatever preparation is used.

**Side Effects.** The major adverse side effect of the nitrates is headache, reported by 30–60% of patients; however, in most cases tolerance to headache develops in a 1- to 2-week period. In the meantime, the patient can be instructed to take an analgesic to relieve the headache produced by nitroglycerin. Rare adverse effects include postural hypotension and even syncope.

**Summary.** The major issues in stable angina are whether to use nitrates preemptively, how to obtain the longest duration of action without tolerance, and how to keep the patient compliant. The effects of nitrates, though physiologically appropriate, attenuate symptoms more than they affect prognosis. With the wide choice of preparations available, nitrates can be given safely with sustained bioavailability on dosing schedules that generally avoid tolerance and promote compliance.

### *β-Blockers*

**Mechanism of Action.** β-receptors are proteins embedded in the lipid bilayer of target cells. They are subdivided into $\beta_1$- and $\beta_2$-receptors. $\beta_1$-receptors predominate in cardiac cells (about 80%). They are also found in adipose tissue and in the kidneys. $\beta_2$-Receptors predominate in the bronchial tree and peripheral arteries.

Activation of β-receptors results in stimulation of adenyl cyclase, which in turn converts cyclic adenosine triphosphate to cyclic adenosine monophosphate (cAMP). Cyclic adenosine monophosphate, as an intracellular messenger, provides positive chronotropic and inotropic effects on the heart by increasing pacemaker current in the sinus node and opening the calcium channels. Blockade of β-receptors, therefore, has negative inotropic and chronotropic effects to decrease contractility and heart rate, respectively.

β-Blockers and agonists are competitive for the receptor site, and the relative concentration of the two determines the degree of cell stimulation or inhibition.

β-Blockers work on both sides of the demand-supply equation to reduce ischemia (Fig. 5.2). On the demand side, they reduce heart rate and contractility, whereas on the supply side, they increase flow to ischemic zones by increasing the diastolic filling period, thus increasing coronary perfusion time (34). They also reduce coronary vasoconstriction during exercise (35).

**β-Blocking Agents.** Table 5.3 outlines the currently available β-blocking agents. Some are relatively $\beta_1$-selective (cardioselective), and others are noncardioselective. Some block all receptors whereas others have intrinsic sympathomimetic activity through partial stimulation of β-receptors. The selection of a specific β-blocker depends on any comorbid conditions that

**Table 5.3**
**Guide to β-Adrenergic Blockade in Therapy for Chronic Stable Angina Pectoris**

| Drug | Cardio-selective | Dosage | Plasma Half-life (h) | Lipid Solubility | Metabolization |
|---|---|---|---|---|---|
| Atenolol<br>Tenormin[a] | Yes | 50–200 mg q.d. | 6–9 | 0 | Kidney |
| Metoprolol<br>*Lopressor*[b] | Yes | 50–200 mg b.i.d. | 3–7 | + | Liver |
| Nadolol<br>*Corgard*[c] | No | 40–80 mg q.d. | 20–24 | 0 | Kidney |
| Propranolol<br>*Inderal*[d] | No | 80–320 mg b.i.d., t.i.d., or q.i.d. | 3–5 | +++ | Liver |
| *Inderal LA*[d] | No | 80–160 mg q.d. | 8–11 | +++ | Liver |

[a] ICI Pharma, Wilmington, Delaware.
[b] GEIGY Pharmaceuticals, Ardsley, New York.
[c] Bristol Laboratories, Evansville, Indiana.
[d] Wyeth-Ayerst Laboratories, Philadelphia, Pennsylvania.
b.i.d. = twice a day; h = hours; q.d. = every day; q.i.d. = four times a day; t.i.d. = three times a day; 0 = not soluble; + = somewhat soluble; +++ = very soluble.
Adapted with permission from Drugs for stable angina pectoris. Medical Letter 1994;36:111–114; and Opie LH, ed. Drugs for the heart. 3rd ed. Philadelphia: WB Saunders, 1991.

may preclude the use of certain β-blockers. For example, cardioselective β-blockers may be useful in patients with diabetes, peripheral vascular disease, or asthma. Caution must be exercised in patients with bronchial asthma, because even the so-called cardioselective β-blockers can induce bronchial constriction. Cardioselectivity is dose related, and at extremely high doses most $\beta_1$-selective compounds lose their cardioselectivity.

The lipid-soluble β-blockers are rapidly absorbed from the gastrointestinal tract, are metabolized in the liver, are highly bound to the plasma protein, are widely distributed in all tissues, and have short half-lives. In contrast, the water-soluble β-blockers are less well absorbed from the gastrointestinal tract, are excreted unchanged by the kidneys, are poorly bound to plasma proteins, are less well distributed, do not cross the blood-brain barrier, and in general have long half-lives. The bioavailability of β-blockers depends upon drug absorption from the gastrointestinal tract—that is, the amount of drug reaching the receptors without being metabolized—and is therefore variable among the β-blockers. Theoretically, lipid-soluble β-blockers are taken up more rapidly by the brain than water-soluble ones.

In choosing a β-blocker, one may select any agent that is tolerated by the patient and suited to any comorbid condition. It is important to note that β-blockers are considered cardioprotective. A metaanalysis of trials including 23,000 patients on long-term β-blocker therapy following MI showed a 22% reduction in the risk of death (36) (Fig. 5.7). The use of β-blockers in patients with chronic stable angina who have not sustained an MI, however, has not been studied. A more recent study of patients with mild or no angina showed that atenolol reduced both daily life ischemia and morbid events over 1 year of follow-up and diminished both the number and duration of ischemic episodes (Fig. 5.8)(37).

β-Blockers are also useful in combination therapy with either nitrates or calcium channel blockers, or both (see below).

**Dose Response and Efficacy.** The responsiveness to β-blocker therapy is evaluated by observation of reduction in heart rate and blood pressure in comparison with previous resting values or in response to exercise. Reduction of exercise-induced tachycardia is an important determinant of effectiveness, especially in exertional angina, with the aim of achieving a rate of less than 100 beats/minute with mild exercise (38).

**Tolerance and Rebound Angina.** If a patient is on β-blocker therapy for more than 4–5 weeks and develops side effects, therapy should be withdrawn gradually, since abrupt β-blocker withdrawal can lead to a rebound effect of increased anginal attacks, tachycardia, and (rarely) myocardial infarction (39).

**Side Effects.** Several adverse effects are linked with β-blockade, including bradycardia, heart block, hypotension, fatigue, dyspnea, cold extremities, impotence, lethargy, depression, and bronchospasm.

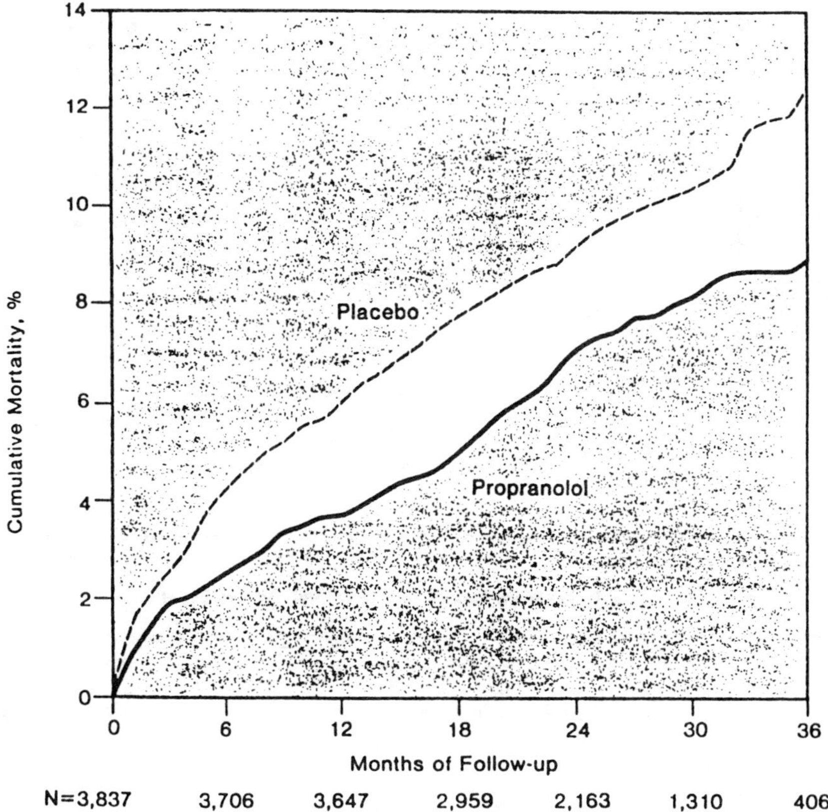


Figure 5.7. β-Blocker Heart Attack Trial Research Group. Cumulative mortality in patients with acute myocardial infarction. Reproduced with permission from β-Blocker Heart Attack Research Group. A randomized trial of propranolol in patients with acute myocardial infarction. I. Mortality results. JAMA 1982;247:1707–1714.

**Summary.** The use of β-blockers in chronic stable angina may be limited because of their side effects. To date, however, these agents are the only class of drugs shown to be cardioprotective; moreover, they are safe when used properly.

### *Calcium Channel Antagonists*

**Mechanism of Action.** Calcium channel antagonists are useful in ameliorating the extent and duration of myocardial ischemia. There are two calcium channels in the cardiac and skeletal muscles that regulate excitation-contraction coupling: dihydropyridine receptors and ryanodine receptors. The dihydropyridine receptors, located on the transverse tubule (T tubule) (Fig. 5.9), are voltage-gated channels (40). During excitation-

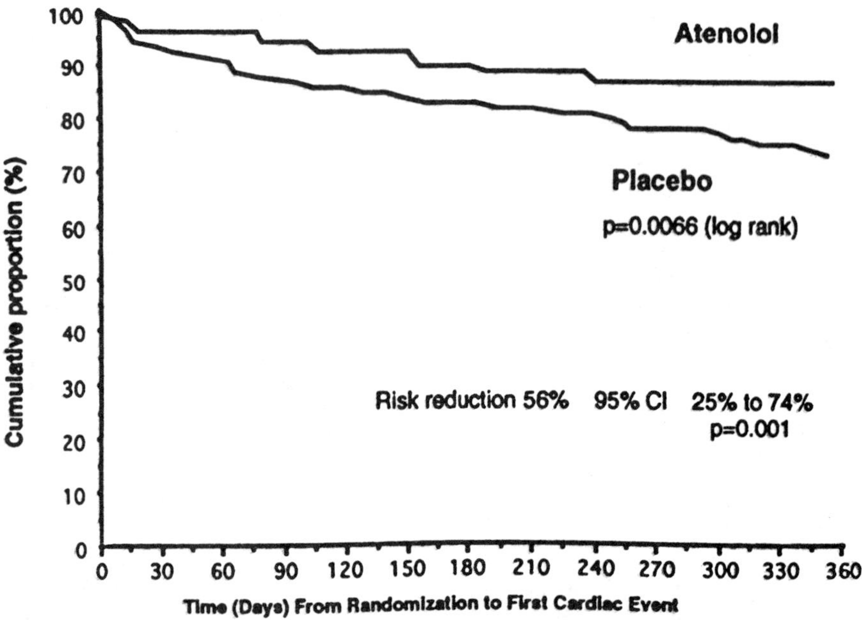


Figure 5.8. Cumulative probability of not experiencing an adverse event among patients with silent ischemia randomized to treatment with atenolol. CI = confidence interval. Reproduced with permission from Pepine CJ, Cohn PF, Deedwania PC, et al. Effects of treatment on outcome in mildly symptomatic patients with ischemia during daily life. The Atenolol Silent Ischemia Study (ASIST). Circulation 1994;90:762–768.

contraction coupling, the voltage-activated calcium channel (dihydropyridine receptor) senses membrane depolarization and activates the ryanodine receptor, a calcium-release channel on the terminal cisternae. The calcium-adenosine triphosphatase (Ca-ATPase) is located in the sarcoplasmic reticulum and is responsible for reuptake of calcium. In cardiac muscle, the dihydropyridine receptor serves two purposes; it is a voltage sensor activated by membrane depolarization, and it is a calcium channel providing the calcium influx required for calcium-induced calcium release.

Inositol 1,4,5-triphosphate ($IP_3$) receptors are the major intracellular calcium release channels that support contraction in vascular smooth muscle cells. These receptors are also expressed in cardiac muscle (41). In contrast to dihydropyridine receptors and ryanodine receptors, $IP_3$ receptors are activated via cell surface receptor (e.g., angiotensin II receptor) activation of G protein–coupled production of the second messenger $IP_3$. $IP_3$ binds to its receptor on the endoplasmic reticulum, the $IP_3$ receptor, and stimulates the release of intracellular calcium that activates smooth muscle cell contraction.

Although the ryanodine receptor is activated by caffeine and the $IP_3$ receptor is blocked by heparin, no therapeutically useful agents have been

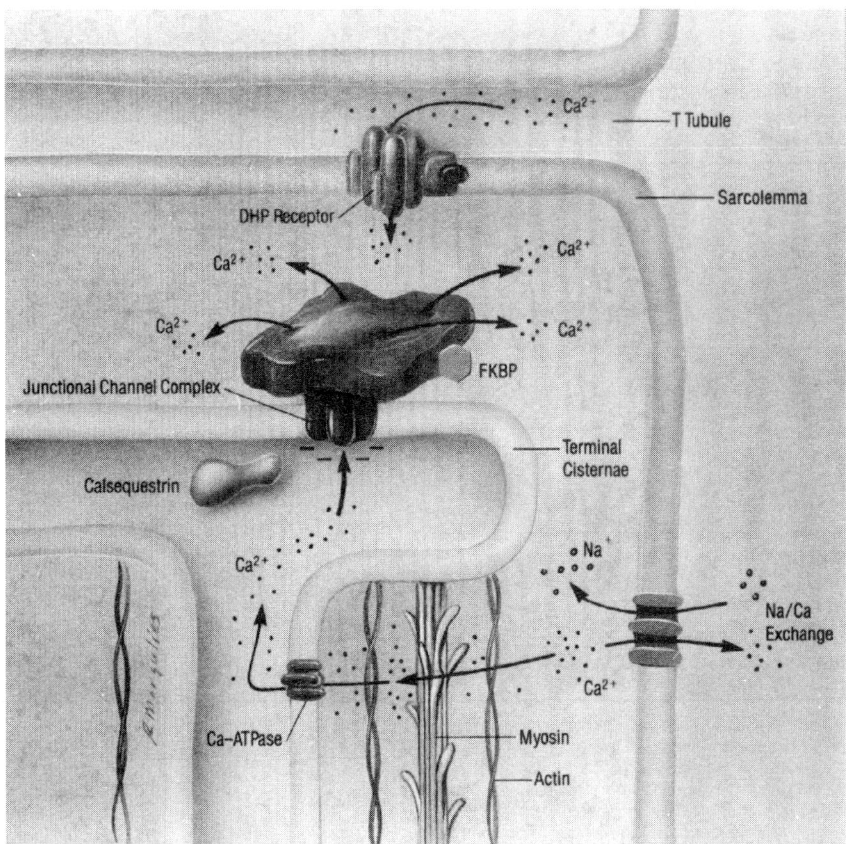


Figure 5.9. The calcium channels involved in excitation-contraction (EC) coupling in skeletal and cardiac muscle are the dihydropyridine (DHP) receptor and the junctional channel complex. The DHP receptor is schematically represented on the transverse tubule, which is an invagination of the plasma membrane of the myocyte. An interaction between the DHP receptor and the junctional channel complex is believed to be the basis for EC coupling in striated muscle. The Ca-adenosine triphosphatase (ATPase) is located in the sarcoplasmic reticulum and is responsible for re-uptake of calcium released through the calcium release channel during EC coupling. Reproduced with permission from Marks AM, Brillantes AMB. The molecular biology of calcium channels. Primary Cardiology 1993;19:33–36, 39–41, 45–46, 49.

found that modulate activity of either intracellular calcium-release channel. In contrast, calcium channel blockers, including nifedipine, verapamil, and diltiazem, that act on dihydropyridine receptors are among the most widely used cardiovascular drugs.

### *Calcium Channel Blocking Agents*

The most frequently used calcium channel blockers are verapamil, nifedipine, and diltiazem, all of which block dihydropyridine receptors (Table 5.4). They affect both the supply and demand components of the is-

**Table 5.4**
**Guide to Calcium Blocker Therapy for Chronic Stable Angina Pectoris**

| Drug | Dosage | Metabolism | Half-life (h) |
|---|---|---|---|
| Nifedipine | | | |
| Immediate release | 10–30 mg t.i.d. or q.i.d. | Kidney | 2–5 |
| Extended release | 30–90 mg q.d. | | — |
| Amlodipine | | | |
| Norvasc[a] | 5–10 mg q.d. | Kidney | — |
| Nicardipine | | | |
| Cardene[b] | 20–40 mg t.i.d. | Kidney | 2–4 |
| Diltiazem | | | |
| Immediate release | 30–120 mg t.i.d. or q.i.d. | Kidney/GI | 4–7 |
| Extended release | 120–480 mg q.d. | Kidney/GI | — |
| Verapamil<br>Calan[c]<br>Isoptin[d] | 80–120 mg t.i.d. or q.i.d. | Kidney/GI | 3–7 |
| Bepridil[e] | 200–400 mg q.d. | | — |

[a] *Pfizer Labs, New York, New York.*
[b] Syntex Laboratories, Inc., Palo Alto, California.
[c] GD Searle and Company, Chicago, Illinois.
[d] Knoll Pharmaceutical Company, Whippany, New Jersey.
[e] Mixed sodium and calcium channel antagonists.
GI = gastrointestinal tract; h = hour; q.d. = every day; q.i.d. = four times a day; t.i.d. = three times a day.
Adapted with permission from Drugs for stable angina pectoris. Medical Letter 1994;36:111–114; and Thadani U. medical therapy of stable angina pectoris. Cardiol Clin 1991;9:73–87.

chemic imbalance by decreasing oxygen consumption, increasing coronary blood flow through primary vasodilation, and dilating large-vessel coronary stenoses (42–45). These agents affect heart rate and contractility differently (Table 5.5). Although they all increase diastolic relaxation and thereby improve coronary perfusion, the atrioventricular nodal delay and decrease in heart rate produced by diltiazem and verapamil limit their use in patients with heart block and sick sinus syndrome. Nifedipine and nicardipine are potent vasodilators and can cause reflex tachycardia and peripheral edema.

Diltiazem protects the myocardium during transient ischemia (46). Some of the newer agents, such as nicardipine, appear to have favorable hemodynamic effects in the ischemic model. This agent dramatically increases coronary blood flow without any effect on left ventricular end-diastolic pressure but decreases systolic blood pressure and heart rate. The new long-acting agent, amlodipine, produces favorable effects during is-

**Table 5.5**
**Pharmacological Effects of Calcium Channel Blocking Therapy for Chronic Stable Angina Pectoris**

| | Verapamil | Diltiazem | Nifedipine |
|---|---|---|---|
| Heart rate | ↓0 | ↓ | ↑ |
| Systemic BP | ↓ | ↓ | ↓↓ |
| AV nodal delay | ↑↑ | ↑↑ | ?0 |
| Contractility | ↓↓ | ↓0 | ?0 |
| Coronary vasodilation | ↑↑ | ↑ | ↑ |
| Diastolic relaxation | ↑ | ↑ | ↑ |

↓ = Decrease; ↑ = increase; 0 = no effect.
Adapted with permission from Thadani U. Medical therapy of stable anginal pectoris. Cardiol Clin 1991;9:73–87.

chemia by improving cardiac compliance and diastolic function (47). These agents have reportedly fewer negative inotropic effects.

Bepridil, a mixed calcium and sodium channel antagonist, has been recommended for patients whose angina is refractory to other forms of therapy and for whom revascularization is not a choice. A major side effect is prolongation of the QT interval, which can pose the risk of torsades de pointes, particularly in the presence of hypokalemia and decreased left ventricular function.

**Dosing and Efficacy.** When the clinical response to calcium blockers is inadequate, increasing the dosage may help, though judging the endpoint of responsiveness is difficult. Symptoms of dizziness, flushing, and fall in diastolic blood pressure, however, may aid in demonstrating adequate calcium channel blockade. Although withdrawal phenomena have been reported, they are rare, and these drugs may be discontinued abruptly when necessary.

**Side Effects.** Calcium channel blockers are usually well tolerated. They may cause flushing, headache, and dizziness due to their vasodilator properties. Dihydropyridines may cause edema, whereas diltiazem and verapamil are associated with constipation and atrioventricular nodal blockade. One of the problems with some of the dihydropyridines is reflex tachycardia and coronary steal, which may provoke angina. Amlodipine, a new agent of this class, generally avoids this effect.

**Summary.** No long-term cardioprotection has been reported with the use of calcium channel blockers, so they are used only for relief of symptoms and control of hypertension when it is present.

### *Combination Therapy*

Patients often require combination therapy for symptom control or treatment of comorbid conditions.

**Plan of Therapy.** All patients should take aspirin unless there are contraindications. In a patient with no other medical problems or risk factors, the first single agent used is a mononitrate. As with any other pharmacologic agent, it is important to instruct the patient carefully in the use of the drug to prevent tolerance and anginal attacks. Sublingual nitroglycerin is always prescribed in addition for use as needed.

**Nitrates with β-Blockers.** After nitrate monotherapy is instituted, β-blockers are usually added, even if symptoms have been relieved by the nitrates. β-Blockers, alone among drugs used to treat chronic stable angina, are beneficial not only in controlling ischemia (48) but also in reducing mortality (49).

**Nitrates, β-Blockers, and Calcium Channel Antagonists.** If the patient remains symptomatic on both nitrates and β-blockers, and both drugs are well tolerated, a calcium channel antagonist may be introduced. It may also be substituted for the nitrate or the β-blocker in some cases. Diltiazem is well tolerated in conjunction with β-blockers. Hung and colleagues (50) showed that the time to onset of angina improved significantly with a combination of propranolol and diltiazem compared with single-drug therapy. Patients had fewer ischemic events as well as increased exercise capacity. The combination of verapamil and β-blockers is less acceptable. Winniford and coworkers compared maximally tolerated verapamil combined with the β-blocker propranolol with placebo (51; 52). This double-blind crossover study showed improvement in exercise duration with less ST depression. Patients on this combination had more heart block and heart failure, however. Akhras and Jackson (53), however, found that in patients who were on atenolol, nifedipine alone, mononitrate alone, or a combination of all three drugs produced only an equivalent reduction in anginal episodes and nitroglycerin usage. There was no additive effect.

The most useful clinical practice is to try to utilize β-blockade first and then to add a calcium blocker. Although the maximum β-blocking dose may benefit the patient, it may have more side effects and limit exercise duration as a result of fatigue.

## Medical Management of Stable Coronary Disease in the Presence of Comorbid Conditions

### *Hypertension*

Patients with angina pectoris secondary to atherosclerosis may have hypertension as well. In these cases, the first line of therapy is with β-blockers. Black patients tolerate calcium channel blockers well and achieve better control of both angina and blood pressure when calcium blockers are used as the first course of treatment. Combination therapy with β-blockers and calcium channel blockers is particularly valuable in patients with both angina and hypertension. As always, sublingual nitroglycerin is prescribed for control of acute anginal attacks. In these patients, angina may also arise solely in relation to hypertension and the associated left ventricular hypertrophy, in which case therapy should focus on treatment of the hypertension and regression of the hypertrophy. Angiotensin-converting enzyme (ACE) inhibitors may be useful in this group.

*Diabetes*

In general, diabetic patients should be started on nitrates. Calcium blockers are also safe and effective. Both classes of agent are direct vascular smooth muscle dilators and are important in the setting of dysfunctional endothelium found in diabetes. In nonbrittle diabetics, β-blockers can be used, although the cardioselective forms are preferred so as not to mask hypoglycemic symptoms.

*Hypertension and Diabetes*

In patients who have hypertension and diabetes in addition to stable angina pectoris, nitrates and calcium blockers are preferred if left ventricular function is normal. ACE inhibitors may also be used to control blood pressure and to attenuate diabetic renal disease.

*Congestive Heart Failure*

In patients with heart failure and stable angina pectoris, nitrates are, again, the first choice. As selective venodilators they reduce preload. When conventional therapy for congestive heart failure has been taken to its limit with digoxin, diuretics, ACE inhibitors, and aspirin, small doses of β-blockers are remarkably effective and safe, if carefully titrated. These agents reduce mortality in patients with congestive heart failure (54–56). Calcium antagonists should be avoided because of their negative inotropic effects and the increased mortality associated with their use (57).

*Silent Ischemia*

When a patient presents with objective evidence of myocardial ischemia by exercise testing or electrocardiographic evidence but without symptoms, the ischemia is "silent." The therapeutic plan is complex and should be aimed at reducing or abolishing the signs of ischemia (58). In general, the prognosis of these patients is good. The therapeutic approach should be directed toward modifying risk factors, limiting strenuous exercise, and identifying the patients with severe demonstrable ischemia (whose prognosis is worse). The aim is to increase the time to demonstrable ischemia during exercise and, if possible, to improve cardiac wall motion in the ischemic zones (59). Several studies of combination therapy with β-blockers and calcium antagonists report reduction of ischemia in these patients (60–64). None of these studies, except the Atenolol Silent Ischemia Study (ASIST) trial (48), indicates improved prognosis, even when ischemia is abolished. β-Blockers should probably be the first course of therapy in this group. If ischemia persists, one may add a calcium channel blocker to the regimen.

### *Advanced Age*

In the elderly, calcium blockers are usually well tolerated. A recent study by de Vries (65) evaluated the efficacy and safety of the calcium blocker felodipine versus isosorbide mononitrate to augment β-blocker therapy in elderly patients. Felodipine, 5 mg daily, improved time to ischemia and increased total exercise time significantly. This was not seen with isosorbide mononitrate. Furthermore, felodipine was better tolerated than isosorbide mononitrate. It should, however, be noted that felodipine is not approved by the US Food and Drug Administration for use in the treatment of angina pectoris.

### *Peripheral Vascular Disease*

In patients with peripheral vascular disease, intermittent claudication may worsen if the patient is on a nonselective β-blocking agent. Therefore, nitrates with calcium blockers or cardioselective β-blockers may be used in this population.

### *Hyperlipidemia*

Nifedipine, nicardipine, and verapamil are among the calcium blockers associated with some retardation of plaque progression but no change in clinical events (66–68). Although some β-blockers may increase low-density lipoprotein (LDL) cholesterol and decrease high-density lipoprotein (HDL) cholesterol, to date no study has shown progression of coronary artery disease in patients on chronic β-blocker therapy. On the contrary, all the β-blocker trials show a reduction in mortality, recurrent MI, and sudden death. Although calcium blockers theoretically may be preferred in this group, use of β-blocking agents should not be avoided. Use of these agents should be judged solely on their cardioprotective and antianginal effects rather than on their possible adverse effects on the lipid profile. Aggressive control of HDL and LDL through diet and pharmacological means should be the mainstay of lipid-lowering therapy (69; 70).

### *Microvascular Angina*

The distal microvasculature plays an important role in the subset of patients who have chest pain but angiographically normal coronary arteries. This group of patients has a reduced vasodilator response to metabolic stimuli, such as exercise (71) and atrial pacing (72). The mechanism may be enhanced sympathetic tone, a disorder of microvascular medial smooth muscle, or abnormal humorally mediated vasoconstrictor influences. Quyyumi and colleagues (73) studied the response of the microvasculature to rapid atrial pacing in patients with chest pain and normal coronary arteries. Endothelial function was tested by arteriography using acetylcholine and nitroprusside. These patients had endothelial dysfunction of the coronary microvasculature in addition to reduced vasodilation in response to atrial pacing.

In this group of patients nitrates and calcium channel blockers are the main forms of therapy because of their effects on the endothelium and the distal microvasculature (74).

### *Summary*

In the selection of therapy for the patient with stable angina, many factors come into play. It is important to start with a single agent and to make the dosing schedule as simple as possible while establishing efficacy. The patient's risk factors and other comorbid conditions guide the physician in choosing the agent best tolerated by the patient. The physician must distinguish between the simple ineffectiveness of medical therapy and a change in the pattern of symptoms. The latter usually signifies progression of disease to an acute coronary syndrome, which has other therapeutic implications.

In this era of awareness of cost-effectiveness, medical therapy should be given a thorough trial before surgical or interventional therapy is prescribed, provided that it does not increase the risk or leave the patient symptomatically disabled.

The combination of nitrates and β-blockers is beneficial in that β-blockers may prevent angina during a nitrate-free period as well as afford cardioprotection. When β-blockers and calcium channel blockers are combined, caution should be taken in using β-blockers with verapamil, as this combination may be associated with heart block and heart failure. Nifedipine and other newer dihydropyridine calcium channel blockers in combination with β-blockers may be more efficacious than monotherapy in reducing ischemia and increasing exercise duration. All patients must be on antiplatelet agents, and when possible, β-blockers should be included in the regimen of patients with stable coronary disease. The choice of other antianginal agents is governed by relief of symptoms, tolerance, and efficacy.

## Revascularization

Although pharmacotherapy is the appropriate first step in treating stable angina pectoris, certain patients should be considered for early revascularization.

### *Coronary Artery Bypass Graft Surgery*

Several clinical trials comparing medical therapy with coronary artery bypass grafting (CABG) in patients with stable angina (75–77) confirm that surgery improves survival in patients with left main coronary disease or severe three-vessel disease and decreased left ventricular function. In all of these studies the benefits outweigh the attendant risks of both surgery and the vulnerability of grafts to subsequent atherosclerosis.

If medical therapy fails to assuage symptoms, is not tolerated, or does not afford the lifestyle sought for, then such patients may be offered direct revascularization. The choice between CABG and percutaneous transluminal coronary angioplasty is driven by the following considerations:

- Both have similar mortality and recurrent MI rates (78; 79).
- Surgery is more suitable in the presence of totally occluded arteries and gives more relief of angina; moreover, repeat procedures are less frequently required.
- Angioplasty is more suitable if the patient wants to avoid surgery, will accept repeated catheterizations, and does not present with pathoanatomic contraindications.

Thus, the patient, his or her personal physician, and the interventional cardiologist must participate in the decision making.

Not infrequently, and particularly during the first decade after surgical revascularization, the patient may develop recurrent ischemic symptoms. Another intervention may be less than desirable or perhaps technically very difficult. Medical therapy returns then as a major cornerstone of treatment.

### *Medical Therapy versus Direct Revascularization*

To date, there has been no true test of medical therapy versus revascularization. In none of the trials including both medicine and surgery was there careful titration of combination therapy to maximal tolerated doses of the current available antianginal drugs.

The only study comparing medical therapy with percutaneous transluminal coronary angioplasty is the Angioplasty Compared to Medicine (ACME) trial (80). In patients with single-vessel coronary artery disease, angioplasty offered better relief of angina with improved exercise performance even though patients were not on maximal medical therapy (Fig. 5.10).

### *The Role of the Nervous System in Angina*

In a subgroup of patients who have chest pain and normal coronary arteries, regardless of the issue of microvascular dysfunction, abnormal visceral nociception may be responsible for the pain (81). Several abnormal functions of the central nervous system have been described in connection with these phenomena. Therapy in this group would be focused on blunting the activation of the efferent limb of the sympathetic nervous system with β-blockers or diminishing smooth muscle cell activation with calcium

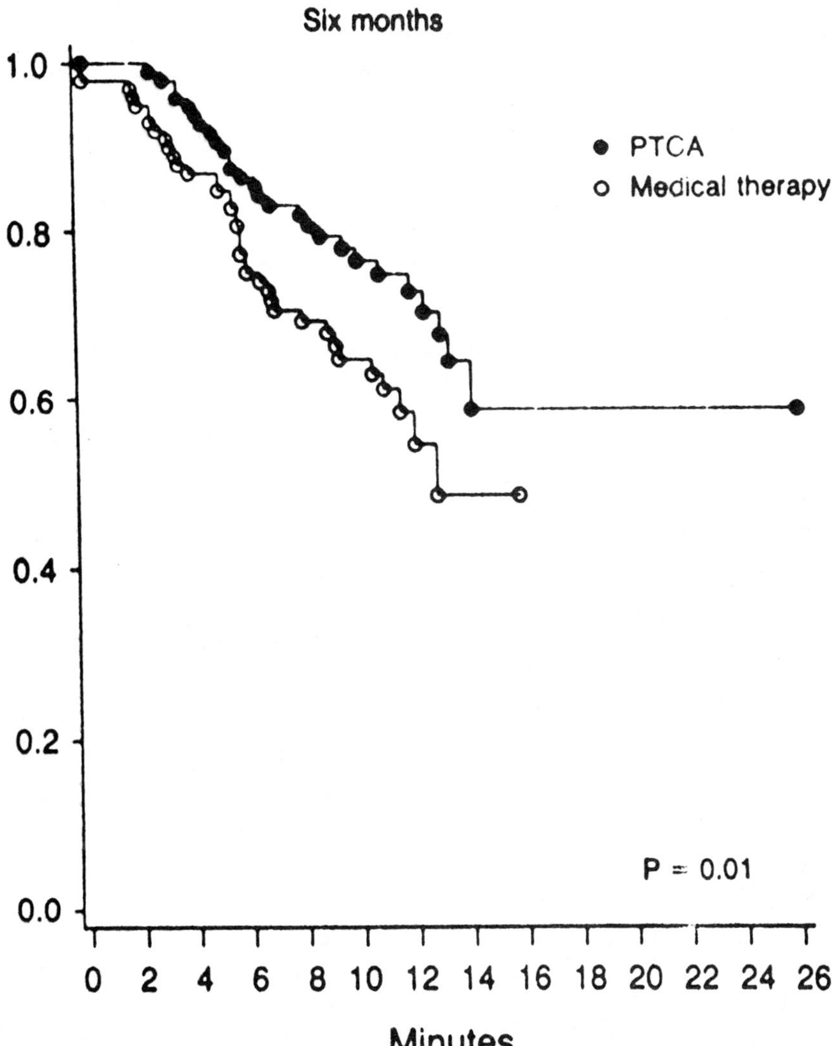


**Figure 5.10.** Duration of angina-free treadmill exercise 6 months after treatment of stable single-vessel coronary artery disease with percutaneous transluminal coronary angioplasty (PTCA) or medical therapy. Reproduced with permission from Parisi AF, Folland ED, Hartigan P, on behalf of the Veterans Affairs ACME Investigators. A comparison of angioplasty with medical therapy in the treatment of single-vessel coronary artery disease. N Engl J Med 1992;326:10–16.

channel blockers. Tricyclic antidepressants also seem to be efficacious in some of these patients (82).

There is another very small subgroup of patients with severe angina who are already on maximal medical therapy for documented coronary artery disease and who are not candidates for revascularization. The treatment options in this group are limited. Recently, the antianginal effects of endoscopic transthoracic sympathectomy have been evaluated in these patients (83). The sympathetic nervous system is important in the perception of pain. The antianginal effects of sympathectomy may be in part due to a direct analgesic effect in addition to alteration of determinants of myocardial oxygen demand (i.e., decrease in heart rate and systolic blood pressure during exercise).

## CONCLUSION

In conclusion, in the management of the patient with chronic stable angina, many factors come into play. An understanding of the pathophysiology of the disease is essential in the formulation of a therapeutic decision tree. Before the establishment of therapy to alleviate symptoms, modification of risk factors should be attempted through cessation of smoking, lipid lowering, increase in exercise, and control of hypertension. Medical therapy should be tailored to the individual patient according to risk factors, comorbid conditions, and tolerance of the agent prescribed. It should both improve the patient's lifestyle and prolong survival. Medical therapy has failed if symptoms continue and interfere with perceived quality of life or if significant myocardial ischemia persists after a thorough trial of therapy. Such a trial should test all three classes of antianginal agent to the point that they are either ineffective or not tolerated.

In summary, patients with severe three-vessel or left main coronary artery disease and decreased left ventricular function probably have a better survival rate with surgical revascularization than with medical therapy. Medical therapy is the choice in all other patients unless symptoms are not controlled. Once medical therapy fails, revascularization should be offered.

### *Acknowledgement*

The authors acknowledge the work of Karen Sadock in editorial review and manuscript preparation.

---

## REFERENCES

1. Heberden W. Some account of a disorder of the breast. Med Trans Coll Physicians (London) 2:59,1772.
2. Griffith TM, Edwards DH, Lewis MJ, et al. The nature of endothelium-derived vascular relaxing factor. Nature 1984;308:645–647.
3. Furchgott RF, Zawadski JV. The obligatory role of endothelial cells in the relaxation of arterial smooth muscle by acetylcholine. Nature 1980;288:373–376.
4. Cocks TM, Angus JA. Endothelium-dependent relaxation of coronary arteries by noradrenaline and serotonin. Nature 1983;305:627–630.
5. Gillispie MN, Owasoyo JO, McMurtry IF, et al. Sustained coronary vasoconstriction provoked by a peptidergic substance released from endothelial cells in culture. J Pharmacol Exp Ther 1986;236:339–343.
6. Vanhoutte PM. Endothelium-dependent contractions in arteries and veins. Blood Vessels 1987;24:141–144.

7. Luckhoff A, Busse R, Winter I, et al. Characterization of vascular relaxant factor released from cultured endothelial cells. Hypertension 1987;9:295–303.
8. Yanagisawa M, Kurihara H, Kimura S, et al. A novel potent vasoconstrictor peptide produced by vascular endothelial cells. Nature 1988;332:411–415.
9. Nabel EG, Selwyn AP, Ganz P. Large coronary arteries in humans are responsive to changing blood flow: an endothelium-dependent mechanism that fails in patients with atherosclerosis. J Am Coll Cardiol 1990;16:349–356.
10. Panza JA, Quyyumi AA, Epstein SE. Abnormal endothelium-dependent vascular relaxation in patients with essential hypertension. N Engl J Med 1990;323:22–27.
11. Nitenberg A, Valensi P, Sachs R, et al. Impairment of coronary vascular reserve and ACh-induced coronary vasodilation in diabetic patients with angiographically normal coronary arteries and normal left ventricular systolic function. Diabetes 1993; 42:1017–1025.
12. Celermajer DS, Sorensen KE, Georgadopoulos D, et al. Cigarette smoking is associated with dose-related and potentially reversible impairment of endothelium-dependent dilation in healthy young adults. Circulation 1993;88(part 1):2149–2155.
13. Levine GN, Keaney JF, Vita JA. Cholesterol reduction in cardiovascular disease. Clinical benefits and possible mechanisms. N Engl J Med 1995;332:512–521.
14. Gould KL. Quantification of coronary artery stenosis in vivo. Circ Res 1985;57: 341–353.
15. Sheldon WC. On the significance of coronary collaterals. Am J Cardiol 1969:24: 303–304.
16. Gorlin R. Physiology of myocardial blood flow and metabolism. In: Gorlin R. Coronary artery disease. Philadelphia: WB Saunders,1976:73–74.
17. Estes EH, Entman ML, Dixon HB, et al. The vascular supply of the left ventricular wall. Am Heart J 1966;71:58–67.
18. Brown BG, Bolson E, Peterson RB, et al. The mechanism of nitroglycerine action: stenosis vasodilation as major component of drug response. Circulation 1981;64: 1089–1097.
19. Brown BG, Lee AB, Bolson EL, et al. Reflex constriction of significant coronary stenosis as a mechanism contributing to ischemic left ventricular dysfunction during isometric exercise. Circulation 1984;70:18–24.
20. Cohn PF, Maddox DE, Holman BL, et al. Effect of coronary collateral vessels on regional myocardial blood flow in patients with coronary artery disease. Am J Cardiol 1980;46:359–364.
21. Kattus AA, Grollman J. Patterns of coronary collateral circulation in angina pectoris: relation to exercise training. In: Russek H, Zohman BL, eds. Changing concepts in cardiovascular disease. Baltimore: Williams & Wilkins, 1972:352–376.
22. Gorlin R. Management of angina pectoris: the evolution of therapy —are there still unresolved needs? Am J Cardiol 1992;69:1D–3D.
23. Ignarro LJ, Ross G, Tillisch J. Pharmacology of endothelium-derived nitric oxide and nitrovasodilators. West J Med 1991;154:51–62.
24. Moncada S, Higgs A. The L-arginine-nitric oxide pathway. N Engl J Med 1993;329: 2002–2012.
25. Abrams J. Newer concepts on using nitrates in angina pectoris. Contemp Intern Med 1991;3:92–102.
26. Gage JE, Hess OM, Muradami T, et al. Vasoconstriction of stenotic coronary arteries during dynamic exercise in patients with classic angina pectoris: reversibility by nitroglycerine. Circulation 1986;73:865–876.
27. Abrams J. Nitrates for acute MI and in post-MI patients. Cardiology 1991;8:37–44, 97.
28. Nitroglycerin patches—do they work? Med Lett Drug Ther 1989;31:65–66.
29. Steering Committee, Transdermal Nitroglycerin Cooperative Study. Acute and chronic antianginal efficacy of continuous twenty-four-hour application of transdermal nitroglycerin. Am J Cardiol 1991;68:1263–1273.
30. Abshagen U, Betzien G, Endele R, et al. Pharmacokinetics and metabolism of isosorbide-dinitrate after intravenous and oral administration. Eur J Clin Pharmacol 1985;27:637–644.
31. Parker JO. Eccentric dosing with isosorbide-5-mononitrate in angina pectoris. Am J Cardiol 1993;72:871–876.

32. Axelsson KL, Andersson RGG. Tolerance towards nitroglycerine induced in vivo is correlated to reduced cGMP response and an alteration in cGMP turnover. Eur J Pharmacol 1983;88:71–79.
33. Packer M, Lee WH, Kessler PD, et al. Prevention and reversal of nitrate tolerance in patients with congestive heart failure. N Engl J Med 1987;317:799–804.
34. Wolfson S, Gorlin R. Cardiovascular pharmacology of propranolol in man. Circulation 1969;40:501–512.
35. Gaglione A, Hess OM, Croin WJ, et al. Is there coronary vasoconstriction after intracoronary beta adrenergic blockade in patients with coronary artery disease? J Am Coll Cardiol 1987;10:299–310.
36. Yusuf S, Wittes J, Friedman L. Overview of results of randomized clinical trials in heart disease. I. Treatments following myocardial infarction. JAMA 1988;260: 2088–2093.
37. Pepine CJ, Cohn PF, Deedwania PC, et al. Effects of treatment on outcome in mildly symptomatic patients with ischemia during daily life. The Atenolol Silent Ischemia Study (ASIST). Circulation 1994;90:762–768.
38. Thadani U. Assessment of "optimal" beta blockade in treating patients with angina pectoris. Acta Med Scand 1985;694 (Suppl):178–187.
39. Frishman WH. Beta-adrenergic blocker withdrawal. Am J Cardiol 1987;59: 26F–32F.
40. Marks AM, Brillantes AMB. The molecular biology of calcium channels. Primary Cardiology 1993;19:33–36, 39–41, 45–46, 49.
41. Moschella MC, Marks AR. Inositol 1,4,5-trisphosphate receptor expression in cardiac myocytes. J Cell Biol 1993;120:1137–1146.
42. Chafman M, Brogden RN. Diltiazem: a review of its pharmacologic properties and therapeutic efficacy. Drugs 1985;29:387–454.
43. Singh B, Ellrodt G, Peter CT. Verapamil: a review of its pharmacological properties and therapeutic uses. Drugs 1978;15:169–197.
44. Sorkin EM, Clissold SP, Brogden RN. Nifedipine: a review of its pharmacodynamic and pharmacokinetic properties and therapeutic efficacy in ischemic heart disease, hypertension and related cardiovascular diseases. Drugs 1985;30:182–274.
45. Subramanian VB. Calcium antagonists in chronic stable angina pectoris. Amsterdam: Excerpta Medica, 1982:79–116, 217–229.
46. Kavanaugh KM, Aisen AM, Fechner KP, et al. Effect of diltiazem and phosphate metabolism in ischemic and reperfused myocardium using P-31 nuclear magnetic resonance spectroscopy in vivo. Am Heart J 1989;118:1210–1219.
47. Lucchesi BR, Tamura Y. Cardioprotective effects of amlodipine in the ischemic-reperfused heart. Am Heart J 1989;118:1121–1122.
48. Pepine C, Cohn PF, Deedwania PC, et al. for the ASIST Study Group. Effect of treatment on outcome in mildly symptomatic patients with ischemia during daily life. The Atenolol Silent Ischemia Study (ASIST). Circulation 1994;90:762–768.
49. Olsson G, Odén A, Johansson L, et al. Prognosis after withdrawal of chronic postinfarction metoprolol treatment: a 2–7 year follow-up. Eur Heart J 1988;9:365–372.
50. Hung J, Lamb IH, Connolly SJ, et al. The effect of diltiazem and propranolol, alone and in combination, on exercise performance and left ventricular function in patients with stable effort angina: a double blind, randomized, and placebo-controlled study. Circulation 1983;68:560–567.
51. Winniford MD, Markham RV, Firth BG, et al. Hemodynamic and electrophysiologic effects of verapamil and nifedipine in patients on propranolol. Am J Cardiol 1082;50:704–710.
52. Winniford MD, Fulton KL, Hillis LD. Symptomatic sinus bradycardia during concomitant propranolol-verapamil administration. Am Heart J 1985;110:498.
53. Akhras F, Jackson G. Efficacy of nifedipine and isosorbide mononitrate in combination with atenolol in stable angina. Lancet 1991;338:1036–1039.
54. Cleland GJF, Henderson E, McLenachan J, et al. Effect of captopril, an angiotensin-converting enzyme inhibitor, in patients with angina pectoris and heart failure. J Am Coll Cardiol 1991;17:733–739.
55. Eichhorn EJ, Heesch CM, Barnett JH, et al. Effect of metoprolol on myocardial function and energetics in patients with nonischemic dilated cardiomyopathy: a randomized, double-blind placebo-controlled study. J Am Coll Cardiol 1994;24:1310–1320.

56. Maisel AS. Beneficial effects of metoprolol treatment in congestive heart failure. Reversal of sympathetic-induced alterations of immunologic function. Circulation 1994;90:1774–1780.
57. The Multicenter Diltiazem Postinfarction Trial Research Group. The effect of diltiazem on mortality and re-infarction after myocardial infarction. N Engl J Med 1988;819:385–392.
58. von Arnim T for the TIBBS Investigators. Medical treatment to reduce total ischemic burden: Total Ischemic Burden Bisoprolol Study (TIBBS), a multicenter trial comparing bisoprolol and nifedipine. J Am Coll Cardiol 1995;25:231–238.
59. Cohn PF, Brown EJ, Swinford R, et al. Effects of beta blockade on silent regional left ventricular wall motion abnormalities. Am J Cardiol 1986;57:521–526.
60. Frishman W, Charlap S, Kimmel B, et al. Diltiazem, nifedipine and their combination in patients with stable angina pectoris: effects on angina, exercise tolerance and the ambulatory electrocardiographic ST segment. Circulation 1988;77:774–786.
61. Théroux P, Baird M, Juneau M, et al. Effect of diltiazem on symptomatic and asymptomatic episodes of ST segment depression occurring during daily life and during exercise. Circulation 1991;84:15–22.
62. Oakley GDG, Fox KM, Dargie HJ, et al. Objective assessment of therapy in severe angina. Br Med J 1979;1:1540.
63. Cohn PF, Vetrovec GW, Neso R, Gerber FR, and the Total Ischemia Awareness Program Investigators. The Nifedipine-Total Ischemia Awareness Program: A national survey of painful and painless myocardial ischemia including results of antiischemic therapy. Am J Cardiol 1989;63:534–539.
64. Stone PH, Gibson RS, Glasser SP, et al. Comparison of propranolol, diltiazem, and nifedipine in the treatment of ambulatory ischemia in patients with stable angina: differential effects on ambulatory ischemia, exercise performance, and anginal symptoms. Circulation 1990;82:1962–1972.
65. de Vries RJM, Dunselman PHJM, van Veldhuisen DJ, et al. Comparison between felodipine and isosorbide mononitrate as adjunct to beta blockade in patients >65 years of age with angina pectoris. Am J Cardiol 1994;74:1201–1206.
66. Henry PD. Calcium antagonists as antiatherogenic agents. Ann NY Acad Sci 1988;522:411–419.
67. Lichtlen PR, Hugenholtz PG, Rafflenbeul W, et al. and the INTACT Group Investigators. Retardation of angiographic progression of coronary artery disease by nifedipine. Lancet 1990;335:1109–1113.
68. Waters D, Lespérance J, Francetich M, et al. A controlled clinical trial to assess the effect of a calcium channel blocker on the progression of coronary atherosclerosis. Circulation 1990;32:1940–1953.
69. Brown BG, Albers JJ, Fisher LD, et al. Regression of coronary artery disease as a result of intensive lipid-lowering therapy in men with high levels of lipoprotein B. N Engl J Med 1990;323:1289–1298.
70. Scandinavian Simvastatin Survival Study Group. Randomised trial of cholesterol lowering in 4444 patients with coronary heart disease: the Scandinavian Simvastatin Survival Study (4S). Lancet 1994;344:1383–1389.
71. Bortone AS, Hess OM, Eberli FR, et al. Abnormal coronary vasomotion during exercise in patients with normal coronary arteries and reduced coronary flow reserve. Circulation 1989;79:516–527.
72. Greenberg MA, Grose RM, Neuburger N, et al. Impaired coronary vasodilator responsiveness as a cause of lactate production during pacing-induced ischemia in patients with angina pectoris and normal coronary arteries. J Am Coll Cardiol 1987;9:743–751.
73. Quyyumi AA, Cannon RO, Panza JA, et al. Endothelial dysfunction in patients with chest pain and normal coronary arteries. Circulation 1992;86:1864–1871.
74. Lanza GA, Cianflone D, Buffon A, et al. Therapy of microvascular angina. Cardiologia 1993;38:169–179.
75. Peduzzi P, Hultgren HN. Effect of medical vs surgical treatment on symptoms in stable angina pectoris. The Veterans Administration Cooperative Study of Surgery for Coronary Arterial Occlusive Disease. Circulation 1979;60:888–899.
76. European Coronary Surgery Study Group. Coronary-artery bypass surgery in stable angina pectoris: survival at two years. Lancet 1979;1:889–893.

77. Myers WO, Marshfield WI, Gersh BJ, et al. Medical versus early surgical therapy in patients with triple-vessel disease and mild angina pectoris: a CASS registry study of survival. Ann Thorac Surg 1987;44:471–486.
78. RITA Trial Participants. Coronary angioplasty versus coronary artery bypass surgery: the Randomised Intervention Treatment of Angina (RITA) trial. Lancet 1993;341:573–580.
79. Hamm CW, Reimers J, Ischinger, et al. A randomized study of coronary angioplasty compared with bypass surgery in patients with symptomatic multivessel coronary disease. German Angioplasty Bypass Surgery Investigation. N Engl J Med 1994;331: 1037–1043.
80. Parisi AF, Folland ED, Hartigan P, on behalf of the Veterans Affairs ACME Investigators. A comparison of angioplasty with medical therapy in the treatment of single-vessel coronary artery disease. N Engl J Med 1992;326:10–16.
81. Cannon RO III, Quyyumi AA, Schenke WH, et al. Abnormal cardiac sensitivity in patients with chest pain and normal coronary arteries. J Am Coll Cardiol 1990;16: 1359–1366.
82. Cannon R. Diagnosis and management of microvascular angina. Primary Cardiology 1990;16:15, 16, 21–23.
83. Wettervik C, Claes G, Drott C, et al. Endoscopic transthoracic sympathectomy for severe angina. Lancet 1995;345:97–98.

CHAPTER 6

# Management of the Acute Phase of Myocardial Infarction and Unstable Angina

Joseph S. Alpert, MD

Myocardial infarction is common in hospitalized patients in technically advanced countries. Approximately 1 million individuals in the United States each year suffer a myocardial infarction (MI). It has been estimated that an average man in North America has approximately a 20% chance of suffering either MI or sudden death (secondary to severe arteriosclerotic heart disease but without acute MI) by age 65 (1). Acute mortality for MI ranges from 5–95%, depending on a variety of demographic and clinical factors. The average hospital mortality is 7–15%. Recently a decline in coronary artery disease–associated mortality has been noted in the United States (2). Possible causes for this observed decline in mortality rate include improved diagnosis and therapy, declining incidence of acute MI, or changes in the affected population.

## ACUTE MYOCARDIAL INFARCTION

Myocardial infarction is myocardial cell death or necrosis resulting from ischemia, secondary to total or near total obstruction of a coronary artery. Coronary arterial obstruction is most often the result of atherosclerosis. Coronary spasm appears to play a role in the initiation of coronary thrombosis in many individuals.

### Pathophysiology of Acute Ischemic Syndromes

In the early years of this century, two Russian physicians, Obraztsov and Strazhesko, realized that coronary arterial thrombosis led to acute MI (1). Shortly thereafter, Herrick made similar observations in the United States (1). Since these initial descriptions, enormous efforts have been expended to understand the pathophysiology of acute MI and its attendant complications.

Although contested in the past, it is now generally agreed that coronary arterial thrombosis is the event that initiates MI. Coronary thrombi are approximately 1 cm in length and are composed of platelets, fibrin, erythrocytes, and leukocytes (2).

Early thrombi are usually nonocclusive and are composed primarily of platelets. Such early thrombi usually overlie a newly generated ulcer or fissure in a long-standing atherosclerotic plaque (3). This fissuring or ulceration of the plaque exposes underlying thrombogenic material to the circulating blood with resultant thrombogenesis. Once thrombus formation is initiated, a series of dynamic reactions is set into motion, with endogenous thrombolysis opposing thrombogenesis. If thrombogenesis prevails, a thrombus totally occludes the coronary arterial lumen.

The process that causes a previously stable atherosclerotic plaque to rupture, fissure, or ulcerate is currently under intense investigation.

## Pathophysiology and Pathology of Acute MI

A number of hypotheses have been suggested to explain the cause of plaque disruption, including the following: (1) coronary arterial vasospasm, (2) stress fracture of the plaque secondary to repetitive bending during ventricular systole, (3) injury to coronary arterial vasa vasorum with resultant intramural hemorrhage or plaque necrosis, or (4) platelet aggregation with release of thromboxanes and other vasoactive substances (2–8). All of these processes may be operative simultaneously or sequentially.

In summary, angiographic, angioscopic, and pathologic studies have repeatedly documented that patients with acute ischemic syndromes (unstable angina, acute MI) have eccentric, irregular lesions in the involved coronary artery. These lesions represent plaque fissures with overlying partially occlusive thrombus. A sequence of events involving coronary arterial vasospasm, platelet activation, and thrombogenesis leads to ever-increasing coronary arterial obstruction. If the intrinsic thrombolytic system fails to counterbalance the forces favoring thrombogenesis, total arterial obstruction results, leading to myocardial ischemia and eventually necrosis.

A number of environmental factors also are apparently involved in the genesis of the coronary arterial events just described. A recent respiratory viral infection is a common precursor of acute MI (9, 10). Moreover, there is a circadian rhythm present in the occurrence of MI: the onset of infarction is most frequent during the early morning hours and least frequent in the evening (11). Platelet aggregatory activity is also increased in the early morning hours, again supporting the role of platelets in the onset of acute MI (12).

After experimental infarction in dogs, the first 7 days of healing are associated with expansion of the infarct zone and dilatation of the left ventricular cavity (13). Thereafter, the infarct zone contracts and thins as collagen is deposited. Similar changes have been observed in humans following acute MI (14–16). Marked infarct expansion and left ventricular cavity dilatation are associated with a poor prognosis, (13). Noninfarcted zones develop volume-overload hypertrophy, thereby further contributing to remodeling of the left ventricle after acute infarction (15). Large infarcts are more likely to expand than small infarcts (16). Expansion of infarction is the result of slippage of intramural fibers within the infarct zone. In addition, infarct expansion contributes to left ventricular aneurysm formation.

Dissolution of coronary arterial thrombus by fibrinolytic agents has become the standard of early therapy for patients with acute MI. The principle of therapy applied here is to eradicate myocardial ischemia as quickly as possible by reopening the obstructed coronary artery. Thrombolytic and associated anticoagulant therapy are discussed extensively in Chapters 8 and 9. Agents aimed at reducing infarct size by diminishing myocardial ischemia are termed *antiischemic*. These pharmaceuticals work by decreasing myocardial oxygen demand (i.e., β-blockers, nitrates) or by improving collateral blood flow (i.e., nitrates, calcium channel blockers); they are discussed in Chapters 4 and 7. The latter agents are employed in many patients regardless of whether they have received prior thrombolytic therapy. This chapter will examine a wide variety of therapeutic interventions, including thrombolytic and antiischemic agents, that are employed in the acute phase of MI and unstable angina (see Chapter 8 for additional information).

## Management of MI

Prognosis after MI is related to the quantity of surviving, functional myocardium. When 40% of the left ventricle is destroyed (by one or more infarcts), cardiogenic shock usually develops. Hospital therapy for MI focuses on the following three therapeutic principles: (1) reestablish myocardial blood flow, (2) decrease the work of the myocardium in order to decrease ischemia and potential infarct extension, and (3) prevent and eradicate life-threatening arrhythmias.

The cornerstone of modern therapy for acute MI is thrombolysis. Reestablishing myocardial blood flow abolishes ischemia and decreases myocardial necrosis. A number of large, randomized trials have confirmed the efficacy of thrombolytic therapy (17–20). Table 6.1 summarizes commonly employed protocols for streptokinase, anisoylated plasminogen streptokinase activator complex (APSAC), and tissue plasminogen activator in patients with acute MI.

Alleviation of pain is also important in patients with ischemic heart disease, since discomfort leads to activation of the sympathetic nervous system with resultant increase in the determinants of myocardial oxygen consumption (heart rate, blood pressure, and myocardial contractility). Moreover, sympathetic nervous stimulation of the heart may lead to life-threatening ventricular arrhythmias. Ischemic pain is usually relieved by coronary arterial reperfusion, secondary to thrombolytic therapy. Residual myocardial necrotic pain can be relieved with a variety of agents. Reassurance and gentle psychological support should be given to all MI patients, as this alone may help to relieve discomfort. In addition to nitrate therapy (see below), narcotic analgesics (morphine or meperidine) relieve the discomfort of myocardial ischemia and necrosis. These agents are administered intravenously, slowly, and in small repeated doses (morphine, 2–5 mg; meperidine, 25–30 mg). Repeat doses may be given at intervals of

**Table 6.1**
**Coronary Thrombolysis Protocols**

Patients should fulfill the following criteria for coronary thrombolysis:

1. Chest pain at rest compatible with acute myocardial ischemia for less than 12 hours.
2. Electrocardiogram that reveals one of the following findings:
   A. New or presumably new ST segment elevation >0.1 mV present in 2 of 3 inferior leads or 2 of 6 precordial leads or in leads 1 and AVL. ST segment elevation is measured 0.02 sec after the S wave.
   B. New or presumably new Q wave of 0.03 seconds' duration and >0.2 mV depth.
   C. Left bundle branch block or idioventricular pacemaker.

**Intracoronary streptokinase** is administered in the cardiac catheterization laboratory after angiography. Intracoronary streptokinase is given as a slow bolus (20,000 U) followed by a dose of 6000 U/minutes for 90 minutes directly into the thrombosed artery. Intracoronary streptokinase is made up by adding 5 mL of saline to 250,000 U of drug to make a reconstituted solution of 50,000 U/mL. A solution of 2000 U/mL is prepared by the addition of 8 mL (400,000 U) streptokinase to 192 mL of saline. With this solution the initial bolus is 10 mL and the intracoronary infusion rate is 3 mL/minute for 90 minutes through a constant infusion pump.

**Intravenous streptokinase** is administered in the coronary care unit as follows: Six vials of streptokinase (250,000 U/vial) are reconstituted with 5 mL of normal saline per vial. The resulting 30 mL is added to 70 mL of saline to make a 100-mL solution with streptokinase at 10,000 U/mL. Over a 10-minute period 750,000 U (50 mL) are infused intravenously; after a pause of 15 minutes, the remaining 750,000 U (50 mL) are infused over 10 minutes.

**Tissue plasminogen activator** is administered according to the following protocol, which may change as new evidence is obtained: 15 mg immediately followed by 0.75 mg/kg body weight over 30 minutes (maximum dose = 1 50 mg), followed by 0.50 mg/kg body weight over 60 minutes (maximum dose = 35 mg): Total maximum dose = 100 mg.

**APSAC** (30 U) is administered as a 5-minute intravenous infusion.

10–15 minutes. The size of the initial dose depends on the size of the patient and the severity of the chest discomfort. Subsequent doses of narcotics may be larger or smaller than the initial dose, depending on the effect of the first dose. Great caution should be exercised in administering narcotic analgesics to patients with severe chronic obstructive pulmonary disease. Intramuscular injections of analgesic agents should not be given because they produce an elevation in serum enzyme values that may result in an incorrect diagnosis of myocardial necrosis.

Hypoxemia is common in patients with myocardial infarction and can accentuate myocardial ischemia. Thus, supplemental inspiratory oxygen is usually indicated in these individuals. Patients should receive supplemental oxygen at 2 L/minute by nasal prongs. Arterial blood gas levels should be determined approximately 5–10 minutes after the initiation of oxygen therapy. If the $PO_2$ in the arterial blood sample is less than 80 mm

Hg, the delivery of supplemental oxygen should be increased to 4 L/minute, and measurement of arterial blood gas levels should be repeated 5–10 minutes later. If the arterial $PO_2$ is still less than 80 mm Hg, supplemental oxygen should be delivered by face mask rather than by nasal prongs. In severely hypoxemic patients, such as those with pulmonary edema, oxygen supplementation should be initiated by the face mask route. Failure to obtain adequate arterial $PO_2$ values with face mask oxygen delivery should result in a switch to a rebreathing face mask apparatus for oxygen supplementation. Oxygen therapy should continue at least as long as the patient is in the coronary care unit and possibly until the fourth or fifth day after infarction.

Hypertension not uncommonly complicates MI. Elevation of arterial blood pressure increases myocardial oxygen consumption unnecessarily. Measures should be taken to lower blood pressures exceeding 140/90 mm Hg.

Residual chest pain may itself lead to elevated blood pressure. Analgesics should be given repeatedly every 10–15 minutes in moderate doses (e.g., morphine, 5 mg) until pain is relieved. Pentazocine should be avoided because it can further elevate blood pressure. Patients who remain hypertensive (blood pressure more than 140/90 mm Hg by cuff) 30–60 minutes after admission to the hospital should be strongly considered for nitrate or β-blocker therapy, or both, if these agents have not already been administered. Commonly employed nitrate protocols include sublingual or chewable isosorbide dinitrate, 5 mg, or intravenous nitroglycerin (25–50 μg/minute); blood pressure should be rechecked in 5 minutes. Intravenous use of nitroglycerine is preferred when patients are refractory or require repeated doses of sublingual nitroglycerine. If an adequate hypotensive effect is obtained, the patient is placed on sublingual or oral isosorbide dinitrate or is continued on intravenous nitroglycerin at sufficient dosage to control the blood pressure. Vascular headaches associated with nitrate therapy can usually be suppressed with acetaminophen, aspirin, or narcotics. Oral antihypertensives (e.g., metoprolol, 25–50 mg twice daily) should be started at moderate doses and increased daily as required. Intravenous nitroprusside infusion is more effective for lowering blood pressure than is intravenous nitroglycerine. Important side effects that may occur as a result of nitroprusside therapy include elevated thiocyanate levels generated during prolonged therapy. Thiocyanate toxicity results in symptoms such as fatigue, anorexia, disorientation, psychosis, and muscle spasms. If toxic symptoms occur or thiocyanate levels exceed 10 mg/100 mL, the drug should be discontinued.

Nitroprusside infusions are initiated at 15 μg/minute, and the drip rate is increased at intervals of 3–5 minutes until the arterial pressure drops to normal levels (systolic blood pressure 100–120 mm Hg). It is rarely necessary to infuse more than 200 μg/minute. Patients who require nitroprusside therapy should be started concomitantly on more aggressive oral antihypertensive drugs if this has not already been done. Oral agents include β-blockers, calcium channel blockers, and angiotensin-converting enzyme (ACE) inhibitors. Clonidine may be contraindicated in the period immediately after infarction (particularly after nitroprusside infusions), since significant hypotension can occur with the combination of these two medicines in the setting of acute MI.

In patients with Q-wave MI, the ACE inhibitor captopril (25–50 mg orally twice daily) has been shown to reduce infarct expansion, congestive heart failure, and long-term mortality in patients with left ventricular ejection fraction 40% or less (see Chapter 12 for additional details).

Episodes of spontaneous or provoked ischemic pain after MI are worrisome since they imply threatened, but as yet viable, residual myocardium. Such individuals have frequently sustained a "non–Q-wave" infarct. Patients with prolonged episodes of ischemic discomfort but without infarction (unstable angina) are similar in many ways to patients with non–Q-wave myocardial infarction. These individuals should receive aggressive antiischemic therapy. Numerous studies have documented the benefit of such therapy (21–26).

β-Blockers, calcium channel-blockers, nitrate therapy, or some combination of these agents should be strongly considered. All anginal episodes should be promptly treated with sublingual or increasing intravenous doses of nitroglycerine. Typical doses (see also Chapters 4 and 7) are propranolol, 20–60 mg orally every 6 hours; metoprolol, 50–100 mg twice daily; verapamil, 80 mg every 8 hours; diltiazem, 60–120 mg every 8 hours; and isosorbide dinitrate, 5–20 mg chewed or sublingually every 2–3 hours. Diltiazem and verapamil should not be used in patients with signs of left ventricular failure.

Intravenous nitroglycerin therapy is administered either by continuous infusion or by intermittent intravenous bolus, the former representing the more popular mode. Continuous infusion is generally begun at 25–50 μg/minute and increased by 10–20 μg/minute every 5–10 minutes until the desired hemodynamic response (drop in systemic or left ventricular filling pressure) or clinical response (relief of chest pain, or reversal of ischemic ECG changes, or both) occurs.

## UNSTABLE ANGINA AND CORONARY ARTERY SPASM

The syndrome of unstable angina consists of an accelerating pattern of ischemic chest pain and identifies a patient subset at substantial risk for MI and sudden death. Patients with unstable angina should receive emergency therapeutic intervention in order to reduce morbidity and mortality.

Not all cardiologists agree as to the appropriate criteria or even the best name for unstable angina or coronary insufficiency (also called *crescendo angina, preinfarction angina,* or *intermediate syndrome*). Patients with unstable angina have recurring anginal chest pain at rest with episodes lasting 20–30 minutes or more. At least one episode occurring within 7 days of the current hospitalization (or during it) is required in order to make the diagnosis. The pain is usually more severe than that in exertional angina. The anginal episode may respond to nitrates (usually more than a single dose) but frequently requires opiates for relief. There are no precipitating factors (e.g., heavy meals, emotion). Patients who simply have a change in the pattern of previously stable angina, angina of recent onset, or angina decubitus are not included in this category unless they meet the preceding criteria. The latter categories of patients, however, frequently have severe coronary artery disease. In the past, patients with unstable angina were frequently considered to have "severe coronary insufficiency."

At least one episode of pain is usually associated with characteristic ischemic ST-T changes on the electrocardiogram (ECG). Many patients will have fluctuating ECG changes; others will develop persistent changes. Serum enzyme changes are not diagnostic of MI.

In recent years, it has become clear that patients with so-called non–Q-wave myocardial infarction (ECG changes limited to the ST-T segments with elevated peak serum CK values) resemble patients with unstable angina with respect to prognosis, complications, and natural history (27, 28). It is my practice to treat such patients in the same way as patients with unstable angina. In fact, there is evidence that many, if not most, episodes of unstable angina are associated with "microinfarction." Hence, these patients should be treated seriously by the practitioner.

Patients with unstable angina often experience infarction, arrhythmias, and even sudden death during the first 6 months after the onset of this syndrome. The cause of episodes of unstable angina resembles that of acute MI (discussed earlier) with plaque rupture and coronary thrombus formation. Activated platelets are also involved in the genesis of this entity. Severe myocardial ischemia develops, with each episode of unstable angina often leading to prolonged myocardial dysfunction, the syndrome of "stunned myocardium." Myocardial stunning that occurs following reperfusion after MI is reversible. Effective therapy is mandatory and should be delivered without delay.

### *Management*

Effective therapy can include various combinations of the following pharmacological agents: calcium channel blockers, β-blockers, and nitrates (29–31). Careful attention should also be paid to coronary artery risk factor reduction (smoking, hypertension, adverse lifestyle patterns) and the patient's psychological state. Thrombolytic therapy for unstable angina has been carefully evaluated in the Thrombolysis in Myocardial Infarction (TIMI)-3 trial; thrombolytic therapy was not beneficial in the patients studied. Intravenous nitroglycerin is extremely efficacious in controlling episodes of unstable angina. Some cardiologists start all patients with unstable angina on intravenous nitroglycerin at the same time that they initiate oral β-blocker, nitrate, and calcium channel blocker therapy (Table 6.2). When an adequate dose of oral medication is achieved, intravenous nitroglycerin is tapered and discontinued.

Some cardiologists avoid using β-blockers in patients with resting angina because of observations suggesting that episodes of unstable angina in these patients are the result of coronary arterial vasospasm (32). These cardiologists prescribe calcium channel blockers and nitrates only. Other cardiologists treat these patients with β-blockers in combination with nitrates or calcium channel blockers, or both (see Chapters 4 and 5 for details). Patients whose anginal attacks continue at rest or with minimal exertion or who have a clearly positive modified exercise test are candidates for catheterization followed by coronary artery bypass surgery or coronary angioplasty. The AHCPR recently presented a number of guidelines for the management of patients with unstable angina (see Table 6.2) (33). Since patients with unstable angina usually have fresh thrombus overlying a ruptured coronary arterial atherosclerotic plaque, use of heparin and aspirin represents a rational therapeutic approach (see below).

**Table 6.2**
**Pharmacologic Management of Unstable Angina**

| Mechanism | Treatment | Dose | Comments |
|---|---|---|---|
| Plaque rupture | Aspirin | 40–325 mg/day | |
| Platelet adhesion and aggregation | Heparin | 50 U/kg i.v. followed by 10–25 U/kg/h i.v. according to PTT | |
| Vasospasm; increased arterial blood pressure | Nifedipine | 10–30 mg t.i.d | Should be combined with a β-blocker |
| | Verapamil | 240–360 mg/day | Contraindicated for overt CHF or symptomatic bradyarrhythmias |
| ↓$M\dot{V}O_2$ | Diltiazem | 60–120 mg q.i.d. | |
| | Nitroglycerin | 10–200 (or more) μg/min i.v. | |
| | Esmolol | 500 μg/kg/min i.v. loading dose followed by 25–300 μg/kg/min | |
| | Propranolol | 1–10 mg i.v.; 10–100 mg t.i.d. p.o. | |
| | Metoprolol | 5–15 mg i.v.; 50–100 mg b.i.d. p.o. | |
| | Atenolol | 5–15 mg i.v.; 25–50 mg q.d. p.o. | |

b.i.d. = twice a day; bpm = beats/minute; CHF = congestive heart failure; h = hour; i.v. = intravenously; min = minute; $MVO_2$ = myocardial oxygen consumption; p.o. = orally; PTT = partial thromboplastin time; q.d. = every day; q.i.d. = four times a day; t.i.d. = three times a day.

In all patients with unstable angina, potentially reversible factors must be sought and treated, if identified. Conditions that result in increased cardiac output may result in an imbalance in oxygen demand and supply, with resulting angina. Such conditions include hyperthyroidism, anemia, or fever. Treating these conditions will frequently result in a marked improvement in the unstable anginal syndrome.

Conditions that increase left ventricular wall tension and hence the ventricular workload can also cause unstable angina, e.g., congestive heart failure. Elevation of arterial blood pressure increases myocardial oxygen demand and may also lead to unstable angina. By controlling systemic hypertension associated with angina, the physician can expect a decrease in myocardial oxygen demand and an improvement in anginal symptoms.

**Nitrate Therapy.** As noted earlier, nitrates are the mainstay of treatment for unstable angina. Nitrates come in three major forms, nitroglycerin, isosorbide dinitrate, and isosorbide mononitrate. These forms can be delivered in a variety of ways including sublingual, chewable, oral (short acting and long acting), transbuccal (34), intravenous, transcutaneous, and oral spray (35). Nitrates are believed to work by increasing blood flow to ischemic areas of myocardium secondary to coronary arterial dilatation and by systemic venous pooling, thereby decreasing ventricular preload and thus leading to a reduction in systolic arterial blood pressure (36–40).

Sublingual nitroglycerin is employed initially in the treatment of an acute anginal attack. Sublingual nitroglycerin comes in different tablet sizes: 0.3, 0.4, and 0.6 mg. The dose used is usually based on the individual's previous exposure. It is often best to treat patients with unstable angina with intravenous nitroglycerin. This agent is easy to administer, extremely effective, and can be titrated minute to minute. Initially patients receive 25–50 μg/minute, which is increased by 10–20 μg/minute every 3–5 minutes until pain is relieved or mean arterial pressure drops 20 mm Hg or below 70 mm Hg. Doses as high as 1 mg/minute can be employed. Not all patients receiving intravenous nitroglycerin require a pulmonary artery (Swan-Ganz) catheter; it is used only if there is concern about left ventricular function. Patients with systolic arterial blood pressure less than 120–130 mm Hg should be considered for intraarterial pressure monitoring. Patients on long-term intravenous nitroglycerin may develop methemoglobinemia, which may result in an exacerbation of angina. Methemoglobinemia should be considered when a patient has been on intravenous nitroglycerin for a prolonged period of time; if it does occur, administration of folic acid or other reducing agents can counterbalance this effect. For a discussion of nitrate tolerance and its avoidance, see Chapter 7.

**β-Blocker Therapy.** Along with nitrates, β-blockers and calcium channel antagonists form the mainstay of treatment for unstable angina.

The blocking of β-adrenergic receptors results in a reduction in heart rate, a diminution in myocardial contractility, and a reduction in blood pressure leading to a reduction in myocardial oxygen demand. Another potential benefit of β-blockers is their antiarrhythmic effect, which may be important in the long-term protective effects of this drug class in patients with ischemic heart disease (41–50) (See Table 6.2).

**Calcium Channel Blocker Therapy.** Another class of drugs useful in the treatment of unstable angina is the calcium channel blockers (Table 6.2). Structurally these drugs are quite diverse; thus, they act with varying selectivity on different organs and tissues. Hemodynamic effects include a reduction in arterial blood pressure, an increase in cardiac output, and in some individuals a reflex increase in heart rate. In patients with congestive heart failure, diltiazem and verapamil should be avoided. Each of the drugs mentioned above is effective in the treatment of unstable angina; the choice of drug is usually based on concomitant therapy and the presence or absence of underlying disease. Occasionally, a combination of two calcium channel blockers may be beneficial when a single drug is unable to stabilize the patient. When two calcium channel blockers are used, the physician should employ a combination of a dihydropteridine, e.g., nifedipine or nicardipine, and either verapamil or diltiazem.

Because of the possible role of thrombus formation in the etiology of acute MI, a strong argument can be made for using anticoagulants in patients with unstable angina in an attempt to limit thrombus production (Table 6.2). Aspirin and heparin have both been shown to be of benefit in patients with unstable angina. In patients awaiting bypass surgery aspirin may be discontinued several days before surgery. Heparin is continued up to the time of surgery.

Heparin therapy for unstable angina and acute myocardial infarction seeks to stabilize the ruptured atherosclerotic plaque and to prevent rethrombosis once coronary arterial patency has been restored with thrombolytic therapy. Anticoagulation also seeks to prevent thrombotic complications such as deep venous thrombosis and arterial embolism from left ventricular mural thrombi (51–55). Intravenous heparin infusion is now considered routine for the overwhelming majority of patients with acute MI and unstable angina.

**Aspirin Therapy.** Aspirin therapy is likewise highly efficacious in preventing rethrombosis after thrombolytic therapy for acute MI. The prognosis of patients with unstable angina is also favorably influenced by aspirin therapy. Most authorities prefer 325 mg of aspirin per day, although beneficial effects have been observed with doses as low as 40 mg/day (56). Recent studies support the concept that aspirin or heparin alone is sufficient for patients with unstable angina (57).

When medical therapy fails to control unstable angina, more aggressive nonpharmacologic interventions must be considered. Intraaortic balloon counterpulsation (IABP) is effective in controlling angina in patients with persistent pain despite maximal β-blocker, nitrate, and calcium channel blocker therapy. Intraaortic balloon counterpulsation provides two important physiologic benefits: increased coronary perfusion pressure and decreased left ventricular workload. In patients who are hemodynamically unstable, intraaortic balloon counterpulsation permits procedures such as cardiac catheterization and angiography to be performed and allows time for surgical or angioplasty intervention if the coronary anatomy is suitable.

The management of patients with unstable angina was studied by the National Cooperative Randomized Study on Unstable Angina. This study prospectively randomized patients with unstable angina to medical and surgical therapeutic groups. The results indicate that patients with unstable angina can be treated initially with intensive medical therapy. In most patients, pain is adequately controlled with no increase in early mortality or myocardial infarction rate as compared with surgically treated patients. In general, patients with impaired left ventricular function or multivessel coronary artery disease, or both, fare better with surgical as compared with medical therapy (31).

**Interventional Therapy.** Emergency coronary bypass surgery or angioplasty is reserved for a small group of patients who have unstable angina and who fall in a high risk subgroup or who fail to respond to initial medical therapy. Because urgent mechanical intervention is not often needed, angiography is often deferred as well, until the patient has stabilized. Coronary angiography is performed emergently when medical therapy is failing and intervention is being considered for control of pain.

In summary, prevention of acute MI and minimization of cardiac mortality remain the goals in the management of unstable angina. The mainstay of treatment is medical: nitrates, β-blockers, calcium channel blockers, and anticoagulation (aspirin, heparin, or both). In some patients, nonpharmacologic treatment will be needed in the form of intraaortic balloon counterpulsation. In a small percent of patients, all attempts at pain control will be partially or totally ineffective. In this subgroup of patients, urgent cardiac catheterization and coronary angiography are needed. Once the coronary anatomy is known, a decision about angioplasty or coronary bypass surgery can be made.

---

## REFERENCES

1. Muller JE. Coronary artery thrombosis: historical aspects. J Am Coll Cardiol 1983; 3:893.
2. Roberts WC. Coronary arteries in fatal acute myocardial infarction. Circulation 1972;45:215.
3. Sherman CT, Litivack F, Grundfest W, et al. Coronary angioscopy in patients with unstable angina pectoris. N Engl J Med 1986;315:913.
4. Dalen JE, Ockene JS, Alpert JS. Coronary spasm, coronary thrombosis and myocardial infarction: a hypothesis concerning the pathophysiology of acute myocardial infarction. Am Heart J 1982;104:1119.

5. Mehta J, Mehta P, Feldman RL. Thromboxane release in coronary artery disease: spontaneous versus pacing-induced angina. Am Heart J 1984; 107:286.
6. Bush LR, Campbell WB, Kern K, et al. The effects of alpha adrenergic and serotonergic receptor antagonists on cyclic blood flow alterations in stenosed canine coronary arteries. Circ Res 1984;55:642.
7. Lewis HD, Davis JW, Archibald DG, et al. Protective effects of aspirin against acute myocardial infarction and death in men with unstable angina. N Engl J Med 1983;309:396.
8. Barger AC, Beeuwkes R, Lainey LL, et al. Hypothesis: vasa vasorum and neovascularization of human coronary arteries, a possible role in the pathophysiology of atherosclerosis. N Engl J Med 1984;310:175.
9. Spodick DH, Flessas AP, Johnson MM. Association of acute respiratory symptoms with onset of acute myocardial infarction: prospective investigation of 150 consecutive patients and matched control patients. Am J Cardiol 1984;53:481.
10. Spodick DH. Acute viral (and other) infection in the onset, pathogenesis, and mimicry of acute myocardial infarction. Am J Med 1986;81:661.
11. Muller JE, Stone PH, Turi ZG, et al. Circadian variation in the frequency of onset of acute myocardial infarction. N Engl J Med 1985;313:1315.
12. Toffler GH, Brezinski D, Schafer AI, et al. Concurrent morning increase in platelet aggregability and the risk of myocardial infarction and sudden cardiac death. N Engl J Med 1987;316:1514.
13. Jugdutt BI, Amy RW. Healing after myocardial infarction in the dog: changes in infarct hydroxyproline and topography. J Am Coll Cardiol 1986;7:91.
14. Eaton LW, Weiss JL, Bulkley BH, et al. Regional cardiac dilatation after acute myocardial infarction. N Engl J Med 1979;300:57.
15. McKay RG, Pfeffer MA, Pasternak RC, et al. Left ventricular remodeling after myocardial infarction: a corollary to infarct expansion. Circulation 1986;74:693.
16. Pirolo JS, Hutchins GM, Moore GW. Infarct expansion: pathologic analysis of 204 patients with a single myocardial infarct. J Am Coll Cardiol 1986;7:349.
17. Midgette AS, O'Connor GT, Baron JA, et al. Effect of intravenous streptokinase on early mortality in patients with suspected acute myocardial infarction: a meta-analysis by anatomic location of infarction. Ann Intern Med 1990;113:961.
18. Mueller HS, Cohen LS, Braunwald E, et al. Predictors of early morbidity and mortality after thrombolytic therapy of acute myocardial infarction. Analyses of patient subgroups in the TIMI Trial, phase II. Circulation 1992;85: 1254.
19. Muller DWM, Topol EJ. Selection of patients with acute myocardial infarction for thrombolytic therapy. Ann Intern Med 1990;113:949.
20. The Gusto Angiographic Investigators. The effects of tissue plasminogen activator, streptokinase, or both, on coronary artery patency, ventricular function, and survival after acute myocardial infarction. N Engl J Med 1993;329:1615.
21. Gerstenblith G, Ouyand P, Achuff SC, et al. Nifedipine in unstable angina: a double-blind, randomized trial. N Engl J Med 1982;306:885.
22. Mehta J, Pepine CJ, Day M, et al. Short-term efficacy of oral verapamil in rest angina—a double-blind placebo-controlled trial in CCU patients. Am J Med 1981; 71:977.
23. Parodi O, Maseri A, Simonetti I. Management of unstable angina at rest by verapamil: a double-blind, cross-over study in the coronary care unit. Br Heart J 1979;41:167.
24. Gottlieb SO, Weisfeldt ML, Ouyand P, et al. Effect of the addition of propranolol to therapy with nifedipine for unstable angina pectoris: a randomized, double-blind, placebo-controlled trial. Circulation 1986;73:331.
25. Parodi O, Simonetti I, Michelassi C, et al. Comparison of verapamil and propranolol therapy for angina pectoris at rest: a randomized multiple-crossover, controlled trial in the coronary care unit. Am J Cardiol 1986;57:899.
26. Singh B H, Nademanee K. Beta-adrenergic blockade in unstable angina pectoris. Am J Cardiol 1986;57:992.
27. Armstrong PW, Chiong MA, Parker JO. The spectrum of unstable angina: prognostic role of serum creatine kinase determination. Am J Cardiol 1982;49:1849.

28. Bertolasi CA, Tronge JE, Carreno CA, et al. Unstable angina—prospective and randomized study of its evolution, with and without surgery. Am J Cardiol 1974;33:201.
29. Crea F, Deanfield F, Crean P, et al. Effects of verapamil in preventing early postinfarction angina and reinfarction. Am J Cardiol 1985;55:900.
30. Gerstenblith G, Ouyand P, Achuff SC, et al. Nifedipine in unstable angina—a double-blind, randomized trial. N Engl J Med 1992;306:885.
31. Unstable Angina Pectoris Study Group. Unstable angina pectoris: national cooperative study group to compare surgical and medical therapy. II. In-hospital experience and initial follow-up results in patients with one, two and three vessel disease. Am J Cardiol 1978;42:839.
32. Parodi O, Uthurralt N, Severi S, et al. Transient reduction of regional myocardial perfusion during angina at rest with S-T segment depression or normalization of negative T waves. Circulation 1981;63:1238.
33. Diagnosing and Managing Unstable Angina. (AHCPR Publication No. 94-0603.) Washington, DC: US Department of Health and Human Services, 1993.
34. Bussmann WD, Passek D, Seidel W, et al. Reduction of CK and CK-MB indexes of infarct size by intravenous nitroglycerin. Circulation 1981;63:615.
35. Flaherty JC, Becker LC, Bulkley BH, et al. A randomized prospective trial of intravenous nitroglycerin in patients with acute myocardial infarction. Circulation 1983;68:576.
36. Jugdutt BL, Sussex BA, Warnica JW, et al. Persistent reduction in left ventricular asynergy in patients with acute myocardial infarction by intravenous infusion of nitroglycerin. Circulation 1983;68:1264.
37. Jaffe AS, Geltman EM, Tiefenbrunn AJ, et al. Reduction of infarct size in patients with inferior infarction with intravenous glyceryl trinitrate. A randomized study. Br Heart J 1983;49:452.
38. Jugdutt BL, Warnica JW. Intravenous nitroglycerin therapy to limit myocardial infarct size, expansion, and complications. Effect of timing, dosage and infarct location. Circulation 1988;78:906.
39. Yusuf S, Collins R, MacMahon S, et al. Effect of intravenous nitrates on mortality in acute myocardial infarction: an overview of the randomized trials. Lancet 1988;2:1088.
40. Curfman GD, Heinsimer JA, Lozner LC, et al. Intravenous nitroglycerin in the treatment of spontaneous angina pectoris. A prospective, randomized trial. Circulation 1983;67:276.
41. Wilcox RG, Roland JM, Banks DC, et al. Randomized trial comparing propranolol with atenolol in immediate treatment of suspected myocardial infarction. Br Med J 1980;280:885.
42. Wilcox RG, Rowley JM, Hampton JR, et al. Randomized placebo-controlled trial comparing propranolol with atenolol in immediate treatment of suspected myocardial infarction. Lancet 1980;2:765.
43. Andersen MP, Bechsgaard P,Fredrickson J, et al. Effect of alprenolol on mortality among patients with definite or suspected acute myocardial infarction, preliminary results. Lancet 1979;2:865.
44. Hjalmarson A, Herlitz J, Holmberg S, et al. The Goteborg Metoprolol Trial: effects on mortality and morbidity in acute myocardial infarction. Circulation 1983;67(Suppl I):26.
45. Yusuf S, Sleight P, Rossi P, et al. Reduction in infarct size, arrhythmias and chest pain by early intravenous beta-blockade in suspected acute myocardial infarction. Circulation 1983;67(Suppl I):32.
46. The International Collaborative Study Group. Reduction of infarct size with the early use of timolol in acute myocardial infarction. N Engl J Med 1984;310:9.
47. Norris RM, Barnaby PF, Brown MD, et al. Prevention of ventricular fibrillation during acute myocardial infarction by intravenous propranolol. Lancet 1984;2:883.
48. Roberts R, Croft C, Gold HK, et al. Effect of propranolol on myocardial infarct size in a randomized blinded multicenter trial. N Engl J Med 1984;311:218.
49. The MIAMI Trial Research Group, Metoprolol in Acute Myocardial Infarction (MIAMI). A randomized placebo-controlled international trial. Eur Heart J 1985;6:199.

50. Salathia KS, Barber JM, McIlmoyle EL, et al. Very early intervention with metoprolol in suspected acute myocardial infarction. Eur Heart J 1985;6:190.
51. Chalmers TC, Matta RJ, Smith H Jr, et al. Evidence favoring the use of anticoagulants in the hospital phase of acute myocardial infarction. N Engl J Med 1977; 297:1091.
52. Mitchell JRA. Anticoagulants in coronary heart disease—retrospect and prospect. Lancet 1981;1:257.
53. Modan R, Shani M, Schor S, et al. Reduction of hospital mortality from acute myocardial infarction by anticoagulant therapy. N Engl J Med 1979;292:1359.
54. Tonascia J, Gordis L, Schmerler H. Retrospective evidence favoring use of anticoagulants for myocardial infarction. N Engl J Med 1975;292:1362.
55. Szklo M, Tonascia JA, Goldbert R, et al. Additional data favoring use of anticoagulant therapy in myocardial infarction: a population-based study. JAMA 1979; 242:1261.
56. Willard JE, Lange RA, Hollis LD. The use of aspirin in ischemic heart disease. N Engl J Med 1992;327:175.
57. Dalen JE, Hirsh J, eds. Third ACCP Consensus Conference on Antithrombotic Therapy. Chest 1992;102 (Suppl):15.

# CHAPTER 7

## Long-Term Management and Secondary Prevention After Myocardial Infarction

Prakash C. Deedwania, MD

Coronary artery disease (CAD) remains a leading cause of death and disability in industrialized nations. Acute myocardial infarction (MI) is one of the major sequelae of CAD, and it carries an adverse prognosis for life. Although there has been a remarkable decline (nearly 50%) in deaths due to CAD during the past two decades, the overall incidence of acute myocardial infarction in the United States has not decreased significantly (1). In the United States each year nearly 1.5 million Americans suffer from an acute MI, and of these, approximately 70% survive the acute event (2).

Considerable progress has been made in the treatment of the acute phase of MI, resulting in significant improvement in survival during this phase. Despite such progress, patients recovering from acute MI remain at increased risk (fourfold to eightfold increase) of reinfarction and sudden cardiac death during the post-MI period. It is estimated that nearly 50% of patients who develop MI have evidence of prior MI. Therefore, one of the most significant risk factors for future risk of MI is history of previous MI. In addition, survivors of MI also remain at increased risk of sudden cardiac death and have increased mortality in the postinfarction period (3–5). A large number of clinical investigations conducted during the past two decades have provided considerable insight regarding the natural history and various prognostic factors that determine survival after MI (3–11). Survivors of MI are a heterogeneous group of patients with varying prognoses and the need for further diagnostic workup and long-term management (3–6). The most important determinants of subsequent prognosis in survivors of MI are the extent and location of MI, left ventricular dysfunction, electrical instability of myocardium, and presence of residual ischemia (8–10).

During the past decade, considerable effort has been made to limit the infarct size by utilizing reperfusion therapy with thrombolytic agents (see Chapter 8). It is now well established that timely administration of thrombolytic agents is beneficial in limiting infarct size and improves subsequent prognosis. Recent data, however, indicate that in the United States only 20 to 30% of patients suffering from acute MI receive thrombolytic therapy. Consequently, the majority of patients surviving the acute phase of MI remain at risk of future coronary events and cardiac death. In this chapter, the practical issues involved in the long-term management of survivors of MI will be described first with subsequent discussion focusing on various therapeutic strategies available for secondary prevention after MI.

## LONG-TERM PROGNOSIS AND RISK STRATIFICATION AFTER MI

A large number of studies conducted during the last two decades have demonstrated that the long-term prognosis in survivors of acute MI varies considerably, with 1-year mortality rates ranging from 2% in the low-risk subset to up to 50% in the highest risk subset (9, 10). Because of this tremendous variability in the prognosis of survivors of MI, it is crucial to first stratify survivors of acute MI into various risk categories before considering therapeutic strategies most suitable for secondary prevention in the postinfarction period (3–5). As shown in Table 7.1, the most important determinants of long-term prognosis after an acute MI are degree of left ventricular dysfunction, presence of residual ischemia, and extent of electrical instability. Based on the results of noninvasive tests that are available for evaluation (Table 7.1) in the postinfarction period, the clinician should be able to stratify the survivors of MI into low-risk, intermediate-risk, or high-risk categories.

Because the status of left ventricular function is the single most powerful determinant of subsequent prognosis in stable patients after MI, it is

**Table 7.1**
**Determinants of Long-Term Prognosis After Myocardial Infarction and List of Diagnostic Tests Used in Postinfarction Period**

- Important Prognostic Factors in the Postinfarction Period
  - Left ventricular dysfunction
  - Residual myocardial ischemia
  - Electrical instability
- Common Diagnostic Tests for Risk Stratification in the Postinfarction Period
  - Evaluation of left ventricular function
    - Echocardiogram
    - Radionuclide ventriculogram
  - Evaluation for residual ischemia
    - Electrocardiogram (ECG) monitoring
      - Treadmill exercise test
      - Ambulatory ECG monitoring
    - Thallium scintigraphy
    - Stress echocardiography
    - Pharmacologic stress testing
    - Dipyridamole thallium scintigraphy
    - Dobutamine echocardiography
  - Evaluation of electrical instability
    - Holter monitoring
      - Arrhythmia detection
      - Heart rate variability
    - Signal-averaged ECG

generally recommended to first evaluate left ventricular systolic function by noninvasive measurement of left ventricular ejection fraction (LVEF) by an echocardiogram or a radionuclide ventriculogram. In general, patients with normal LVEF (40% or more) are considered to be at relatively low risk of mortality in the postinfarction period, especially if they have no evidence of residual ischemia on a symptom-limited treadmill exercise test (3, 4, 8–10). In contrast, the patients with left ventricular dysfunction (LVEF less than 40%) are at substantially increased risk of future coronary events and cardiac death (4, 7). It is, therefore, essential to further stratify these patients by evaluation for residual ischemia and electrical instability (3–6). Most experts in the field recommend a cardiac stress imaging study (such as exercise thallium scintigraphy or stress echocardiography) to define the presence and extent of residual myocardial ischemia (3, 10). If the results of stress imaging study reveal significant residual myocardial ischemia in patients with markedly compromised left ventricular function (i.e., LVEF less than 35%), most experts would recommend further evaluation by coronary angiography to better define the severity and extent of CAD (3). Because this group constitutes a high-risk subset, based on the anatomic severity of CAD, myocardial revascularization might indeed be required in many of these patients to reduce the risk of subsequent coronary events and cardiac death.

The largest number (more than 50%) of patients after MI, however, actually belong to the intermediate-risk category, which comprises patients who have some evidence of left ventricular dysfunction but who have minimal or no residual ischemia on stress testing (7). These patients seem to derive the most benefit from the treatment prescribed for secondary prevention after MI (11). In these patients various therapeutic strategies designed for cardioprotection after MI appear to be most cost-effective and provide the greatest long-term benefit. Because of the large size of this group of postinfarction patients and the obvious effectiveness of treatment prescribed for secondary prevention in these patients, it is important for the primary care physician to be familiar with the available therapies used for secondary prevention after MI and their usefulness. This is particularly important because not all available therapeutic choices are beneficial and cost-effective, and some drugs might even be harmful (11). Furthermore, the treatment prescribed for secondary prevention after MI generally needs to be administered for a long period of time, and with the evolution of health care reform, it is more than likely that a great majority of these patients will be cared for by the primary care provider and not the specialist.

## SECONDARY PREVENTION AFTER MI: WHAT IS IT AND WHY IS IT NEEDED?

Secondary prevention after MI can be best defined as the therapeutic strategy designed to enhance survival and reduce cardiac morbidity and mortality in survivors of MI. Because of the magnitude of the problem, during the last three decades a large number of clinical studies have been conducted to define the safest and most effective therapeutic modalities suitable for secondary prevention after MI. The results of these studies have provided a wide array of results that have been both exciting (e.g., cardioprotection with aspirin and β-blockers) and disappointing (e.g., adverse impact of antiarrhythmic drugs). These studies have taught us important lessons and emphasize the need for the clinician to be fully aware of the pros and cons of the various therapeutic choices available for secondary prevention after MI (11, 12).

Recent studies have also emphasized that, despite the well-documented cardioprotective effects of drugs such as β-blockers, aspirin, and angiotensin-converting enzyme (ACE) inhibitors, these drugs are not prescribed for many patients after MI (11–17). This might indeed be one of the reasons for recent observations indicating that, despite the remarkable improvement in short-term prognosis after MI observed during the past 30 years, no improvement in long-term prognosis after MI can be demonstrated (16, 17). Although some recent data indicated that there is a trend toward increased use of proven therapies for secondary prevention after MI, there is considerable room for improvement (12–15). Some of the recent statistics have indeed demonstrated that the use of aspirin and β-blockers after MI has increased in the last 5 years; however, there is still considerable underutilization of these drugs in the elderly, in women, and in high-risk patients with left ventricular dysfunction (11–15). It is important for clinicians to recognize that elderly and high-risk patients are the very patients in whom the benefit of these drugs (especially β-blockers and aspirin) is most evident; therefore, not prescribing these drugs in such patients is depriving them of good medical care. Clinicians also need to recognize that it is not only important to prescribe the appropriate therapy but also essential to emphasize the significance and benefit of such therapy to their patients through proper patient education. Recent studies have shown that adherence to prescribed therapy is much better with inpatient education, and it is an important determinant of subsequent survival in the postinfarction period (18, 19).

## CHOICES OF THERAPY FOR SECONDARY PREVENTION AFTER MI

During the past 25 years, a large number of clinical trials have been conducted to define the most effective therapeutic strategies for secondary prevention in survivors of MI. These studies have evaluated the role of β-blockers (20–31), calcium channel blockers (32–42), ACE inhibitors (43–53), antiplatelet agents and antithrombotic therapy (54–58), antiarrhythmic drugs (59–61), and risk factor modification, including the use of aggressive lipid-lowering therapy (62–71).

Despite the large number of studies and the huge investments made to conduct these trials, it is disappointing to note that there has been considerable delay in the clinical implementation of the findings and changes in physicians' practice patterns (72). In many cases even the experts have taken a long time to make specific recommendations for use of effective therapies (e.g., β-blockers), and in other cases (e.g., calcium channel blockers) clinicians have been using therapy not ever proven to be effective for secondary prevention after MI (11, 12, 72). Although a large number of review articles have been written on the subject of secondary prevention in survivors of MI, these reviews have lacked specific recommendations with clear directions for physicians to use in clinical practice (72). Because the survivors of MI constitute such a large group of patients who are encountered by the clinician on a frequent basis, it is crucial to clearly define the effects of various therapeutic strategies and establish the guidelines for use of effective therapies for secondary prevention after MI. In the following section, all of the major therapeutic choices that have been utilized for secondary prevention after MI will be discussed with special emphasis on the detailed description of current practice guidelines in this area.

## Role of β-Blockers in Secondary Prevention *After MI*

Several clinical trials have demonstrated that treatment with β-blockers provides unquestionable benefit in reducing the rate of reinfarction and cardiac death in survivors of MI (20–31). Many of these clinical trials have evaluated benefits of β-blocker therapy during the acute phase of MI (21–23) as well as in the period after MI (24–27). A recent analysis (20) of 27 available randomized clinical trials totaling approximately 27,000 patients indicated that treatment with β-blockers reduced mortality by 13% in the first week ($P < 0.02$). Early treatment with β-blockers also significantly reduced the risk of nonfatal reinfarction and nonfatal cardiac arrest in the hospital (19% and 16%, respectively). These data provide strong evidence in support of early treatment with β-blockers in patients with MI. Of the numerous mechanisms that could be responsible for the beneficial effects of β-blockers in the acute phase of MI, the factors that are most likely are listed in Table 7.2.

The long-term use of β-blockers for secondary prevention after MI has also been extensively studied. Over 23,000 patients recovering from MI have been evaluated in 25 randomized clinical trials (20). In the vast majority of these trials (24–26), treatment with oral β-blockers began within the first few days to several weeks after the index MI and continued during the period after MI. As shown in Figure 7.1, there was a significant reduction (22%) in cardiac death rate among patients randomized to β-blocker therapy compared to those receiving placebo (7.6% versus 9.4% mortality, respectively, $P < 0.001$). The greatest benefit seems to be related

**Table 7.2**
**Potential Beneficial Effects of Short-Term β-Blocker Therapy on Infarct in Acute Evolving Myocardial Infarction**

| |
|---|
| Reduction in oxygen demands as a result of decreased heart rate, blood pressure, and possible contractility |
| Counteraction of the cardiotoxic effects of excessive catecholamines |
| Counteraction of indirect effects of high levels of catecholamines (prevention of increases in free fatty acids and in uptake of excess free fatty acids) |
| Redistribution of blood from epicardial areas to more ischemic subendocardial tissue |
| Reduction in the frequency of complex ventricular arrhythmias and possibly an elevation in ventricular fibrillation thresholds |
| Reduction in the incidence of cardiac rupture |
| Reduction in the frequency of recurrent ischemia and infarct extension |

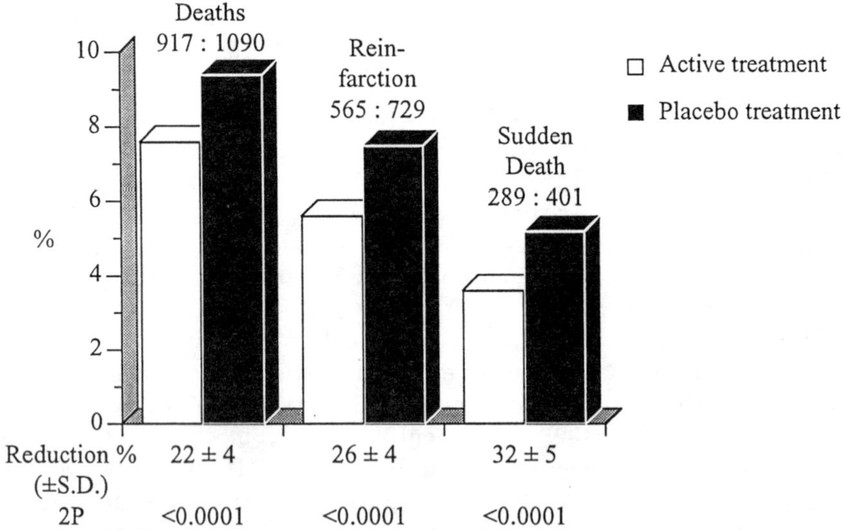


Figure 7.1 Cumulative results of 25 clinical trials of long-term therapy with β-blockers after myocardial infarction. The findings clearly illustrate the significant reduction in overall mortality, reinfarction rate, and the number of sudden cardiac deaths in patients receiving long-term β-blocker therapy.

to a significant reduction in the risk of sudden cardiac death (32%) and a marked reduction (26%) in the rate of nonfatal reinfarctions during the follow-up period (20). Patients with evidence of electromechanical complications (e.g., arrhythmias or congestive heart failure) during the acute phase of infarction received the greatest benefit with β-blockade. This is critical to note because many clinicians are hesitant to prescribe β-blocker therapy in such high-risk patients due to the fear of exacerbating congestive heart failure. Indeed, the results of randomized, controlled trials clearly indicate that β-blockers should be prescribed after MI for all patients who have no obvious contraindication for their use.

Thus, the results of secondary prevention trials with β-blockers clearly demonstrate the unquestionable benefits of these agents in reducing the risk of coronary events and cardiac death in the postinfarction period. Although a variety of factors might be responsible, these beneficial effects have been thought to occur largely due to the heart rate lowering effect of these agents (Table 7.2). It has been shown that β-blocking agents, devoid of such effects on heart rate (e.g., pindolol), do not have beneficial effects on survivors of MI. Therapy with β-blockers also reduces myocardial oxygen demand by counteracting the adverse effects of catecholamines and by preventing the increases in heart rate and blood pressure during periods of mental or physical stress. Additionally, β-blockers have been shown to increase the threshold for ventricular fibrillation in experimental animals and suppress ventricular arrhythmias in humans (30).

Despite the well-demonstrated efficacy of β-blockers, it is disconcerting to note that fewer than 50% of survivors of MI currently receive β-blocker therapy for secondary prevention. This is in contrast to the recent evidence showing widespread use of calcium channel blockers in as many as 50 to 60% of patients after MI. This is particularly disturbing because β-blockers are quite inexpensive and provide one of the most cost-effective therapies currently available for secondary prevention after MI. These data emphasize the need for reappraisal of the current practice patterns for secondary prevention in the postinfarction period.

### *Practical Guidelines About Use of β-blockers for Secondary Prevention*

β-Blockers are simple to use and do not require any special preparation except for evaluation for obvious contraindications. The major contraindications for use of β-blockers include presence of significant bronchopulmonary obstructive disease, advanced atrioventricular block, or profound sinus bradycardia, hypotension, and advanced decompensated congestive heart failure. Based on the available data, it is estimated that approximately 20% of patients after MI might not be able to tolerate β-blockade. Although in selected patients early use of β-blockers during the acute phase of MI might be necessary, for the vast majority of patients administration of oral agents 24–48 hours after onset of MI appears to be reasonable and achieves cardioprotective benefits during the postinfarction period. Early use of intravenous or oral β-blockade is most beneficial in patients with persistent sinus tachycardia or uncontrolled hypertension during the acute phase of MI. Patients with continuing or recurrent ischemic pain and tachyarrhythmias will also benefit from acute β-blockade. For all other patients, therapy with one of the approved oral β-blockers can be started after the first 24 hours of MI (Table 7.3). Although for obvious safety reasons the initial dose should be small, it is crucial to recognize that, after the first few doses, the dose of β-blocker being used should be rapidly increased to the recommended range or the maximum tolerated dose to achieve the cardioprotective effects demonstrated in the clinical trials (Table 7.3). This is especially important because it is a common observation that, when β-blockers are prescribed, many survivors of MI are not given the doses used in the controlled clinical trials. There is no way to guarantee that without comparable doses patients would gain a similar degree of cardioprotection. In addition, it is also important to educate patients regarding the danger of β-blocker withdrawal should they abruptly stop the β-blocker. Patients should be advised to always keep a reserve supply of β-blockers and communicate with family members and other health care workers about the importance of continued therapy with β-blockers to avoid the dangers of β-blocker withdrawal reactions.

Some of the other practical questions that are frequently asked deal with selection of an agent, duration of therapy, and the degree of benefit when other therapies are being used for secondary prevention after MI. Although comparative studies are lacking, there is no reason to believe that any of the approved and previously proved agents (Table 7.3) differ significantly from one another. Obviously, if the patient has mild chronic obstructive pulmonary disease, peripheral vascular disease, or diabetes, use of a cardioselective β-blocker such as metoprolol or atenolol is preferred. Also, whenever compliance is an issue, the long-acting (once-a-day) β-blockers are preferred over the short-acting agents, which require frequent administration. As far as the duration of therapy is concerned, there are no established guidelines, except that some recent observations do indicate that cardioprotective benefits of β-blockers can be demonstrated up to 3–5 years after MI. The precise duration of therapy in a given patient obviously varies depending upon the physician's clinical judgment and the size, location, and complications of acute MI as well as the patient's tolerance of the prescribed agent. Finally, although the results of recent trials with ACE inhibitors (47–49) showed that therapy with these agents was beneficial regardless of the concomitant use of β-blockers, it is important to note that, to date, there has not been any study that has made head-to-head comparison of the two treatments.

Based on the available data, it appears reasonable to conclude that

**Table 7.3**

**Pharmacologic Properties of β-Blockers for Secondary Prevention After Myocardial Infarction[a]**

| | Dose (mg/d) | Onset of Action (h) | Peak Effect (h) | Duration of Action (h) | Plasma Half-life (h) | Bioavailability (%) | Protein Binding (%) |
|---|---|---|---|---|---|---|---|
| Propranolol | 180–240 | 2 | 1.0–1.5 | 6–24 | 3–5 | 30–40 | 80–95 |
| Timolol | 20 | 0.5 | 1–2 | 12–24 | 4 | 50 | <10 |
| Atenolol | 100 | 1 | 2–4 | 24 | 6–7 | 50 | 5–15 |
| Metoprolol | 150–200 | 1 | 1–2 | 12 | 3–7 | 95 | 12 |

[a]Drugs shown have been approved by the US Food and Drug Administration for this use.
d = day; h = hour.

treatment with β-blockers is unquestionably effective in reducing the cardiovascular mortality and the rate of recurrent infarctions in survivors of MI. β-Blockers are cheap, easy to use, and appear to be safe for long-term use. Indeed, secondary prevention with β-blockade in survivors of MI is one of the most efficacious and cost-effective therapies currently available for clinical use.

## Role of Calcium Channel Blockers in Secondary Prevention

Calcium channel blockers are among the most popular cardiovascular drugs used in clinical practice today. Although most calcium channel blockers are well tolerated by patients and they produce few or no significant adverse side effects, their usefulness (especially dihydropyridines such as nifedipine or nicardipine) in secondary prevention after MI has not been well documented. As a matter of fact, some recent studies have shown deleterious effects of calcium channel blockers used for secondary prevention (11, 32–34). The increased early mortality secondary to nifedipine treatment recently reported in the second Secondary Prevention Reinfarction Israeli Nifedipine Trial (SPRINT-2) emphasized the need for clinicians to reevaluate the current therapeutic strategies in the management of patients during the postinfarction period (11, 32).

Despite little evidence to support the use of calcium channel blockers in the postinfarction period (Fig. 7.2), recent data from several large clinical trials evaluating patients after MI showed that a large number of these patients were being treated with calcium blockers (11–15). It is important to note that the SPRINT-2 study was actually terminated prematurely based on results of the interim analysis that revealed increased mortality in the nifedipine group during the early titration period (32). Furthermore, in the SPRINT-2 study, of the 826 patients who continued treatment with nifedipine, there was no difference in mortality, rate of nonfatal MI, or hospitalization for unstable angina during the 6-month follow-up period (32). Based on these results, the authors emphasized that early routine administration of nifedipine in acute MI might be hazardous and contraindicated. A recent review of 13 published clinical trials with nifedipine, including 9990 patients with acute MI, revealed no evidence of treatment-related beneficial effect on mortality, reinfarction rate, or overall incidence of ischemic events (35). Many of these trials demonstrated a trend towards harmful effects similar to those reported in SPRINT-2 study (32, 35).

The precise reason for the lack of efficacy and the potentially harmful effects of dihydropyridine calcium channel blockers is not known. It has been suggested that, in general, calcium channel blockers may produce adverse effects in patients with congestive heart failure by worsening left ventricular function (11, 39). The other possible explanation for lack of efficacy of calcium channel blockers might be related to reflex tachycardia, which is commonly seen in patients treated with nifedipine or other dihydropyridine

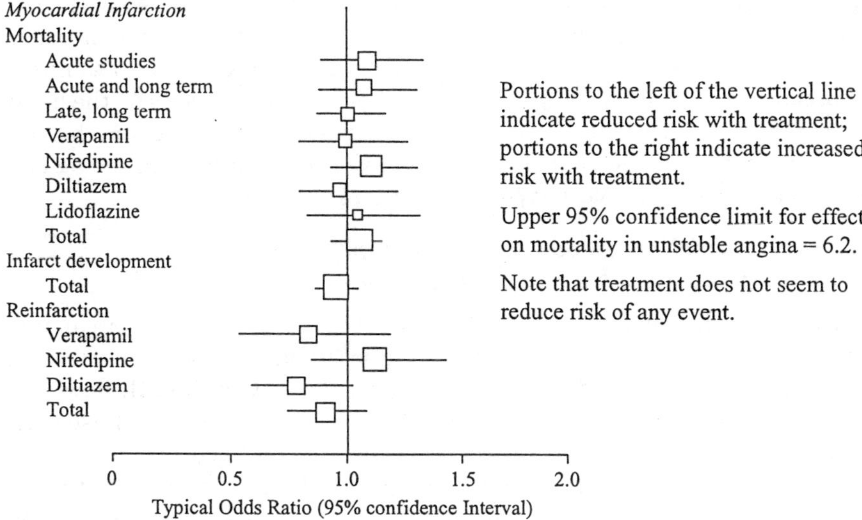


Figure 7.2 Results of the metaanalysis of clinical trials using calcium channel blockers after acute myocardial infarction. The first column describes the effects on mortality of acute and long-term therapy with various calcium channel blockers. The cumulative results indicate that there is no mortality benefit secondary to treatment with calcium channel blockers. The reinfarction rate was, however, reduced by verapamil and diltiazem, the two calcium channel blockers that do not cause reflex tachycardia. Adapted with permission from Held P, Yusuf S, Furberg C. Calcium channel blockers in acute myocardial infarction and unstable angina: an overview. Br Med J 1989;299:1187–1192.

calcium channel blockers. It is well known that a significant increase in heart rate can trigger myocardial ischemia. It is conceivable that the increased mortality observed during the first 6 days after administration of nifedipine in the SPRINT-2 study could be related to the extension of MI or recurrent ischemia in the postinfarction period. The cumulative results of previous trials with dihydropyridines have demonstrated similar trends. A recent metaanalysis (38) of data available from published trials of dihydropyridine calcium channel blockers also revealed a trend toward increased death and reinfarction in patients with acute MI treated with dihydropyridine calcium channel blockers in the postinfarction period.

It is, however, important to note that in contrast to the above-mentioned effects of dihydropyridine calcium channel blockers, a recent study reported beneficial effect of verapamil in survivors of acute MI (40). In the Second Danish Verapamil Infarction Trial (DAVIT2) of 1775 patients after MI, the patients treated with verapamil had a significantly lower reinfarction rate compared with those receiving placebo (11% versus 13.2%, respectively, $P = 0.04$). Similar results have been reported previously with diltiazem in the Diltiazem Reinfarction Study (41) in patients with non–Q wave MI (Fig. 7.2). Compared to placebo, treatment with diltiazem was associated with a significant reduction in the rate of reinfarction (9.3% versus 5.2%, $P < 0.02$)

as well as reduced frequency of postinfarction angina and ischemic electrocardiographic changes. The different outcome with verapamil and diltiazem compared to the dihydropyridine calcium channel blockers (Fig. 7.2) might be predominantly related to the differing effects of these agents on the heart rate. Based on these findings, it can be suggested that calcium channel blockers that lower the heart rate might have the potential of reducing risk of coronary events in selected patients after MI (38–41).

### *Practical Guidelines About Use of Calcium Channel Blockers for Secondary Prevention*

Based on the available scientific evidence, the routine use of calcium channel blockers is not recommended for secondary prevention after MI. The benefits of diltiazem use in patients with non–Q wave MI, however, appear well substantiated at least for short-term (up to 14 days) use (Fig. 7.3). Whether diltiazem would be efficacious during long-term use in patients with non–Q wave MI is not known. It is also important to note that administration of diltiazem has been shown to have deleterious effects and increased mortality in postinfarction patients with evidence of congestive heart failure or depressed left ventricular function. Therefore, the use of first-generation calcium channel blockers, including diltiazem, verapamil, and nifedipine, is not recommended for postinfarction patients with left ventricular dysfunction.

In patients who cannot tolerate β-blockers, it might be reasonable to con-

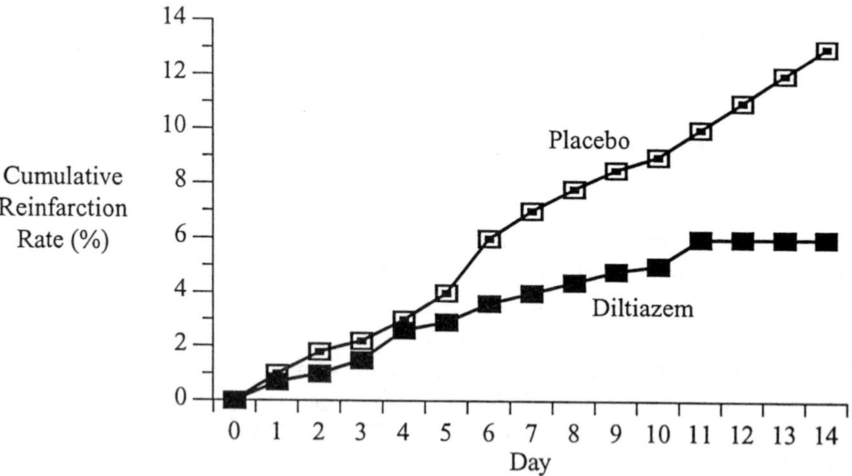


Figure 7.3 Kaplan-Meier survival curves for the cumulative rates of reinfarction for patients with non–Q-wave myocardial infarction assigned to placebo or diltiazem in the Diltiazem Reinfarction Study (DRS). The results show a significant reduction in the rate of reinfarction with diltiazem during the 14-day follow-up period. Adapted with permission from Gibson R, Boden W, Theroux P, et al. Diltiazem and reinfarction in patients with non-Q-wave myocardial infarction. N Engl J Med 1986;315:423–429.

sider using calcium channel blockers such as verapamil or diltiazem (which do not produce reflex tachycardia), especially when an effective antiischemic treatment is indicated. One of the largest groups that clinicians are usually faced with consists of patients who were being treated with the dihydropyridine calcium channel blockers nifedipine or nicardipine before their MI. The question arises as to whether these drugs should be discontinued in these patients after they have had an acute MI because of the adverse effects demonstrated in SPRINT-2 and other studies. Although there is no clear-cut answer to this question, it seems reasonable to recommend that, whenever possible, therapy with other agents that are safe and effective in the postinfarction setting should be considered. Alternatively, one might also consider adding an effective dose of a β-blocker to negate the reflex tachycardia produced by the dihydropyridine calcium channel blockers. Clinicians have to make such decisions empirically, based largely on their best clinical judgment, because no data are currently available in this area.

## Role of ACE Inhibitors in Secondary Prevention

As discussed earlier, the presence of left ventricular dysfunction is one of the most important determinants of prognosis and survival after MI in patients with left ventricular systolic dysfunction (LVEF less than 40%). In addition, it has become evident that those with left ventricular dilatation are at significantly greater risk of subsequent mortality than those who have normal sized left ventricles (43, 45). Because it is now possible to treat and prevent the progression of left ventricular dysfunction and dilatation with ACE inhibitors, it is quite important to examine the role of ACE inhibitors in secondary prevention after MI. Although this topic is discussed in detail elsewhere in this text (see Chapter 12), it will be described briefly in the present context.

In order to properly understand the role of ACE inhibitors in improving left ventricular function after MI, it is important to discuss the pathophysiologic process involved in left ventricular dysfunction after MI.

Left ventricular dilatation after MI occurs primarily by the process of remodeling. In postinfarction patients, the process of left ventricular dilatation begins rapidly (usually within the first few weeks) after infarction and continues to progress unless specific measures are taken to interrupt the process by altering the increased wall stress. During the healing phase of myocardial infarction, the infarcted area of the myocardium is replaced by a noncontractile, thin scar that is susceptible to further elongation and thinning due to infarct expansion. Patients with large anteroapical transmural MI are particularly at high risk of infarct expansion. Echocardiographic examination during the early phase of acute MI can identify the areas of infarct expansion. Patients with evidence of infarct expansion have a significantly increased risk of cardiovascular events. In addition to the infarct expansion that occurs early after myocardial infarction, the process of left ventricular dilatation continues to progress in the weeks and months after myocardial infarction (44–46). The progressive left ventricular dilatation after myocardial infarction occurs due to the scar and thinning of the infarcted area, and it progresses further because of the morphologic and geometric changes that affect the adjacent normal myocardium during the process of ventricular remodeling (44, 45). Although the precise mechanism of left ventricular remodeling after myocardial infarction remains to be established, the available evidence suggests that increased wall stress secondary to the altered neurohormonal axes, including activation of the renin-angiotensin system, plays a key role (46). These neurohormonal systems are activated during the acute phase of myocardial infarction, as demonstrated by the elevated levels of circulating angiotensin II and plasma catecholamines within a few days after a large MI (46). These neurohormonal changes in combination with the altered shape of the left ventricle lead to increased wall stress on the remaining normal muscle. The increased wall stress along with the need for the remaining normal myocardium to compensate for loss of function due to infarction leads to myocardial hypertrophy, which helps to maintain stroke volume. Initially, left ventricular hypertrophy and chamber dilatation may act as a compensatory mechanism and maintain stroke volume by the Frank-Starling mechanism. If no corrective measures are taken, however, the continued stimulation of sympathoadrenal and renin-angiotensin systems secondary to left ventricular dysfunction leads to progressive morphologic and geometric changes that result in further left ventricular dilatation. There is considerable evidence suggesting that continued high levels of angiotensin II lead to an increase in ACE activity. The increased tissue ACE activity can facilitate the adrenergic system and may also lead to coronary vasoconstriction. These neurohormonal changes along with the increased ventricular volume lead to further increases in wall stress by Laplace's law, and this vicious circle continues to induce further left ventricular dilatation.

Because the renin-angiotensin system (RAS) plays such a critical role in the process of postinfarction left ventricular remodeling, it seems logical to think that the use of ACE inhibitors would be beneficial to alter this process and prevent the progression of left ventricular dysfunction and dilatation after MI. It was not until the pioneering work of Pfeffer and coworkers in experimental animals, however, that the benefit of treatment with ACE inhibition in the postinfarction model was established (44–46). The initial work by Pfeffer et al. demonstrated that, in animals with similar extent of experimentally induced MI, treatment with captopril was associated with higher ejection fraction, lower left ventricular volume, and improved survival (44). These experimental observations were subsequently confirmed by Pfeffer and coworkers in a small group of patients with first anterior wall MI (45). Subsequently, several large-scale clinical

**Table 7.4**
**ACE Inhibitors for Left Ventricular Remodeling After Myocardial Infarction[a]**

| | Number | ACE I | F/U (months) | Outcome |
|---|---|---|---|---|
| Early (Nonselective) Trials | | | | |
| CONSENSUS II | 6,090 (all) | Enalapril | 6 | Neutral |
| GISSI-3 | 20,000 (all) | Lisinopril | 1.5 | Weak + |
| ISIS-4 | 60,000 (all) | Captopril | 1.2 | Weak + |
| Chinese | 10,000 (all) | Captopril | 1 | +/neutral |
| SMILE | 1,556 (no thrombolysis) | Zofenopril | 1.5 | +/combined |
| Late (Selective) Trials | | | | |
| SAVE | 2,231 (EF<40%) | Captopril | 42 | +/↓MI |
| TRACE | 1,749 (EF<35%) | Trandolapril | >12 | Strong + |
| AIRE | 2,006 (CHF) | Ramipril | 15 | Strong + |

[a]Early trials are those in which treatment with ACE inhibitors was begun early (within 24–48 hours) after myocardial infarction. In most of these early trials, patients were enrolled regardless of the status of left ventricle function. Late trials are those in which patients were selected based on the evidence of left ventricular dysfunction or CHF after myocardial infarction, and treatment was begun usually 2–3 days after myocardial infarction. In contrast to the results of the early nonselective trials, which were neutral or weakly positive, the benefit of treatment with ACE inhibitors was more evident in the late trials, which included mostly high-risk patients.
ACE = angiotensin-converting enzyme; AIRE = Acute Infarction Ramipril Efficacy study; CHF = congestive heart failure; CONSENSUS II = Cooperative New Scandinavian Enalapril Survival Study; EF = ejection fraction; F/U = follow-up; GISSI-3 = Gruppo Italiano per lo Studio della Sopravvivenza nell'Infarcto Miocardico; ISIS-4 = Fourth International Study of Infarct Survival; MI = myocardial infarction; SAVE = Survival and Ventricular Enlargement trial; SMILE = Survival of Myocardial Infarction Long-Term Evaluation; TRACE = Trandolapril Cardiac Evaluation; + = positive; ↓ = decreased.

trials (Table 7.4) have been conducted across the world to evaluate the clinical benefits of ACE inhibition after MI in patients with and without left ventricular dysfunction (46–53). The first published study in the area was the Survival and Ventricular Enlargement (SAVE) trial, which compared the effects of captopril to those of placebo in patients with a recent MI and depressed left ventricular function (LVEF less than 40%) during a 4-year treatment period (47). The group receiving captopril had a significantly lower (21% decrease, $P = 0.01$) risk of death from cardiovascular causes as well as reduced risk (37% decrease, $P < 0.001$) of developing severe congestive heart failure and also reduced number (22% decrease, $P = 0.019$) of hospitalizations for congestive heart failure. Treatment with captopril also reduced the risk (25% decrease, $P < 0.015$) of recurrent MI and hospitalization for unstable angina. The beneficial effects of captopril were observed in all subgroups of patients regardless of the location of MI or use of concomitant drugs such as aspirin or β-blockers (Fig. 7.4). The results of SAVE have been confirmed by the findings reported from several other large-scale clinical trials (Table 7.5), in some of which treatment with ACE inhibitors was started within the first 24 hours of acute MI. Some trials

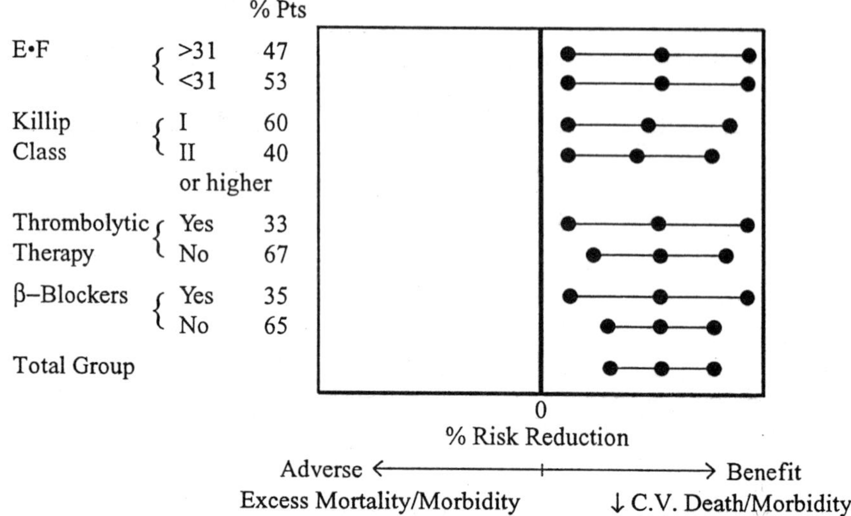


Figure 7.4 Breakdown of therapeutic benefits observed in the SAVE trial in terms of reduction in morbidity and mortality in various subgroups of patients after myocardial infarction. The benefit of treatment with captopril was evident in all subgroups regardless of whether patients had received thrombolytic therapy and were receiving concomitant β-blocker therapy. Adapted with permission from Pfeffer MA, Braunwald E, Moye LA, et al. Effect of captopril on mortality and morbidity in patients with left ventricular dysfunction after myocardial infarction: results of the survival and ventricular enlargement trial. N Engl J Med 1992;327:669–677.

have included patients with clinically overt congestive heart failure as well as those without left ventricular dysfunction (48–53). Although the benefits of ACE inhibition after MI can be demonstrated across all studies, the results of the largest clinical studies, including Gruppo Italiano per lo Studio della Sopravvivenza nell'Infarcto miocardio (GISSI-3) and the Fourth International Study of Infarct Survival (ISIS-4), suggest that when ACE inhibitors are given to unselected patients with MI (regardless of left ventricular function), the demonstrable survival benefit is of significantly lesser magnitude than that observed in the SAVE and other trials that included only patients with left ventricular dysfunction (Table 7.4). These findings suggest that the greatest benefit of treatment with an ACE inhibitor would be seen in the high-risk subset of patients with reduced LVEF. In addition, a closer look at the results of these studies also demonstrates that the benefits are evident as early as 6 months and could be demonstrated throughout the duration of the trials, as evidenced by the continued separation of the survival curves throughout the follow-up periods. Although it is quite apparent that the beneficial effects of ACE inhibition are secondary to the favorable hemodynamic actions of these drugs,

**Table 7.5**
**Details of Clinical Trials with ACE Inhibitors for Secondary Prevention After Myocardial Infarction**

| Study | No. of Patients | Drug Used | Final Dose | Time of Initiation[a] | Follow-up | Outcome (% Risk Reduction)[b] | *P* value |
|---|---|---|---|---|---|---|---|
| SAVE | 2,231 | Captopril | 50 mg t.i.d. | 3–16 days | 42 mon | 19 (3–32) | 0·019 |
| CONSENSUS II | 6,090 | Enalapril | I.V. infusion followed by 10–20 mg q.d. | Immediately; average 15h | 6 mon | 10 (7% reduction–29% increase) | 0·26 |
| AIRE | 2,006 | Ramipril | 5 mg b.i.d. | 3–10 days; average 5 days | Average 15 mon; minimum 6 mon | 27 (11–40) | 0·002 |
| ISIS-4 | 54,824 | Captopril | 50 mg b.i.d. | <24 h | 35 days | 6 (<1–12) | 0·04 |
| GISSI-3 | 18,985 | Lisinopril | 10 mg q.d. | <24 h | 6 weeks | 11 (1–20) | 0·03 |
| Chinese Captopril Study | 11,345 | Captopril | 12.5 mg t.i.d. | <36 h | 28 days | No change | NS |

[a]Time after myocardial infarction to start of treatment.
[b]Confidence interval 95%.
ACE = angiotensin-converting enzyme; AIRE = Acute Infarction Ramipril Efficacy study; b.i.d. = twice a day; CONSENSUS II = Cooperative New Scandinavian Enalapril Survival Study; GISSI-3 = Gruppo Italiano per lo Studio della Sopravvivenza nell'Infarcto miocardio; h = hours; ISIS-4 = Fourth International Study of Infarct Survival; I.V. = intravenous; mon = months; NS = not significant; q.d. = every day; t.i.d. = three times a day.

**Table 7.6**
**Potential Mechanisms of Beneficial Effects of ACE Inhibitor Therapy**

| |
|---|
| Hemodynamic Actions |
| Afterload reduction |
| Reduced preload |
| Decreased LV wall stress |
| Effects on Neurohormones |
| Decreased levels of circulating angiotensin II |
| Decreased tissue ACE activity |
| Reduced degradation of bradykinin |
| Decreased levels of plasma aldosterone |
| Decreased levels of plasma catecholamines |
| Improved baroreceptor function |
| Effects on LV Structure and Functions |
| Reduced LV chamber size |
| Reduced intracavitary pressures |
| Reduced risk of infarct expansion |
| Improved LV geometric shape |
| Reduced mitral regurgitation |
| Improved ventricular performance |
| Antiischemic Effects |
| Improvement in coronary blood flow and its distribution |
| Plaque stabilization and vascular protection |

ACE = angiotensin-converting enzyme; LV = left ventricular.

there are several other potential mechanisms that could be playing a role (Table 7.6).

### *Practical Guidelines About Use of ACE Inhibitors for Secondary Prevention*

Based on the preceding discussion and the available scientific evidence, all patients with a recent MI and left ventricular dysfunction with or without evidence of congestive heart failure should be treated with an ACE inhibitor after MI. The benefits of ACE inhibition in these patients are evident and such therapy is cost-effective because it not only improves survival but also reduces the risk of developing congestive heart failure and rate of hospitalization for congestive heart failure. It is, however, less compelling to recommend routine ACE inhibition in the postinfarction patients without clinical evidence of left ventricular dysfunction because the benefit in these patients is small, less well defined, and does not appear to be cost-effective.

The other important practical questions regarding the use of ACE inhibitors in patients after MI are the timing of initiation of therapy, the duration of therapy, and the use of concomitant medications. Although after the results of the Cooperative New Scandinavian Enalapril Survival Study (CONSENSUS II) there was some concern about the safety of early administration of an ACE inhibitor in the postinfarction period, the results of GISSI-3 and ISIS-4 have clearly established that an ACE inhibitor can be safely administered as early as 24 hours after MI. Because of the changing hemodynamic milieu during the acute phase of MI, however, it appears reasonable to start treatment with an ACE inhibitor on the second or third day after MI. As with other drugs that have significant hemodynamic effects, ACE inhibitors should be started with a small test dose and increased gradually as tolerated. In order to achieve the degree of benefit demonstrated in the clinical trials, however, it is absolutely essential that the dose of the ACE inhibitor be titrated so that it is comparable to that used in the studies, or the maximum tolerated dose of the given agent should be used (Table 7.5). Based on the results of these clinical trials, the benefits of ACE inhibition were observed regardless of the concomitant use of aspirin or β-blockers, so it is recommended that ACE inhibitors be used in conjunction with these drugs for secondary prevention after MI. The longest duration of therapy in the clinical studies was 4 years in the SAVE trial. Based on the continued benefits observed throughout the duration of that trial, it seems reasonable to recommend continuation of treatment with the ACE inhibitor for up to 4 years. This question deserves further examination, however, because it is conceivable that after a certain period of time the process of left ventricular remodeling might cease to occur in some patients, and if these patients had stable left ventricular function with no evidence of clinical congestive heart failure, it might be reasonable to consider stopping treatment with the ACE inhibitor in such patients. In the meantime, clinicians have to make that decision based on their clinical impression and their judgment on a case-by-case basis.

## Role of Antiplatelet Drugs in Secondary Prevention

A variety of antiplatelet agents have been evaluated for secondary prevention after MI. Several large-scale clinical trials have evaluated the role of treatment with aspirin, dipyridamole, sulfinpyrazone, and ticlodipine in the long-term management of patients with MI (54–56). Of these, aspirin is the most extensively studied antiplatelet drug for secondary prevention after MI (54). The results of these trials have demonstrated that aspirin definitely reduces the risk of recurrent MI and cardiac death. Although some of these trials showed only marginal benefit of treatment with aspirin, the results of the metaanalysis of 25 trials with antiplatelet drugs involving a total of 29,000 patients with prior MI revealed unquestionable and statistically significant benefits of antiplatelet therapy. Table 7.7 shows the results of the metaanalysis and demonstrates that treatment with antiplatelet drugs was associated with a 32% reduction in recurrent MI, a 27% reduction in nonfatal stroke, and a 15% reduction in death due to any vascular event. When all important vascular events (nonfatal MI, nonfatal stroke, and vascular death) were combined, there was an im-

**Table 7.7**
**Metaanalysis of 25 Trials of Antiplatelet Therapy for Secondary Prevention of Cardiovascular Disease**

| Endpoint | Risk Reduction Among Those Assigned Antiplatelet Therapy (% ± standard deviation) |
|---|---|
| Nonfatal myocardial infarction | 32 ± 5 |
| Nonfatal stroke | 27 ± 6 |
| Total vascular mortality | 15 ± 4 |
| Combined vascular events | 25 ± 3 |

pressive 25% reduction in combined vascular events. All of these reductions were statistically significant (54). A comparison of different antiplatelet agents used in various trials did not demonstrate the superiority of any agent over the effects of aspirin in secondary prevention. The comparison of various doses of aspirin used in these studies also revealed that the higher doses of aspirin (900–1500 mg/day) were no more effective than the 300-mg dose (the lowest dose tested). It was also found that the incidence of side effects was much less with the lower dose (300 mg/day). Based on these results, it seems prudent to recommend the use of aspirin, 300–325 mg/day, for secondary prevention after MI in all survivors of MI. Because of the adverse effects of aspirin on gastric mucosa and the rare occurrence of gastritis or gastric ulcer, use of enteric-coated aspirin, which will avoid the gastric side effects, is now generally recommended. For patients who are known to be allergic to aspirin and those who cannot tolerate aspirin, the use of ticlopidine is recommended. Based on the cost comparison of all therapies in patients with cardiovascular disorders, the treatment with aspirin appears to be one of the cheapest and most effective therapies for prevention of future coronary events and cardiac death. Indeed, aspirin is one of the most effective therapies in medicine, especially in cardiac patients, and should be prescribed for all survivors of MI.

## Role of Anticoagulants in Secondary Prevention

Based on the results of recent investigations, it is now well established that an occluding coronary thrombus is responsible for the vast majority of transmural MI. It is also known that survivors of MI are at an increased risk of future MI. Because coronary thrombosis plays such a critical role in the pathogenesis of MI, it seems logical to think that anticoagulant therapy would be effective in reducing the risk of future coronary events in survivors of MI. Due to the potential therapeutic efficacy of anticoagulants in secondary prevention, several clinical trials during the past two decades have evaluated their role in survivors of MI (57, 58). Although the use of anticoagulants was considered standard therapy in the 1960s and early

1970s, their use later declined. In the 1980s, however, when the concept of total thrombotic occlusion of the infarct-related artery became well established, there was renewed interest in the use of anticoagulants after MI. In addition, with the advent of echocardiography and its routine use in patients with acute MI, it became apparent that as many as one third of patients with anterior wall MI had evidence of left ventricular mural thrombus that had the potential for systemic embolization.

The high risk of potential thromboembolic complications in survivors of MI has led to renewed interest in the use of anticoagulant therapy for secondary prevention. Although some earlier studies focused on initiation of anticoagulant therapy with heparin within the first few days after MI followed by long-term treatment with warfarin, most recent studies have focused on the use of warfarin for secondary prevention (58). Although several of these trials with warfarin have shown favorable effects, the most striking results were observed in the Warfarin Reinfarction Study (WARIS). This was a randomized, double-blind, placebo-controlled trial in which 1214 patients were enrolled and followed for an average of 37 months after initiation of anticoagulant therapy. The dose of warfarin was adjusted to achieve an international normalized ratio (INR) of 2·5 to 4·8. The intention-to-treat analysis of the WARIS data revealed that a total of 94 (15%) patients in the warfarin group had died compared with 123 (20%) in the placebo group ($P = 0.026$). When the analysis was performed for patients who maintained treatment for at least 28 days, a total of 60 patients had died in the warfarin group compared with 92 deaths in the placebo group (35% risk reduction, $P = 0.005$). The combined risk of fatal and nonfatal MI was also reduced by 43% ($P = 0.0001$). Thus, the results of WARIS are extremely encouraging and suggest that treatment with an oral anticoagulant might indeed be beneficial in secondary prevention after MI.

There are several questions, however, that remain to be answered regarding the use of oral anticoagulants in survivors of MI. The first important question is how does use of aspirin compare with administration of warfarin after MI? This issue has been evaluated in two clinical trials, neither of which revealed a significant difference between aspirin and coumadin; however, it should be noted that both of these trials were open labeled and, as such, the results may not be entirely reliable (58). Additionally, the level of anticoagulation achieved might not have been sufficient to produce the desired benefit. A second important question deals with the relevance of results obtained in trials with oral anticoagulant therapy in patients who have received thrombolytic therapy for acute MI. Because most previous trials, including WARIS, enrolled a majority of patients who did not receive thrombolytic therapy, it seems inappropriate to apply the results of these trials to patients who have been treated with thrombolytic agents. There is also the issue of safety of oral anticoagulants during the initial phase of MI after thrombolysis. Because of these remaining questions, the concern for long-term safety, and the need for constant monitoring of anticoagulant activity, the routine use of long-term oral anticoagulants is not widely recommended for secondary prevention after MI. The use of an oral anticoagulant should be strongly considered in patients with anterior wall MI who have significant wall motion abnormality or left ventricular mural thrombus, or both.

## Role of Antiarrhythmic Drugs in Secondary Prevention

Electrical instability and the presence of ventricular arrhythmias are predictive of increased mortality in survivors of MI. Because ventricular arrhythmias have such a strong predictive value, it has been postulated that treatment with antiarrhythmic drugs would be beneficial for secondary prevention after MI. Although physicians had been empirically prescribing antiarrhythmic drugs for suppression of ventricular arrhythmias in survivors of MI, the results of two large clinical trials sponsored by the National Heart, Lung and Blood Institute have revealed that antiarrhythmic drug therapy is not beneficial in the setting of MI (59–61). The Cardiac Arrhythmia Suppression Trials I and II (CAST I and CAST II) were both conducted to evaluate the benefit of arrhythmia suppression with antiarrhythmic drugs in survivors of MI with frequent premature ventricular contractions (10 premature ventricular contractions/hour) in the postinfarction period (60, 61). The results of both CAST I and CAST II revealed that, although the drugs (encainide, flecainide, and ethmozine) used in the study were effective in adequately suppressing arrhythmias, there was an increased mortality (60). The most disturbing aspect of the findings was that the mortality in the antiarrhythmic drug group was increased largely due to arrhythmic deaths (60). These findings have led the experts in the area to conclude that the proarrhythmic effects of these drugs are quite deleterious, especially in patients with MI. Presently, most antiarrhythmic drugs are not recommended for secondary prevention after MI. It is important to emphasize here that β-blockers do have antiarrhythmic actions and results of several studies with β-blockers in postinfarction patients do provide indirect evidence to support the concept that treatment with β-blockers might indeed reduce the risk of arrhythmic deaths in survivors of MI with ventricular arrhythmias (30, 31).

## Role of Risk Factor Modification in Secondary Prevention

Based on the above discussion, it is evident that considerable attention has been focused on evaluating the role of various drug therapies for secondary prevention after MI. However, clinicians pay little attention to risk factor modification in the management of patients in the postinfarction period. It is generally assumed that because the atherosclerotic process is already established, such treatment is unlikely to provide any significant benefit. The available evidence, however, suggests that treatment directed toward risk factor modification can indeed alter the risk of future coronary events and cardiac death. Currently, risk factor modification strategies include lowering of elevated serum cholesterol levels, control of hypertension, smoking cessation, weight reduction, and behavior modification (62).

### *Role of Lipid-Lowering Therapy*

The benefit of lowering raised serum cholesterol in survivors of acute MI has been well demonstrated in several large clinical studies (63–67). Although until recently there was doubt about the benefit of lipid-lowering therapy because of the small numbers of patients evaluated in most prior studies, the results of the recently published Scandinavian Simvastatin Survival Study (4S) in which 4444 patients were enrolled leave little doubt in this area. Even when the results of previously available studies were pooled, there remained little doubt regarding the benefits of lipid-lowering therapy in secondary prevention (63–65). A metaanalysis of the combined data from 7837 patients in eight randomized trials of cholesterol-lowering therapies for secondary prevention indicated that there were significant reductions in the rate of fatal and nonfatal reinfarctions (63).

Despite the favorable results observed in a majority of secondary prevention trials, evidence shows that most physicians (generalist as well as specialist) have not adopted the use of lipid-lowering therapy in patients with clinically manifested congestive heart disease. Recent evidence suggests that no more than one third of the patients with established congestive heart disease are receiving treatment to lower their cholesterol levels with either diet or drug therapy. Although the precise reasons for the lack of attention in this area are difficult to determine, various possibilities exist. It has been suggested that many physicians do not yet believe that survival after MI can be improved by cholesterol-lowering drugs. Also, patients resist significant lifestyle changes over a prolonged period of time and tend to expect a "quick fix" to the problem. In addition, most health care workers, including physicians, are not well trained in preventive measures; thus, they feel uncomfortable in giving advice in this area. More recently, the pressure on physicians' time and cost-containment issues in the managed care era have prevented even able and willing physicians to pursue preventive strategies actively. Although one or many of these reasons have prevented institution of measures for secondary prevention in the past, it is becoming increasingly evident that lipid-lowering drugs in conjunction with dietary modification are highly effective in reducing the morbidity and mortality in patients with established congestive heart disease (62). Such therapies are highly cost-effective, and it is likely that with increasing awareness of patients, as a result of wide publicity by the National Cholesterol Eduction Program (NCEP), physicians will be forced to participate actively in the evaluation and management of abnormal lipid levels in patients with congestive heart disease (66).

A large number of studies have been conducted during the last two decades to evaluate the role of lipid-lowering drugs in secondary prevention (63–67). Although most of these trials have demonstrated a significant reduction in the rate of cardiovascular events, many earlier studies failed to show an improvement in overall survival rates. The lack of survival benefit has been a major concern raised by many clinicians, and this might well have contributed to the lukewarm response on the part of the clinician to routine use of lipid-lowering drugs in patients with congestive heart disease. Data from the Scandinavian Simvastatin Survival Study, however, have provided convincing evidence of the benefit of lipid-lowering therapy in improving overall survival (65).

The Coronary Drug Project was the first large secondary prevention trial that evaluated the effects of a variety of drugs in 8341 survivors of MI (64). Although initially the drugs chosen included estrogen conjugates, dextrothyroxine, clofibrate, and nicotinic acid, treatment with dextrothyroxine and estrogen conjugates was discontinued before completion of the trial owing to an excess mortality observed in the groups receiving these drugs. The 5-year trial was completed for the groups assigned to clofibrate or nicotinic acid. Although treatment with clofibrate or nicotinic acid did not significantly reduce cardiovascular mortality, the combined end point of cardiovascular deaths and nonfatal MI was reduced by 9% with clofibrate and 15% with nicotinic acid during the 5-year trial period (64). A subsequent report of a survey performed 10 years after termination of the trial revealed that the group that received nicotinic acid during the trial had an 11% lower all-cause mortality compared with the group randomized to placebo (52% versus 58%, $P = 0.004$) (64). This benefit was largely attributed to a presumed slower rate of progression of atherosclerotic lesions resulting in a lower rate of MI secondary to intervention with nicotinic acid.

The results of the Scandinavian Simvastatin Survival Study (4S) have provided the most compelling evidence in favor of the beneficial role of cholesterol-lowering drugs in secondary prevention of congestive heart disease. A total of 4444 patients with angina pectoris or MI were enrolled in the 4S and randomized to receive 3-hydroxy-3-methyl-glutaryl (HMG) coreductase inhibitor, simvastatin, or a matching placebo (65). As shown in Table 7.8, after 6 weeks of therapy with simvastatin, there was a 38% decrease in low-density lipoprotein (LDL) cholesterol, a 28% reduction in total serum cholesterol, and an 8% increase in high-density lipoprotein (HDL) cholesterol. The predefined primary end point in the 4S study was the effect of simvastatin versus placebo on overall mortality. During the 5.4-year median follow-up period, compared with placebo treatment, simvastatin treatment was associated with a 30% reduction in all-cause mortality (Table 7.8). The improvement in overall survival was chiefly attributed to the reduction in fatal coronary events, which were reduced by an impressive 42%. Compared with placebo treatment, there was a 34% reduction in risk of a major coronary event and a 37% decrease in the need

**Table 7.8**
**Summary Results of the Scandinavian Simvastatin Survival Study**

| End Point | Relative Risk (%) | Comment |
|---|---|---|
| Overall risk of death | ↓ 30 | Only trial to date with cholesterol-lowering agent to show definitely reduction in total or coronary mortality |
| Risk of coronary death | ↓ 42 | Cardiovascular disease is the world's leading cause of death, accounting for one-fourth of all deaths |
| Risk of major coronary events | ↓ 34 | Includes death from coronary disease and nonfatal heart attacks |
| Risk of revascularization procedures | ↓ 37 | Includes percutaneous coronary angioplasties and coronary artery bypass grafts |
| Event-free survival | ↑ 26 | Finished the study without suffering any coronary events or other atherosclerotic events such as stroke |
| LDL cholesterol | ↓ 38 | Human atherosclerotic plaques primarily contain LDL |
| HDL cholesterol | ↑ 8[a] | High concentrations of HDL may protect against coronary heart disease |
| Total cholesterol | ↓28[a] | Simvastatin is the most effective cholesterol-lowering agent available at recommended doses |

[a] After 6 weeks of treatment with 20 mg. HDL = high-density lipoprotein; LDL = Low-density lipoprotein
↓ = decreased; ↑ = increased
Adapted with permission from Scandinavian Simvastatin Survival Study Group: Randomized trial of cholesterol lowering in 4,444 patients with coronary heart disease: The Scandinavian Simvastatin Survival Study (4S) (65).

for revascularization procedures during the study period (Table 7.8). There was a reduction in all cardiovascular events, which accounted for an overall 35% reduction in combined cardiovascular mortality in the simvastatin group when compared with the placebo group (65).

These findings of the 4S study are intriguing because it is the first study of lipid-lowering drug therapy in secondary prevention of congestive heart disease that has shown a significant decline in all-cause mortality (65). There are several reasons for these exciting results. First, the trial enrolled a sufficiently large number of patients who were at risk of developing congestive heart disease during the study period (65, 67). Second, the treatment used was highly effective in reducing total as well as LDL cholesterol levels, and it increased HDL cholesterol levels. Also, the highly effective lipid-lowering therapy with simvastatin was continued for a sufficient period (median duration 5.4 years) to allow significant beneficial effect on atherosclerotic plaques. Finally, in contrast to treatment with other lipid-lowering drugs, the use of simvastatin was extremely safe and did not result in an increase in deaths owing to noncardiovascular causes, such as cancer, suicide, or trauma. These results should indeed put to rest the concern raised about an association between low cholesterol and risk of cancer. Although it is premature to draw too many conclusions from the 4S study, it seems reasonable to think that the previously reported increase in cancer owing to various other drugs might indeed be agent specific or relate to the mechanism of action of those drugs, and it appears that HMG coreductase inhibitors do not produce such harmful effects (65–67). Based on the results of these studies, it is strongly recommended that survivors of MI be carefully evaluated for elevated lipids and aggressive lipid-lowering therapy be prescribed for secondary prevention after MI with the goal of reducing LDL cholesterol below 100 mg/dL (67).

### *Role of Blood Pressure Control in Hypertensive Patients After MI*

Although there is much less direct evidence regarding the benefits of blood pressure control, smoking cessation, and weight reduction in secondary prevention after MI, the available data (62) indicate that such treatment strategies have the potential to alter the adverse prognosis. There is indirect evidence from the results of several large clinical trials that the treatment of hypertension in patients with a history of MI significantly lowers total mortality (68–71). In general, the treatment with β-blockers recommended for secondary prevention after MI should be sufficient for control of blood pressure. If β-blockers are contraindicated or another agent is required, however, it would be preferable to select an ACE inhibitor for the added benefit of controlling blood pressure as well as preventing left ventricular remodeling and associated chamber dilatation.

## SUMMARY

Acute MI is a major sequela of coronary artery disease. Each year approximately 1.5 million Americans suffer from MI, and of those, nearly 800,000 patients survive the acute phase. However, the survivors of MI remain at increased risk of future coronary events and cardiac death. A large number of investigations during the last three decades have identified the presence of left ventricular dysfunction, electrical instability, and residual ischemia as the most important determinants of long-term outcome in survivors of MI.

During the past two decades, considerable effort has been made to develop therapeutic strategies for secondary prevention after MI. Numerous clinical trials have been conducted to evaluate the role of β-blockers, calcium channel blockers, ACE inhibitors, antiplatelet agents, oral anticoagulants, antiarrhythmic drugs, lipid-lowering agents, and antihypertensive drugs for secondary prevention after MI. Of all these therapies, treatment with aspirin, β-blockers, and ACE inhibitors appears to be the most useful and cost-effective for secondary prevention after MI. The results of some recent studies suggest that lipid-lowering therapy is also highly effective in reducing the risk of future coronary events, cardiac death, and overall mortality. Although, because of cost considerations, lipid-lowering drugs cannot be routinely recommended for secondary prevention after MI, sufficient evidence exists to support their use in patients with elevated LDL cholesterol (more than 100 mg/dL) who are at significant increased risk of future coronary events. In addition, it is important to recognize that risk-factor modification, including treatment of hypertension, smoking cessation, and regular exercise prescription, is also an important and integral part of secondary prevention after MI.

Based on the review of the available data, the clinician now has several cost-effective therapeutic choices that are useful for secondary prevention after MI. It is, however, disconcerting to note that, despite these data and a number of choices available to the clinician, many survivors of MI do not receive adequate therapy for secondary prevention. Because of the long-term prognostic implication and the cost-effectiveness of the appropriate therapy for secondary prevention, it is imperative that the clinician become familiar with the therapeutic strategy for secondary prevention and prescribe the effective therapy as appropriate for all survivors of MI. It is probably more appropriate here than in any other clinical setting to remind ourselves that an ounce of prevention is better than a pound of cure.

---

## REFERENCES

1. Morbidity and mortality: chartbook on cardiovascular, lung, and blood diseases. Bethesda, MD: National Heart, Lung, and Blood Institute, US Department of Health and Human Services, 1992.
2. Heart and stroke facts: 1995 statistical supplement. Dallas: American Heart Association, 1995.
3. Epstein SE, Palmari ST, Patterson RE. Evaluation of patients after acute myocardial infarction: indications for cardiac catheterization and surgical intervention. N Engl J Med 1982;307:1487.
4. Nicod P, Gilpin E, Dittrich H, et al. Influence on prognosis and morbidity of left ventricular ejection fraction with and without signs of left ventricular failure after acute myocardial infarction. Am J Cardiol 1988;61:1165–1171.
5. Mattioni, TA. Long-term prognosis after myocardial infarction. Postgrad Med 1992;92:107–114.
6. DeBusk RF, Glomqvist CG, Kouchoukos NT, et al. Identification and treatment of low-risk patients after acute myocardial infarction and coronary-artery bypass graft surgery. N Engl J Med 1986;314:161–166.
7. The Multicenter Postinfarction Research Group. Risk stratification and survival after myocardial infarction. N Engl J Med 1983;309:331–336.

8. Deedwania P. Silent myocardial ischemia and its relationship to acute myocardial infarction. Cardiol Clin 1986;4:643–658.
9. Moss AJ, Benhorin J. Prognosis and management after a first myocardial infarction. N Engl J Med 1990;322:743–753.
10. Krone RJ. The role of risk stratification in the early management of a myocardial infarction. Ann Intern Med 1992;116:223–237.
11. Deedwania PC, Carbajal EV. Secondary prevention after myocardial infarction: too many choices, which ones work. (Editorial). Arch Intern Med 1993;153:285–288.
12. Lamas GA, Pfeffer MA, Hamm P, et al. Do the results of randomized clinical trials of cardiovascular drugs influence medical practice? N Engl J Med 1992;327:241–247.
13. Heller RF, Dobson AJ, Alexander HM, et al. Changes in drug treatment and case fatality of patients with acute myocardial infarction. Med J Aust 1992;157:83–86.
14. Whitford DL, Southern AJ. Audit of secondary prophylaxis after myocardial infarction. Br Med J 1994;309:1268–1269.
15. Agusti A, Arnau JM, Laporte JR. Clinical trials versus clinical practice in the secondary prevention of myocardial infarction. Eur J Clin Pharmacol 1994;46:95–99.
16. Naylor CD. Population-wide mortality trends among patients hospitalized for acute myocardial infarction: the Ontario experience, 1981 to 1991. J Am Coll Cardiol 1994;24:1431–1438.
17. DeVreede JJM, Gorgels APM, Verstraaten GMP, et al. Did prognosis after acute myocardial infarction change during the past 30 years? A meta-analysis. J Am Coll Cardiol 1991;18:698–706.
18. Gallagher EJ, Viscoli CM, Horwitz RI. The relationship of treatment adherence to the risk of death after myocardial infarction in women. JAMA 1993;270;742–744.
19. Duryee R. The efficacy of inpatient education after myocardial infarction. Heart Lung 1992;21:217–227.
20. Yusuf S, Wittes J, Friedman L. Overview of results of randomized clinical trials in heart disease. I. Treatments following myocardial infarction. JAMA 1988;260: 2088–2093.
21. ISIS-1 Collaborative Group. A randomized trial of intravenous atenolol among 16,027 cases of suspected acute myocardial infarction. Lancet 1986;2:57–66.
22. The MIAMI Trial Research Group. Metoprolol in acute myocardial infarction (MIAMI): a randomized placebo-controlled international trial. Eur Heart J 1985;6: 199–226.
23. Roberts R, Rogers W, Mueller H, et al. Immediate versus deferred beta-blockade following thrombolytic therapy in patients with acute myocardial infarction. Circulation 1991;83:422–437.
24. Hansteen V. Beta blockage after myocardial infarction: the Norwegian propranolol study in high-risk patients. Circulation 1983;67(Suppl I):I57–I60.
25. Beta-blocker Heart Attack Trial Research Group. A randomized trial of propranolol in patients with acute myocardial infarction. 1. Mortality results. JAMA 1982; 247:1707–1714.
26. The Norwegian Multicenter Study Group. Timolol-induced reduction in mortality and reinfarction in patients surviving acute myocardial infarction. N Engl J Med 1981;304:801–807.
27. Yusuf S, Peto R, Lewis J, et al. Beta blockade during and after myocardial infarction: an overview of the randomized trials. Prog Cardiovasc Dis 1985;27:335–371.
28. Yusuf S. The use of beta-adrenergic blocking agents, i.v. nitrates and calcium channel blocking agents following acute myocardial infarction. Chest 1988;93: 25S–28S.
29. Yusuf S, Sleight P, Hels P, et al. Routine medical management of acute myocardial infarction. Lessons from overviews of recent randomized controlled trials. Circulation 1990;82(Suppl II):II-117–II-134.
30. Anderson J. Effects of beta-blockers on ventricular fibrillation threshold. In: Deedwania P, ed. Beta-blockers and cardiac arrhythmias. New York: Marcel Dekker, 1992:31–53.
31. Lichstein E. Effects of beta-blockers on cardiac arrhythmia in acute myocardial infarction: the BHAT experience. In: Deedwania P, ed. Beta-blockers and cardiac arrhythmias. New York: Marcel Dekker, 1992:133–149.

32. The Israeli SPRINT Study Group. Early administration of nifedipine in suspected acute myocardial infarction. The SPRINT-2 Study. Arch Intern Med 1993;153: 345–353.
33. The Israeli SPRINT Study Group. Secondary prevention reinfarction Israeli nifedipine trial (SPRINT). A randomized intervention trial of nifedipine in patients with acute myocardial infarction. Eur Heart J 1988;9:354–364.
34. Wilcox R, Hampton J, Banks D, et al. Trial of early nifedipine in acute myocardial infarction: the TRENT study. Br Med J 1986;293:1204–1208.
35. Gibson R. Current status of calcium channel-blocking drugs after Q wave and non-Q wave myocardial infarction. Circulation 1989;80(Suppl IV):IV–107–IV–119.
36. Muller J, Morrison J, Stone P, et al. Nifedipine therapy for patients with threatened and acute myocardial infarction: a randomized double-blind, placebo-controlled comparison. Circulation 1984;69:740–747.
37. Report of the Holland Interuniversity Nifedipine/Metoprolol Trial (HINT) Research Group. A randomized, double blind, placebo controlled comparison of recurrent ischemia in patients treated with nifedipine or metoprolol or both. Br Heart J 1986; 56:400–413.
38. Yusuf S, Held P, Furberg C. Update of effects of calcium antagonists in myocardial infarction or angina in light of the second Danish Verapamil Infarction Trial (DAVIT-II) and other recent studies. Am J Cardiol 1991;67:1295–1297.
39. The Multicenter Diltiazem Postinfarction Trial Research Group. The effect of diltiazem on mortality and reinfarction after myocardial infarction. N Engl J Med 1988;319:385–392.
40. The Danish Study Group on Verapamil in Myocardial Infarction. Effect of verapamil on mortality and major events after acute myocardial infarction (the Danish Verapamil Infarction Trial II-DAVIT II). Am J Cardiol 1990;66:779–785.
41. Gibson R, Boden W, Theroux P, et al. Diltiazem and reinfarction in patients with non-Q-wave myocardial infarction. N Engl J Med 1986;315:423–429.
42. Held P, Yusuf S, Furberg C. Calcium channel blockers in acute myocardial infarction and unstable angina: an overview. Br Med J 1989;299:1187–1192.
43. White MD, Norris RM, Brown MA, et al. Left ventricular end-systolic volume as the major determinant of survival after recovery from myocardial infarction. Circulation 1987;76:44–51.
44. Pfeffer MA, Pfeffer J, Steinberg C, et al. Survival after an experimental myocardial infarction: beneficial effects of long-term therapy with captopril. Circulation 1985; 72:406–412.
45. Pfeffer MA, Lamas GA, Vaughan DE, et al. Effect of captopril on progressive ventricular dilatation after anterior myocardial infarction. N Engl J Med 1988;319: 80–86.
46. Pfeffer MA, Braunwald E. Ventricular remodeling after myocardial infarction. Circulation 1990;81:1161–1172.
47. Pfeffer MA, Braunwald E, Moye LA, et al. Effect of captopril on mortality and morbidity in patients with left ventricular dysfunction after myocardial infarction: results of the survival and ventricular enlargement trial. N Engl J Med 1992;327:669–677.
48. Acute Infarction Ramipril Efficacy (AIRE) Study Investigators. Effects of ramipril on mortality and morbidity of survivors of acute myocardial infarction with clinical evidence of heart failure. Lancet 1993;342:821–828.
49. Gruppo Italiano per lo Studio della Sopravvivenza nell'Infarcto Miocardico. GISSI-3: effects of lisinopril and transdermal glyceryl trinitrate singly and together on 6-week mortality and ventricular function after acute myocardial infarction. Lancet 1994; 343:1115–1122.
50. Swedberg K, Held P, Kjekshus J, et al. on behalf of the CONSENSUS II Study Group. Effects of the early administration of enalapril on mortality in patients with acute myocardial infarction. Results of the Cooperative New Scandinavian Enalapril Survival Study II (CONSENSUS II). N Engl J Med 1992;327:678–684.
51. Ambrosioni E, Borghi C, Magnani B. The effect of the angiotensin-converting enzyme inhibitor zofenopril on mortality and morbidity after anterior myocardial infarction. N Engl J Med 1995;332:80–85.
52. ISIS-4 (Fourth International Study of Infarct Survival) Collaborative Group. ISIS-

4: a randomised factorial trial assessing early oral captopril, oral mononitrate, and intravenous magnesium sulphate in 58,050 patients with suspected acute myocardial infarction. Lancet 1995;345:669–685.
53. Chinese Cardiac Study Collaborative Group. Oral captopril versus placebo among 13,634 patients with suspected acute myocardial infarction: interim report from the Chinese Cardiac Study (CCS-1). Lancet 1995;345:686–687.
54. Antiplatelet Trialists' Collaboration. Secondary prevention of vascular disease by prolonged anti-platelet therapy. Br Med J 1988;296:320–332.
55. Hennekens CH, Buring JE, Peto R. Antioxidant vitamins—benefits not yet proved. N Engl J Med 1994;330:1080–1081.
56. Antiplatelet Trialists' Collaboration. Collaborative overview of randomized trials of antiplatelet treatment. Part I: Prevention of vascular death, myocardial infarction and stroke by prolonged antiplatelet therapy in different categories of patients. Br Med J 1994;308:81–106.
57. Chalmers TC, Matta RJ, Smith H, et al. Evidence favoring the use of anticoagulants in the hospital phase of acute myocardial infarction. N Engl J Med 1977;297: 1091–1096.
58. Smith P. Oral anticoagulant therapy in the chronic phase of myocardial infarction. Arch Pathol Lab Med 1993;117:97–101.
59. The Cardiac Arrhythmia Suppression Trial (CAST) Investigators. Preliminary report: effect of encainide and flecainide on mortality in a randomized trial of arrhythmia suppression after myocardial infarction. N Engl J Med 1989;321:406–412.
60. Echt D, Liebson P, Mitchell L, et al. Mortality and morbidity in patients receiving encainide, flecainide, or placebo. The cardiac arrhythmia suppression trial. N Engl J Med 1991;324:781–788.
61. Greene H, Roden D, Katz R, et al. The cardiac arrhythmia suppression trial: first CAST . . ., then CAST-II. J Am Coll Cardiol 1992;19:894–898.
62. Siegel D, Grady D, Browner W, et al. Risk factor modification after myocardial infarction. Ann Intern Med 1988;109:213–218.
63. Rossouw J, Lewis B, Rifkind B. The value of lowering cholesterol after myocardial infarction. N Engl J Med 1990;323:112–119.
64. Canner PL, Berge KG, Wenger NK, et al. Fifteen-year mortality in Coronary Drug Project patients: long-term benefit with niacin. J Am Coll Cardiol 1986;8:1245–1255.
65. Scandinavian Simvastatin Survival Study Group. Randomised trial of cholesterol lowering in 4,444 patients with coronary heart disease: the Scandinavian Simvastatin Survival Study (4S). Lancet 1994;344:1383–1389.
66. The Expert Panel. Report of the National Cholesterol Education Program (NCEP) Expert Panel on Detection, Evaluation, and Treatment of High Blood Cholesterol in Adults (Adult Treatment Panel II). JAMA 1993;23:3015–3023.
67. Deedwania PC. Clinical perspectives on primary and secondary prevention of coronary atherosclerosis. Med Clin North Am 1995;79:973–998.
68. Kannel WB, Sorlie P, Castelli WP, et al. Blood pressure and survival after myocardial infarction: the Framingham Study. Am J Cardiol 1980;45:326–330.
69. The Coronary Drug Project Research Group. Blood pressure in survivors of myocardial infarction. J Am Coll Cardiol 1984;4:1135–1147.
70. Herlitz J, Karlson BW, Richter A, et al. Prognosis in hypertensives with acute myocardial infarction. J Hypertens 1992;10:1265–1271.
71. Connolly DC, Elveback OR, Oxman HA. Coronary heart disease in residents of Rochester, Minnesota 1950–1975 III. Effect of hypertension and its treatment on survival of patients with coronary artery disease. Mayo Clin Proc 1983;58:249–254.
72. Antman EM, Lau J, Kupelnick B, et al. A comparison of results of meta-analyses of randomized control trials and recommendations of clinical experts. JAMA 1992;268: 240–248.

# PART IV

# Thrombolytics, Anticoagulant and Antiplatelet Therapy

CHAPTER 8

# Thrombolytics

Robert M. Califf

The development and use of thrombolytic therapy for the treatment of acute myocardial infarction provides a rich template for contemplating the issues that confront modern medicine. The development of thrombolytic therapy emanated from laboratory study of bacterial products (1), advanced through pioneering clinical investigation, and now is moving into an era of genetic engineering and modification of molecules. Clinical trials in this field have provided a paradigm for the development of an empirical basis for the practice of medicine, including detection of modest treatment effects, assessment of differential cost-effectiveness, and worldwide dissemination of effective therapy. In this chapter we will review the basis for thrombolytic treatment, the characteristics of available molecules, the basis for clinical decision making, and the direction of future research.

## PATHOPHYSIOLOGY OF ACUTE EVENTS

In order to understand the mechanisms for the efficacy of thrombolytic therapy, it is necessary to review the pathophysiology of acute ischemic heart disease events. In Western society, a variety of factors converge to produce focal, discrete lesions in the epicardial coronary arteries, often in the context of a diffusely abnormal arterial wall. These lesions initially tend to be nonocclusive, composed of a core of cholesterol and a large component of smooth muscle cells, connective tissue, and a fibrous cap (2, 3). The identity of the factors that precipitate the conversion of an asymptomatic atherosclerotic plaque to a lesion causing a symptomatic manifestation or sudden death is one of the great medical mysteries of the past several decades. Conceptually, the precipitating factors can be divided into intrinsic characteristics of the plaque that produce susceptibility, systemic factors that lead to plaque disruption, and coagulation activation, which leads to thrombus formation and propagation.

Detailed pathologic studies have provided substantial insight into the type of atherosclerotic plaque susceptible to an acute event. Although the majority of a cardiovascular specialist's time is spent dealing with high-grade stenoses that limit coronary blood flow, the most common "culprit" lesion in acute coronary syndromes is a low-grade lesion that is not flow limiting (4). Multiple studies of atherosclerosis progression have found that high-grade lesions are more likely to progress to complete obstruction than low-grade lesions, but low-grade lesions that progress to complete occlusion are much more likely to produce a clinical event.

Younger lesions that are susceptible tend to have a larger lipid pool and less fibrous tissue. Those that develop a fissure tend to have a thinned fibrous cap, often with an infiltration of macrophages. These findings suggest that an inciting agent attracts the macrophages, leading to thinning of the plaque and a higher risk of plaque rupture. Leading candidates as the inciting agent thus far have been oxidized low-density lipoprotein (LDL) cholesterol and viral infection. Finally, lesions at branch points in the coronary circulation are thought to be at increased risk of fissuring and thrombus propagation because of the increased shear force.

Given a susceptible plaque, a variety of systemic factors, labeled ischemic *triggers,* are associated with a higher likelihood of acute ischemic events (5). The first major clue to ischemic triggers came from the observation that acute myocardial infarction, unstable angina, and sudden death seemed to have a circadian pattern with an early morning peak in incidence. Pursuit of this concept led to the observation that the major issue in the early morning hours seems to be the presence of a hypercoagulable state and the assumption of an upright posture after a night of recumbency (6). Aspirin and β-adrenergic blocking agents both block this early morning peak in incidence.

More detailed epidemiologic investigation has now confirmed that behavioral and biological processes that lead to a surge of catecholamines are the key ischemic triggers. These include vigorous exercise in someone not aerobically fit, sexual activity, cigarette smoking, and even exposure to war (7).

Once a vulnerable plaque has developed a fissure, the major issue in determining whether an acute myocardial infarction will result is whether the thrombus propagates to produce a totally occluded vessel. In addition to the degree of stenosis prior to thrombus development, the intensity of the stimulus to clot propagation relative to inhibitors of clot formation is the major determinant of the likelihood of progression to occlusion. Of course, if the myocardium supplied by the vessel is well collateralized by other vessels, the damage may be minimal (8).

The fundamental process of thrombus development as currently understood is depicted in Figure 8.1. The fissured plaque exposes tissue factor to factor VII complex, which interacts with factors IXa and VIIIa to form prothrombinase complex. Activated protein C and protein S block this reaction, which is oriented toward the conversion of prothrombin to thrombin. The final steps involve the conversion of prothrombin to thrombin, leading to the formation of fibrin from fibrinogen, and the cross-linking of fibrin to stabilize the clot.

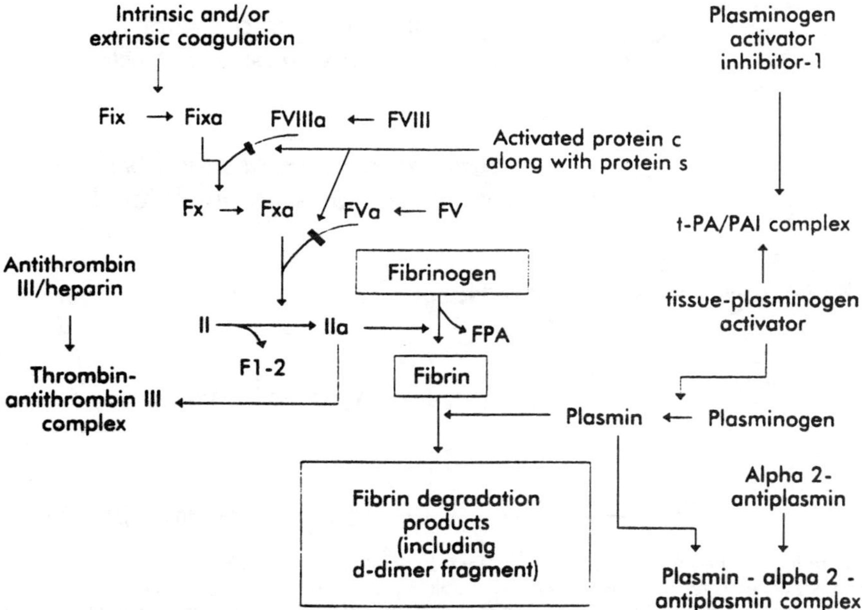


Figure 8.1 Schematic overview of coagulation and fibrinolysis. This diagram is meant to put several key factors in the context of the overall process of clot formation and resolution. The coagulation factors, factor V, factor VII, factor VIII, factor IX, and factor X, are abbreviated as FV, FVII, FVIII, FIX, and FX, respectively. II = prothrombin; PAI = plasminogen activator inhibitor; t-PA = tissue plasminogen I activator. Active forms of the coagulation zymogens include the suffix a (see also Figure 3, Chapter 9). Reprinted with permission from Tracy RP, Bovill EG. Hemostasis and risk of ischemic disease: epidemiologic evidence with emphasis on the elderly. In Califf RM, Mark DB, Wagner GS, eds. Acute coronary care. St. Louis: Mosby-Year Book, Inc., 1995;27–43.

## MECHANISMS OF CLOT LYSIS

### General Mechanisms

The fundamental components of the lysis of clot include the conversion of plasminogen to plasmin by plasminogen activators and the dissolution of fibrin to fibrin degradation products by plasmin (Fig. 8.2). Plasminogen is a glycoprotein including five triple-loop structures, termed *kringles*. The conversion of plasminogen to plasmin occurs via cleavage of a single peptide bond. The binding of plasminogen to fibrin and the mediation of the interaction of plasminogen with inactivators occurs via lysine binding sites, which interact with lysine and similar amino acids.

A variety of inhibitors of plasminogen have been described (9). α-2 Antiplasmin is a member of the serpin or serine proteinase inhibitor protein family. It forms a one-to-one complex with plasmin, which inactivates the serine protease activity of plasmin. Plasminogen activator inhibitor-1 (PAI-1) is also a serpin family member that is released from multiple cells

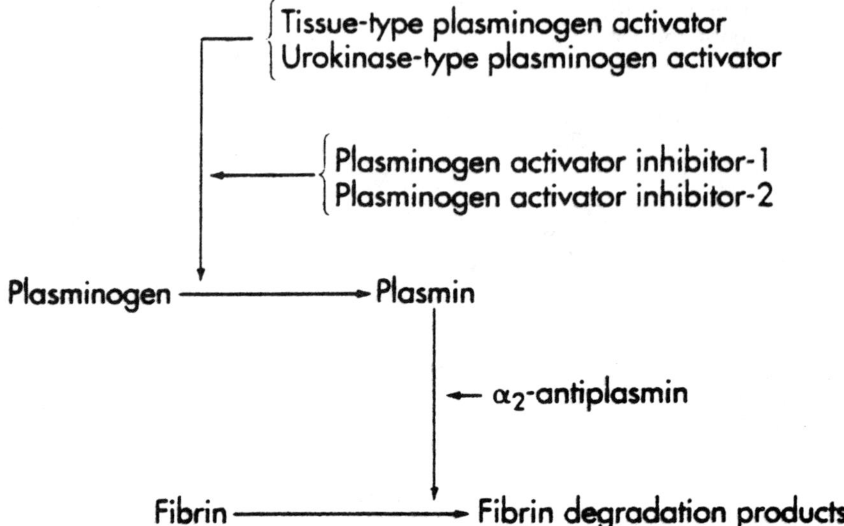


Figure 8.2 Schematic representation of the fibrinolytic system. The proenzyme plasminogen is activated to the active enzyme plasmin by tissue or urokinase plasminogen activator. Plasmin degrades fibrin into soluble fibrin degradation products. Inhibition of the fibrinolytic system may occur at the level of the plasminogen activators, by plasminogen activator inhibitors, or at the level of plasmin, mainly by $\alpha_2$-antiplasmin. Reprinted with permission from Collen D, Lijnen HR. Fibrinolytic system: implications for thrombolytic therapy. In: Califf RM, Mark DB, Wagner GS, eds. Acute coronary care. St. Louis: Mosby Year-Book, Inc., 1995;85–95.

with regulatory control now demonstrated by a variety of stimuli including thrombin, endotoxin, and tumor necrosis factor. Multiple pathophysiologic entities, including coronary artery disease, venous thrombosis, obesity, and sepsis have been associated with elevated levels of PAI-1 (10). PAI-1 is thought to be the major physiologic inhibitor of both tissue plasminogen activator (t-PA) and urinary plasminogen activator (u-PA). PAI-2, another serpin, has a less well described role in inhibiting plasminogen activators. To date it has been described most often in elevated levels in pregnancy, and no specific associations with disease states have been identified (11).

## Characteristics

Plasminogen activators can be characterized by their physiologic characteristics, including half-life, clearance, stability, and affinity for fibrin and plasminogen. Table 8.1 displays these data for comercially available agents. Fibrin specificity, the characteristic of greatest interest, is the ability of a plasminogen activator to convert plasminogen to plasmin on the fibrin surface in preference to conversion in the systemic circulation. Interestingly, the mechanisms by which fibrin specificity is conferred vary with different activators. To the extent that an activator is not fibrin spe-

**Table 8.1**
**Comparison of US Food and Drug Administration–Approved Thrombolytic Agents**

| | SK | APSAC | Alteplase |
|---|---|---|---|
| Dose | 1.5 million U (30–60 min) | 30 mg (5 min) | Weight-adjusted (90 min)[a] |
| Circulating half-life (min) | 20 | 100 | 6 |
| Clearance | Hepatic | Hepatic | Hepatic |
| Antigenic | Yes | Yes | No |
| Allergic reactions | Yes | Yes | No |
| Systemic fibrinogen depletion | Substantial | Substantial | Moderate, variable |
| Intracerebral hemorrhage | ~0.4% | ~0.6% | 0.6% |
| 90–min recanalization rate[b] | ~40% | ~63% | ~79% |
| TIMI 2 and 3 combined[c] | 60% | NA | 81% |
| TIMI 3[c] | 32% | NA | 54% |
| Lives saved per 100 | ~2.5 | ~2.5 | ~3.5[d] |
| Cost per dose (approximate $US) | 200 | 1700 | 2200 |
| Cost per life saved ($US) | 8,000 | 68,000 | 62,857 |
| Cost per year of life saved ($US) | <1000 | NA | 25,000–35,000[e] |

[a]Accelerated t-PA is given as follows: 15 mg bolus, then 0.75 mg/kg over 30 min (maximum 50 mg), then 0.50 mg/kg over 60 min (maximum 35 mg).
[b]Based on published data and assuming that 20% of arteries are already open prior to therapy.
[c]These data are from the GUSTO-I angiographic substudy.[37]
[d]Based on the finding from the GUSTO-I trial that accelerated t-PA saves one more additional life per 100 than does SK.
[e]Incremental cost per year of life saved for alteplase compared with streptokinase.
APSAC = anisoylated plasminogen streptokinase activator complex; GUSTO-I = Global Utilization of Streptokinase and t-PA for Occluded Coronary Arteries; min = minute; NA = not available; SK = streptokinase; TIMI = Thrombolysis in Myocardial infarction; t-PA = tissue plasminogen activator.
Adapted with permission from Califf RM: Acute myocardial infarction. In: Smith TW, ed. Cardiovascular Therapeutics. Philadelphia: W.B. Saunders, 1996, in press.

cific, it will create a systemic fibrinolytic state in order to lyse a specific thrombus in an epicardial coronary vessel. In theory, a highly fibrin-specific activator could lyse a coronary thrombus while causing no disturbance of the systemic circulation.

All currently described activators are cleared by the liver. Probably more importantly, these activators are also bound to a variety of cells and tissues, making it difficult to determine the duration of biological activity with certainty. The half-life of plasminogen activators may be important, although the concept of a half-life with these compounds is complicated by the binding of these agents. Thus, the measured activity in plasma samples may not accurately reflect the ongoing activity of bound plasminogen activator. Nevertheless, in concept, an agent with a short half-life should be given as an infusion, whereas an agent with a longer half-life may be given as a bolus. This concept will be tested in the Global Use of Strategies to Open Occluded Coronary Arteries (GUSTO)-III Trial, which will evaluate reteplase given as a double bolus compared with alteplase in an accelerated infusion in a mortality trial.

## MECHANISMS OF INDIVIDUAL AGENTS

### Streptokinase

Streptokinase is produced by several strains of hemolytic streptococci. Brand names of streptokinase in use are Streptase (Astra, Westborough, Massachusetts) and Kabikinase (KabiVitrum, Stockholm, Sweden). It is a single polypeptide chain that must form a complex with plasminogen before it can convert plasminogen to plasmin. After a complex is formed with plasminogen, the complex changes its conformation, allowing the active site to be exposed. The active site catalyzes the conversion of plasminogen to plasmin, and a streptokinase-plasmin complex is formed. α-2 Antiplasmin cannot inhibit the streptokinase-plasminogen complex.

Since streptokinase does not have greater affinity for fibrin-bound plasminogen than for circulating plasminogen, it must degrade plasma coagulation proteins to lyse coronary thrombus when given systemically (12, 13). Circulating neutralizing antibodies are prevalent given the frequency of infections with β-hemolytic streptococci in the general population (14). The dose of streptokinase currently used exceeds the concentration of these antibodies in almost all cases. However, a dose of streptokinase will produce neutralizing antibodies for at least 3–4 years (15).

Detailed dose response studies with intermediate physiologic end points have not been done with streptokinase. Based on small, incomplete studies, however, a regimen of 1.5 million U given over 60–90 minutes has become the standard (16), and this dose has been used in the mortality trials that have shown benefit. The recommended duration of the infusion is based on a concern about hypotension with more rapid administration and a dosing study suggesting higher patency with rapid infusion (17). Nevertheless, dramatic clinical results achieved in one small placebo-controlled trial (18), coupled with the success of the accelerated regimen of streptokinase, have stimulated interest in an even more rapid infusion of streptokinase.

The major side effects of streptokinase are hypotension, allergic reactions, and bleeding. The average drop in systolic blood pressure during the infusion is 10–20 mm Hg. The blood pressure usually responds rapidly when the patient's legs are raised and intravenous fluids are given; occasionally intravenous vasopressor support is needed. Allergy with streptokinase takes a variety of forms, including rash, pulmonary infiltrates, and a syndrome resembling serum sickness with arthritis.

### Urokinase

Prourokinase exists in nature as a single-chain glycoprotein (scu-PA), which is readily converted to two-chain urokinase plasminogen activator (tcu-PA). It is thought that tcu-PA has most of the plasminogen-activating activity, although the details of the fibrinolytic effect of scu-PA remain controversial.

Urokinase, commercially available as a tcu-PA product (Abbokinase; Abbott, Chicago, Illinois), is used extensively in the treatment of peripheral vascular thrombosis. It has never been studied in an adequately sized mortality trial for treatment of acute myocardial infarction, although smaller comparative trials with physiologic end points have found it to be similar to streptokinase (19). Recombinant scu-PA is currently in phase II clinical trials with promising results regarding coronary perfusion and reocclusion (20). When two-chain urokinase has been used for intravenous thrombolysis, a dose of 3,000,000 U over 3 hours has been used.

### Anistreplase

Anisoylated plasminogen-streptokinase activator complex (APSAC) (generic name anistreplase; brand name Eminase; SmithKline Beecham, Philadelphia, Pennsylvania) essentially consists of a complex of plasminogen and streptokinase with a p-anisoyl group added to protect the catalytic center from activation (21). Deacylation results in regeneration of the catalytic center of the complex, allowing the conversion of plasminogen to plasmin. This process initially was thought to occur preferentially on the fibrin surface, yielding a relatively fibrin-specific streptokinase; it is clear, however, that no significant fibrin specificity occurs, since deacylation occurs in the systemic circulation also.

Modestly sized dosing studies with anistreplase arrived at a dose of 30 U intravenously as a push over 2–5 minutes (22, 23). Just as with streptokinase, special attention is required because of the drop in blood pressure seen in many patients. The allergic manifestations are similar to those seen with streptokinase.

### Alteplase

t-PA (alteplase is the form of t-PA in use, the brand name is Activase; Genentech, South San Francisco, California) is a serpin with five domains: an NH2 region homologous with the finger domain; an "E domain" that is homologous with human epidermal growth factor; two disulfide-rich residues; a serine protease domain; and a COOH terminal. The structure of t-PA has been elucidated and the molecule itself and several mutants can now be manufactured. In the absence of fibrin, t-PA is a poor plasminogen activator, but in the presence of fibrin, t-PA becomes a potent fibrinolytic agent.

The $\alpha$ half-life of alteplase, the commercial form of t-PA, is 4.3 minutes, with a $\beta$ half-life of 46.2 minutes. The molecule is cleared primarily by hepatocytes. It is neutralized by PAI-1. Alteplase is now given as a dose of 15 mg by intravenous bolus, followed by 0.75 mg/kg over 30 minutes (not to exceed 50 mg), then followed by 0.50 mg/kg for 60 minutes (not to exceed 35 mg). This dose was arrived at through a series of angiographic trials and confirmed in the large Global Utilization of Streptokinase and t-PA for Occluded Coronary Arteries (GUSTO)-I mortality trial (24). Other doses have been tried with less successful results. The previous standard infusion was 60 mg over 1 hour (with 6–10 mg as a bolus), followed by 20 mg/hour for 2 hours, but this regimen was found to cause a higher intracranial bleeding rate than streptokinase with no apparent reduction in mortality (25, 26). A double bolus of alteplase recently demonstrated exciting perfusion data in one small study (27), and a mortality trial (Continuous Infusion versus Double-Bolus Administration of Alteplase; COBALT) has recently been mounted to test this regimen against the accelerated alteplase regimen.

### Reteplase

Reteplase (r-PA) is a relatively fibrin-specific thrombolytic agent derived from human t-PA. It is engineered from E. coli with the critical differences including lack of the finger, epidermal growth factor, and kringle-1 domains, and absence of carbohydrate side chains. These differences in structure allow r-PA to have a longer half life (four to eight times that of alteplase), making it a reasonable candidate for bolus administration. Although in most ways r-PA acts in a manner similar to that of alteplase, modest differences include somewhat less fibrin specificity and less hepatic uptake. r-PA is given in a dose of 10 MU as a bolus, followed by another 10 MU as a bolus 30 minutes later. This agent is in the final stages of clinical testing before becoming available for clinical use in the United States.

### Mutant TNK

Mutant TNK is a genetically engineered molecule with the basic structure of t-PA, altered by a series of mutations to provide it with enhanced fibrin specificity and a longer half-life (28). The molecule is also resistant to inhibition by PAI-1. In theory this combination of properties may permit the drug to be administered as a bolus with little disturbance of the coagulation system and less patient-to-patient variability engendered by differences in levels of inhibitors. Initial basic studies (28) and studies in rabbit cerebral thrombus models (29) have demonstrated that clot lysis is preserved and perhaps even enhanced compared with results of alteplase use and that the coagulation system can be relatively unperturbed with successful clot lysis. This compound has entered into phase II clinical trials.

### Bat-PA

The vampire bat Desmodus rotundus produces a plasminogen activator in its saliva that is similar to human t-PA but lacks the second kringle domain and the plasmin cleavage site for conversion to the two-chain form (30, 31). These differences result in a highly fibrin-specific molecule. The ability of bat-PA to lyse clot is increased 45,000 times on the fibrin surface. Studies in humans have not yet started.

### Staphylokinase

Staphylokinase is a compound produced by Staphylococcus aureus; its fibrinolytic potential has been known for many years (32). Although staphylokinase must form a complex with plasminogen to become a plasminogen activator, the active site is readily inhibited by α-2 antiplasmin, whereas with streptokinase this inhibition does not occur. Accordingly, staphylokinase is highly fibrin specific. Initial clinical trials in very small numbers of patients have been encouraging (33).

## MODEL FOR CLINICAL BENEFIT

The general model for clinical benefit was developed from seminal animal experiments by Reimer and Jennings (34) and concisely described by Rentrop (Fig. 8.3) in 1979 (35). The three critical elements are time from occlusion to reperfusion, the amount of myocardium at risk, and the extent of collateral flow. When an epicardial coronary vessel is occluded, the myocardium begins to necrose from the endocardium out towards the epicardium in a "wavefront of ischemic cell death" (34). Different species are subject to different time courses once occlusion occurs, predominantly due to differences in collateral flow. Infarction in the pig can be complete within 45 minutes since collaterals are usually minimal, whereas an infarction in a rat may not be transmural, even if reperfusion never occurs. Humans can fall anywhere within this spectrum, and no clinically useful predictive model has been developed.

For research purposes, technetium sestamibi has been helpful in demonstrating the applicability of this model to the human condition (36). This imaging agent, if injected early in the course of coronary occlusion, can provide an estimate of the amount of myocardium at risk; a follow-up study can provide evidence of final infarct size. In essence, the model as developed in the animal by Reimer and Jennings and as posed by Rentrop has been validated in clinical populations. Most recently, findings from sestamibi infarct sizing have been found to predict mortality in clinical populations (8).

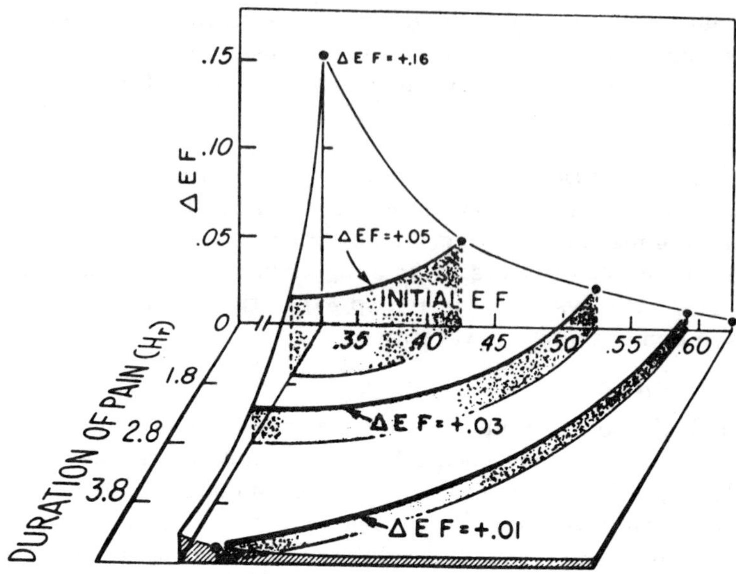


Figure 8.3 A conceptual model relating changes of ejection fraction (ΔEF) from preintervention to chronic angiography, duration of infarct symptoms (hours), and preintervention EF (initial EF). The two key factors are the duration of symptoms before reperfusion and the size of the infarction. Reprinted with permission from Rentrop P, Smith H, Painter L, et al. Changes in left ventricular ejection fraction after intracoronary thrombolytic therapy: results of the Registry of the European Society of Cardiology. Circulation 1983;68(Suppl I):I-55–I-60.

## PATHOPHYSIOLOGIC END POINTS

### General Description

Given the structural and physiologic properties of plasminogen activators and an understanding of the disease, the physiologic mechanisms for clinical benefit seem straightforward. Fundamentally, reperfusion therapy improves clinical outcome in acute myocardial infarction by opening occluded coronary arteries and perfusing downstream myocardium (37, 38). These effects lead to a reduction in myocardial infarct size and an improvement in left ventricular systolic function. Evidence is accumulating that reperfusion also improves the healing process.

Measurement of these intermediate pathophysiologic end points provides insight into expected clinical benefit. Higher rates of early and sustained reperfusion would be expected to produce more clinical benefits. Unfortunately, the fine balance between improvement in survival and risk of bleeding requires measurement of the end points themselves, since small differences can change the balance enough to alter the selection of one regimen versus another.

### Perfusion

In early trials of thrombolysis, the Thrombolysis in Myocardial Infarction (TIMI) Study Group (39) developed a grading system for coronary flow that has become the standard for assessing perfusion in clinical trials and clinical practice. TIMI grade 0 flow denotes a totally occluded artery at the point of the culprit lesion. TIMI grade 1 flow refers to the penetration of angiographic contrast beyond the culprit lesion but failure of the contrast to fill the artery. TIMI grade 2 flow is defined as complete filling of the artery at a slower rate than observed in normal arteries. When the artery fills normally angiographically, the flow is designated TIMI grade 3.

In the aggregated clinical trial data with thrombolytic therapy, the early attainment of TIMI grade 3 flow has been the dominant prognostic factor (38, 40). Patients with TIMI grade 3 flow at initial angiography have half the mortality of patients with TIMI grade 0 or 1 flow, with TIMI grade 2 flow in an intermediate mortality position. Additionally, patients with TIMI grade 3 flow have less heart failure or cardiogenic shock, better systolic left ventricular function, and fewer other clinical complications related to left ventricular function.

Prior to 1992, angiographic patency rates had been measured in 13,728 patients treated with streptokinase, alteplase administered at 100 mg over 3 hours, accelerated alteplase, APSAC, or conservative care (Fig. 8.4). Even without thrombolytic therapy, 20% of patients had a patent infarct-related artery within 60 minutes of enrollment in one study and close to 70% were patent beyond 3 days. Both alteplase and APSAC had more favorable patency profiles than control or streptokinase. Accelerated alteplase had the most favorable profile. Beyond 2–3 hours, no differences remained, but few observations were available between 2–3 hours and 24 hours.

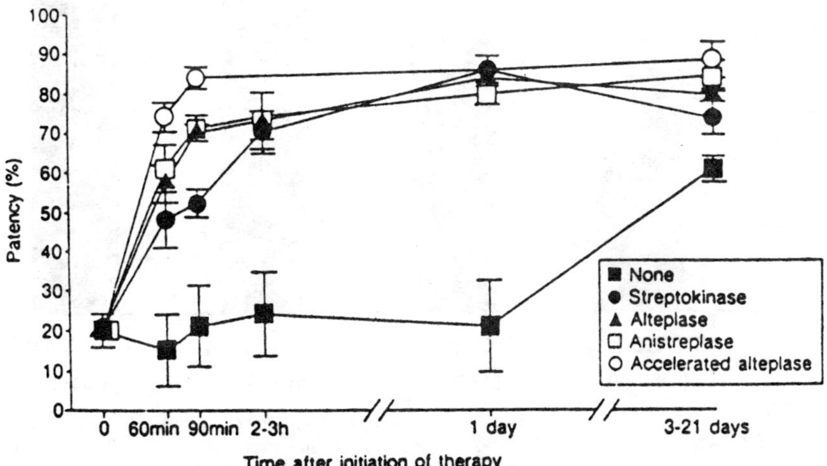


Figure 8.4 Pooled analysis of angiographic patency rates over time after various thrombolytic agents. Patency rates are highest after treatment with accelerated tissue plasminogen activator (alteplase). Early rates with conventional alteplase and anistreplase therapy are strikingly similar, and the patency rate after streptokinase treatment has "caught up" to that of conventional alteplase and anistreplase within 2 to 3 hours; includes 13,728 angiographic observations. Reprinted with permission from Granger CB, Califf RM, Topol EJ. Thrombolytic therapy for acute myocardial infarction. A review. Drugs 1992;44:293–325.

The GUSTO-I Trial randomly allocated the timing of angiography in a 2400-patient substudy to provide a "snapshot" of perfusion rates 90 minutes, 3 hours, 24 hours, and 1 week after entry into the study (37). The results prospectively confirmed the findings of the overview by Granger and colleagues (41). Accelerated alteplase was associated with a significantly higher patency rate at 90 minutes, but no difference was observed beyond that time point (Fig. 8.5).

The second important finding from the GUSTO angiographic substudy was that the major angiographic difference among the four treatment strategies was in TIMI grade 3 flow at 90 minutes (54% with accelerated alteplase versus 30–33% with streptokinase). Further analyses demonstrated that the mortality rates observed in the mortality trial were predicted accurately by calculating the relationship between the rate of TIMI grade 3 flow for each treatment regimen and mortality for that TIMI grade in the angiographic trial and extrapolating these findings to the mortality trial (38). The direct relationship between mortality and TIMI grade has been found in all angiographic studies to date (Fig. 8.6) (40).

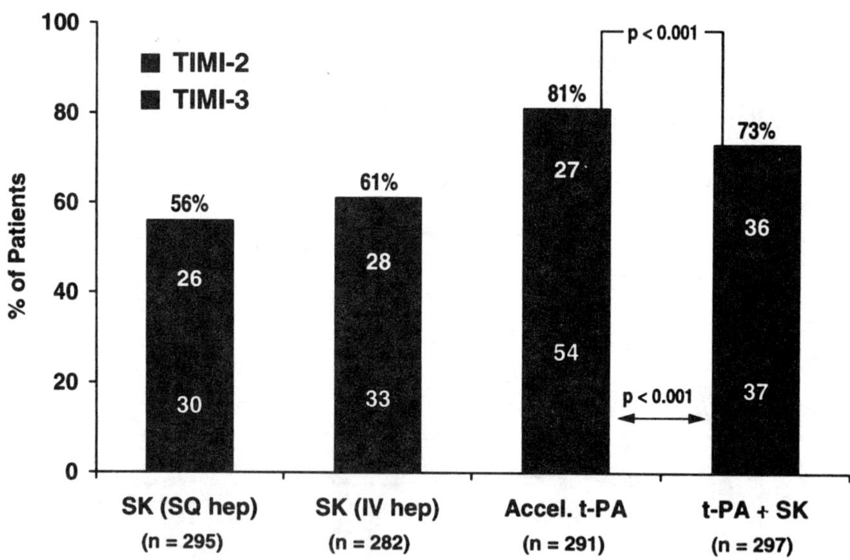


Figure 8.5 Patients randomized to receive accelerated (Accel.) tissue plasminogen activator (t-PA) who underwent angiography after 90 minutes had significantly higher rates of patency (Thrombosis in Myocardial Infarction [TIMI] grade 2 and 3 flow) than patients in the other three arms of the Global Utilization of Streptokinase and t-PA for Occluded Coronary Arteries (GUSTO)-I trial, and the difference in TIMI grade 3 flow was significant. IV hep = intravenous heparin; SK = streptokinase; SQ hep = subcutaneous heparin. Reprinted with permission from Califf RM, Topol EJ. The paradigm of acute reperfusion and the GUSTO-I trial. In: Califf RM, Mark DB, Wagner GS, eds. Acute coronary care. St. Louis: Mosby-Year Book, Inc., 1995;69–83.

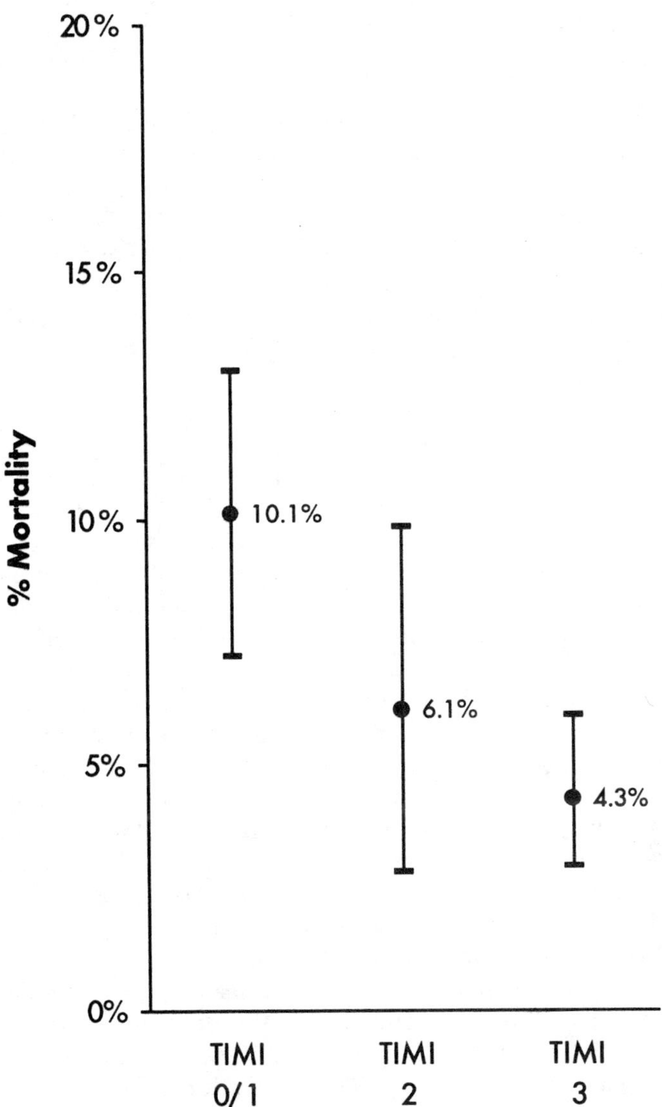


**Figure 8.6** In-hospital clinical outcome in patient groups defined by 90-minute coronary blood flow in the Thrombolysis in Myocardial Infarction (TIMI) trial. Values are displayed as percentage of patients with 95% confidence intervals. Adapted with permission from Lincoff AM, Topol EJ, Califf RM, et al., for the Thrombolysis and Angioplasty in Myocardial Infarction Study Group. Significance of a coronary artery with thrombolysis in myocardial infarction grade 2 flow "patency" (outcome in the Thrombolysis and Angioplasty in Myocardial Infarction Trials). Am J Cardiol 1995;75:871–876.

The higher TIMI 3 perfusion rate observed with accelerated alteplase in GUSTO-I has been confirmed by a review of previous studies. In small angiographic studies, TIMI grade 3 flow has been observed in 10–15% more cases of accelerated dosing with alteplase than with the older dosing regimen (42).

The newer thrombolytic agents and adjunctive therapies have demonstrated promising improvements in achievement of TIMI grade 3 flow. In comparisons with both 3-hour (RAPID-1) and accelerated dosing (RAPID-2) of alteplase, reteplase has demonstrated superior TIMI grade 3 flow at 60 and 90 minutes (20, 43). When added to either alteplase or streptokinase, both hirudin (44) and hirulog (45) have been associated with better TIMI grade 3 rates than heparin. Integrelin, a glycoprotein IIb/IIIa inhibitor, has resulted in very high rates of TIMI grade 3 flow when combined with alteplase (46).

## Reocclusion

With substantial focus on reperfusion in the literature, the importance of reocclusion has been underestimated. The first detailed report on the clinical consequences of reocclusion noted a doubling of mortality (11% versus 5%) (47) and most other major complications of infarction in patients with angiographically documented reocclusion compared with patients with sustained perfusion. Thus, reocclusion can offset the benefits gained by early reperfusion and in some cases may actually cause detriment beyond the clinical state observed in the absence of reperfusion. Unfortunately, some patients who are stable prior to administration of a thrombolytic suddenly deteriorate with reocclusion. Causative mechanisms are speculative, but two concepts are prominent. One is that the combination of reperfusion injury and failure to maintain nutrient flow creates an especially adverse situation. The other is that collateral blood flow, which may have developed prior to the acute occlusion causing the index infarction, is rapidly decreased when reperfusion occurs, leading to a more profound loss of tissue perfusion with reocclusion.

Efforts to determine which patients are at risk of reocclusion have not yielded satisfactory results. In one study (47), only inferior infarction, bradycardia at the time of thrombolytic administration, and the use of a 3-hour alteplase infusion predicted reocclusion from information readily available to the clinician. From angiographically available data, surprisingly, the degree of residual stenosis and perfusion status are only weakly related (48, 49) if at all (50), to the likelihood of reocclusion.

Initial reports demonstrated that standard dose alteplase was associated with a higher rate of reocclusion than was streptokinase. The change to accelerated dosing of alteplase has been associated with a much lower risk of reocclusion (Fig. 8.7). In GUSTO-I, the rates of reocclusion were not different among the four thrombolytic regimens. Reocclusion rates with

## Reocclusion Rates

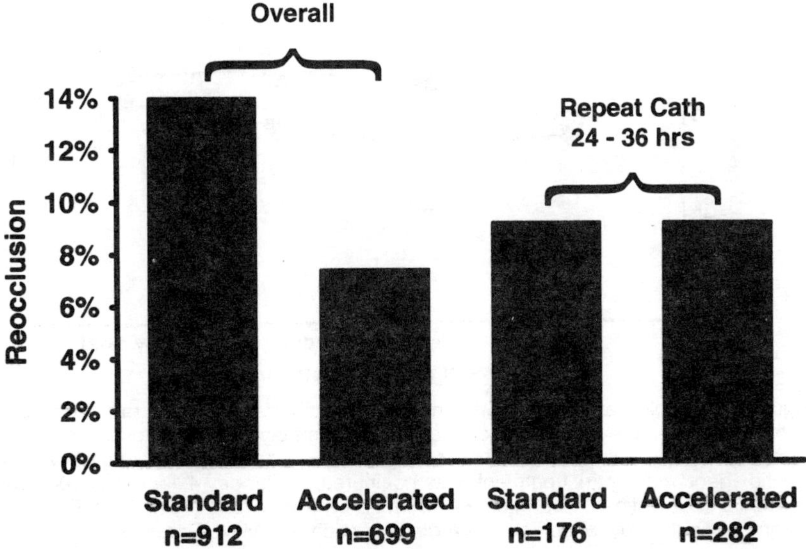


Figure 8.7 Patients given accelerated tissue plasminogen activator (t-PA) are less likely to have a reocclusion than patients given standard t-PA. Cath = catheterization. Reprinted with permission from Califf RM, Topol EJ. The paradigm of acute reperfusion and the GUSTO-I trial. In: Califf RM, Mark DB, Wagner GS, eds. Acute coronary care. St. Louis: Mosby-Year Book, Inc., 1995;69–83.

anistreplase appear to be similar to those of streptokinase (13), whereas the reocclusion rates with new regimens have not been established with certainty. The new antithrombin and antiplatelet agents have shown promising results with regard to reocclusion, but larger trials are needed to establish reliable estimates.

### Left Ventricular Function

In a pooled analysis of 3066 ventriculographic observations comparing a thrombolytic agent versus control treatment, a modest improvement in ejection fraction with thrombolytic therapy was demonstrated by Granger and colleagues (Fig. 8.8) (41). This effect was most substantial on day 4 and seemed to erode over the next several weeks. At 2–3 weeks after entry into the studies, the difference was only several ejection fraction points. This apparently small difference could have arisen partially from the higher mortality in patients with poor ejection fractions in the control groups, thus artifactually raising the ejection fraction values for the surviving control patients; since thrombolysis allows better survival, particularly in high-risk patients, many patients with poor left ventricular function survive,

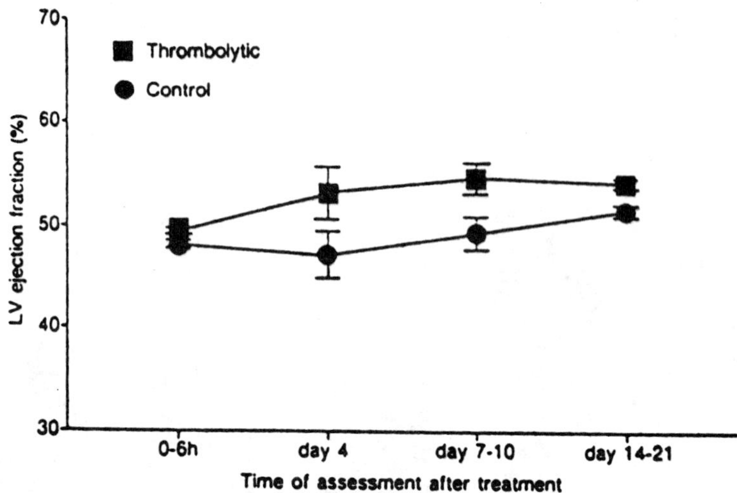


Figure 8.8 Pooled analysis of left ventricular ejection fraction from randomized trials of thrombolytic therapy versus control treatment. Thrombolytic therapy results in significantly higher ejection fraction ($P \leq 0.001$ for each time point), and the difference between thrombolytic agent and control treatment does not increase after day 4. Includes 3,066 ventriculographic observations. Reprinted with permission from Granger CB, Califf RM, Topol EJ. Thrombolytic therapy for acute myocardial infarction. A review. Drugs 1992;44:293–325.

tending to lower the average ejection fraction in the group treated with thrombolytic.

Given the small differences in ejection fraction comparing thrombolytic therapy with conservative care, it is not surprising that no significant difference was observed comparing one thrombolytic agent with another until accelerated alteplase was tested in large groups of patients. In both GUSTO-I37 and TIMI 4 (51), accelerated alteplase resulted in modestly better global function than did streptokinase or APSAC. In GUSTO-I, multiple measures of regional systolic function and ventricular volumes also were better with accelerated alteplase.

## Coagulation Factors

The fibrin-specific agents produce less disturbance of the coagulation system, but the relevance of this to clinical outcome is uncertain. In studies of nonspecific thrombolytic agents (streptokinase, APSAC, urokinase), coronary thrombolysis does not occur unless a systemic lytic effect is present. When fibrin-specific agents are tested, bleeding is greater with more fibrinogen breakdown, but reocclusion is more frequent when fibrinogen is spared (52, 53). Thus, coagulation measures are critical in the development of a profile of drug activity but cannot be used alone to provide insight into the balance from a total picture of clinical outcomes.

## CLINICAL END POINTS

### Death

The most important clinical outcome with acute myocardial infarction is death. Currently in patients with ST-segment elevation who qualify for thrombolytic therapy, the expected mortality is 6–8% over the first 30 days. Each of the currently available drugs has been evaluated in a trial designed to demonstrate effect on mortality. Although it is tempting to compare the mortality reductions in these different trials, no valid conclusions can be drawn from such indirect comparisons.

A substantial effort has been devoted to developing an understanding of factors predictive of mortality in patients eligible for thrombolytic therapy. More than 80% of the information about prognosis is contained in five simple clinical variables: age, blood pressure, Killip class, heart rate, and location of infarction. As one might anticipate, age and blood pressure are not linearly related to the risk of death. As shown in Figures 8.9–8.11 (from GUSTO-I), the risk of death increases dramatically in individuals more than 65 years of age and in those with a systolic pressure of less than 110 mm Hg or a diastolic pressure of less than 70 mm Hg (54). Interestingly, both a slow heart rate and tachycardia are associated with an increasing risk of death. Anterior myocardial infarction is associated with a doubling of mortality compared with inferior myocardial infarction.

A more sophisticated view of the electrocardiogram (ECG) demonstrates that the sum of ST-segment deviation and the presence of conduction

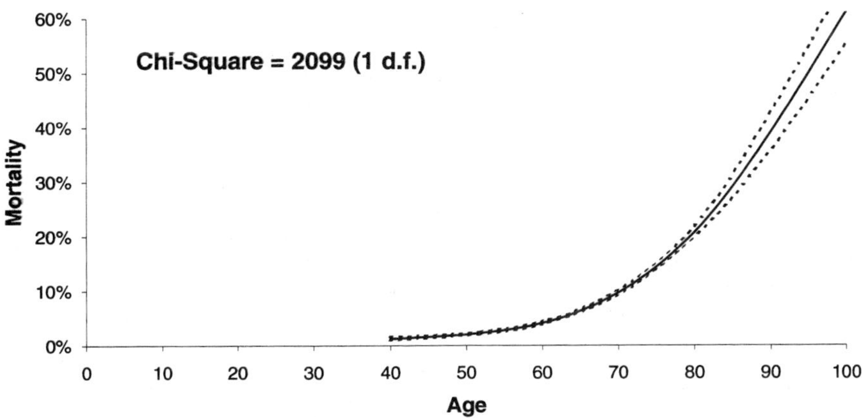


Figure 8.9 Graph shows unadjusted (univariate) relations between age and 30-day mortality from GUSTO-I. Dotted curves show 95% confidence intervals. d.f.= degrees of freedom. Reprinted with permission from Lee KL, Woodlief LH, Topol EJ, et al., for the GUSTO-I Investigators. Predictors of 30-day mortality in the era of reperfusion for acute myocardial infarction: results from an international trial of 41,021 patients. Circulation 1995;91:1659–1668.

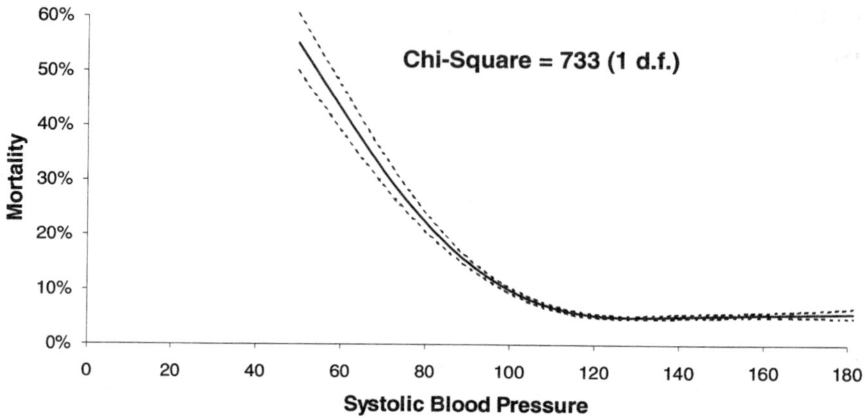


Figure 8.10 Graph shows unadjusted (univariate) relations between systolic blood pressure and 30-day mortality. d.f. = degrees of freedom. Reprinted with permission from Lee KL, Woodlief LH, Topol EJ, et al., for the GUSTO-I Investigators. Predictors of 30-day mortality in the era of reperfusion for acute myocardial infarction: results from an international trial of 41,021 patients. Circulation 1995;91:1659–1668.

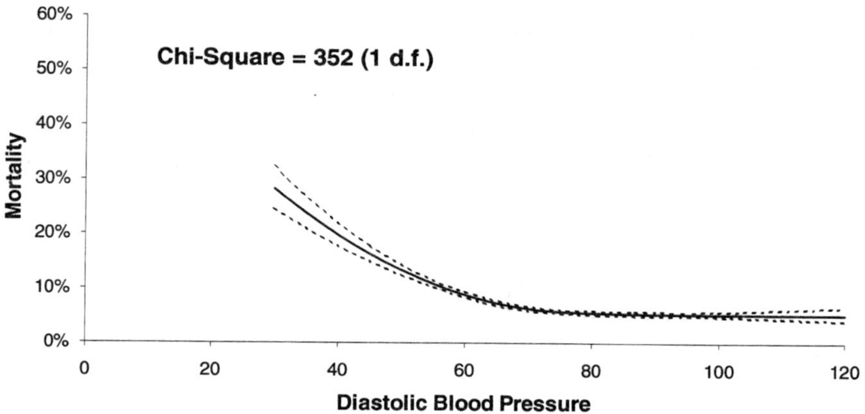


Figure 8.11 Graph shows unadjusted (univariate) relations between diastolic blood pressure and 30-day mortality. d.f. = degrees of freedom. Reprinted with permission from Lee KL, Woodlief LH, Topol EJ, et al., for the GUSTO-I Investigators. Predictors of 30-day mortality in the era of reperfusion for acute myocardial infarction: results from an international trial of 41,021 patients. Circulation 1995;91:1659–1668.

system abnormalities add substantial information (55). A number of other factors are much less important in predicting acute outcome. When angiographic information is available, ejection fraction, number of diseased vessels, and severity of mitral regurgitation are important predictors of outcome.

Through a collaborative effort termed the Fibrinolytic Therapy Trialists' (FTT) Collaboration, data from the major trials comparing thrombolytic agents with a control group have been combined in an electronic database (56). The summary of the data demonstrates a reduction in risk of death of 18% overall and 25% for patients with ST-segment elevation or bundle branch block treated within 6 hours of symptom onset. In general, the higher the risk category of the patient if treated with conservative treatment the greater the benefit of thrombolytic therapy. The relative reduction in risk is constant across subgroups, making the absolute reduction in risk via thrombolytic therapy linearly related to the underlying risk without thrombolytic therapy.

The relationship of thrombolytic benefit to age is fascinating. Patients under the age of 55 years have an underlying risk of death of less than 5%, making the absolute benefit of treatment very small. Between the ages of 55 and 75 the underlying risk of death constantly increases, as does the benefit of thrombolytic therapy when measured in absolute terms. After the age of 75, the risk of death continues to accelerate, but the observed benefit of thrombolytic therapy is attenuated, although still measurable. Whether this attenuation of relative benefit is a valid reflection of the effect of the treatment or simply a statistical artifact cannot be determined because the number of patients randomized over age 75 is quite small (56). An identical pattern of a trend toward a reduction in relative benefit in patients over age 75 was observed in the GUSTO-I trial comparing accelerated alteplase with streptokinase (38).

In a similar manner both the relative benefit and the absolute benefit of thrombolytic therapy in patients who have inferior myocardial infarction appear to be diminished compared with the benefit in patients who have anterior myocardial infarction. Again, a similar pattern was observed comparing accelerated alteplase with streptokinase in GUSTO-I. Further analysis revealed, however, that this effect predominantly related to inferior myocardial infarction without other electrocardiographic changes such as precordial ST-segment depression myocardial infarction (57). For patients who have inferior myocardial infarction with precordial ST-segment depression or ST-segment elevation in the apical or lateral leads, factors associated with higher risk, the benefit of accelerated alteplase is apparent.

Patients with cardiogenic shock pose a problem of substantial proportions. These patients have a very high mortality if treated conservatively, yet the randomized trials fail to show a benefit, violating the general principle that patients with higher baseline risk have greater benefit. The confidence limits for the observed effect included a 25% reduction in the risk of death. Furthermore, in the International Study of Infarct Survival (ISIS)-2 cohort with hypotension and tachycardia, a substantial treatment effect was observed. Thus, the lack of observed benefit simply may reflect inadequate numbers of patients randomized. Alternatively, there is ample evidence that reperfusion rates may be markedly reduced in the absence of adequate systolic pressure. Controlled trials comparing thrombolytic agents continue to report mortality rates of over 60% in patients with cardiogenic shock, and alteplase appears to be no more effective than streptokinase in this setting. Direct angioplasty may be a preferable strategy (58, 59), although thrombolytic therapy is recommended when direct angioplasty cannot be performed expeditiously.

Time to treatment has been a major issue for research efforts, predominantly because the concept that more myocardium can be salvaged with earlier reperfusion has been a cornerstone of the therapeutic strategy. Indeed, a direct relationship exists between the time to randomization in the clinical trials of thrombolytic therapy and the benefit of thrombolytic treatment, with approximately 1.6 additional lives saved per 100 patients treated for each hour earlier that treatment is instituted (56). The issue has been clouded because only time to randomization has been recorded in clinical trials thus far, not time from symptom onset to *treatment.* In particular, interest has focused on the first hour after symptom onset (17), with some evidence that treatment in this time frame can result in substantially greater savings of life and preservation of left ventricular function. The FTT data are controversial on this point, and different authorities have come to different conclusions.

A major focus has been placed on shortening the time to treatment in practice. Prehospital thrombolysis has been tested in randomized trials and was found to be feasible (60–62). Although some improvement in outcome is evident when this approach is implemented, the cost of maintaining a prehospital system is a major impediment in many communities; prehospital electrocardiography offers an alternative that many communities can implement. Each hospital should have a protocol for thrombolysis administration that reduces the door to needle time to less than 45 minutes, although 30 minutes is the desirable goal (63, 64). One such protocol is shown in Figure 8.12. Tracking the components of time to treatment can provide a useful instrument for improvement (Fig. 8.13).

Streptokinase (65–67), APSAC (68), and alteplase given as 100 mg over 3 hours (69) have all been shown to reduce mortality compared with placebo or open control therapy. Unfortunately, indirect comparisons cannot be used to determine which approach leads to the greatest reduction in mortality, since differences in the baseline characteristics of the patients and underlying associated therapies influence the observed mortality rates in an uncontrolled fashion.

The FTT overview provides the most comprehensive picture of the relationship between baseline characteristics and the benefit of thrombolytic therapy. A benefit was observed in all groups of patients except those without ST-segment elevation or bundle branch block on the ECG (Fig. 8.14) (56).

Two large trials, ISIS-3 and Gruppo Italiano per lo Studio della Sopravvivenza nell'Infarto Miocardico (GISSI)-2/International have definitively shown that streptokinase and alteplase given over an extended period yield

# Sample Standing Orders for the Acute MI Patient

☐ Patient screened, 12-lead ECG obtained

☐ Aspirin: 160 mg chewed STAT; then ASA 325 mg po qd

☐ Patient has no known contraindications to thrombolytic therapy

☐ Start 2 – 3 IV lines

☐ Prior to beginning infusion, draw CCU MI admission labs including aPTT

☐ Heparin:
a. 80 u/kg bolus (rounded to nearest 50 units) = ______________ units
b. 15 u/kg/hr starting infusion (rounded to nearest 50 units) = ______________ units/hr
c. draw aPTT at 2 hrs and q6h x 24 hrs; then qd while heparinized
d. follow heparin protocol for aPTT< 60 only, for first 24 hours
→ DO NOT ADJUST FOR aPTT > 100 DURING FIRST 24 HOURS
e. follow heparin protocol for aPTT < 60 or > 100 after first 24 hours

Notify pharmacy to mix, deliver drug and administer when applicable:

## Thrombolytic Agent (check one)

| | |
|---|---|
| ☐ "front loaded" rt-PA (100 mg/100 ml IV PB) | 15 mg bolus over 1–2 minutes<br>0.75 mg/kg over 30 minutes (NTE 50 mg)<br>0.50 mg/kg over 60 minutes (NTE 35 mg) |

| ☐ rt-PA reconstitute 1 mg/ml | pts > 65 kgs (143 lbs) 100 mg total dose | pts < 65 kgs (143 lbs) 1.25 mg/kg total dose |
|---|---|---|
| | 6 mg bolus over 1–2 minutes | 6 mg bolus over 1–2 minutes |
| | 54 mg IVPB over 1 hour | 54% IVPB over 1 hour |
| | 40 mg IVPB over 2 hours | 40% IVPB over 2 hours |

| | |
|---|---|
| ☐ streptokinase (SK) | 1.5 million units diluted in 50 ml D5W IVPB over 60 minutes |

☐ Administer thrombolytic infusion via controlled infusion pump. At end of infusion (bag empty), add 30 cc NS to the bag and continue infusing to flush tubing

☐ Repeat 12-lead ECG at 3, 6, 12 and 24 hours after admission or if any chest pain reoccurs

☐ Vital signs with neuro checks every 15 mins x 4; then every 30 mins x 2; then every 2 hours x 18; then routine, CCU vital signs

☐ Guiac all stools and emesis x 2 days

☐ Heme-test urine x 24 hours

☐ No radial artery or femoral artery punctures

☐ No subclavian or I.J. lines

☐ Notify MD STAT if evidence of significant internal bleeding occurs or there is a change in neurologic status. Stop heparin and thrombolytic agents

☐ Notify MD STAT if chest pain reoccurs

MD signature: ______________________________ Date: ________________

Figure 8.12 Sample standard orders and thrombolytic protocol for patients with acute myocardial infarction (MI). Reprinted with permission from Kline E, Smith D, Martin J, et al. Strategies to decrease treatment delays in patients receiving thrombolytic therapy for acute myocardial infarction. In: Califf RM, Mark DB, Wagner GS, eds. Acute coronary care. St. Louis: Mosby Year-Book, Inc., 1995; 265–279.

# Emergency Department Thrombolytic Worksheet

## Treatment Criteria

BP ______________

Weight ______________

☐ Ongoing chest pain > 30 min and < 6 hrs

☐ ST elevation > 2 mm in two anterior leads or > 1 mm in two inferior leads

## Contraindications

☐ SBP < 90 (unresponsive to fluid or vasopressors) or > 180 mmHg

☐ DBP > 110 mmHg

Within the previous two weeks:

- ☐ GI bleed
- ☐ Surgery, biopsies
- ☐ Non-compressible central lines
- ☐ Trauma
- ☐ Recent internal bleeding

Medical history of:

- ☐ CVA, TIA, Hx of head injury/surgery
- ☐ Recent CPR > 10 minutes
- ☐ Hemorrhagic retinopathy
- ☐ Recent pericarditis
- ☐ Terminal illness
- ☐ Left heart thrombus

## Time to Treatment Evaluation

| Note Time | Initials | |
|---|---|---|
| ___:___ | ______ | Arrival in ER |
| ___:___ | ______ | Triage nurse evaluation |
| ___:___ | ______ | Nursing H/P |
| ___:___ | ______ | ASA given |
| ___:___ | ______ | ECG obtained |
| ___:___ | ______ | ED physician H/P |
| ___:___ | ______ | MD consult, if ordered |
| ___:___ | ______ | Drug ordered from Pharmacy |
| ___:___ | ______ | Standing orders signed |
| ___:___ | ______ | IV access |
| ___:___ | ______ | Baseline labs drawn: CBC, PTT, FDP, Fibrinogen, CK, CK-MB, Chem Panel |
| ___:___ | ______ | Heparin ______ u bolus and infusion begun |
| ___:___ | ______ | Thrombolytic infusion begun |
| ___:___ | ______ | CCU bed arranged |
| ___:___ | ______ | Transferred to CCU |

## Decision to Treat

With lytic: ______________ (type) ☐ Yes ☐ No

**WARNINGS** The risks of thrombolytic therapy may be increased and should be weighed against the anticipated benefits in any condition in which bleeding constitutes a significant hazard or would be particularly difficult to manage because of its location.

Figure 8.13 Checklist of inclusion and exclusion criteria for thrombolysis. Reprinted with permission from Kline E, Smith D, Martin J, et al. Strategies to decrease treatment delays in patients receiving thrombolytic therapy for acute myocardial infarction. In: Califf RM, Mark DB, Wagner GS, eds. Acute coronary care. St. Louis: Mosby Year-Book, Inc., 1995; 265–279.

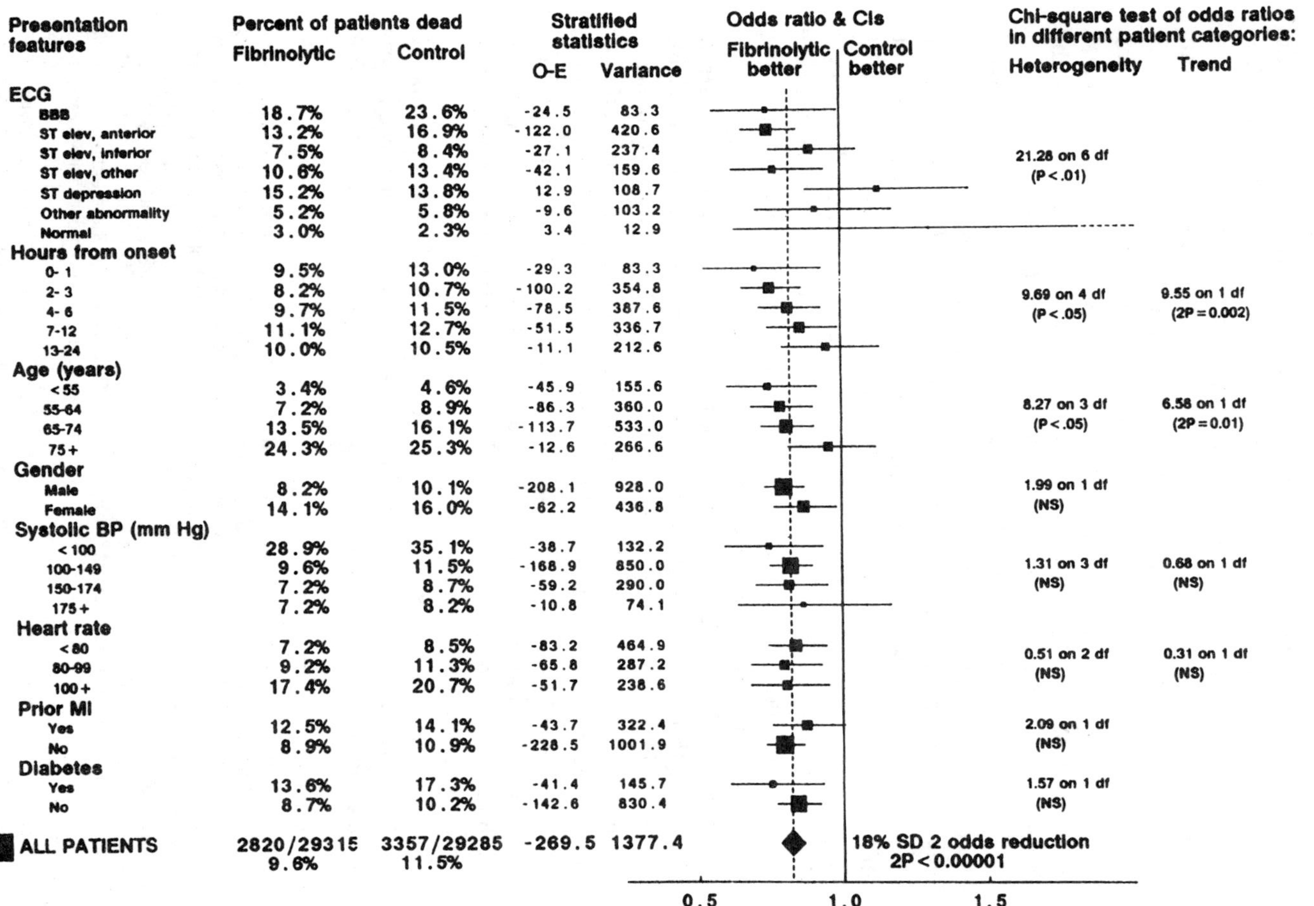
Presentation features
Percent of patients dead
Fibrinolytic Control
Stratified statistics
O-E Variance
Odds ratio & CIs
Fibrinolytic better | Control better
Chi-square test of odds ratios in different patient categories:
Heterogeneity Trend
ECG
BBB 18.7% 23.6% -24.5 83.3
ST elev, anterior 13.2% 16.9% -122.0 420.6
ST elev, inferior 7.5% 8.4% -27.1 237.4
ST elev, other 10.6% 13.4% -42.1 159.6
ST depression 15.2% 13.8% 12.9 108.7
Other abnormality 5.2% 5.8% -9.6 103.2
Normal 3.0% 2.3% 3.4 12.9
21.28 on 6 df (P < .01)
Hours from onset
0- 1 9.5% 13.0% -29.3 83.3
2- 3 8.2% 10.7% -100.2 354.8
4- 6 9.7% 11.5% -78.5 387.6
7-12 11.1% 12.7% -51.5 336.7
13-24 10.0% 10.5% -11.1 212.6
9.69 on 4 df (P < .05)
9.55 on 1 df (2P = 0.002)
Age (years)
< 55 3.4% 4.6% -45.9 155.6
55-64 7.2% 8.9% -86.3 360.0
65-74 13.5% 16.1% -113.7 533.0
75 + 24.3% 25.3% -12.6 266.6
8.27 on 3 df (P < .05)
6.58 on 1 df (2P = 0.01)
Gender
Male 8.2% 10.1% -208.1 928.0
Female 14.1% 16.0% -62.2 436.8
1.99 on 1 df (NS)
Systolic BP (mm Hg)
< 100 28.9% 35.1% -38.7 132.2
100-149 9.6% 11.5% -168.9 850.0
150-174 7.2% 8.7% -59.2 290.0
175 + 7.2% 8.2% -10.8 74.1
1.31 on 3 df (NS)
0.68 on 1 df (NS)
Heart rate
< 80 7.2% 8.5% -83.2 464.9
80-99 9.2% 11.3% -65.8 287.2
100 + 17.4% 20.7% -51.7 238.6
0.51 on 2 df (NS)
0.31 on 1 df (NS)
Prior MI
Yes 12.5% 14.1% -43.7 322.4
No 8.9% 10.9% -228.5 1001.9
2.09 on 1 df (NS)
Diabetes
Yes 13.6% 17.3% -41.4 145.7
No 8.7% 10.2% -142.6 830.4
1.57 on 1 df (NS)
ALL PATIENTS 2820/29315 9.6% 3357/29285 11.5% -269.5 1377.4
18% SD 2 odds reduction
2P < 0.00001
0.5
1.0
1.5

almost identical mortality rates (Fig. 8.15) (70, 71). Given the fact that these two trials included almost 50,000 patients, the accuracy of the results for the thrombolytic regimens as given in the trials is beyond doubt. The disparity between the observed mortality rates and the expected outcomes based on differences in early perfusion with the regimens caused substantial controversy. Several explanations for these findings have been put forward. Neither trial routinely used intravenous heparin. ISIS-3 used a different form of t-PA (duteplase) that has never been commercially developed. The prolonged dosing of alteplase resulted in lower perfusion rates and higher reocclusion rates compared with accelerated dosing.

These concerns led to the design and conduct of the GUSTO-I trial, which was undertaken to test the hypothesis that early and sustained perfusion would decrease mortality and morbidity. The 30-day and 1-year follow-up results are displayed in Figure 8.16. The use of accelerated alteplase led to a saving of 11 lives per 1000 patients treated compared with standard streptokinase dosing. The combination of the mortality results with the perfusion and left ventricular function results discussed above provides the linkage among perfusion, left ventricular function, and mortality that confirms the initial concepts of Rentrop.

In the ISIS-3 trial, APSAC was found to have no advantage over streptokinase with regard to mortality. Subsequent smaller studies comparing APSAC with accelerated alteplase found evidence for superiority of accelerated alteplase when APSAC was used with intravenous heparin (51) or without heparin (23). Neither of these studies had the statistical power to evaluate mortality, but the evidence with regard to left ventricular function, perfusion, bleeding, and morbid outcomes in conjunction with the ISIS-3 results has markedly slowed, if not terminated, further large-scale studies with anistreplase.

The subgroup analyses comparing accelerated alteplase with streptokinase from GUSTO-I are quite similar to the comparisons of thrombolytic therapy and conservative care from the FTT analysis (Figs. 8.17–8.21) (56).

←

Figure 8.14 Proportional effects of fibrinolytic therapy on mortality during days 0 to 35, subdivided by presentation features. "Observed minus expected" (O-E) number of events among fibrinolytic-allocated patients (and its variance) is given for subdivisions of presentation features, stratified by trial. This is used to calculate odds ratios (ORs) of death among patients allocated to fibrinolytic therapy versus that among those allocated control therapy. ORs (black squares with areas proportional to amount of "statistical information" contributed by the trials) are plotted with their 99% confidence intervals (CIs) (horizontal lines). Squares to the left of the solid vertical line indicate benefit (significant at 2 $P < 0.01$ only where entire CI is to left of vertical line). Overall result and 95% CI is represented by the diamond, with overall proportional reduction in the odds of death and statistical significance given alongside. Chi-square tests for evidence of heterogeneity of, or trends in, size of ORs in subdivisions of each presentation feature are also given. BBB = bundle branch block; BP = blood pressure; MI = myocardial infarction; SD = standard deviation. Reprinted with permission from Fibrinolytic Therapy Trialists (FTT) Collaborative Group. Indications for fibrinolytic therapy in suspected acute myocardial infarction: collaborative overview of early mortality and major morbidity results from all randomised trials of more than 1000 patients. Lancet 1994;343:311–322.

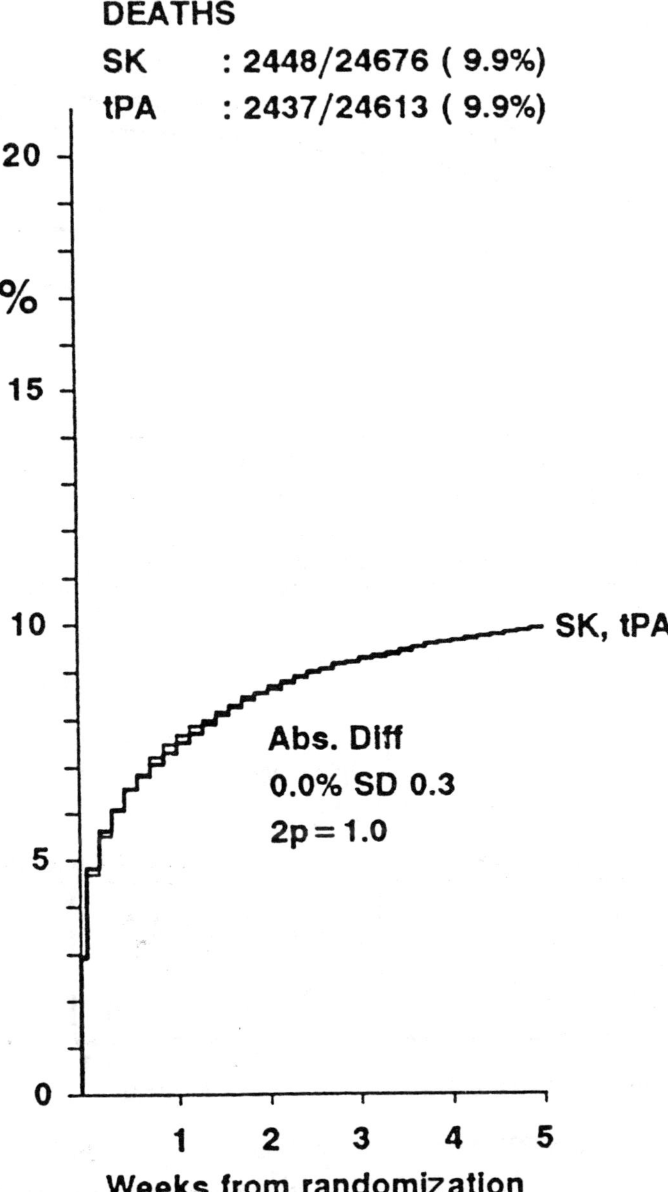


Figure 8.15 Cumulative percentage of deaths in days 0 to 35 shows no difference between patients treated with streptokinase (SK) and those treated with tissue-plasminogen activator (t-PA) in the ISIS-3 and GISSI-2 trials. SD = standard deviation. Reprinted with permission from Califf RM, Topol EJ. The paradigm of acute reperfusion and the GUSTO-I trial. In: Califf RM, Mark DB, Wagner GS, eds. Acute coronary care. St. Louis: Mosby-Year Book, Inc., 1995;69–83. Data from ISIS-3 (Third International Study of Infarct Survival) Collaborative Group. ISIS-3: a randomised comparison of streptokinase vs tissue plasminogen activator vs anistreplase and of aspirin plus heparin vs aspirin alone among 41,299 cases of suspected acute myocardial infarction. Lancet 1992;339:753–770.

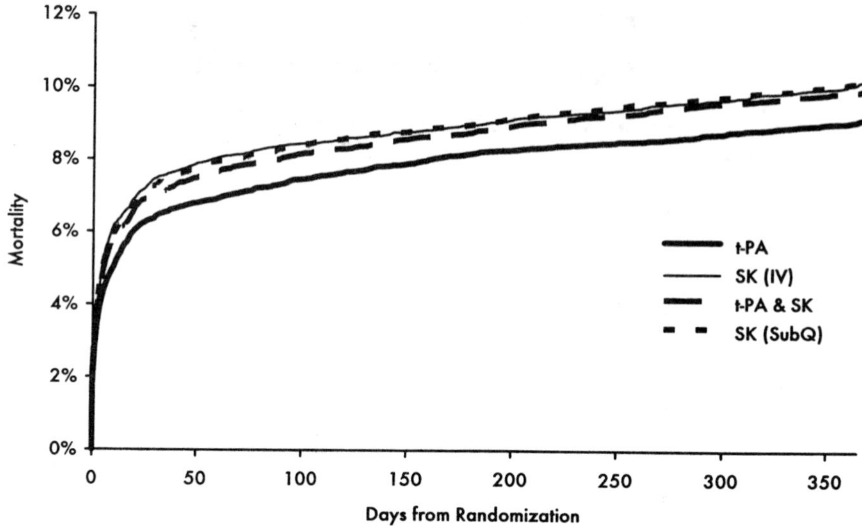


Figure 8.16 After 1 year the mortality rate among patients who received tissue plasminogen activator (t-PA) was significantly lower than that among patients who received one of the other three strategies. IV = intravenous heparin; SK = streptokinase; SubQ = subcutaneous heparin.

## Prior MI

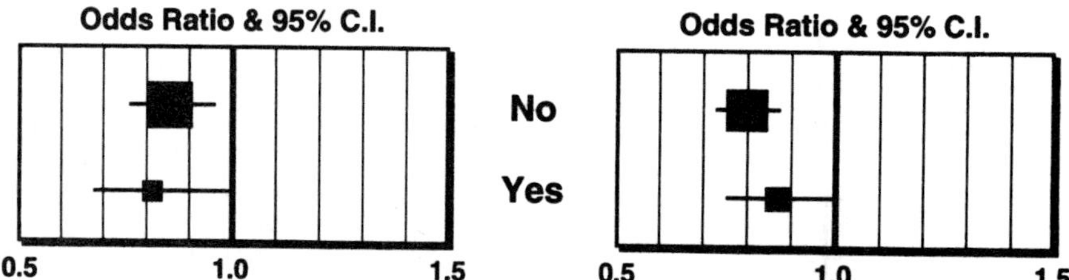


*GUSTO* *FTT*

Figure 8.17 This figure and Figures 8.18 through 8.22 present data from the GUSTO-I trial and the Fibrinolytic Therapy Trialists (FTT), showing odds ratios and 95% confidence intervals (C.I.) for accelerated tissue-plasminogen activator (t-PA) versus streptokinase (SK) in GUSTO-I and for thrombolytic therapy (TT) versus control in the FTT data. Thrombolytic therapy is clearly better than control therapy for patients with and without a previous myocardial infarction (MI), as is accelerated t-PA in comparison with SK. Reprinted with permission from Califf RM, Topol EJ. The paradigm of acute reperfusion and the GUSTO-I trial. In: Califf RM, Mark DB, Wagner GS, eds. Acute coronary care. St. Louis: Mosby-Year Book, Inc., 1995;69–83.

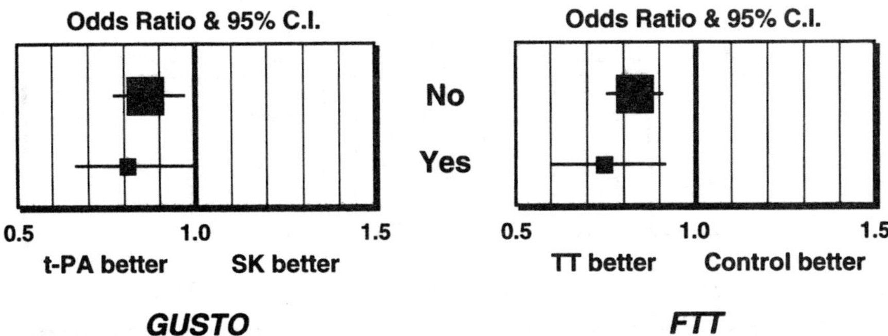


Figure 8.18 Among patients with and without diabetes, thrombolytic therapy is better than no therapy and accelerated tissue-plasminogen activator (t-PA) is superior to streptokinase (SK). C.I. = confidence interval; FTT = Fibrinolytic Therapy Trialists; TT = thrombolytic therapy. Reprinted with permission from Califf RM, Topol EJ. The paradigm of acute reperfusion and the GUSTO-I trial. In: Califf RM, Mark DB, Wagner GS, eds. Acute coronary care. St. Louis: Mosby-Year Book, Inc., 1995;69–83.

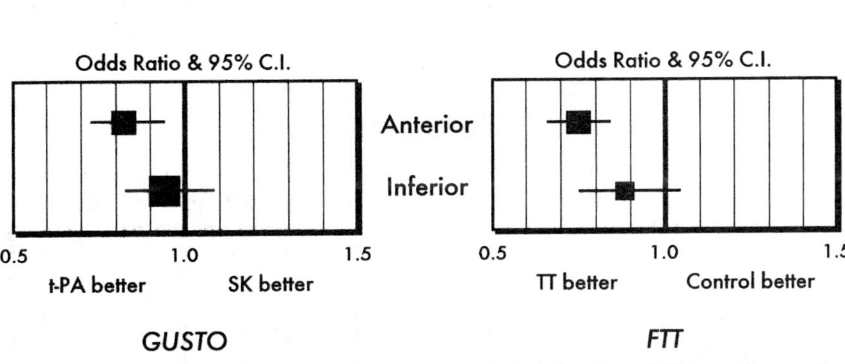


Figure 8.19 Patients with anterior or inferior myocardial infarctions (MI) benefit more from thrombolytic therapy (TT) and from tissue plasminogen activator (t-PA) among thrombolytics. C.I. = confidence interval; FTT = Fibrinolytic Therapy Trialists; SK = streptokinase. Reprinted with permission from Califf RM, Topol EJ. The paradigm of acute reperfusion and the GUSTO-I trial. In: Califf RM, Mark DB, Wagner GS, eds. Acute coronary care. St. Louis: Mosby-Year Book, Inc., 1995;69–83.

The degree of benefit of accelerated alteplase is proportional to the underlying risk of the patient. Figure 8.22 demonstrates a simple method to find patients most likely to benefit from accelerated alteplase compared with streptokinase. As with the FTT analysis, the most uncertainty about the general conclusion that sicker patients do better with more aggressive therapy lies with patients over age 75 (38) and those with cardiogenic shock (72).

**Systolic Blood Pressure**

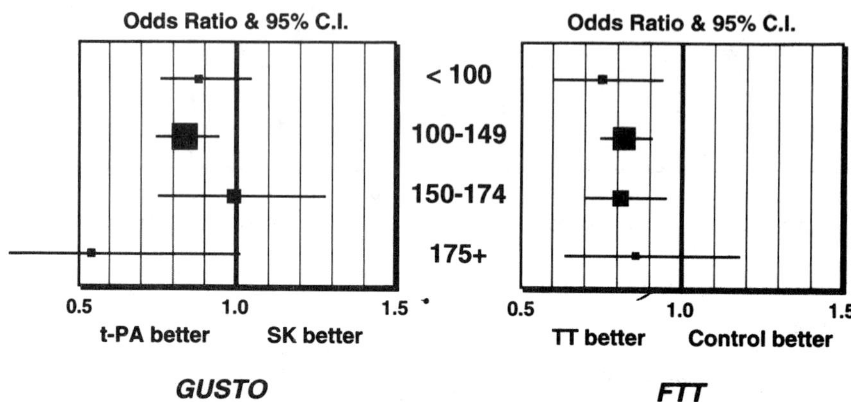


Figure 8.20 From the Fibrinolytic Therapy Trialists (FTT) data, patients within all ranges of systolic blood pressure do best with thrombolytic therapy (TT). The same is true for GUSTO-I patients who received accelerated tissue plasminogen activator (t-PA), although results for those with systolic blood pressure in the range of 150 to 174 mm Hg were equivocal, probably representing the "play of chance." C.I. = confidence interval; SK = streptokinase. Reprinted with permission from Califf RM, Topol EJ. The paradigm of acute reperfusion and the GUSTO-I trial. In: Califf RM, Mark DB, Wagner GS, eds. Acute coronary care. St. Louis: Mosby-Year Book, Inc., 1995;69–83.

**Heart Rate**

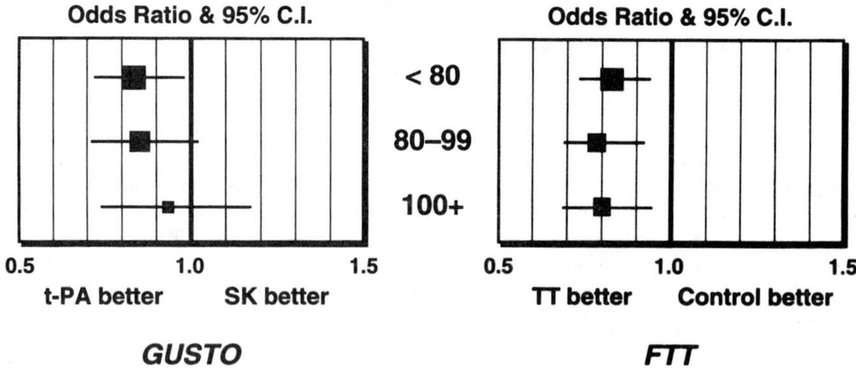


Figure 8.21 Regardless of heart rate, patients do better with thrombolytic therapy (TT) than control therapy, and the patterns for accelerated tissue plasminogen activator (t-PA) versus streptokinase (SK) are similar. C.I. = confidence interval; FTT = Fibrinolytic Therapy Trialists. Reprinted with permission from Califf RM, Topol EJ. The paradigm of acute reperfusion and the GUSTO-I trial. In: Califf RM, Mark DB, Wagner GS, eds. Acute coronary care. St. Louis: Mosby-Year Book, Inc., 1995;69–83.

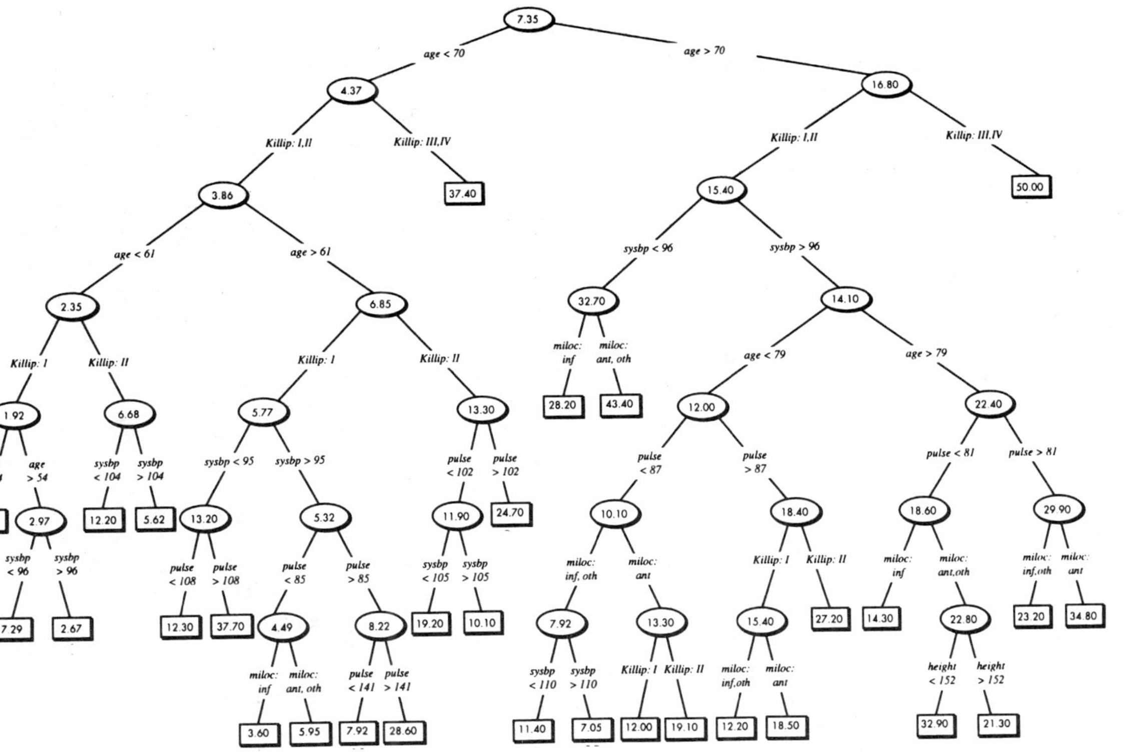


**Figure 8.22** This figure depicts the results of a statistical analysis of the GUSTO-I data in which patients were split into groups based on the estimation of risk of death if treated with streptokinase (*ovals* and *rectangles, rectangles* represent end of sequence). Since the degree of benefit with alteplase was directly related to the extent of underlying risk with streptokinase, the figure also points out the patients who receive the most benefit when alteplase is chosen rather than streptokinase. The most important determinants are age, Killip class, systolic blood pressure, heart rate, and myocardial infarction location. Reprinted with permission from Califf RM. Acute myocardial infarction. In Smith TW, ed. Cardiovascular therapeutics. Philadelphia: WB Saunders, 1996, in press.

## Stroke

Stroke remains the complication of thrombolytic therapy that is feared as much or more than death. Generally, stroke in association with myocardial infarction can be classified into one of two types, hemorrhagic or nonhemorrhagic. In 10–15% of primarily nonhemorrhagic strokes, hemorrhage occurs into the area of cerebral necrosis and a "hemorrhagic conversion" can be diagnosed.

Prior to the advent of thrombolytic therapy, stroke occurred in 1–4% of patients during the acute myocardial infarction hospitalization. The overwhelming majority of these events were nonhemorrhagic and were presumed to emanate from thrombotic emboli from the left ventricle (73). A major conceptual issue that was debated prior to the availability of large trials was the possibility that thrombolytic therapy would *reduce* the risk of nonhemorrhagic stroke, thus offsetting the increased risk of hemorrhagic stroke. The FTT analysis clearly demonstrated that thrombolytic therapy was associated with an increase in the overall risk of stroke of 2 per 1000 patients treated, including a dramatic increase in the likelihood of hemorrhagic stroke coupled with a modest decrease in the risk of nonhemorrhagic stroke (56).

### *Hemorrhagic Stroke*

Hemorrhagic stroke is rare in myocardial infarction patients who have not been treated with thrombolytic therapy. All thrombolytic agents increase the risk of hemorrhagic stroke, and the increase in risk appears to be related to the potency of the thrombolytic regimen in lysing thrombus. Table 8.2 gives the overall rates of intracranial hemorrhage reported in the large trials published to date. Although the relative proportions reported in the ISIS and GISSI studies are unbiased and probably reliable, the absolute rates probably somewhat underestimate the true incidence because systematic brain imaging was not part of the protocols.

In the GUSTO-I trial, brain images were obtained systematically as an integral part of the protocol and the results were reviewed by a Stroke Committee (74). Figure 8.23 displays the time until stroke in patients with a hemorrhagic stroke. These events are most likely to occur in the first 24 hours after treatment is initiated. Table 8.3 demonstrates the type of stroke as a function of thrombolytic agent. The majority of strokes are parenchymal, although a significant number of events are both parenchymal and subdural. The risk of hemorrhagic stroke is not evenly distributed across the patient population treated with thrombolytic therapy. The major risk factors are listed in Table 8.4. The common risk factors have been evaluated systematically in the GUSTO-I trial.

A regression analysis has allowed the prediction of the risk of stroke in the individual patient. Age is the most important factor, followed by diastolic blood pressure, then a history of cerebrovascular disease. In a case-

**Table 8.2**
**Incidence of Stroke and Intracerebral Hemorrhage in Randomized Clinical Trials[a]**

| Clinical Trial (N) | Total Stroke | Intracerebral Hemorrhage |
|---|---|---|
| GISSI-1 | | |
| Streptokinase (5,852) | 54 (0.92%) | 8 (0.13%) |
| Control (5,860) | 45 (0.77%) | 0 |
| ISIS-2 | | |
| Streptokinase (8,592) | 61 (0.71%) | 7 (0.08%) |
| Control (8,595) | 67 (0.78%) | 0 |
| ISIS-3 | | |
| Streptokinase (13,607) | 141 (1.03%) | 25 (0.18%) |
| Duteplase (13,569) | 188 (1.39%) | 76 (0.56%) |
| Anistreplase (13,599) | 172 (1.26%) | 54 (0.39%) |
| GISSI-2/International | | |
| Alteplase (10,372) | 138 (1.33%) | 44 (0.42%) |
| Streptokinase (10,396) | 98 (0.94%) | 30 (0.29%) |
| GUSTO-I | | |
| Alteplase (10,268) | 161 (1.57%) | 73 (0.71%) |
| Streptokinase with i.v. heparin (10,314) | 144 (1.40%) | 59 (0.57%) |
| Streptokinase with s.c. heparin (9,709) | 117 (1.21%) | 45 (0.46%) |
| Streptokinase and alteplase (10,248) | 170 (1.66%) | 91 (0.88%) |

[a]Based on published data (24, 25, 132–134).
GISSI-2 = Gruppo Italiano per lo Studio della Sopravvivenza nell'Infarto Miocardico; GISSI-I = Gruppo Italiano per lo Studio della Streptochinasi nell'Infarto Miocardico; GUSTO-I = Global Utilization of Streptokinase and t-PA for Occluded Coronary Arteries; ISIS = International Study of Infarct Survival; i.v. = intravenous; N = number; s.c. = subcutaneous.

control study, a recent history of head trauma and alcohol consumption were associated with a higher risk of intracranial hemorrhage and a strong trend was observed for history of Alzheimer's disease (75).

To date the rate of hemorrhagic stroke has been directly related to the intensity of the fibrinolytic regimen. In GUSTO-I, a stepwise increase in the risk of hemorrhagic stroke was observed going from the streptokinase-subcutaneous heparin regimen to the streptokinase-intravenous heparin regimen to the accelerated alteplase-intravenous heparin regimen to the streptokinase/alteplase-intravenous heparin regimen. Whether this increase in hemorrhagic stroke rate will be the limiting factor in defining more effective regimens for lysis of coronary thrombus remains a major issue in the design of new thrombolytic regimens. Since the majority of patients with hemorrhagic stroke die, the risk of nonfatal disabling stroke does not go up directly as a function of the risk of stroke (76); therefore it can be difficult to determine the risk/benefit trade-off, and in formal decision analysis a substantial increase in the risk of stroke is required to offset a mortality benefit.

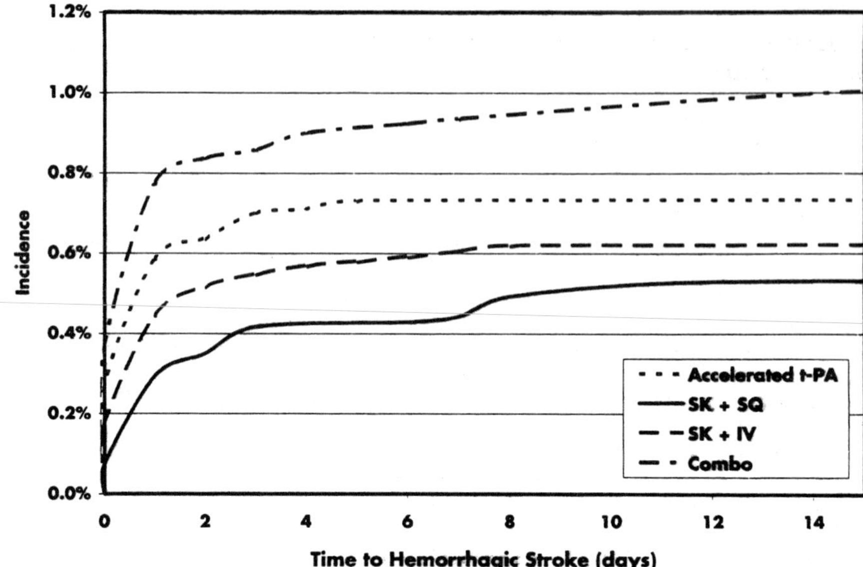


Figure 8.23 Timing of primary hemorrhagic stroke per treatment assignment. SK + SQ = streptokinase plus subcutaneous heparin; SK + IV = streptokinase plus intravenous heparin; t-PA = accelerated tissue plasminogen activator plus intravenous heparin; Combo = streptokinase and t-PA plus intravenous heparin. Reprinted with permission from Gore JM, Granger CB, Sloan MA, et al., for the GUSTO-I Investigators. Stroke after thrombolysis: mortality and functional outcomes in the GUSTO-I trial. Circulation 1995;92:2811–2818.

**Table 8.3.**
**Incidence of Stroke per Treatment Assignment in GUSTO-I**

| | SK + s.c. (n = 117) | SK + i.v. (n = 144) | t-PA (n = 161) | Combo (n = 170) | Total (n = 592) |
|---|---|---|---|---|---|
| Primary intracranial hemorrhage | 45[a] | 59 | 73 | 91 | 268 |
| Subdural | 4 | 2 | 1 | 5 | 12 |
| Subdural + intracerebral | 3 | 7 | 7 | 11 | 28 |
| Intracerebral | 38 | 50 | 65 | 75 | 228 |
| Nonhemorrhagic infarct | 55 | 67 | 69 | 56 | 247 |
| Hemorrhagic conversion of infarct | 7 | 6 | 10 | 11 | 34 |
| Unknown | 10 | 12 | 9 | 12 | 43 |

[a]Values are numbers of patients in each category; total number of study, 41,021.
SK + s.c. = streptokinase plus subcutaneous heparin; SK + i.v. = streptokinase plus intravenous heparin; t-PA = accelerated tissue plasminogen activator plus intravenous heparin; Combo = streptokinase and t-PA plus intravenous heparin.

**Table 8.4.**
**Risk Factors for Stroke Following Thrombolytic Therapy in Acute Myocardial Infarction[a]**

| Risk Factor | Cerebral Infarction | Intracranial Hemorrhage |
|---|---|---|
| Age | +++ | +++ |
| Head trauma | | + |
| Elevated systolic and diastolic blood pressure | | +++ |
| History of cerebral vascular disease | +++ | +++ |
| Lower body weight | | +++ |
| History of hypertension | +++ | +++ |
| Dementia | | + |
| Thrombolytic therapy type (alteplase and APSAC > SK) | | +++ |
| Heparin | | ++ |
| Elevated pulse pressure | | ++ |
| Thrombolytic therapy dose | | +++ |
| Calcium blocker | | + |
| Female gender | | + |
| Diabetes mellitus | | + |
| Atrial fibrillation | +++ | |
| History of anticoagulation | | + |
| Hemodynamic compromise | +++ | |
| Anterior myocardial infarction | +++ | |
| Higher Killip class | +++ | |

Adapted with permission from O'Connor CM. Stroke during acute myocardial infarction. In: Califf RM, Mark DB, Wagner GS, eds. Acute coronary care. 2nd ed. St. Louis: CV Mosby, 1995: 635–650.
[a] Listed in order of importance for risk of intracranial hemorrhage. APSAC = anisoylated plasminogen = streptokinase activator complex; SK = streptokinase; +++ = definite risk factor identified in multiple studies; ++ = likely risk factor; + = questionable risk factor, needs verification.

### *Nonhemorrhagic Stroke*

As in the prethrombolytic era, nonhemorrhagic stroke predominantly reflects the embolic substrate emanating from a large infarction and dysrhythmia or underlying cerebrovascular disease in patients with acute myocardial infarction. Accordingly, atrial fibrillation, extensive anteroapical infarction, and prior cerebrovascular disease are the major risk factors for nonhemorrhagic stroke. Given the presumed thromboembolic nature of most of these events, it is somewhat surprising that thrombolytic therapy and associated anticoagulation do not reduce the risk of nonhemorrhagic stroke even further. The lower rate of nonhemorrhagic stroke in thrombolytic trials compared with the prethrombolytic era should not be attributed to the therapy, since many of the highest risk patients are excluded from thrombolytic trials because of prior cerebrovascular disease or other comorbidity.

### *Hemorrhagic Conversion*

In 5–15% of initially nonhemorrhagic strokes, conversion to a hemorrhagic stroke occurs during the same hospitalization (77, 78). The exact incidence of conversion is difficult to estimate because of the rapidly improving ability to image small amounts of blood in the brain. It is thought that hemorrhagic conversion is frequently associated with clinical deterioration because of the larger volume of brain tissue consumed by the stroke and the greater frequency of cerebral edema. Large infarct volume, midline shift on brain imaging, and older age have been associated with hemorrhagic conversion.

### *Consequences of Stroke*

The clinical outcomes of stroke were carefully assessed in the GUSTO-I trial, including a prospective assessment of quality of life (Fig. 8.24). Approximately 60% of patients with hemorrhagic stroke died in the initial hospitalization, and 19% were left with moderate or severe disability. In comparison, only 15% of patients with nonhemorrhagic stroke died in the same hospitalization and 45–50% were left with moderate or severe disability.

### *Treatment of Stroke*

Since hemorrhagic stroke occurs most frequently in the first 24 hours after thrombolytic treatment, careful surveillance of the patient for neurologic status is essential in the first day after therapy. Any new focal neurologic deficit must be addressed by discontinuation of thrombolytic therapy and other antithrombotic therapy while an emergency imaging study is obtained. Commonly, the patient becomes confused, disoriented, nauseated, or lethargic before clear evidence of a focal deficit is present; given one of these findings, a detailed neurologic examination is indicated. Once

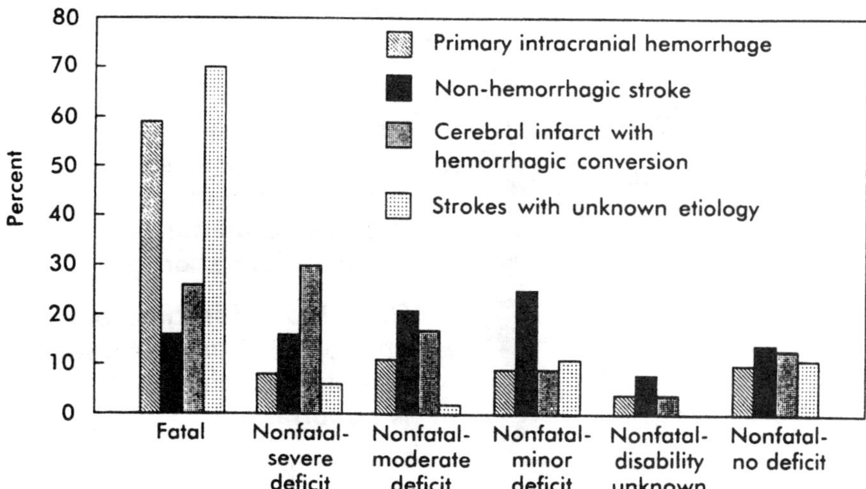


Figure 8.24 Among 41,021 patients randomized in the GUSTO-I trial, 592 had strokes. This figure shows how the strokes were distributed according to resultant disability and type of stroke. Reprinted with permission from O'Connor CM. Stroke during acute myocardial infarction. In: Califf RM, Mark DB, Wagner GS, eds. Acute coronary care. St. Louis: Mosby Year-Book, Inc., 1995;635–650.

an intracranial hemorrhage occurs, the emergency bleeding should be addressed as described in Figure 8.25.

In some cases immediate neurosurgical evacuation should be instituted. In a recent analysis, Mahaffey and colleagues demonstrated that after an attempt to adjust for differences in baseline characteristics, patients with intracranial hemorrhage treated with neurosurgical evacuation fared better than patients treated conservatively (79). Unfortunately, criteria identifying candidates for evacuation are unclear.

## Systemic Bleeding

Thrombolytic agents cannot distinguish between pathologic thrombus occluding a coronary artery and physiologic thrombus preventing hemorrhage in a damaged blood vessel. Most systemic bleeding caused by thrombolytic agents is at the site of a physiologic hemostatic plug. Accordingly, the risk of systemic bleeding is directly related to the recent exposure to vascular punctures or pathologic conditions (ulcer, hemorrhoids, etc.) that have been associated with spontaneous bleeding. Indeed, in the absence of cardiac catheterization, percutaneous revascularization, and surgery, the risk of significant extracranial bleeding is less than 5%. The major sources

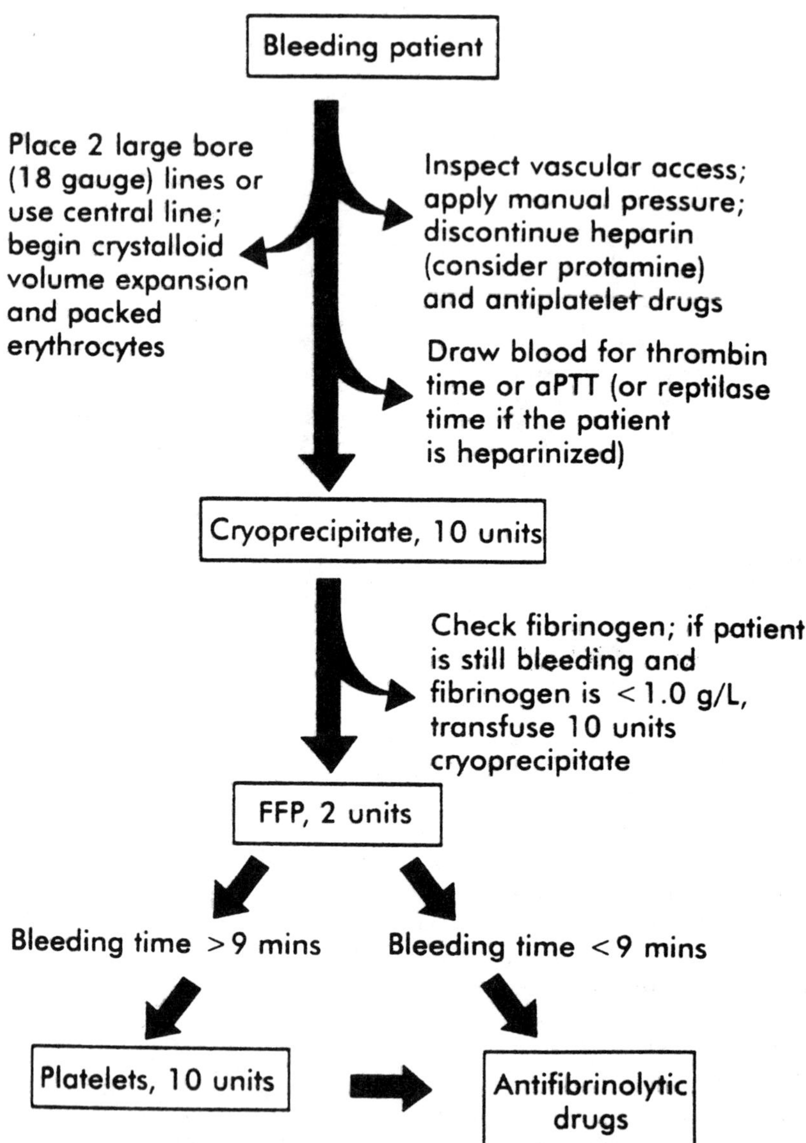


Figure 8.25 A typical strategy for the management of major bleeding causing hemodynamic compromise that is not immediately life-threatening. aPTT = activated partial thromboplastin time; FFP = fresh frozen plasma. Reprinted with permission from Sane DC, Califf RM, Topol EJ, et al. Bleeding during thrombolytic therapy for acute myocardial infarction: mechanisms and management. Ann Intern Med 1989;111:1010–1022.

**Table 8.5**
**Frequency of Extracranial Hemorrhage by Site**

| Site | % |
|---|---|
| Catheterization site hematoma | 25–45 |
| Other puncture sites | 1–5 |
| Gastrointestinal tract | 4–10 |
| Genitourinary tract | 1–5 |
| Retroperitoneum | ≤1 |
| Epistaxis | ≤1 |
| Unknown site | ≤5 |

Reprinted with permission from Sane DC. Extracranial hemorrhagic complications of thrombolytic therapy. In: Califf RM, Mark: DB, Wagner GS, eds. Acute coronary care. St. Louis: Mosby-Year Book, Inc. 1995:625–633.

of bleeding are listed in Table 8.5. As with intracranial hemorrhage, the risk is directly related to old age and to the occurrence of hypertension. Patients with lower body weight are at higher risk of bleeding, and women have an additional risk for unclear reasons. In contrast to findings in intracranial hemorrhage, alteplase is associated with a modestly lower risk of extracranial bleeding than is streptokinase (80).

## Failure to Reperfuse

Since thrombolytic therapy benefits the patient by achieving reperfusion of the occluded artery, failure to reperfuse is a major clinical issue. Observation of the patient for resolution of symptoms provides an improved probabilistic assessment of the likelihood of reperfusion, but the discrimination of symptom assessment is not sufficient for clinical decision making (81). "Reperfusion arrhythmias," although commonly observed with reperfusion, are also commonly observed in patients with persistently occluded arteries (81). A number of studies have now shown that electrocardiographic assessment provides a much more reliable prediction of which patients have a perfused vessel. A standard ECG taken 60–90 minutes after initiation of thrombolytic therapy provides not only a probabilistic assessment of perfusion (81–85) but also an excellent stratification of risk of death and pump dysfunction (86).

More sophististicated efforts have been undertaken using cardiac enzymes and continuous monitoring of either the 12-lead ECG or the vectorcardiogram. Although peak levels of cardiac enzymes and the timing of the peak provide interesting prognostic information, the results are not available soon enough to lead to successful myocardial salvage by reopening an occluded artery (87). On-line measurements in the first 60–90 minutes could provide useful information (88, 89), but such measurements are not available in most hospitals. Both 12-lead ECG measurements on a continuous basis (90) and vectorcardiographic measurements (91) provide more information than either enzymes or routine electrocardiography, but the complexity of these measurements has delayed their introduction into clinical practice.

Our practice is to use 12-lead continuous monitoring when available or a second 12-lead recording 60 minutes after initiating thrombolytic therapy to evaluate whether reperfusion has occurred. A simple guideline is that failure to resolve the ST segment by at least 50% in the lead with the maximum ST-segment elevation at baseline is associated with a substantial probability of failure to reperfuse.

When failure to reperfuse is detected, a major question remains about whether further intervention will improve prognosis. Multiple studies have demonstrated the feasibility of "rescue" coronary angioplasty to restore perfusion (92), but only one randomized trial has been completed (93). This study demonstrated that rescue angioplasty in proximal left anterior descending occlusion resulted in a reduction in the combined end point of death and symptomatic congestive heart failure. Based on this limited information, we proceed to coronary angiography when there is noninvasive evidence of failure to reperfuse and the infarction is judged to be large (anterior, multiple leads, clinical evidence of heart failure, second infarction).

### Cardiac Rupture/Early Hazard

The FTT overview provides evidence that in the first 24 hours after administration of thrombolytic therapy, the risk of death is higher than it is in control populations in the first 24 hours after admission (56). The presumed reason for this "early hazard" is an increased risk of cardiac rupture, especially in patients treated later and elderly patients. In at least one systematic overview including all available autopsy data, Honan and colleagues found that patients treated early were protected from myocardial rupture, whereas patients treated later had an excess risk of myocardial rupture (94). Whether the same early hazard also exists in patients treated with alteplase remains uncertain, raising the question of whether the hypotension produced by streptokinse and APSAC could produce the incremental risk. In the GUSTO-I study, early mortality was most directly related to failure to reperfuse, with no evidence for rupture as a major problem, but the vast majority of patients were treated within 6 hours of symptom onset in this trial (95).

### Nonfatal End Points

Patients treated with thrombolytic therapy continue to have a number of secondary complications that are targets for further intervention (Table 8.6). These may be conveniently divided into several categories.

**Table 8.6**
**Secondary End Points in the GUSTO-I Trial**

| Complications | SK and s.c. heparin (n = 8,669) | SK and i.v. heparin (n = 9,260) | Accelerated t-PA and i.v. heparin (n = 9,235) | t-PA + SK and i.v. heparin (n = 9,193) | *P* value, accelerated t-PA vs. both SK groups |
|---|---|---|---|---|---|
| Percentage of patients with | | | | | |
| Allergic reaction | 5.7 | 5.8 | 1.6 | 5.4 | <0.001 |
| Anaphylaxis | 0.7 | 0.6 | 0.2 | 0.6 | <0.001 |
| Congestive heart failure | 17.5 | 16.8 | 15.2 | 16.8 | <0.001 |
| Cardiogenic shock | 6.9 | 6.3 | 5.1 | 6.1 | <0.001 |
| Sustained hypotension | 13.3 | 12.5 | 10.1 | 12.4 | <0.001 |
| Atrioventricular block[a] | 9.5 | 8.7 | 7.3 | 8.4 | <0.001 |
| Sustained ventricular tachycardia | 6.8 | 6.5 | 5.6 | 6.1 | 0.001 |
| Ventricular fibrillation | 7.1 | 6.9 | 6.3 | 6.9 | 0.02 |
| Asystole | 6 | 6.4 | 5.3 | 6.4 | 0.003 |
| Atrial fibrillation or flutter | 9.9 | 9.8 | 8.6 | 9.1 | 0.001 |
| Reinfarction | 3.4 | 4 | 4 | 4 | 0.26 |
| Recurrent ischemia | 19.9 | 19.6 | 19 | 18.8 | 0.14 |
| Acute mitral regurgitation | 1.6 | 2.6 | 1.3 | 1.4 | 0.11 |
| Acute VSD | 0.5 | 0.4 | 0.4 | 0.6 | 0.59 |

[a] Refers to second-degree or third-degree block.
GUSTO = Global Utilization of Streptokinase and t-PA for Occluded Coronary Arteries; i.v. = intravenous; n = number; s.c. = subcutaneous; SK = streptokinase; t-PA = tissue plasminogen activator; VSD = ventricular septal defect.
Reprinted with permission from Califf RM, Topol EJ. The paradigm of acute reperfusion and the GUSTO-I trial. In: Califf RM, Mark DB, Wagner GS, eds. Acute coronary care. St. Louis: Mosby-Year Book, 1995:69–83.

Arrhythmias were thought to be a major concern in patients treated with thrombolytics because of "reperfusion arrhythmias" observed in animal models. Indeed, among patients reperfused early and patients with large infarctions, sudden arrhythmias do seem to occur more frequently at the time of reperfusion. Accelerated idioventricular rhythm, a ventricular tachycardia with a rate of less than 120 beats/minute, is statistically more likely to occur with reperfusion, but the differences are too modest to be clinically useful. Over the course of the hospitalization, ventricular tachycardia, ventricular fibrillation, high degree atrioventricular block, and atrial fibrillation are less likely to occur in patients treated with thrombolytics than in control populations and less likely to occur after accelerated alteplase than after streptokinase (24).

Mechanical complications, including pulmonary edema, congestive heart failure, and acute mitral regurgitation, are also less likely to occur with thrombolysis than with control therapy. Additionally, these complications are less common with accelerated alteplase administration than with use of streptokinase (24).

Recurrent ischemia is more common with thrombolytic therapy than with control therapy. This observation fits in with the concept that achieving early reperfusion with viable tissue downstream and an unstable atherosclerotic plaque leaves the patient at special risk. As with reocclusion, recurrent ischemia cannot be easily predicted; therefore, careful observation of the patient is required in the first several hours. Recurrent ischemia is considered particularly dangerous when it is associated with electrocardiographic changes or evidence of hemodynamic instability (96, 97).

Reinfarction almost always results from recurrent total occlusion of the vessel, as discussed above. The treatment of reinfarction remains highly controversial. Several series have been reported of repeat thrombolytic therapy administration, generally with alteplase since neutralizing antibodies develop to streptokinase (98, 99). A patency rate of more than 60% has been demonstrated with acceptable bleeding and mortality rates, but no controlled trials have been done. Many practitioners proceed to angiography when reinfarction is suspected.

## COMPARISONS WITH DIRECT PERCUTANEOUS TRANSLUMINAL CORONARY ANGIOPLASTY

The clinician evaluating a patient who has acute myocardial infarction with ST-segment elevation must make a decision not only about which thrombolytic agent to use but also about whether to use thrombolytic therapy or direct coronary angioplasty. Until recently, many experts assumed that angioplasty was not suited for the disrupted atherosclerotic plaque or that it would be too expensive and not generalizable. Recently, a series of observational studies and randomized clinical trials have challenged this notion.

Direct coronary angioplasty is clearly feasible, and the literature has a large number of reports on thousands of patients. The carefully controlled Primary Angioplasty Registry (PAR) study demonstrated that more than 90% of patients identified in the emergency department could be treated with direct angioplasty and the occlusion could be reduced to less than 70% stenosis in more than 90% of those treated (100). The majority of patients who were not treated either had no significant residual stenosis or had spontaneous reperfusion, with less than 2% of patients not treated with angioplasty because of unsuitable lesion morphology. Six-month follow-up in these patients showed restenosis in a large proportion of patients but a dramatic improvement in left ventricular function (101).

A series of small clinical trials comparing thrombolytic therapy with direct angioplasty have recently been reported, including more than 600 patients (Table 8.7). In these studies direct angioplasty resulted in lower rates of death, reinfarction, recurrent ischemia, and stroke. There was no difference in transfusion rates. Analyses seemed to demonstrate a lower cost for patients treated with direct angioplasty, mostly because of the longer length of stay and greater use of ancillary procedures and tests in patients treated with thrombolytics.

**Table 8.7**
**Outcomes in Recent Randomized Trials of Direct PTCA versus Thrombolytic Therapy**

| | PAMI | | Mayo | | Dutch | | Total | | *Odds ratio*[a] |
|---|---|---|---|---|---|---|---|---|---|
| | PTCA (n = 195) | TT (n = 200) | PTCA (n = 47) | TT (n = 50) | PTCA (n = 72) | TT (n = 70) | PTCA (n = 314) | TT (n = 320) | (95% CI) |
| Death | 5 | 13 | 2 | 2 | 0 | 4 | 7 | 19 | 2.7 (1.2–6.4) |
| Reinfarction | 5 | 8 | 0 | 2 | 0 | 9 | 5 | 19 | 5.0 (2.1–12) |
| Recurrent ischemia | 20 | 56 | — | — | 6 | 27 | 26 | 83 | 4.1 (2.6–6.5) |
| Stroke | 0 | 4 | 0 | 0 | 0 | 2 | 0 | 6 | 7.0 (0.8–57.6) |
| Transfusion | 24 | 16 | — | — | 2 | 6 | 26 | 22 | 0.8 (0.5–1.5) |

[a]Odds of outcome for thrombolytic therapy relative to direct PTCA.
CI = confidence interval; n = number; PAMI = Primary Angioplasty in Myocardial Infarction; PTCA = percutaneous transluminal coronary angioplasty; TT = thrombolytic therapy.
Reprinted with permission from Harrington RA, Califf RM, Phillips HR, et al. Primary angioplasty for acute myocardial infarction. In: Califf RM, Mark DB, Wagner GS, eds. Acute coronary care. St. Louis: Mosby-Year Book, 1995:305–313.

The lack of convincing evidence of the benefit of thrombolytic therapy in the setting of cardiogenic shock was reviewed above. In the first major prospective study of cardiogenic shock, Hochman and colleagues demonstrated that undergoing cardiac catheterization in the setting of shock seemed to be more important for prognosis than having an angioplasty procedure (102). Accordingly, some concern must be expressed that the seeming benefit of angioplasty for cardiogenic shock could simply represent selection of healthier patients for the procedure rather than the benefits of the procedure itself. A major randomized trial is underway to resolve this issue.

The demonstration of feasibility in observational studies and superiority in randomized clinical trials has made direct angioplasty the preferable treatment when it can be performed expeditiously in experienced hands. The available studies raise important questions about whether generalizations can be drawn from the results, however. These trials were performed by experienced centers with considerable expertise in the practice of direct angioplasty. Whether the results would be the same in less experienced centers remains unclear. Recent evidence from Jollis and coworkers indicates that the relationship between procedural volume and outcome is substantial with angioplasty, especially in patients with myocardial infarction (103). Until the final results of larger ongoing trials are available, a reasonable policy is to employ direct angioplasty when it is anticipated that the infarct-related artery can be visualized within an hour by an experienced operator in a high-volume center. Direct angioplasty is the preferred mode of reperfusion when a relative contraindication to thrombolytic therapy is present, such as previous stroke, or when the patient is in cardiogenic shock.

## CONJUNCTIVE THERAPY

Thrombolytic therapy is one of many treatment strategies for acute myocardial infarction. Associated therapies have been a major focus of ongoing investigation, particularly antithrombotic therapy. For the purpose of simplification, these conjunctive therapies may be divided into those primarily oriented toward inhibiting platelets, those primarily aimed at inhibiting thrombin, and other antithrombotic compounds.

Antiplatelet agents are clearly beneficial in the setting of thrombolytic therapy. Convincing evidence for this came from the ISIS-2 study (65), which randomized patients in a factorial design to aspirin (160 mg/day), streptokinase, both, or neither. Aspirin reduced mortality independently of streptokinase but when given in addition to streptokinase provided an additive benefit. The first dose of aspirin is given in chewable form to ensure absorption. The maintenance doses advocated by experts range from 30–325 mg, but the best data emanate from the ISIS-2 trial using 160 mg/day. In aspirin-allergic patients, ticlopidine is recommended, although no specific data exist on the combination of this agent with thrombolytic therapy.

Whether the new antiplatelet agents that inhibit the glycoprotein IIb/IIIa receptor (104) will add further benefit remains uncertain, although pilot studies indicate substantial improvement in patency with the combination of a thrombolytic agent and a glycoprotein IIb/IIIa inhibitor (46). Of course, the translation of these angiographic findings into clinical practice requires demonstration of clinical benefit without excess hemorrhage at a reasonable cost.

The use of direct antithrombin agents with thrombolytic therapy has an excellent rationale; thrombin is thought to play a central role in both the classic coagulation pathway and platelet activation and aggregation. Thrombin bound to fibrin is inaccessible to heparin, which is a large molecule that is made even more unwieldy by the requirement that it form a complex with antithrombin III in order to inactivate thrombin. Heparin also provides an unpredictable level of anticoagulation because of its inactivation by a variety of plasma proteins and vascular surfaces. Critical studies with hirudin, the prototypical direct antihrombin agent, are now underway.

Heparin had been considered to be essential in conjunction with thrombolytic therapy until recent controlled trials were completed. The ISIS-3 and GISSI 2/International trials enrolled more than 60,000 patients in direct comparisons of subcutaneous heparin and placebo therapy in conjunction with streptokinase and anistreplase. No differences were observed in mortality or other major clinical end points, although there was an increase in bleeding with subcutaneous heparin. The GUSTO-I trial randomized almost 20,000 patients treated with streptokinase to either intravenous or subcutaneous heparin (24). Again, no differences in major clinical outcomes were evident, although intravenous heparin caused more bleeding than subcutaneous heparin. From these data and a small supporting study comparing anistreplase with intravenous heparin versus placebo, it is reasonable to conclude that there is no empirical basis for the use of heparin with nonspecific fibrinolytic agents.

The appropriate role of heparin with alteplase remains unclear. A series of small studies that used angiography to determine the perfusion status of the infarct-related artery proved beyond question that intravenous heparin improves the infarct-related artery's perfusion status. Unfortunately, these studies did not prove that the clinical status of the patients was enhanced; a statistically nonsignificant 18% mortality reduction was observed, and there was a paradoxical increase in reinfarction and stroke (105). GUSTO-I did not randomize the alteplase-treated patients to intravenous or subcutaneous heparin, but the GISSI 2/International study found no advantage to subcutaneous heparin in conjunction with the 3-hour alteplase infusion. Until further data are available, it is reasonable to continue using intravenous heparin with alteplase.

## ADJUNCTIVE THERAPY

In addition to receiving antithrombotic therapy, patients with acute myocardial infarction undergo a variety of other therapies designed to reduce mortality and improve quality of life. A full discussion of these therapies is beyond the scope of this chapter except as they relate to thrombolytic therapy.

### β-Blockers

Although the acute use of β-blockers in myocardial infarction was shown to reduce mortality in ISIS-1 and other trials reviewed in a systematic overview (106), few studies have evaluated β-blockers in the setting of thrombolytic therapy. Only the TIMI-2 study provides direct evidence with a commonly used β-blocker; this trial demonstrated a reduction in reinfarction but no effect on mortality in a comparison of intravenous β-blocker given acutely with oral β-blocker started at the time of hospital discharge (107). With only 1390 patients enrolled, this trial was not adequately powered to make a statement about mortality. The other benefits of β-blockade before the thrombolytic era included reduction in recurrent ischemia as well as in ventricular and supraventricular arrhythmias and improved left ventricular function. TIMI-2 also found that intravenous metoprolol had no effect on systolic left ventricular function.

Until further evidence is available, most experts recommend routine use of β-blockade in patients treated with thrombolytic therapy unless a contraindication is present. In the GUSTO-I trial (108), 42% of patients were treated with acute intravenous β-blocker and 32% with oral β-blocker without initiation via the intravenous route; substantial variation was observed from region to region and from country to country (109).

### Nitrates

A series of small clinical trials initially indicated a substantial benefit from the early use of nitrates in acute myocardial infarction (110). Two large studies have recently evaluated the role of nitrates in clinical trials in which a large proportion of the population was treated with thrombolytic therapy (111, 112). Neither trial observed a significant benefit, although both were weakened by the use of nitrates in more than 50% of the control group. A theoretical advantage of nitrates resides in the prevention of coronary vasospasm, which could enhance reperfusion; alternatively, concern has been raised about an interaction between nitrates and heparin (113). Given the uncertain advantages of routine nitrate therapy, it seems reasonable to use nitrates for episodes of recurrent ischemia or pump failure unless the clinician has a strong belief in routine use of nitrates.

## Angiotensin-Converting Enzyme Inhibitors

Several small trials have demonstrated that early angiotensin-converting enzyme (ACE) inhibition can reduce left ventricular dilation when used in combination with thrombolytic therapy (114). Both the GISSI-3 and ISIS-4 trials evaluated ACE inhibitors in populations in which a high proportion of thrombolytic therapy was used, and a modest mortality benefit was observed (112, 115). A reasonable policy is to institute ACE inhibitors in patients with anterior myocardial infarction, extensive myocardial infarction judged by a large number of leads with ST-segment elevation or second myocardial infarction, or as soon as left ventricular dysfunction is observed.

## Revascularization

The use of coronary angiography and revascularization after thrombolytic therapy has been controversial. Invasive procedures might be considered in one of four possible time frames: immediately after lysis, in the early cardiac care unit phase, prior to discharge, or only after demonstration of recurrent ischemia.

A series of clinical trials has evaluated the use of coronary angiography and angioplasty immediately after successful lysis. Despite the theoretical attractiveness of eliminating the residual stenosis after successful lysis, the policy of routine angioplasty in this situation has not led to improved outcomes (116–118). Failure to improve outcomes probably results from the higher rate of complications associated with angioplasty of lesions with a high thrombus burden. The TAMI-5 trial evaluated a policy of immediate catheterization with angioplasty only of totally occluded vessels (119). Although the trial was small, this approach seemed to lead to improved clinical outcomes and improved left ventricular function.

The TIMI group also evaluated routine catheterization and revascularization 18–48 hours after thrombolytic therapy (107). Compared with conservative care, this strategy provided no advantage with regard to death or nonfatal myocardial infarction; a lower rate of recurrent ischemia was observed. On balance, the cost of follow-up care appeared somewhat higher with the routine angiography strategy, although a formal analysis was not done. Routine predischarge catheterization followed by revascularization was evaluated in several trials with essentially the same results.

In all clinical trials to date, selective angiography has led to a rate of death and nonfatal myocardial infarction equivalent to that of more aggressive approaches. This selective angiography strategy involves careful evaluation of the patient with clinical measures and a predischarge provocative test for ischemia. Under this scheme, angiography is recommended in patients with clinical findings of pump dysfunction or recurrent ischemia. The TIMI group found that this strategy led to a 33% rate of coronary angiography during the initial hospitalization and a 60% rate over the first year (107). Interestingly, the rates of bypass surgery and angioplasty were quite similar between the selective and aggressive strategies over the first year.

Our practice is to evaluate patients carefully in the period immediately following administration of thrombolytic therapy. If there is evidence of failure to reperfuse and the infarction is large, immediate angiography is performed. If there is no evidence of failure to reperfuse, pump dysfunction, or recurrent ischemia, conservative management is pursued until the fourth hospital day. Because of increasing evidence that revascularization improves survival in patients with impaired left ventricular function and multivessel disease (120, 121), we routinely advocate catheterization if left ventricular dysfunction is present on noninvasive testing or physical examination. In other patients a strategy of either angiography or provocative testing is followed; if angiography is performed, revascularization is reserved for patients with high-grade proximal left anterior descending stenosis or multivessel disease or those with evidence of ischemia.

## CLINICAL RISK STRATIFICATION

Risk assessment after administration of thrombolytic therapy is a continuous process beginning with assessment for evidence of failure to reperfuse, arrhythmia, stroke, pump dysfunction, and recurrent ischemia, as described above. At approximately 24 hours the patient with no complications should be assessed again for transfer from the cardiac care unit. Patients without stroke, sustained ventricular arrhythmia, advanced atrioventricular block, recurrent ischemia, or heart failure can be safely transferred to a lower level of care and observation. Recent data indicate that if none of these adverse events occurs, safe discharge can be allowed after day 4 in the typical patient (122). Prior to discharge, either coronary angiography or provocative testing is recommended, as described above.

## COST-EFFECTIVENESS

The general cost-effectiveness of thrombolytic therapy has been addressed by several studies using modeling of economic costs and clinical outcomes. None of the mortality trials comparing a fibrinolytic agent with placebo or conventional therapy measured cost prospectively. Streptokinase therapy meets all criteria for acceptability from the point of view of the benefit in lives saved relative to the cost. Naylor and colleagues have provided perhaps the most complete analysis with a finding that the cost-effectiveness ratio for streptokinase is approximately $2000–4000 per year of life saved (123). Several other studies have found essentially the same result, making streptokinase a "bargain" compared with many other frequently used therapies (Table 8.8).

**Table 8.8**
**League Table of Cost-Effectiveness Ratios**

| New Rx | Comparison Rx | Patient Condition | CE ratio ($) |
|---|---|---|---|
| CABG | Medicine | Left main coronary artery disease | 7000 |
| Medical Rx | No Rx | Severe HBP | 20,000 |
| Dialysis | No dialysis | Chronic renal failure | 35,000 |
| Medical Rx | No Rx | Moderate HBP | 40,000 |
| Cholestyramine | No Rx | Cholesterol > 265 in men 45–60 | 180,000 |
| Nonionic contrast | Ionic contrast | Low-risk patients | 22,000 |
| Streptokinase | No thrombolytic | Acute myocardial infarction | 2,000–4,000 |

CABG = coronary artery bypass surgery; CE = cost effectiveness; HBP = hypertension; Rx = treatment. Adapted with permission from Mark DB. Economic analysis methods and endpoints. In: Califf RM, Mark DB, Wagner GS, eds. Acute coronary care. St. Louis: Mosby Year-Book, 1995;167–182. Data from Goldman L. Cost-effective strategies in cardiology. In: Braunwald E, ed. Heart disease: a textbook of cardiovascular medicine. 4th ed. Philadelphia: WB Saunders, 1992; and Goel V, Deber RB, Detsky AS. Nonionic contrast media: a bargain for some, a burden for many. Can Med Assoc J 1990; 143:480–481.

The incremental value of substituting accelerated alteplase for streptokinase was prospectively addressed by Mark and colleagues (124). The best estimate of the cost of an incremental year of life saved was $32,678, again within the realm of societally accepted therapies in the United States. Of course, the cost-effectiveness varies depending upon the type of patient. Using age and location of infarction to characterize patients, Mark and colleagues demonstrated that the cost-effectiveness ratio ranged from $13,410 in patients over age 75 with anterior myocardial infarction to $203,071 in patients under age 40 with inferior myocardial infarction (Table 8.9). It is important not to confuse the *incremental* cost-effectiveness of accelerated alteplase with the cost-effectiveness data for streptokinase alone. A direct comparison of these two dollar figures would be inappropriate, since one is evaluating the cost per year of life saved and the other is evaluating the additional cost per additional year of life saved.

## THE FUTURE

Although substantial progress has been made with new approaches to coronary reperfusion, much room is left for improvement. Today, one of every 16 patients dies, and many more have major complications such as shock, heart failure, stroke, and major arrhythmia. Patients who are not candidates for thrombolytic therapy have an even higher mortality. More

**Table 8.9**
**Cost-Effectiveness Ratios for Tissue Plasminogen Activator as Compared with Streptokinase in the Primary Analysis and for Selected Subgroups of Patients**

| Group of Patients[a] | Increased Life Expectancy with t-PA (year of life saved) | | Cost-Effectiveness Ratio ($)[b] |
|---|---|---|---|
| | Undiscounted | Discounted | |
| Primary analysis | 0.14 | 0.09 | 32,678 |
| Inferior MI, age ≤40 | 0.03 | 0.01 | 203,071 |
| Anterior MI, age ≤40 | 0.04 | 0.02 | 123,609 |
| Inferior MI, age 41–60 | 0.07 | 0.04 | 74,816 |
| Anterior MI, age 41–60 | 0.10 | 0.06 | 49,877 |
| Inferior MI, age 61–75 | 0.16 | 0.10 | 27,873 |
| Anterior MI, age 61–75 | 0.20 | 0.14 | 20.601 |
| Inferior MI, age >75 | 0.26 | 0.17 | 16,246 |
| Anterior MI, age >75 | 0.29 | 0.21 | 13,410 |

[a] All patients in each treatment group were included in the primary analysis.
[b] Cost-effectiveness ratios show the cost in dollars per year of life saved (both discounted at 5%) in 1993 dollars; these calculations were based on the assumption that patients treated with t-PA had costs in the first year that were $2,845 higher than those for patients treated with streptokinase.
MI = myocardial infarction; t-PA = tissue plasminogen activator.
Reprinted with permission from Mark DB, Hlatky MA, Califf RM, et al. Cost effectiveness of thrombolytic therapy with tissue plasminogen activator as compared with streptokinase for acute myocardial infarction. N Engl J Med 1995; 332:1418–1424.

effective plasminogen activators that are easier to administer are on the horizon. The new thrombin inhibitors and glycoprotein IIb/IIIa inhibitors will soon be clinically available. The rudimentary understanding of how to combine thrombolysis with other effective therapies will continue to evolve. Patients with acute myocardial infarction have much continued improvement in store over the next decade.

## REFERENCES

1. Sherry S, Fletcher AP, Alkjaersig N. Fibrinolysis and fibrinolytic activity in man. Physiol Rev 1959;39:343–382.
2. Fuster V, Badimon L, Badimon JJ, et al. The pathogenesis of coronary artery disease and the acute coronary syndromes. N Engl J Med 1992;326:242–250.
3. Falk E. Morphologic features of unstable atherothrombotic plaques underlying acute coronary syndromes. Am J Cardiol 1989;63:114E–120E.

4. Little WC, Constantinescu M, Applegate RJ, et al. Can coronary angiography predict the site of a subsequent myocardial infarction in patients with mild to moderate coronary artery disease? Circulation 1988;78:1157–1166.
5. Tofler GH, Stone PH, Maclure M. Analysis of possible triggers of acute myocardial infarction (MILIS Study). Am J Cardiol 1990;66:28–30.
6. Muller JE, Ludmer PL, Willich SN, et al. Circadian variation in the frequency of sudden cardiac death. Circulation 1987;75:131–138.
7. Muller JE, Abela GS, Nesto RW, et al. Triggers, acute risk factors and vulnerable plaques: the lexicon of a new frontier. J Am Coll Cardiol 1994;23:809–813.
8. Christian TF, Schwartz RS, Gibbons RJ. Determinants of infarct size in reperfusion therapy for acute myocardial infarction. Circulation 1992;86:81–90.
9. Kruithof EKO. Plasminogen activator inhibitors—a review. Enzyme 1988;40: 113–121.
10. Wiman B, Hamsten A. The fibrinolytic enzyme system and its role in the etiology of thromboembolic disease. Semin Thromb Hemost 1990;16:207–216.
11. Lee C, Mann K. Activation/inactivation of human factor V by plasmin. Blood 1989;73:185–190.
12. Marder VJ, Sherry S. Thrombolytic therapy: current status (first of two parts). N Engl J Med 1988;318:1512–1520.
13. Marder VJ, Sherry S. Thrombolytic therapy: current status (second of two parts). N Engl J Med 1988;318:1585–1595.
14. Lynch M, Littler WA, Pentecost BL, et al. Immunoglobulin response to intravenous streptokinase in acute myocardial infarction. Br Heart J 1991;66:139–142.
15. Elliott JM, Cross DB, Cederholm-Williams SA, et al. Neutralizing antibodies to streptokinase four years after intravenous thrombolytic therapy. Am J Cardiol 1993;71: 640–645.
16. Six AJ, Louwerenburg HW, Braams R, et al. A double-blind randomized multicenter dose-ranging trial of intravenous streptokinase in acute myocardial infarction. Am J Cardiol 1990;65:119–123.
17. Weaver DW, Cerquerira M, Hallstrom AP, et al. Pre-hospital-initiated vs hospital-initiated thrombolytic therapy: the Myocardial Infarction and Triage Intervention trial. JAMA 1993;1211–1216.
18. White HD, Norris RM, Brown MA, et al. Effect of intravenous streptokinase on left ventricular function and early survival after acute myocardial infarction. N Engl J Med 1987;317:850–855.
19. Wall TC, Phillips HR III, Stack RS, et al. Results of high dose intravenous urokinase for acute myocardial infarction. Am J Cardiol 1990;65:124–131.
20. Weaver WD, Bode C, Burnett C, et al. for the RAPID-2 Investigators. Reteplase vs Alteplase Patency Investigation During myocardial infarction trial (RAPID 2). J Am Coll Cardiol 1995;25:87A (Abstract).
21. Smith RAG, Dupe RJ, English PD, et al. Fibrinolysis with acyl-enzymes: a new approach to thrombolytic therapy. Nature 1981;290:505–508.
22. O'Connor CM, Meese R, Carney R, et al. for the DUCCS Group. A randomized trial of intravenous heparin in conjunction with anistreplase (anisoylated plasminogen streptokinase activator complex) in acute myocardial infarction: the Duke University Clinical Cardiology Study (DUCCS) 1. J Am Coll Cardiol 1994;23:11–18.
23. O'Connor CM, Meese RB, McNulty S, et al. for the DUCCS-II Investigators. A randomized factorial trial of reperfusion strategies and aspirin dosing in acute myocardial infarction. Am J Cardiol 1996; in press.
24. The GUSTO Investigators. An international randomized trial comparing four thrombolytic strategies for acute myocardial infarction. N Engl J Med 1993;329:673–682.
25. ISIS-3 Collaborative Group. ISIS-3: a randomised comparison of streptokinase vs tissue plasminogen activator vs anistreplase and of aspirin plus heparin vs aspirin alone among 41,299 cases of suspected acute myocardial infarction. ISIS-3 (Third International Study of Infarct Survival) Collaborative Group. Lancet 1992;339:753–770.
26. Gruppo Italiano per lo Studio della Sopravvivenza nell'Infarto Miocardico. GISSI-2: a factorial randomised trial of alteplase versus streptokinase and heparin versus no heparin among 12,490 patients with acute myocardial infarction. Lancet 1990; 336:65–71.

27. Purvis JA, McNeill AJ, Siddiqui RA, et al. Efficacy of 100 mg of double-bolus alteplase in achieving complete perfusion in the treatment of acute myocardial infarction. Am J Cardiol 1994;2:6–10.
28. Keyt BA, Paoni NF, Refino CJ, et al. A faster-acting and more potent form of tissue plasminogen activator. Proc Natl Acad Sci USA 1994;91:3670–3674.
29. Thomas GR, Thibodeaux H, Errett CJ, et al. A long-half-life and fibrin-specific form of tissue plasminogen activator in rabbit models of embolic stroke and peripheral bleeding. Stroke 1994;25:2072–2079.
30. Montoney M, Gardell SJ, Marder VJ. Comparison of the bleeding potential of vampire bat salivary plasminogen activator versus tissue plasminogen activator in an experimental rabbit model. Circulation 1995;91:1540–1544.
31. Witt W, Maass B, Baldus B, et al. Coronary thrombolysis with Desmodus salivary plasminogen activator in dogs: fast and persistent recanalization by intravenous bolus administration. Circulation 1994;90:421–426.
32. Lack CH. Staphylokinase: an activator of plasma protease. Nature 1948;161: 559–560.
33. Collen D, Van de Werf F. Coronary thrombolysis with recombinant staphylokinase in patients with evolving myocardial infarction. Circulation 1993;87:1850–1853.
34. Reimer KA, Lowe JE, Rasmussen MM, et al. The wave-front phenomenon of ischemic cell death: myocardial infarct size versus duration of coronary occlusion in dogs. Circulation 1977;56:786–794.
35. Rentrop KP, Blanke H, Karsch KR, et al. Acute myocardial infarction: intracoronary application of nitroglycerin and streptokinase. Clin Cardiol 1979;2:354–363.
36. Christian TF, Gibbons RJ. Myocardial perfusion imaging in myocardial infarction and unstable angina. Cardiol Clin 1994;12:247–260.
37. The GUSTO Angiographic Investigators. The effects of tissue plasminogen activator, streptokinase, or both on coronary-artery patency, ventricular function, and survival after acute myocardial infarction. N Engl J Med 1993;329:1615–1622.
38. Simes RJ, Topol EJ, Holmes DR Jr, et al. for the GUSTO-I Investigators. Link between the angiographic substudy and mortality outcomes in a large randomized trial of myocardial reperfusion: importance of early and complete infarct artery reperfusion. Circulation 1995;91:1923–1928.
39. Chesebro JH, Knatterud G, Roberts R, et al. Thrombolysis in Myocardial Infarction (TIMI) Trial, Phase I: a comparison between intravenous tissue plasminogen activator and intravenous streptokinase. Circulation 1987;76:142–154.
40. Lincoff AM, Topol EJ, Califf RM, et al. for the Thrombolysis and Angioplasty in Myocardial Infarction Study Group. Significance of a coronary artery with thrombolysis in myocardial infarction grade 2 flow "patency" (outcome in the Thrombolysis and Angioplasty in Myocardial Infarction Trials). Am J Cardiol 1995;75:871–876.
41. Granger CB, Califf RM, Topol EJ. . Thrombolytic therapy for acute myocardial infarction. A review. Drugs 1992;44:293–325.
42. Barbagelata A, Pieper K. TIMI 3 flow and reocclusion rates following thrombolysis in acute myocardial infarction. Results of an angiographic pooled analysis. Circulation 1994;90 (Suppl I):I-221 (Abstract).
43. Bode C, Smalling RW, Sen S, et al., the RAPID Investigators. Recombinant plasminogen Activator angiographic Phase II International Dose finding study (RAPID): patency analysis and mortality endpoints. Circulation 1993;88(Suppl II):I-562 (Abstract).
44. Neuhaus KL, Niederer W, Wagner J, et al. HIT (Hirudin for the Improvement of Thrombolysis): results of a dose escalation study. Circulation 1993;88(Suppl I):I-292 (Abstract).
45. Lidon RM, Theroux P, Bonan R, et al. Hirulog as adjunctive therapy to streptokinase in acute myocardial infarction. J Am Coll Cardiol 1993;21(Suppl A):419A (Abstract).
46. Ohman EM, Kleiman NS, Talley JD, et al. for the IMPACT-AMI Study Group. Simultaneous platelet glycoprotein IIb/IIIa integrin blockage with accelerated tissue plasminogen activator in acute myocardial infarction. Circulation 1994;90 (Suppl I):I-564 (Abstract).

47. Ohman EM, Califf RM, Topol EJ, et al., the TAMI Study Group. Consequences of reocclusion after successful reperfusion therapy in acute myocardial infarction. Circulation 1990;82:781–791.
48. Ellis SG, Roubin GS, King SB, et al. Angiographic and clinical predictors of acute closure after native vessel coronary angioplasty. Circulation 1988;77:372–379.
49. Wall TC, Mark DB, Califf RM, et al. Prediction of early recurrent myocardial ischemia and coronary reocclusion after successful thrombolysis: a qualitative and quantitative angiographic study. Am J Cardiol 1989;63:423–428.
50. Reiner JS, Lundergan CF, Boland J, et al. for the GUSTO Investigators. Post thromboytic angiographic features do not predict coronary reocclusion; observations from The GUSTO Angiographic Study. Circulation 1993;88 (Suppl I):I-209 (Abstract).
51. Cannon CP, McCabe CH, Diver DJ, et al., the TIMI 4 Investigators. Comparison of front-loaded recombinant tissue-type plasminogen activator, anistreplase and combination thrombolytic therapy for acute myocardial infarction: results of the Thrombolysis in Myocardial Infarction (TIMI) 4 trial. J Am Coll Cardiol 1994;24: 1602–1610.
52. Stump DC, Califf RM, Topol EJ, et al., the TAMI Study Group. Pharmacodynamics of thrombolysis with recombinant tissue-type plasminogen activator. Correlation with characteristics of and clinical outcomes in patients with acute myocardial infarction. Circulation 1989;80:1222–1230.
53. Bovill EG, Terrin ML, Stump DC, et al., for the TIMI Investigators. Hemorrhagic events during therapy with recombinant tissue-type plasminogen activator, heparin, and aspirin for acute myocardial infarction. Ann Intern Med 1991;115:256–265.
54. Lee KL, Woodlief LH, Topol EJ, et al., for the GUSTO-I Investigators. Predictors of 30-day mortality in the era of reperfusion for acute myocardial infarction: results from an international trial of 41,021 patients. Circulation 1995;91:1659–1668.
55. Hathaway WR, Zabel KM, Peterson ED, et al., GUSTO Investigators. Incremental prognostic value of electrocardiographic findings when added to baseline clinical variables in patients with acute myocardial infarction. J Am Coll Cardiol 1995;25:60A (Abstract).
56. Fibrinolytic Therapy Trialists' (FTT) Collaborative Group. Indications for fibrinolytic therapy in suspected acute myocardial infarction: collaborative overview of early mortality and major morbidity results from all randomised trials of more than 1000 patients. Lancet 1994;343:311–322.
57. Peterson ED, Hathaway WR, Zabel KM, et al. The prognostic importance of anterior ST-segment depression in inferior myocardial infarctions: results in 16,185 patients. J Am Coll Cardiol 1995;25:342A (Abstract).
58. O'Neill WW: Angioplasty therapy of cardiogenic shock: are randomized trials necessary? J Am Coll Cardiol 1992;19:915–917.
59. Bengtson JR, Kaplan AJ, Pieper KS, et al. Prognosis in cardiogenic shock after acute myocardial infarction in the interventional era. J Am Coll Cardiol 1992;20:1482–1489.
60. European Myocardial Infarction Project (EMIP) Subcommittee. Potential time saving with pre-hospital intervention in acute myocardial infarction. Eur Heart J 1988;9:118–124.
61. The GREAT Group. Feasibility, safety, and efficacy of domiciliary thrombolysis by general practitioners: Grampian Region Early Anistreplase Trial. Br Med J 1992;305:548–553.
62. European Myocardial Infarction Project Group. Prehospital thrombolytic therapy in patients with suspected acute myocardial infarction. N Engl J Med 1993;329:383–389.
63. Martin JS, Novotny-Dinsdale V, Jensen SK, et al. Early triage and treatment of the acute myocardial infarction patient: how fast is fast? J Emerg Nurs 1990;16:195–202.
64. Kline EM, Smith DD, Martin JS, et al. In-hospital treatment delays in patients treated with thrombolytic therapy: a report of the GUSTO time to treatment substudy. Circulation 1992;86(Suppl I):I-702 (Abstract).
65. ISIS-2 (Second International Study of Infarct Survival) Collaborative Group. Randomised trial of intravenous streptokinase, oral aspirin, both, or neither among 17,187 cases of suspected acute myocardial infarction: ISIS-2. Lancet 1988;2:349–360.

66. Gruppo Italiano per lo Studio della Streptochinasi nell'Infarto Miocardico (GISSI): Effectiveness of intravenous thrombolytic treatment in acute myocardial infarction. Lancet 1986;1:397–402.
67. EMERAS (Estudio Multicentrico Estreptoquinasa Republicas de America del Sur) Collaborative Group. Randomised trial of late thrombolysis in patients with suspected acute myocardial infarction. Lancet 1993;342:767–772.
68. Julian DG. The APSAC interventional mortality study (AIMS) trial: mortality data. Clin Cardiol 1990;13(Suppl 5):V20.
69. Wilcox RG, von der Lippe G, Olsson CG, et al. Trial of tissue plasminogen activator for mortality reduction in acute myocardial infarction. Anglo-Scandinavian Study of Early Thrombolysis (ASSET). Lancet 1988;2:525–530.
70. GISSI-2. Six-month survival in 20,891 patients with acute myocardial infarction randomised between alteplase and streptokinase with or without heparin. GISSI-2 and International Study Group. Gruppo Italiano per lo Studio della Sopravvivenza nell'Infarto Miocardico. Eur Heart J 1992;13:1692–1697.
71. ISIS-3 (Third International Study of Infarct Survival Collaborative Group). ISIS-3: a randomised comparison of streptokinase vs tissue plasminogen activator vs anistreplase and of aspirin plus heparin vs aspirin alone among 41,299 cases of suspected acute myocardial infarction. Lancet 1992;339:753–770.
72. Tracy RP, Bovill EG: Hemostasis and risk of ischemic disease: epidemiologic evidence with emphasis on the elderly. In: Califf RM, Mark DB, Wagner GS, eds. Acute Coronary Care. St. Louis: Mosby-Year Book, 1995:27–43.
73. Komrad MS, Coffey CE, Coffey KS, et al. Myocardial infarction and stroke. Neurology 1984;34:1403–1409.
74. Frye RL, King SB, III, Sopko G, et al. Introduction. Am J Cardiol 1995;75:1C–2C.
75. Granger C, White H, Simoons M, et al., for the GUSTO Investigators. Risk factors for stroke following thrombolytic therapy: case-control study from the GUSTO trial. J Am Coll Cardiol 1995;25:232A (Abstract).
76. Hillegass WB, Jollis JG, Granger CB, et al. Intracranial hemorrhage risk and new thrombolytic therapies in acute myocardial infarction. Am J Cardiol 1994;73: 444–449.
77. Uglietta JP, O'Connor CM, Boyko OB, et al. CT patterns of intracranial hemorrhage complicating thrombolytic therapy for acute myocardial infarction. Radiology 1991;181:555–559.
78. Oppenheimer S, Hachinski V. Complications of acute stroke. Lancet 1992;339: 721–724.
79. Mahaffey KW, White HD, Granger CB, et al., GUSTO Investigators. Neurosurgical evacuation for intracranial hemorrhage associated with improved outcome in GUSTO. J Am Coll Cardiol 1995;25:232A–233A (Abstract).
80. Berkowitz SD, Granger CB, Pieper KS, Califf RM, for the Global Use of Strategies to Open Occluded Coronary Arteries (GUSTO) I Invesetigators. Hemorrhagic non-CNS complications associated with four thrombolytic strategies for acute myocardial infarction. Circulation 1995;92(Suppl I):I-460 (Abstract).
81. Califf RM, O'Neill W, Stack RS, et al. Failure of simple clinical measurements to predict perfusion status after intravenous thrombolysis. Ann Intern Med 1988;108:658–662.
82. Hackworthy RA, Vogel MB, Harris PJ. Relationship between changes in ST segment elevation and patency of the infarct-related coronary artery in acute myocardial infarction. Am Heart J 1986;112:279–284.
83. Clemmensen P, Ohman EM, Sevilla DC, et al. Changes in standard electrocardiographic ST-segment elevation predictive of successful reperfusion in acute myocardial infarction. Am J Cardiol 1990;66:1407–1411.
84. von Essen R, Schmidt W, Uebis R, et al. Myocardial infarction and thrombolysis: electrocardiographic short-term and long-term results using precordial mapping. Br Heart J 1985;54:6–10.
85. Saran RK, Been M, Furniss SS, et al. Reduction in ST segment elevation after thrombolysis predicts either coronary reperfusion or preservation of left ventricular function. Br Heart J 1990;64:113–117.

86. Barbash GI, Roth A, Hod H, et al. Rapid resolution of ST elevation and prediction of clinical outcome in patients undergoing thrombolysis with alteplase (recombinant tissue-type plasminogen activator): results of the Israeli Study of Early Intervention in Myocardial Infarction. Br Heart J 1990;64:241–247.
87. Christenson RH, Ohman EM, Clemmensen P, et al. Characteristics of creatine kinase-MB and MB isoforms in serum after reperfusion in acute myocardial infarction. Clin Chem 1989;35:2179–2185.
88. Ohman EM, Christenson RH, Califf RM, et al., the TAMI 7 Study Group. Non-invasive detection of reperfusion after thrombolysis based on serum creatine kinase MB changes and clinical variables. Am Heart J 1993;126:819–826.
89. Puleo PR: Detection of coronary artery patency after thrombolytic therapy of acute myocardial infarction using creatine kinase-MB subforms. Coron Artery Dis 1992;3:468–474.
90. Veldkamp RF, Green CL, Wilkins ML, et al., the Thrombolysis and Angioplasty in Myocardial Infarction (TAMI) 7 Study Group. Comparison of continuous ST-segment recovery analysis with methods using static electrocardiograms for noninvasive patency assessment during acute myocardial infarction. Am J Cardiol 1994;73:1069–1074.
91. Dellborg M, Steg PG, Simoons M, et al. Increased rate of evolution of QRS changes in patients with acute myocardial infarction: results from the Vermut Study. J Electrocardiol 1993;26:244–248.
92. Abbottsmith CW, Topol EJ, George BS, et al. Fate of patients with acute myocardial infarction with patency of the infarct-related vessel achieved with successful thrombolysis versus rescue angioplasty. J Am Coll Cardiol 1990;16:770–778.
93. Ellis SG, da Silva ER, Heyndrickx GR, et al. for the RESCUE Investigators. Final results of the randomized RESCUE study evaluating PTCA after failed thrombolysis for patients with anterior infarction. Circulation 1993;88(Suppl I):I-106 (Abstract).
94. Honan MB, Harrell FE, Jr., Reimer KA, et al. Cardiac rupture, mortality and the timing of thrombolytic therapy: a meta-analysis. J Am Coll Cardiol 1990;16: 359–367.
95. Kleiman NS, White HD, Ohman EM, et al., The GUSTO Investigators. Mortality within 24 hours of thrombolysis for myocardial infarction: the importance of early reperfusion. Circulation 1994;90:2658–2665.
96. Barbagelata A, Granger CB, Topol EJ, et al. for the TAMI Study Group. Frequency, significance, and cost of recurrent ischemia after thrombolytic therapy for acute myocardial infarction. Am J Cardiol 1995;76:1007–1013.
97. Betriu A, Califf RM, Granger C, for the GUSTO Investigators. Importance of clinical findings during post-infarction angina in determining prognosis: results from the GUSTO trial. J Am Coll Cardiol 1994;23:27A (Abstract).
98. Simoons ML, Arnout J, van den Brand M, et al. Retreatment with alteplase for early signs of reocclusion after thrombolysis. The European Cooperative Study Group. Am J Cardiol 1993;71:524–528.
99. Barbash GI, Hod H, Roth A, et al. Repeat infusions of recombinant tissue-type plasminogen activator in patients with acute myocardial infarction and early recurrent myocardial ischemia. J Am Coll Cardiol 1990;16:779–783.
100. O'Neill WW, Brodie BR, Ivanhoe R, et al. Primary coronary angioplasty for acute myocardial infarction (the Primary Angioplasty Registry). Am J Cardiol 1994;73:627–634.
101. Brodie BR, Grines CL, Ivanhoe R, et al. Six-month clinical and angiographic follow-up after direct angioplasty for acute myocardial infarction: final results from the primary angioplasty registry. Circulation 1994;90:156–162.
102. Hochman JS, Boland J, Sleeper LA, et al., the SHOCK Registry Investigators. Current spectrum of cardiogenic shock and effect of early revascularization on mortality: results of an international registry. Circulation 1995;91:873–881.
103. Jollis JG, Peterson ED, DeLong ER, et al. The relation between the volume of coronary angioplasty procedures at hospitals treating Medicare beneficiaries and short-term mortality. N Engl J Med 1994;331:1625–1629.

104. Lefkovits J, Plow EF, Topol EJ. Platelet glycoprotein IIb/IIIa receptors in cardiovascular medicine. N Engl J Med 1995;332:1553–1559.
105. Mahaffey KW, Granger CB, O'Connor CM, et al. Overview of randomized trials of intravenous heparin in patients with acute myocardial infarction treated with thrombolytic therapy. Am J Cardiol 1996; in press.
106. Yusuf S, Peto R, Lewis J, et al. Beta blockade during and after myocardial infarction: an overview of the randomized trials. Prog Cardiovasc Dis 1985;27:335–371.
107. TIMI Study Group. Comparison of invasive and conservative strategies after treatment with intravenous tissue plasminogen activator in acute myocardial infarction. Results of the Thrombolysis In Myocardial Infarction (TIMI) phase II trial. The TIMI Study Group. N Engl J Med 1989;320:618–627.
108. Brener SJ, Cox JL, Pfisterer ME, et al., for the GUSTO Investigators. The potential for unexpected hazard of intravenous beta-blockade for acute myocardial infarction: results from the GUSTO trial. J Am Coll Cardiol 1995;Special Edition:5-A–6-A (Abstract).
109. Pilote L, Califf RM, Sapp S, et al. Regional variation across the United States in the management of acute myocardial infarction. N Engl J Med 1995;333:565–572.
110. Yusuf S, Collins R, MacMahon S, et al. Effect of intravenous nitrates on mortality in acute myocardial infarction: an overview of randomised trials. Lancet 1988;1:1088–1092.
111. Ventura B. Findings on the efficacy and safety of thrombolytic therapy. An analysis of key clinical trials. Crit Care Nurs Clin North Am 1990;2:663–671.
112. Gruppo Italiano per lo Studio della Sopravvivenza nell'Infarto Miocardico. GISSI-3: effects of lisinopril and transdermal glyceryl trinitrate singly and together on 6-week mortality and ventricular function after acute myocardial infarction. Lancet 1994;343:1115–1121.
113. Becker RC, Corrao JM, Bovill EG, et al. Intravenous nitroglycerin-induced heparin resistance: a qualitative antithrombin III abnormality. Am Heart J 1990;119: 1254–1261.
114. Nabel EG, Topol EJ, Galeana A, et al. A randomized placebo-controlled trial of combined early intravenous captopril and recombinant tissue-type plasminogen activator therapy in acute myocardial infarction. J Am Coll Cardiol 1991;17:467–473.
115. ISIS-4 (Fourth International Study of Infarct Survival) Collaborative Group. ISIS-4: a randomised factorial trial assessing early oral captopril, oral mononitrate, and intravenous magnesium sulphate in 48,050 patients with suspected acute myocardial infarction. Lancet 1995;345:669–685.
116. Simoons ML, Arnold AE, Betriu A, et al. Thrombolysis with tissue plasminogen activator in acute myocardial infarction: no additional benefit from immediate percutaneous coronary angioplasty. Lancet 1988;1:197–203.
117. TIMI Study Group. Immediate versus delayed catheterization and angioplasty following thrombolytic therapy for acute myocardial infarction. N Engl J Med 1988;260:2849–2858.
118. Topol EJ, Califf RM, George BS, et al. and the TAMI Study Group. A randomized trial of immediate versus delayed elective angioplasty after intravenous tissue plasminogen activator in acute myocardial infarction. N Engl J Med 1987;317: 581–588.
119. Califf RM, Topol EJ, Stack RS, et al., for the TAMI Study Group. Evaluation of combination thrombolytic therapy and timing of cardiac catheterization in acute myocardial infarction. Results of thrombolysis and angioplasty in myocardial infarction—phase 5 randomized trial. Circulation 1991;83:1543–1556.
120. Yusuf S, Zucker D, Peduzzi P, et al. Effect of coronary artery bypass graft surgery on survival: overview of 10-year results from randomised trials by the coronary artery bypass graft surgery trialists collaboration. Lancet 1994;344:563–570.
121. Mark DB, Nelson CL, Califf RM, et al. Continuing evolution of therapy for coronary artery disease: initial results from the era of coronary angioplasty. Circulation 1994;89:2015–2025.
122. Newby LK, Califf RM, for the GUSTO Investigators. Redefining uncomplicated myocardial infarction in the thrombolytic era. Circulation 1994;90 (Suppl I):I-110 (Abstract).

123. Mark DB: Medical economics and health policy issues for interventional cardiology. In: Topol EJ, ed. Textbook of interventional cardiology. Philadelphia: W.B.Saunders, 1993:1323–1353.
124. Mark DB, Hlatky MA, Califf RM, et al. Cost effectiveness of thrombolytic therapy with tissue plasminogen activator as compared with streptokinase for acute myocardial infarction. N Engl J Med 1995;332:1418–1424.
125. Collen D, Lijnen HR. . Fibrinolytic system: implications for thrombolytic therapy. In: Califf RM, Mark DB, Wagner GS, eds. Acute coronary care. St. Louis: Mosby Year-Book, 1995:85–95.
126. Rentrop P, Smith H, Painter L, et al. Changes in left ventricular ejection fraction after intracoronary thrombolytic therapy: results of the Registry of the European Society of Cardiology. Circulation 1983;68(Suppl I):I-55–I-60.
127. Califf RM, Topol EJ. The paradigm of acute reperfusion and the GUSTO-I trial. In: Califf RM, Mark DB, Wagner GS, eds. Acute coronary care. St. Louis: Mosby-Year Book, 1995:69–83.
128. Kline E, Smith D, Martin J, et al. Strategies to decrease treatment delays in patients receiving thrombolytic therapy for acute myocardial infarction. In: Califf RM, Mark DB, Wagner GS, eds. Acute coronary care. St. Louis: Mosby Year-Book, 1995:265–279.
129. Califf RM: Acute myocardial infarction. In: Smith TW, ed. Cardiovascular therapeutics. Philadelphia: WB Saunders, 1996, in press.
130. Gore JM, Granger CB, Sloan MA, et al. for the GUSTO-I Investigators. Stroke after thrombolysis: mortality and functional outcomes in the GUSTO-I trial. Circulation 1995;92:2811–2818.
131. O'Connor CM: Stroke during acute myocardial infarction. In: Califf RM, Mark DB, Wagner GS, eds. Acute coronary care. St. Louis: Mosby Year-Book,1995:635–650.
132. Maggioni AP, Franzosi MG, Santoro E, et al., The Gruppo Italiano per lo Studio della Sopravvivenza nell'Infarto Miocardico II (GISSI-2), The International Study Group. The risk of stroke in patients with acute myocardial infarction after thrombolytic and antithrombotic treatment. N Engl J Med 1992;327:1–6.
133. Maggioni AP, Franzosi MG, Farina ML, et al. Cerebrovascular events after myocardial infarction: analysis of the GISSI trial. Br Med J 1991;302:1428–1431.
134. ISIS-2. Randomized trial of intravenous streptokinase, oral aspirin, both, or neither among 17,187 cases of suspected acute myocardial infarction: ISIS-2. J Am Coll Cardiol 1988;12:3A–13A.

CHAPTER 9

# Platelet-Active Drugs and Anticoagulants

Kenneth A. Schwartz, MD

The clotting system is important in a wide variety of cardiovascular diseases. For example, the pathophysiology of occlusive atherosclerotic vascular disease involves the combined processes of atherosclerosis and thrombosis. Initially, deposits of lipids result in atheromatous injury to endothelial cells of the vessel wall; thrombosis associated with the atheroma probably develops as a secondary process (1). Histologic investigations of diseased vessels as well as direct observation of coronary arteries in symptomatic patients demonstrate that the combined processes of atherosclerosis and thrombosis ("atherothrombosis") are present in diseased arteries (2). Autopsy studies commonly show rupture, cracking, or ulcerations of atherosclerotic plaques (3). Hemorrhage and thrombosis of the ruptured atherosclerotic plaque can further compromise the vessel lumen and result in critical stenosis (4–6). Direct observation of the coronary arteries via coronary angioscopy shows acute thrombi in conjunction with atherosclerotic plaques in patients with preinfarction angina; atherosclerotic narrowing of the coronary arteries without thrombosis is present in patients with stable angina (2). These observations suggest that the accelerated symptoms observed in some patients with preinfarction angina are secondary to the formation of atherosclerosis-associated thrombi (2).

## PHYSIOLOGY OF PLATELET ACTIVATION

Since platelets as well as humoral coagulation factors are instrumental in clot formation, medications that inhibit platelet function help to protect against vascular thrombosis. An understanding of the sequence of platelet activation and the mechanisms involved in platelet stimulation aids in comprehension of the attributes and limitations of drugs that inhibit platelet function and are efficacious in cardiovascular diseases.

In normal, nonatherosclerotic vasculature, activation of platelets and coagulation factors is limited to loci where the protective inhibitory effects of the endothelial cells are removed. Here platelets as well as humoral coagulation factors become exposed to agonists (such as collagen) that are present in the subendothelial tissues. In this way the specificity of clot formation is controlled. Normal platelet activation is commonly divided into four phases: adhesion, aggregation, secretion, and enhancement of humoral coagulation (Fig.9.1) (7).

## Adhesion

The first phase occurs when endothelial cells are removed from blood vessels, and platelets thereby adhere to and spread upon the exposed subendothelial lining. This process of initial contact of platelets with tissues is known as *platelet adhesion.* In the vessel wall, collagen appears to be the most platelet-reactive material. In the arterial circulation where high shear rates are present, platelet adherence also requires von Willebrand factor, a protein synthesized and secreted by endothelial cells (8, 9). Von Willebrand factor is mainly secreted into the bloodstream, but some is also deposited in the subendothelial tissues. The main platelet binding site for von Willebrand factor is glycoprotein Ib, but binding also occurs via glycoprotein IIb-IIIa complex (GPIIb-IIIa) (10). The adhesion of platelets to tissues is the critical first step in the control of bleeding and in the formation of the platelet thrombus.

## Aggregation

Platelet *aggregation* (the second phase), defines the process in which platelets stick to each other and form the hemostatic plug. The normal resting platelet is disc shaped; with activation, it is transformed into a spiny sphere and aggregates, a process that is conveniently investigated

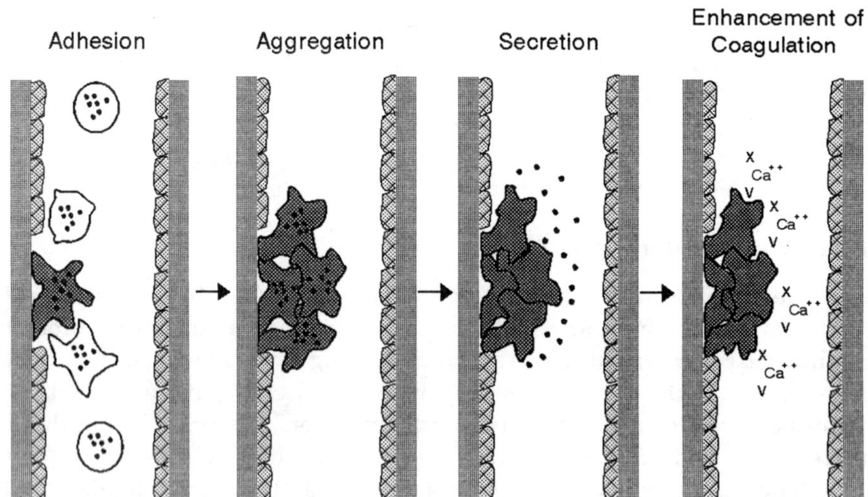


Figure 9.1 Initial platelet activation causes the platelets to become sticky and *adhere* to the vessel wall at loci where the protective endothelium has become damaged or lost. Continued activation results in platelet *aggregation,* which is mediated via multiple intraplatelet pathways. With progressive stimulation, platelets *secrete* their internal granules. During the final phase of platelet activation, *enhancement of coagulation,* aggregated platelets provide a surface for the activation of humeral coagulation factors.

using a platelet aggregometer. Optical aggregometers sense the changes that occur in the transmission of light through a glass cuvette filled with a cloudy appearing, platelet-rich suspension. As the platelets aggregate, the platelet-rich plasma becomes clearer and the increase in transmission of light is recorded. Complex interactions of platelet agonists and inhibitors, such as aspirin, are investigated using the platelet aggregometer.

There are several agonists for platelet aggregation, which can be conveniently divided into strong agonists, such as thrombin and collagen, and weak agonists, such as adenosine diphosphate (ADP) and epinephrine. The interaction of a platelet agonist with the platelet surface generates a signal that is transmitted internally by several signal transduction pathways and that ultimately stimulates aggregation.

Platelet activation increases the production of prostaglandins via activation of phospholipases and generation of arachidonic acid from the platelet membrane phospholipids (11). In platelets and endothelial cells, prostaglandin G/H synthase, possessing both cyclooxygenase and peroxidase functions, produces the common intermediate prostaglandin $H_2$ ($PGH_2$) (11) (Fig. 9.2). In platelets, the enzyme thromboxane synthase converts $PGH_2$ to the predominant platelet prostaglandin product thromboxane $A_2$ ($PGA_2$), a potent platelet stimulator and vasoconstrictor. Prostacyclin ($PGI_2$), a strong inhibitor of platelet function and a vasodilator, is the main product of $PGH_2$ in endothelial cells (not platelets) via the enzyme prostacylin synthase (12).

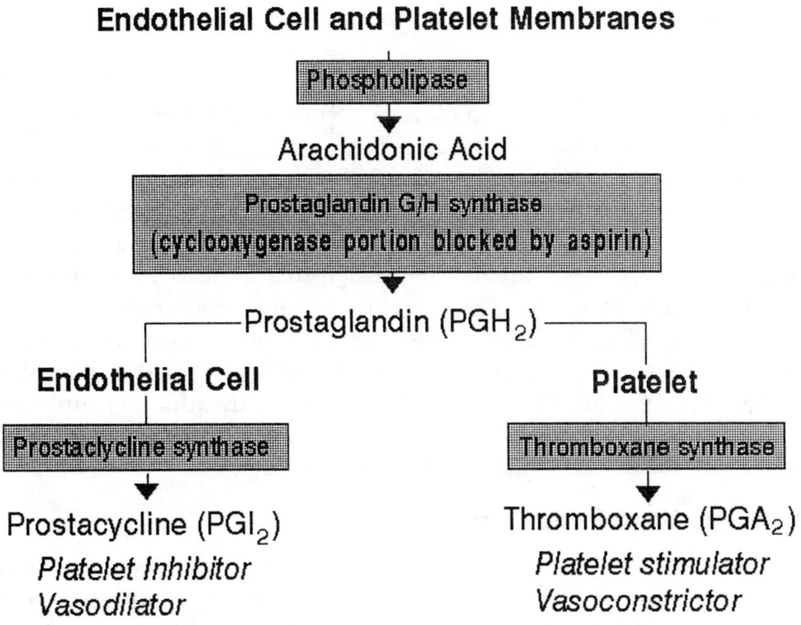

**Endothelial Cell and Platelet Membranes**

Phospholipase

Arachidonic Acid

Prostaglandin G/H synthase
(cyclooxygenase portion blocked by aspirin)

Prostaglandin ($PGH_2$)

**Endothelial Cell**

Prostacycline synthase

Prostacycline ($PGI_2$)
*Platelet Inhibitor*
*Vasodilator*

**Platelet**

Thromboxane synthase

Thromboxane ($PGA_2$)
*Platelet stimulator*
*Vasoconstrictor*

Figure 9.2 Prostaglandin pathways inhibited by aspirin.

Increased concentrations of cyclic adenosine monophosphate (cAMP) inhibit platelet aggregation. This contrasts with an activation effect commonly observed in other cellular systems with increasing concentrations of cAMP. cAMP is increased through increased production by adenyl cyclase, the enzyme located in the platelet membrane that generates cAMP, or via inhibition of phosphodiesterase, the enzyme responsible for the degradation of cAMP. The platelet agonists thrombin, ADP, epinephrine, and collagen are associated with decreased levels of cAMP and increased activity of phosphodiesterase. In contrast, increased levels of cAMP and activity of adenyl cyclase are observed with the strong platelet inhibitor prostaglandin $E_1$ ($PGE_1$) (13).

The inositol pathway also is involved in aggregation in the intraplatelet transfer of signals after agonist-induced receptor activation. In this pathway, activation of phospholipase C results in the production of membrane bound diacylglycerol (DAG) and cytoplasmic inositol 1,4,5 trisphosphate ($IP_3$) from phosphatidylinositol 4,5-bisphosphate ($PIP_2$). $IP_3$ releases calcium from internal platelet stores. DAG is phosphorylated to form phosphatidic acid, which activates protein kinase C. Granule secretion from platelets (see below) is also facilitated by activation of protein kinase C and by increases in calcium (14).

Because three metabolic processes (involving prostaglandins, cyclic AMP, and inositol) are involved in platelet signal transduction, blockade of a single pathway (for example, aspirin blockade of prostaglandin production) does not produce complete inhibition of platelet function (11).

## Secretion

Secretion is the third phase of platelet activation. Platelets contain morphologically distinct types of granules, dense granules and alpha granules, as well as lysosomes that can be regarded as a third type of granule. Extrusion of these granules constitutes platelet *secretion.* Electron microscopic investigation of platelets after stimulation shows that the granules have moved from a near random dispersion to a location in the center of the platelet where they are surrounded by a ring of microtubules (15). After granule secretion, the ADP released from the dense granules serves as an agonist, possibly recruiting additional platelets into the hemostatic plug. Among the multiple constituents present in the alpha granules is a protein termed *P-selectin* that is present on the surface of activated platelets but not platelets in the resting state (16–18).

## Enhancement of Coagulation

The fourth and final phase of platelet activation is enhancement of coagulation. In the past, platelet-induced enhancement of humoral coagulation was termed *platelet factor 3 activity.* Platelets, by providing a phospholipid membrane surface, enhance the formation of several key intermediates in the coagulation cascade. These intermediates include prothombinase complex and, in the contact phase of coagulation, activation of factor XI (19–21). Although fibrinogen does not bind to resting platelets, it does bind to GPIIb-IIIa on the platelet surface with platelet activation. Platelet-bound fibrinogen acts as a bridge connecting platelets to foreign surfaces and other platelets (7).

Detailed understanding of platelet activation has facilitated investigations of the mechanisms of action of platelet inhibitory medications as well as stimulated the development of new platelet inhibitory drugs.

## ANTIPLATELET DRUGS

Antiplatelet drugs and their mechanisms of action are listed in Table 9.1.

**Table 9.1**
**Medications and Mechanisms of Action**

| Medications | Half-Life | Mechanism of Action |
|---|---|---|
| Aspirin | 30–45 min[a] | Blocks cyclooxygenase portion of prostaglandin $H_2$ synthase |
| Dipyridamole | [b] | Increases concentration of platelet cAMP |
| Prostacyclin and prostacyclin analogue iloprost | 30 min | Increases concentration of platelet cAMP |
| Blockers of platelet glycoprotein IIb-IIIa | Variable[c] | Blocks fibrinogen binding to platelet glycoprotein IIb-IIIa |
| Ticlopidine | 20–50 h | Global inhibitor of platelet function—mechanism is unknown |
| Heparin | | |
| Ultrafractionated heparin | | Combines with AT–III to inhibit serine proteases (mainly prothrombin and factor Xa) |
| i.v. | 1.0–1½ h | |
| s.c. | 3 h | |
| Low–molecular weight heparin | | |
| i.v. and s.c. | 4–6 h[d] | Combines with AT-III to mainly inhibit Xa |
| Warfarin | 36–42 h | Inhibits production of vitamin K |

[a] See Table 9.2.
[b] Dipyridamole has a biexponential decay half-life of 1 and 16 hours (43, 44).
[c] Half-life of murine monoclonal antibody varies depending upon host immune response.
[d] See Table 9.3.
AT-III = antithrombin III; cAMP = cyclic adenosine monophosphate; h = hours; i.v. = intravenous; min = minutes; s.c. = subcutaneous.

## Aspirin (Acetylsalicylate)

Aspirin's role in clotting is via selective blockade of cyclooxygenase function of prostaglandin G/H synthase (Fig. 9.2) (by acetylation of the serine residue at position 529) (22). This selective blockade of prostaglandin production occurs in both platelets and endothelial cells. Since platelets lack a nucleus and consequently the metabolic capacity to synthesize new, nonacetylated enzyme, the inhibitory effect of aspirin on platelet function is permanent. Endothelial cells are capable of producing enzymes; hence the aspirin-induced blockade of the cyclooxygenase in these nucleated cells is only temporary (23–25).

The main product of arachidonic acid metabolism in platelets is thromboxane ($PGA_2$) (Fig. 9.2), a potent platelet stimulator and vasoconstrictor. Aspirin-induced blockade here inhibits clotting. In contrast, endothelial cells metabolize arachidonic acid via the prostaglandin pathway to produce prostacyclin ($PGI_2$), a strong inhibitor of platelet function and a vasodilator. This creates a potential dichotomy in the effects of aspirin on clotting. In theory, the inhibitory effect of aspirin on platelet thromboxane could be partially mitigated or even reversed by blockage of endothelial cell production of the platelet inhibitor prostacyclin.

Therefore, a pharmacologic goal of aspirin administration is to selectively inhibit cyclooxygenase in platelets while sparing it in endothelial cells. This result would inhibit platelet production of the platelet stimulator thromboxane while allowing continued endothelial cell production of the platelet inhibitor prostacyclin. The timing of recovery from the cyclooxygenase-inhibiting effect differs among these cells, as shown by various data. After exposure to aspirin, endothelial cells have the capacity to synthesize new nonacylated cyclooxygenase and regain the capacity to produce prostacyclin. A single 300-mg dose of aspirin initially decreases both platelet production of thromboxane and endothelial production of prostacyclin by more than 80%. Within 6 hours after the dose of aspirin, normal endothelial cell production of prostacyclin has resumed; platelet production of thromboxane, on the other hand, remains inhibited for 48 hours after aspirin is given (23). Endothelial cell cyclooxygenase is as sensitive initially to aspirin inhibition as is cyclooxygenase in platelets, but later differences occur. As little as 6.2 μM aspirin blocks cultured endothelial cell production of prostacyclin. Ten minutes after 650 mg of oral aspirin, the plasma level is much higher at 128 μM, but 24 hours after aspirin is removed from cultured endothelial cells, production of prostacyclin returns to preaspirin levels (24). In contrast, after administration of 35 mg of aspirin for 7 days, blood obtained only 12 hours after the last dose of aspirin had significantly decreased concentrations of both thromboxane and prostacyclin (25). In patients treated with 20 mg per day of aspirin for 7 days before open heart surgery, production of thromboxane was inhibited by more than 90% (26). When measured using tissue samples from the aorta and the saphenous vein obtained during open heart surgery, endothelial cell production of prostacyclin was reduced by more than 50%. However, 24 hours after removal of aspirin from the cultured vascular tissues, production of prostacyclin had returned to normal. No difference in surgically related blood loss or in transfusion requirements was demonstrated between the aspirin-treated and control groups (26). These data confirm that both platelet and endothelial cell cyclooxygenase are inhibited by aspirin, but endothelial cells have a much faster recovery from the aspirin blockade.

Oral aspirin is rapidly absorbed by the stomach and small intestine but undergoes first-pass metabolism to salicylate in liver (and also in bowel wall, lung, and red blood cells). Over a dose range of 20–1300 mg, systemic bioavailability is 46–51% (27). Timed studies following oral administration of aspirin demonstrate that the decrease of thromboxane $B_2$ formation (the stable metabolite of thromboxane) precedes the detection of aspirin in blood. Thus, aspirin may inhibit platelet cyclooxygenase in the presystemic portal circulation (27).

In this regard, comparing the pharmacodynamics of controlled-release aspirin (in the form of 75-mg capsules designed to release 10 mg/hour) with those of conventional aspirin is of interest (28). After 28 days, both aspirin formulations produced equivalent prolongations of bleeding times and depression of thromboxane concentrations in platelets. However, systemic synthesis of prostacyclin in endothelium after stimulation with bradykinin was preserved in those receiving controlled-release aspirin but depressed in those taking the conventionally formulated aspirin (28). In theory, low doses of aspirin could inhibit platelets in the portal circulation and be metabolized in the liver so that a minimal amount would be present in the systemic circulation. This strategy would allow for selective inhibition of the cyclooxygenase in platelets while the activity of the enzyme is maintained in endothelial cells.

Regarding other aspirin formulations, both low-dose enteric-coated aspirin and aspirin delivered transdermally inhibited cyclooxygenase activity in platelets. Administration of as little as 27 mg of granular, enteric-coated aspirin blocked formation of thromboxane, inhibited in vitro platelet aggregation, and prolonged bleeding times (29). Both conventional aspirin and enteric-coated aspirin at doses of 325 mg blocked vascular production of prostacyclin, and the latter also inhibited the increased morning reactivity of platelets to standard aggregating agents (30). Comparison of every-other-day administration of 325 mg of conventionally formulated aspirin with enteric-coated aspirin showed no differences in prolongation of bleeding times, inhibition of platelet aggregation, or decreased production of thromboxane (31). Low-dose (20–45 mg/day) and high dose (900 mg/day) aspirin regimens resulted in similar inhibition of platelet function as demonstrated by prolongation of bleeding times, inhibition of platelet aggregation, and decreased production of thromboxane in both normal and hyperlipidemic subjects (32). Administration of aspirin transdermally (which results in release at a slow rate) at a dose of 750 mg/day blocked thromboxane production without affecting prostacyclin synthesis (33). Hence, low doses of aspirin administered as an enteric-coated formulation or transdermally appeared to selectively inhibit platelet cyclooxygenase and production of thromboxane while sparing endothelial cell cyclooxygenase and production of prostacyclin.

Table 9.2 shows the kinetics of various preparations of aspirin (34) and the fact that there is a certain amount of variability among preparations. Elimination is by both liver and kidney (where it is greater at increased urinary pH) (35). It is important to note that although half-lives in blood are short, effects of aspirin on platelets is permanent and lasts for the 7- to 10-day life of that particular platelet. In addition, high-dose aspirin has instantaneous effects whereas a lower dose may take several days for onset of action. When immediate action is needed, as in myocardial infarction, the rapidly absorbed and rapidly acting chewable aspirin should be administered.

Upper gastrointestinal bleeding is the main toxicity associated with aspirin administration; the larger the dose of aspirin, the higher the incidence of gastrointesinal bleeding (6, 36, 37). Since blockade of platelet prostaglandin production occurs with very small doses of aspirin, the upper gastrointestinal toxicity appears to be a direct effect of the aspirin on the gastrointestinal mucosa. In various clinical trials, an increase in hemorrhagic stroke has also occurred along with the more substantial decrease in thrombotic stroke.

Although prostaglandins are important in platelet activation, other intraplatelet systems such as cAMP and the inositol pathway may be able to

**Table 9.2**
**Mean (± SD) Pharmacokinetic Parameters of Various Formulations of Single-Dose Aspirin (Acetylsalicylic Acid) in Healthy Volunteers**

| | Dose (mg) | | | | | |
|---|---|---|---|---|---|---|
| Parameter | 100 (RR) | 100 (RR) | 100 (EC)[a] | 100 (EC) | 325 (PL) | 325 (BU) |
| $C_{max}$ (μg/L) | 1979 ± 580 | 2721 ± 791 | 411 ± 133 | 186 ± 202 | 4860 ± 1330 | 5770 ± 1160 |
| $t_{max}$ (h) | 0.48 ± 0.35 | 0.35 ± 0.10 | 3.73 ± 0.94 | 6.84 ± 2.71 | 0.63 ± 0.31 | 0.46 ± 0.13 |
| $t_{1/2}$ (h) | 0.35 ± 0.04 | 0.37 ± 0.05 | 0.45 ± 0.10 | N/A | 0.45 ± 0.21 | 0.37 ± 0.07 |

[a] Note the variability in different formulations of both RR and EC forms.
BU = buffered formulation; $C_{max}$ = maximal plasma concentration; EC = enteric-coated tablet; h = hours; N/A = not available; PL = plain or conventional-release tablet; RR = rapid-release tablet; $t_{1/2}$ = elimination half-life; $t_{max}$ = time taken to achieve $C_{max}$.
Adapted with permission from Lutomski DM, Bottorff M, Sangha K. Pharmacokinetic optimisation of the treatment of embolic disorders. Clin Pharmacokinet 1994;28:67–92.

compensate when the generation of prostaglandins is pharmacologically blocked by agents such as aspirin. This may explain why aspirin induces only partial blockade of platelet aggregation (38).

Overall, low doses of aspirin are appealing for clinical studies because of a lower incidence of gastrointestinal symptoms and bleeding and because they may be relatively selective in blocking platelet cyclooxygenase and production of the platelet stimulator thromboxane while sparing endothelial cells and production of the platelet inhibitor prostacyclin. However, doses employed in the various clinical trials showing the efficaciousness of aspirin have been variable (see Chapter 10).

## Dipyridamole

Several mechanisms resulting in an increased platelet concentration of cAMP have been proposed to explain dipyridamole's inhibition of platelet function (39). Degradation of cAMP by the enzyme phosphodiesterase is prevented by dipyridamole (39). Intraplatelet cAMP concentrations therefore increase, and platelet activation is inhibited. Additional increases in cAMP may be mediated by the interaction of dipyridamole with platelet inhibiting eicosanoids such as $PGI_2$, $PGD_2$, and $PGE_1$. By inhibiting the uptake of adenine by erythrocytes and endothelial cells, dipyridamole may increase adenine concentration in the microenvironment of clot formation. Adenine inhibits platelet function by stimulating adenyl cyclase and the formation of cAMP (39–41). Dipyridamole may also potentiate the vasodilating and platelet inhibitory effects of the endothelium-derived relaxation factor, nitric oxide (NO) (42).

Bioavailability of dipyridamole appears to be variable (27–88%) (43, 44) with Persantine (Boehringer Ingelheim Pharmaceuticals, Ridgefield, Connecticut), a commercial product, having in one study two times the bioavailability of other products (45). The drug is 99% bound to plasma proteins (mainly α-1 acid glycoprotein). Maximum concentration is acheived in 2.0–2.5 hours, and serum levels have a biexponential decay half-life of 1 and 16 hours (43, 44). Elimination is hepatic with some entrohepatic circulation (44). Maximum and minimum serum levels are in the range of 1.2–1.9 and 0.25–0.8 mg/L, respectively (34). Dose is 75–100 mg four times a day. Dipyridamole's primary indication is as adjunctive therapy to coumadin in patients with artificial cardiac valves.

## Prostacyclin and the Prostacyclin Analogue Iloprost

Both prostacyclin ($PGI_2$) and its stable analogue iloprost (ZK36374) inhibit platelets by stimulating adenyl cyclase and increasing platelet cAMP (46). These medications should be considered experimental, but Iloprost shows promise because it has a longer half-life (30 minutes) than prostacyclin and it does not produce the decrease in blood pressure that prostacyclin does (47, 48).

## Blockade of Platelet Glycoproteins (IIb-IIIa or Ib)

Monoclonal antibodies, specific snake venoms, and some particular types of nonprotein chemicals inhibit platelet function via blockade of platelet glycoproteins. Fibrinogen binding to the platelet GPIIb-IIIa is an important step for attachment of platelets to foreign surfaces or to other platelets. Blockade of platelet GPIIb-IIIa decreases the binding of radiolabeled fibrinogen to platelets, inhibits platelet aggregation as measured by platelet aggregometry, and significantly prolongs bleeding times. When compared with aspirin using animal models, medications that block platelet GPIIb-IIIa produced a greater inhibition of platelet function and a greater protection from thrombosis than did aspirin (49–51).

Several monoclonal antibodies with specificity for platelet GPIIb-IIIa or platelet glycoprotein Ib (GPIb) have been evaluated using artificial systems and animal models. In one study, platelet deposition on artificial surfaces under laminar flow or oscillatory flow conditions was almost completely inhibited by the monoclonal antibody, 10ES, which is specific for platelet GPIIb-IIIa. Antibody 6D1, with specificity for platelet glycoprotein Ib, also inhibits platelet deposition, apparently by blocking the attachment of platelets to the platelets that have already formed the initial layer on the artificial surface (52). In another study, the $F(ab')_2$ fragment of the murine monoclonal antibody 7E3, which binds to GPIIb-IIIa, blocked new thrombosis formation in the partially stenosed circumflex arteries of both dogs and monkeys (53). Further testing of the $F(ab')_2$ of 7E3 in a canine balloon angioplasty model showed that the monoclonal antibody fragment was superior to aspirin in preventing thrombosis (49). In a third study, another monoclonal antibody, P37, with specificity for platelet GPIIb-IIIa, inhibited $^{111}$indium-labeled platelet deposition on electrically injured canine carotid arteries (54). In a fourth study, two anti-GPIIb-IIIa monoclonal antibodies, AP-2 and LJ-CP8, blocked platelet deposition on Dacron grafts in baboons. Both antibodies were more effective as antithrombotic agents than was aspirin, but infusion of AP-2, or its $F(ab')_2$ fragments resulted in decreased platelet concentrations (51). Finally, in a fifth study, infusion of $F(ab')_2$ fragments of 7E3 into a "newly dead" patient being maintained on a respirator inhibited ADP-stimulated platelet aggregation (55).

Hence, blockade of platelet glycoproteins with specific monoclonal antibodies resulted in significant inhibition of platelet function; however, these antibodies have the potential for induction of immune-mediated platelet destruction. In addition, patients who have been treated with murine monoclonal antibodies may produce antibodies to them that may limit their repeated administration (56).

Specific snake venoms and chemicals also inhibit platelet function by blocking GPIIb-IIIa. Triflavin is a snake venom that inhibits fibrinogen binding to platelet GPIIb-IIIa. In addition, it inhibits platelet aggregation and prevents pulmonary thromboembolism in mice treated with ADP (57,

58). DMP 728, a chemical developed to specifically block binding to platelet GPIIb-IIIa, inhibits platelet aggregation and fibrinogen binding to either platelets or purified GPIIb-IIIa receptors, and it increases the bleeding time in dogs. In addition, the antithrombotic effects of DMP 728 have been demonstrated in canine models of coronary and femoral arterial thrombosis (59). Investigations in dogs undergoing open heart surgery showed that another platelet GPIIb-IIIa blocker, R0 44-9883, prolonged the bleeding time, inhibited platelet aggregation, and prevented initial decreases in platelet concentrations without increasing blood loss (60). Thus, nonantibody compounds with specific anti-GPIIb-IIIa activity are under development for possible use as antithrombotic agents in cardiovascular diseases.

## Ticlopidine

Ticlopidine is an inhibitor of platelet function whose exact mechanism of action remains incompletely understood. The drug must be given orally to be effective. Maximal effect is seen after several days of therapy. Current theory suggests that a metabolite of ticlopidine is the active agent rather than the drug itself (61). Ticlopidine inhibits ADP-stimulated platelet aggregation and prolongs the bleeding time in a dose-dependent fashion. Since return of platelet function takes several days, ticlopidine's effect on platelets may be permanent, and return of platelet function may occur via production of new, nonticlopidine-exposed platelets.

Gastrointestinal side effects are common with ticlopidine. Diarrhea is a frequent complaint, but the most severe side effects are hematologic. These include agranulocytosis, leukopenia, and pancytopenia secondary to marrow aplasia. The agranulocytosis usually occurs during the first 3 months of treatment and is reversible when the drug is discontinued. Blood counts are recommended at 2-week intervals for the first 3 months of therapy (61).

Pharmacokinetically, ticlopidine has a bioavailability of about 80%, more if drug is given with meals, and has 98% binding to plasma proteins. Maximum concentration after oral administration occurs approximately 2 hours after the first dose, but half-life is 20–50 hours, with steady-state concentrations taking 5–10 days to develop. The drug is mainly metabolized by the liver. Dose is 250 mg twice a day.

Currently ticlopidine is useful as a backup medication in patients with transient ischemic attacks, strokes, or preinfarction angina who, because of allergies or gastric irritation, cannot take aspirin. It is used as primary therapy, however, along with aspirin, in patients with coronary artery stents.

## Thrombin Inhibitors

Over the past several years, there has been interest in a new class of agents called thrombin inhibitors (62). These agents bind with and block thrombin and therefore have many potenial uses, as for example, adjunctive therapy after coronary angioplasty and in acute coronary syndromes. Thrombin inhibitors neutralize both clot-bound and free thrombin. Their development has also been fostered by the concept that they may theoretically block some of the prothrombotic effects of the thrombolytics (i.e., the latter enhance exposure of fibrin-bound thrombin, thus increasing free thrombin). They do not, however, suppress thrombin generation, which is a potential drawback.

The most studied thrombin inhibitor is hirudin, derived from leech saliva. A number of synthetic thrombin inhibitors also exist, including hirugen, hirulog, PPACK (D-phenylalanyl-L-prolyl-L-arginyl chloromethylketone), argatroban, and thrombin aptamers (62). Hirudin inhibits thrombin formation; prevents activation of factors V, VIII, and XIII; and prevents thrombin-mediated platelet activation in vitro (63, 64). It may have more effect on thrombi composed mainly of platelets than on those composed mainly of fibrin (65). In animal studies, hirudin and hirulog have been found to accelerate thrombolysis and prevent reocclusion after coronary angioplasty (66–70), with a beneficial effect when angioplasty using other balloons and stents is performed.

Although there has been enthusiasm about the theoretical advantages and basic experimental results with hirudin, clinical trials of hirudin have thus far been variable and several more are underway. At present, no thrombin inhibitor has US Food and Drug Administration approval. Lack of suppression of thrombin generation, lack of a clear dose-response curve, lack of a reliable specific laboratory test for antithrombin behavior, potentially severe bleeding, and possible rebound after withdrawal (which has not, however, been proved) are important limitations (62). Investigative effort in this general area is underway, however, and molecular refinements as well as other advances may bring these or similar agents into medical practice.

## HUMORAL ANTICOAGULANTS

Humoral anticoagulants are shown in Figure 9.3.

### Heparin

Heparin anticoagulation prevents the formation of fibrin from fibrinogen by combining with and activating antithrombin III (AT-III). The combination of heparin and AT-III inhibits the activated serine proteases in the coagulation cascade. The two most important of these are thrombin (factor IIa) and factor Xa. After binding to AT-III, heparin accelerates the inhibitory activity of AT-III 100 to 1000 fold (71–73).

Heparin is prepared from either bovine lung or porcine intestine and is composed of complex, highly sulfated, linear polysaccharides of variable molecular weights. The molecular weights of unfractionated heparin (UFH)

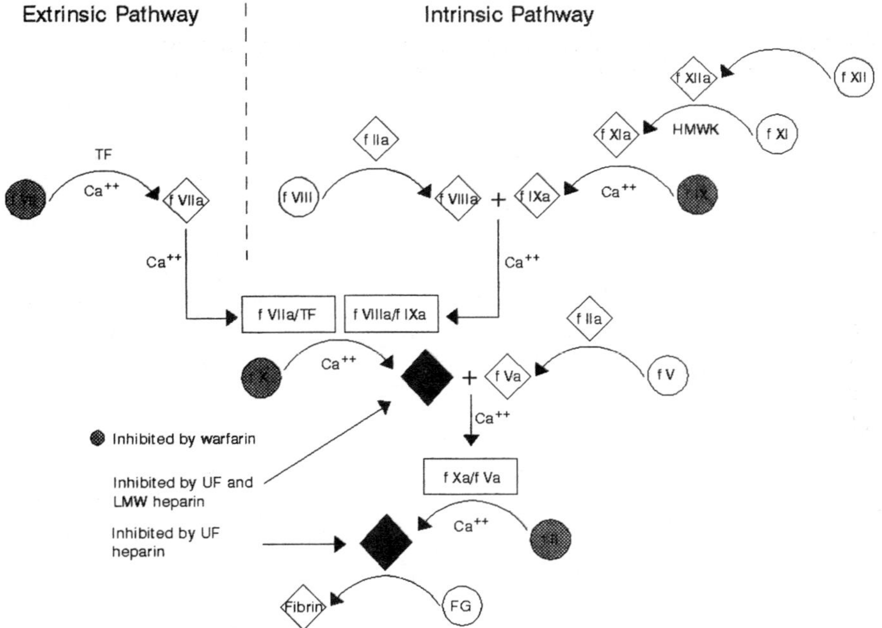


**Figure 9.3** Intrinsic and extrinsic components of the coagulation cascade. Roman numerals denote coagulation factors. Vitamin K dependent proteins (factors II, VII, IX, and X) with decreased activity following warfarin administration are indicated by *shaded diamonds.* Unfractionated (UF) heparin when combined with antithrombin III inhibits both factor IIa (thrombin) and factor Xa. After binding to antithrombin III, low molecular weight (LMW) heparin inhibits predominantly factor Xa. Suffix a = active forms of coagulation zymogens; HMWK = high molecular weight kininogen; TF = tissue factor.

range from 3000–30,000 daltons with an average of 15,000. By comparison, the molecular weights of the polysaccharides in low–molecular weight heparin (LMWH) are smaller, ranging from 1000–10,000 with an average of 4000 to 5000. A specific pentasaccharide sequence of heparin binds to AT-III, and the combination of AT-III and the pentasaccharide sequence is sufficient to inhibit factor Xa. Inhibition of thrombin, however, requires a longer minimum chain length of 18 saccharide units that include the specific pentasaccharide sequence. Because of the requirement for the 18-chain polysaccharide to inhibit thrombin, the smaller LMWHs predominately inhibit activated factor Xa (71, 74) (Table 9.3), whereas the ratio of inhibition of thrombin to factor Xa with the larger UFH is approximately 1 (Fig. 9.3).

UFH also produces significant decreases in platelet counts in a third of normal volunteers (75). Frank thrombocytopenia with UFH is observed in 1–5% of recipients, with a smaller percentage of patients progressing to the life-threatening complication of thrombocytopenia and occlusive thrombi. The thrombi may be located in either arteries or veins and are associated

**Table 9.3**
**Pharmacokinetic Parameters of Low-Molecular Weight Heparins**

| Agent | AFXa:AFIIa | Bioavailability after s.c. (%) | $V_d$ (L) | $\beta t_{1/2}$ after i.v. (h) | $\beta t_{1/2}$ after SC (h) |
|---|---|---|---|---|---|
| Enoxaparin sodium | 2.7 : 1 | 91 | 5.24–9.3 | 4.48–4.58 | 3.46–5.9 |
| Tinzaparin sodium | 1.9 : 1 | 90 | 3.9 | 1.4 | |
| Dalteparin sodium (tedelpurin) | 2.0 : 1 | 87 | 7.74 | 2.0 | 2.81–4.0 |
| Nadroparin calcium | 3.2 : 1 | 98 | 6.77 | 2.16–3.55 | 2.30–5.55 |
| Danaparoid sodium | 20.0 : 1 | 89–101 | 9.1 | 24.5 | |

AFXa = anti-factor Xa activity; AFIIa = anti-factor IIa activity; h = hours; i.v. = intravenous administration; s.c. = subcutaneous administration; $\beta t_{1/2}$ = beta half-life; $V_d$ = volume of distribution
Adapted with permission from Lutomski DM, Bottorff M, Sangha K. Pharmacokinetic optimisation of the treatment of embolic disorders. Clin Pharmacokinet 1995;28:67–92.

with preexisting cardiovascular disease or cardiovascular surgery, or both (76). Major risk factors for bleeding with heparin therapy (both UFH and LMWH) include a poor performance status as measured using the World Health Organization performance score, a total body surface area of less than 2 $M^2$, a history of a bleeding tendency, and recent trauma or surgery (77). Long-term heparin treatment such as that given to prevent thrombi in pregnancy is associated with osteopenia (78).

Heparins are poorly absorbed orally and are given intravenously or subcutaneously (the latter at times for a prolonged period). Since UFH binds in a saturable manner to plasma proteins as well as to the surface of endothelial cells, the bioavailability is limited to approximately 20%. UFH has a volume of distribution of 70–80 mL/kg (approximating whole blood), and after subcutaneous administration a peak plasma concentration of 2–3 hours (both time to peak is shorter and peak concentration is higher with the sodium rather than the calcium salt) (34, 79). After administration of UHF, there is a rapid decline in blood level because of distribution followed by saturable elimination via binding by endothelial cells and macrophages. This is in turn followed by nonsaturable elimination, which is at least partly renal (80). Because of the saturable phase of elimination, half-life can vary from approximately one-half hour at 25 units/kg to 2½ hours at 400 units/kg. At the usual clinical doses, however, half-life is about 1.0–1½ hours (80, 81). Obese individuals have a higher peak concentration and, because of concentration dependence, a longer half-life (82). In smokers, half-life is shorter (34).

Various dosing regimens of UHF have been suggested, e.g., for intravenous administration 5000–10,000 units of UHF loading dose with 1000–2000 units/hour depending upon body weight to keep partial thromboplastin time at about 1.5–2.5 control (or heparin levels of 0.2–0.4 U/mL by protamine titration). For subcutaneous UFH, the initial dose should be about 2000–4000 U higher and steady-state the same (34). Dose should be decreased by about 20% in renal failure (34) and will, of course, depend somewhat on the disease state under treatment.

Kinetics of LMVH, which unlike those for UFH are not dose dependent (83), are given in Table 9.3 for the various preparations. Note that half-life is generally longer than that of UFH, up to 4–6 hours. LMWH does not bind to plasma proteins and intraveneously has a measured bioavailability of more than 90% (84).

Although LMWH may be simpler to administer and may have a lower incidence of associated thrombocytopenia, it is much more expensive than UFH. Current studies continue to support the use of conventional UFH in patients with cardiovascular indications for heparinization. Studies using LMWH in patients with deep venous thrombosis or for prophylaxis after orthopedic surgery, however, suggest that future studies may demonstrate the efficacy of LMWH in patients with occlusive cardiovascular diseases (85–89).

## Warfarin

Warfarin, a widely used anticoagulant, inhibits production of activated vitamin K through partial blockade of vitamin K epoxide reductase. Dicumarol (bishydroxycoumarin), another drug in the category, is far less commonly used. Activation of the vitamin K–dependent proteins (prothrombin, factors VII, IX, and X) occurs in the liver via the posttranslational carboxylation of the gamma chain of the n-terminal glutamines (90). The des-carboxylated coagulation proteins are present in blood as dysfunctional proteins (90). Since production of proteins C and S (thrombin-activated anticoagulant and fibrinolytic cofactors; see Figure 8.1, Chapter 8) are also dependent on vitamin K, a warfarin-induced decrease in the activity of these proteins that serve to inhibit coagulation has the potential for creating a hypercoagulable state.

Warfarin is rapidly absorbed from the gastrointestinal tract into the blood where 99% is bound to albumin. Volume of distribution is close to the size of the albuminic space and thus small. Peak concentration is at approximately 2 hours and the measured half-life is 36–42 hours.

Warfarin is composed of approximately equal amounts of a racemic mixture of two optically active isomers, R and S. Since these isomers have both different metabolic pathways and different anticoagulant potency, interaction with concomitantly administered drugs may selectively affect the metabolism of a specific isomer (91). Both are eliminated by the liver, but R-warfarin undergoes mainly keto reduction and S-warfarin, hydroxylation.

Sulfinpyrazone, phenylbutazone, trimethoprim-sulfamethoxazole, and metronidazole selectively prolong the half-life of the S isomer (92–95). Compared to the R isomer, the S isomer is five times more potent as an anticoagulant (96) and is on the shorter end of the half-life range. Hence, medications that selectively prolong the half-live of the S isomer may greatly potentiate the anticoagulation effect of warfarin.

Bleeding is the main complication of warfarin therapy, especially in the gastrointestinal and urinary tracts. Bleeding may point to lesions at these sites, especially when anticoagulant tests are not above target ranges. Bleeding risk is greatest in the first 3 months of warfarin usage and is treated with vitamin K. Patchy skin necrosis due to thrombi is a rare complication seen especially after large loading doses and probably associated with depletion of protein C. Liver toxicity has also occurred and the drug is also teratogenic. Because of this last property, the common anticoagulant regimen in pregnancy is administration of subcutaneous heparin. Coumadin is usually started again at 3–6 days post partum (97).

Warfarin's anticoagulation can be potentiated or inhibited by a variety of medications (Table 9.4) interacting through multiple mechanisms (96). Cholestyramine decreases the anticoagulant effect of warfarin by decreasing absorption through the gastrointestinal tract. Vitamin K–dependent decarboxylases are inhibited by third generation cephalosporins potentiating warfarin anticoagulation. Amiodarone increases the survival of both the S and R warfarin isomers, increasing anticoagulation. Although aspirin increases the amount of free, nonalbumin bound warfarin, the free warfarin is metabolized more rapidly. The net effect is that aspirin does not directly affect warfarin anticoagulation. Aspirin does, however, inhibit platelet function so that gobal anticoagulation with concomitant administration of both aspirin and warfarin is greater than that with just coumarin alone. Before beginning warfarin anticoagulation, cardiovascular patients should have their current medications checked for possible warfarin interactions.

Warfarin therapy is monitored using the prothrombin time, which is sensative to three of the four coagulant proteins (prothrombin, factors VII and X) that are dependent on vitamin K–induced carboxylation for activation. Since very high doses of heparin are required to influence prothrombin time, this test can be used to evaluate coumadin anticoagulation while the patient is still on heparin. Reagents used to activate coagulation in determinations of the prothrombin time vary with respect to their strength of coagulation stimulation depending on their tissue of origin and method of preparation. The international normalized ratio (INR) is used to standardize the results of the prothrombin time obtained with different reagents used in different institutions (98). Use of the INR allows clinicians to compare strength of anticoagulation using prothrombin times obtained in different laboratories.

**Table 9.4**
**Drug and Food Interactions with Warfarin by Level of Supporting Evidence and Type of Interaction**

| Level of Evidence[a] | Potentiation | Inhibition | No Effect |
|---|---|---|---|
| 1 | Alcohol (if concomitant liver disease), amiodarone, cimetidine[b], clofibrate, cotrimoxazole, erythromycin, fluconazole, isoniazid (600 mg daily), metronidazole, miconazole, omeprazole, phenylbutazone[c], piroxicam, propafenone, propranolol, sulfinpyrazone[c] | Barbiturates, carbamazepine, chlordiazepoxide, cholestyramine, griseofulvin[c], nafcillin, rifampin, sucralfate, high vitamin K–content foods and enteral feeds, large amounts of avocado | Alcohol, antacids, atenolol, bumetanide, diflunisal, enoxacin, famotidine, felodipine, fluoxetine, ketorolac, metoprolol, moricizine, naproxen, nitrazepam, nizatidine, psyllium, ranitidine[d] |
| 2 | Acetaminophen, anabolic steroids, aspirin, chloral hydrate, ciprofloxacin, dextropropoxyphene, disulfiram, itraconazole, quinidine, phenytoin, simvastatin, tamoxifen, tetracycline, influenza vaccine | Dicloxacillin | Ibuprofen, ketoconazole, ketoprofen |
| 3 | Disopyramide, 5-fluorouracil, ifosfamide, lovastatin, metolazone, nalidixic acid, norfloxacin, ofloxacin, topical salicylates, sulindac, tolmetin | Azathioprine, cyclosporine, etretinate, trazodone | |
| 4 | Cefamandole, cefazolin, gemfibrozil, heparin, indomethacin, sulfisoxazole | | Diltiazem, tobacco, vancomycin |

[a] 1, highly probable; 2, probable; 3, possible; 4, doubtful. Further details in original paper.
[b] In a small number of volunteers, an inhibitory drug interaction occurred.
[c] Supporting level 1 evidence from patients and volunteers.
[d] Level 2 evidence of potentiation in patients also exists.
Reprinted by permission of the American College of Physicians from Wells PS, Holbrook AM, Crowther NR, et al. Interactions of warfarin with drugs and food. Ann Intern Med 1994;121:676–683.

Initiation of anticoagulation with warfarin at high doses, 20–40 mg/day, will accelerate prolongation of the prothombin time (99). Because factor VII has a shorter half-life (5 hours) than prothombin or factor X, initial prolongation of the prothrombin time with high doses of warfarin will reflect decreased factor VII activity and not represent optimal anticoagulation produced by comparable decreases in activities of all the vitamin K–dependent coagulation proteins (100). Patients should be started on low doses of warfarin, 5–10 mg/day, with full anticoagulation anticipated after several days of therapy. Since the anticoagulant effect of warfarin can be affected by concomitant administration of many different medications, it is important to monitor patients carefully with serial prothrombin times (INRs). The target INR level of course depends on condition treated (see Chapter 10).

## Nitroglycerine and Calcium Channel Blockers

Patients with cardiovascular diseases are commonly treated with nitroglycerine or calcium channel blockers, or both. Both of these medications inhibit platelet function. Clinically achievable concentrations of nitroglycerine inhibit ADP-stimulated platelet aggregation and induce platelet disaggregation (101). At therapeutic concentrations, the calcium channel blocker diltiazem inhibits platelet aggregation mediated by calcium fluxes and also stimulates endothelial cell prostacylin synthesis (102). Unless investigative study groups are balanced with respect to these additional platelet inhibitory medications, comparative studies on the effects of specific platelet inhibitory drugs in cardiovascular diseases could be biased.

## CONCLUSIONS

As can be seen, physicians have potent anticlotting methods at their disposal. Future therapeutic strategies will be aimed at changing the dose or combinations of currently available medications, or developing new therapeutics capable of inhibiting platelet function and providing even greater protection from vascular occlusion without increasing the risk of bleeding or other side effects.

Chapter 10 reviews the widespread clinical uses and studies on anticlotting agents to date.

*Acknowledgements*

I wish to thank Michael Scott, DVM, for his expert reading and editorial suggestions and Ms. Deborah Howe for help in preparing the manuscript.

---

REFERENCES

1. Buja LM, Willerson JT. Clinicopathologic correlates of acute ischemic heart disease syndromes. Am J Cardiol 1981;47:343–356.
2. Sherman CT, Litvack F, Grundfest W, et al. Coronary angioscopy in patients with unstable angina pectoris. N Engl J Med 1986;315:913–919.

3. Falk E. Unstable angina with fatal outcome: dynamic coronary thrombosis leading to infarction and/or sudden death. Autopsy evidence of recurrent mural thrombosis with peripheral embolization culminating in total vascular occlusion. Circulation 1985;71:699–708.
4. Hellstrom HR. Evidence in favor of the vasospastic cause of coronary artery thrombosis. Am Heart J 1979;97:449–452.
5. Ridolfi RL, Hutchins GM. The relationship between coronary artery lesions and myocardial infarcts: ulceration of atherosclerotic plaques precipitating coronary thrombsosis. Am Heart J 1977;93:468–486.
6. Horie T, Sekiguchi M, Hirosawa K. Coronary thrombosis in pathogenesis of acute myocardial infarction. Br Heart J 1978;40:153–161.
7. Bennett JS, Shattil SJ. Platelet function. In: Williams J, Beutler E, Erslev AJ, et al., eds. Hematology. 4th ed. New York: McGraw-Hill, 1990:1233–1250.
8. McCarroll DR, Levin EG, Montgomery RR. Endothelial cell synthesis of von Willebrand antigen II, von Willebrand factor and von Willebrand factor/von Willebrand antigen II complex. J Clin Invest 1985;75:1089–1095.
9. Wagner DD, Marder VJ. Biosynthesis of von Willebrand protein by human endothelial cells: processing steps and their intracellular localization. J Cell Biol 1984; 99:2123–2130.
10. Ruggeri ZM, Zimmerman TS. von Willebrand Factor and von Willebrand Disease. Blood 1987;70:895–904.
11. Roth GJ, Calverley DC. Aspirin, platelets, and thrombosis: theory and practice. Blood 1994;83:885–898.
12. Miller KP, Frishman WH. Platelets and antiplatelet therapy in ischemic heart disease. Med Clin North Am 1988;72:117–184.
13. Salzman EW. Cyclic AMP and platelet function. N Engl J Med 1972;286:358–363.
14. Holmsen H. Platelet secretion and energy metabolism. In: Colman RW, Hirsh J, Marder VJ, et al., eds. Hemostasis and thrombosis. 3rd ed. Philadelphia: Lippincott-Raven, 1994:524–541.
15. Zucker-Franklin D. Platelet morphology and function. In: Williams WJ, Beutler E, Erslev AJ, et al., eds. Hematology. 4th ed. New York: McGraw-Hill, 1990: 1172–1181.
16. Isenberg WM, McEver PR, Shuman MA, et al. Topographic distribution of a granule membrane protein (GMP-140) that is expressed on the platelet surface after activation: an immunogold-surface replica study. Blood Cells 1986;12:191–204.
17. Berman CL, Yeo EL, Wencel-Drake JD, et al. A platelet alpha granule membrane protein that is associated with the plasma membrane after activation. J Clin Invest 1986;78:130–137.
18. Stenberg PE, McEver RP, Shuman MA, et al. A platelet alpha-granule membrane protein (GMP-140) is expressed on the plasma membrane after activation. J Cell Biol 1985;101:880–886.
19. Hultin MB. Role of human factor VIII and factor X activation. J Clin Invest 1982; 69:950–958.
20. Tracy PB, Mann KG. A model for assembly of coagulation factor complexes on cell surfaces: prothrombin activation on platelets. In: Phillips DR, Shuman MA, eds. Biochemistry of platelets. Orlando, FL: Academic Press, 1986:296–318.
21. Walsh PN, Griffin JH. Contributions of human platelets to the proteolytic activation of blood coagulation factors XII and XI. Blood 1981;57:106–118.
22. Funk CD, Funk LB, Kennedy ME, et al. Human platelet/erythroleukemia cell prostaglandin G/H synthase: cDNA cloning, expression and gene chromosomal assignment. FASEB J 1991;5:2304–2313.
23. Preston FE, Whipps S, Jackson CA, et al. Inhibition of prostacyclin and platelet thromboxane A2 after low-dose aspirin. N Engl J Med 1981;304:76–79.
24. Jaffe EA, Weksler BB. Recovery of endothelial cell prostacyclin production after inhibition by low doses of aspirin. J Clin Invest 1979;63:532–535.
25. Kyrle PA, Eichler HG, Jager U, Lechner K. Inhibition of prostacyclin and thromboxane A2 generation by low-dose aspirin at the site of plug formation in man in vivo. Circulation 1987;75:1025–1029.
26. Weksler BB, Tack-Goldman K, Subramanian VA, Gay WA. Cumulative inhibitory

effect of low-dose aspirin on vascular prostacyclin and platelet thromboxane production in patients with atherosclerosis. Circulation 1985;71:332–340.
27. Pedersen AK, FitzGerald GA. Dose-related kinetics of aspirin: Presystemic acetylation of platelet cyclooxygenase. N Engl J Med 1984;311:1206–1211.
28. Clarke RJ, Mayo G, Price P, FitzGerald GA. Suppression of thromboxane A2 but not of systemic prostacyclin by controlled-release aspirin. N Engl J Med 1991;325: 1137–1141.
29. Jakubowski JA, Stampfer MJ, Vaillancourt DF, et al. Low-dose enteric-coated aspirin: a practical approach to continuous-release low-dose aspirin and presystemic acetylation of human platelet cyclooxygenase. J Lab Clin Med 1986;108:616–621.
30. McCall NT, Tofler GH, Schafer AI, et al. The effect of enteric-coated aspirin on the morning increase in platelet activity. Am Heart J 1991;121:1382–1388.
31. Stampfer MJ, Jakubowski JA, Deykin D, et al. Effect of alternate-day regular and enteric-coated aspirin on platelet aggregation, bleeding time, and thromboxane A2 levels in bleeding-time blood. Am J Med 1986;81:400–404.
32. Zucker ML, Trowbridge C, Woodroof J, et al. Low vs high-dose aspirin: effects on platelet function in hyperlipoproteinemic and normal subjects. Arch Intern Med 1986;146:921–925.
33. Keimowitz RM, Pulvermacher G, Mayo G, et al. Transdermal modification of platelet function: a dermal aspirin preparation selectively inhibits platelet cyclooxygenase and preserves prostacyclin biosynthesis. Circulation 1993;88:556–561.
34. Lutomski DM, Bottorff M, Sangha K. Pharmacokinetic optimisation of the treatment of embolic disorders. Clin Pharmacokinet1995;28:67–92.
35. Smith PK, Gleason HL, Stoll CG, et al. Studies on the pharmacology of salicylates. J Pharmacol Exp Ther 1946;87:237–255.
36. Lanas A, Sekar MC, Hirschowitz BI. Objective evidence of aspirin use in both ulcer and nonulcer upper and lower gastrointestinal bleeding. Gastroenterology 1992;103: 862–869.
37. Levy M. Aspirin use in patients with major upper gastrointestinal bleeding and peptic-ulcer disease. N Engl J Med 1974;290:1158–1162.
38. Zucker MB, Rothwell KG. Differential influences of salicylate compounds on platelet aggregation and serotonin release. Current Therapeutic Research 1978;23:194–199.
39. Oates JA, Wood AJJ, FitzGerald GA. Drug therapy: dipyridamole. N Engl J Med 1987;316:1247–1257.
40. Saniabadi AR, Tomiak RHH, Lowe GDO, et al. Dipyridamole inhibits red cell-induced platelet activation. Atherosclerosis 1989;76:146–154.
41. Soderback U, Sollevi A. Effect of dipyridamole-like compound (R-E 244) on aggregation and cyclic amp accumulation in human platelets. Thromb Res 1991;64:355–362.
42. Bult H, Fret HRL, Jordeans FH, Herman AG. Dipyridamole potentiates platelet inhibition by nitric oxide. Thrombosis and Haemostasis 1991;66:343–349.
43. Bjornsson TD, Mahony C. Clinical pharmacokinetics of dipyridamole. Thromb Res 1983;Suppl.4:93–104.
44. Mahony C, Wolfram KM, Cocchetto DM, et al. Dipyridamole kinetics. Clin Pharmacol Ther 1982;31:330–338.
45. Lehmann CR, Locke K, Shaffer PJ. Persantine bioavailability problems [letter]. Clin Pharm 1984;3:14–15.
46. Jakubowski JA, Adler B, Thompson CB, et al. Influence of platelet volume on the ability of prostacyclin to inhibit platelet aggregation and the release reaction. J Lab Clin Med 1985;105:271–276.
47. Addonizio VP, Fisher CA, Jenkin BK, et al. Iloprost (ZK36374), a stable analogue of prostacyclin, preserves platelets during simulated extracorporeal circulation. J Thorac Cardiovasc Surg 1985;89:926–933.
48. Malpass TW, Amory DW, Harker LA, et al. The effect of prostacyclin infusion on platelet hemostatic function in patients undergoing cardiopulmonary bypass. J Thorac Cardiovasc Surg 1984;87:550–555.
49. Bates ER, McGillem MJ, Mickelson JK, et al. A monoclonal antibody against the platelet glycoprotein IIb/IIIa receptor complex prevents platelet aggregation and thrombosis in a canine model of coronary angioplasty. Circulation 1991;84:2463–2469.

50. Yasuda T, Gold HK, Fallon JT, et al. Monoclonal antibody against the platelet glycoprotein (GP) IIb/IIIa receptor prevents coronary artery reocclusion after reperfusion with recombinant tissue-type plasminogen activator in dogs. J Clin Invest 1988; 81:1284–1291.
51. Hanson SR, Pareti FI, Ruggeri ZM, et al. Effects of monoclonal antibodies against the platelet glycoprotein IIb/IIIa complex on thrombosis and hemostasis in the baboon. J Clin Invest 1988;81:149–158.
52. Sheppeck RA, Bentz M, Dickson C, et al. Examination of the roles of glycoprotein Ib and glycoprotein IIb/IIIa in platelet deposition on an artificial surface using clinical antiplatelet agents and monoclonal antibody blockade. Blood 1991;78:673–680.
53. Coller BS, Folts JD, Scudder LE, et al. Antithrombotic effect of a monoclonal antibody to the platelet glycoprotein IIb/IIIa receptors in an experimental animal model. Blood 1986;68:783–786.
54. Escudero C, Alvarez L, deHaro J, et al. Prevention of arterial thrombosis by a monoclonal antibody against the 100 to 109 amino acid sequence stretch of the beta-subunit of the human platelet fibrinogen receptor: A comparative study with low dose aspirin. J Am Coll Cardiol 1994;23:483–486.
55. Coller BS, Scudder LE, Berger HJ, et al. Inhibition of human platelet function in vivo with a monoclonal antibody: with observations on the newly dead as experimental subjects. Ann Intern Med 1988:635–638.
56. Coller BS, Scudder LE, Beer J, et al. Monoclonal antibodies to platelet glycoprotein IIb/IIIa as antithrombotic agents. Ann NY Acad Sci 1991;614:193–213.
57. Huang TF, Sheu JR, Teng CM. A potent antiplatelet peptide, triflavin, from Trimeresurus Flavoviridis snake venom. Biochem J 1991;277:351–357.
58. Sheu JR, Huang TF. Ex-vivo and in-vivo antithrombotic effect of triflavin, an RGD-containing peptide. J Pharm Pharmacol 1994;46:58–62.
59. Mousa SA, Bozarth JM, Forsythe MS, et al. Antiplatelet and antithrombotic efficacy of DMP 728, a novel platelet GPIIb/IIIa receptor antagonist. Circulation 1994;89: 3–12.
60. Carteaux JP, Roux S, Kuhn H, et al. Ro 44-9883, a new nonpeptide glycoprotein IIb/IIIa antagonist, prevents platelet loss during experimental cardiopulmonary bypass. J Thorac Cardiovasc Surg 1992;106:834–841.
61. Desager JP. Clinical pharmacokinetics of ticlopidine. Clin Pharmacokinet 1994; 26:347–355.
62. Lefkovits J, Topol EJ. Direct thrombin inhibitors in cardiovascular medicine. Circulation 1994;90:1522–1536.
63. Courtney M, Loison G, Lemoine Y, et al. Production and evaluation of recombinant hirudin. Semin Thromb Hemost 1989;15:269–282.
64. Fenton JW, Villanueva GB, Ofosu FA, et al. Thrombin inhibition by hirudin: how hirudin inhibits thrombin. Haemostasis 1991;21(suppl):27–31.
65. Heras M, Chesebro JH, Webster MWI, Mruk JJ, et al. Hirudin, heparin and placebo during deep arterial injury in the pig: the in vivo role of thrombin in platelet-mediated thrombosis. Circulation 1990;82:1476–1484.
66. Mruk JS, Chesbro KJ, Webster MWI, et al. Hirudin markedly enhances thrombolysis with rt-PA. Circulation 1990;82(Suppl III):III-135. (Abstract).
67. Klement P, Hirsh J, Maraganore J, et al. Effects of heparin and hirulog on t-PA induced thrombolysis in a rat model. Thromb Haemost 1992;68:64–68.
68. Buchwald AB, Sandrock D, Unterberg C, et al. Platelet and fibrin deposition on coronary stents in minipigs: effect of hirudin versus heparin. J Am Coll Cardiol 1993;21:249–254.
69. Stringer KA, Lindenfeld J. Hirudins: antithrombin anticoagulants. Ann Pharmacother 1992;26:1535–1540.
70. Fox I, Dawson A, Loynds P, et al. Anticoagulant activity of hirulog, a direct thrombin inhibitor, in humans. Thromb Haemost 1993;69:157–163.
71. Weitz J. New anticoagulant strategies, current status and future potential. Drugs 1994;48:485–497.
72. Pineo GF, Hull RD. Classical anticoagulant therapy for venous thromboembolism. Progress Cardiovasc Dis 1994;37:59–70.

73. Kondo NI, Maddi R, Ewenstein BM, et al. Anticoagulation and hemostasis in cardiac surgical patients. J Card Surg 1994;9:443–461.
74. Messmore HL, Wehrmacher WH. Therapeutic use of low molecular weight heparins. Semin Thromb Hemost 1993;19:97–100.
75. Schwartz KA, Royer G, Kaufman DB, et al. Complications of heparin administration in normal individuals. Am J Hematol 1985;19:355–363.
76. Boshkov LK, Warkentin TE, Hayward CPM, et al. Heparin-induced thrombocytopenia and thrombosis: clinical and laboratory studies. Br J Haematol 1993;84: 322–328.
77. Nieuwenhuis HK, Albada J, Banga JD, et al. Identification of risk factors for bleeding during treatment of acute venous thromboembolism with heparin or low molecular weight heparin. Blood 1991;78:2337–2343.
78. Dahlman T, Lindvall N, Hellgren M. Osteopenia in pregnancy during long-term heparin treatment: a radiological study post partum. Br J Obstet Gynaecol 1990;97: 221–228.
79. Low J, Biggs JC. Comparative plasma heparin levels after subcutaneous sodium and calcium heparin. Thromb Haemost 1978;40:397–406.
80. Kandrotas RJ. Heparin pharmacokinetics and pharmacodynamics. Clin Pharmacokinet 1992;22(5):359–374.
81. Talstad I. Heparin therapy adjusted for body weight. Am J Clin Pathol 1985;83: 378–381.
82. Beermann B, Lahnborg G. Pharmacokinetics of heparin in healthy and obese subjects and in combination with dihydroergotamine. Thromb Haemost 1981;45: 24–26.
83. Fejgin MO, Lourwood DL. Low molecular weight heparins and their use in obstetrics and gynecology. Obstet Gynecol Surv 1994;49:424–431.
84. Wolf H. Low-molecular-weight heparin. Med Clin North Am 1994;78:733–743.
85. Hull RD, Pineo GF. Low molecular weight heparin treatment of venous thromboembolism. Prog Cardiovasc Dis 1994;37:71–78.
86. Nurmohamed MT, Rosendaal FT, Buller HR, et al. Low-molecular-weight heparin versus standard heparin in general and orthopaedic surgery: a meta-analysis. Lancet 1992;340:152–156.
87. Hull RD, Raskob GE, Pineo GF, et al. Subcutaneous low-molecular-weight heparin compared with continuous intravenous heparin in the treatment of proximal-vein thrombosis. N Engl J Med 1992;326:975–982.
88. Turpie AGG, Gent M, Cote R, et al. A low-molecular-weight heparinoid compared with unfractionated heparin in the prevention of deep vein thrombosis in patients with acute ischemic stroke. Ann Intern Med 1992;117:353–357.
89. Turpie AGG, Levine MN, Hirsh J, et al. A randomized controlled trial of a low-molecular-weight heparin (enoxaparin) to prevent deep-vein thrombosis in patients undergoing elective hip surgery. N Engl J Med 1986;315:925–929.
90. Suttie JW. Vitamin K antagonist. In: Colman RW, Whirsh J, Marder VJ, et al., eds. Hemostasis and thrombosis: basic principles and clinical practice. 3rd ed. Philadelphia: Lippincott-Raven, 1994:1562–1566.
91. Breckenridge A, Orme M, Wesseling H, et al. Pharmacokinetics and pharmacodynamics of the enantiomers of warfarin in man. Clin Pharmacol Ther 1973;15:424–430.
92. O'Reilly RA. Stereoselective interaction of trimethoprism-sulfamethoxazole with the separated enantiomorphs of racemic warfarin in man. N Engl J Med 1980;302: 33–35.
93. Lewis RJ, Trager WF, Chan KK, et al. Warfarin. Stereochemical aspects of its metabolism and the interaction with phenylbutazone. J Clin Invest 1974;53:1607–1617.
94. Toon S, Low LK, Gibaldi M, et al. The warfarin-sulfinpyrazone interaction: stereochemical considerations. Clin Pharmacol Ther 1986;39:15–24.
95. O'Reilly RA. The stereoselective interaction of warfarin and metronidazole in man. N Engl J Med 1976;295:354–357.
96. Wells PS, Holbrook AM, Crowther NR, et al. Interactions of warfarin with drugs and food. Ann Intern Med 1994;121:676–683.
97. Greaves M. Anticoagulants in pregnancy. Pharmacol Ther 1993;59:311–327.

98. Hirsh J, Poller L. The international normalized ratio. Arch Intern Med 1994;154: 282–288.
99. Breckenridge A. Oral anticoagulant drugs: pharmacokinetic aspects. Semin Hematol 1978;15:19–26.
100. Hellemans J, Vorlat M, Verstraete M. Survival time of prothrombin and factors VII, IX and X after completely synthesis blocking doses of coumarin derivatives. Br J Haematol 1963;9:506–512.
101. Chirkov YY, Naujalis JI, Sage E, et al. Antiplatelet effects of nitroglycerin in healthy subjects and patients with stable angina pectoris. J Cardiovasc Pharmacol 1993;21:384–389.
102. Mehta J, Mehta P, Ostrowski N. Calcium blocker diltiazem inhibits platelet activation and stimulates vascular prostacyclin synthesis. Am J Med Sci 1986;291: 20–24.

CHAPTER 10

# Management of Cardiac Disorders with Antithrombotic Agents

Jonathan L. Halperin, MD

Thrombosis in the circulatory system has been recognized since the early part of this century as the principal mechanism responsible for cardiovascular morbidity and mortality, and antithrombotic drugs have found an expanding role for both disease prevention and treatment. The vast literature is riddled with controversy, however, leading to confusion among clinicians confronted with decisions regarding patient management. Although consensus is reached from time to time regarding specific therapeutic approaches (1), sound integration of emerging information requires a conceptual framework based upon pathogenetic mechanisms and an understanding of the relative risks of morbid clinical events. In this chapter management of cardiac disorders with antithrombotic drugs is reviewed (characteristics and mechanisms of action of these drugs are discussed in Chapter 9). The review combines a perspective on pathogenesis with stratification of thromboembolic risk in an attempt to provide a rational approach to the clinical application of antithrombotic therapy in patients with cardiovascular disease. Although limited to cardiac syndromes, the same principles apply to peripheral circulatory and cerebrovascular diseases.

## PATHOGENESIS OF THROMBOSIS AND EMBOLISM

### Coronary Arteries

The entire intimal surface of the cardiovascular system is lined with endothelial cells highly resistant to thrombus formation. This property is lost with even superficial vascular injury, as demonstrated in hyperlipidemic animal experiments, resulting in adhesion of a platelet monolayer to the damaged endothelium or exposed subendothelium. When more severe arterial wall injury occurs, as in the case of atherosclerotic plaque rupture, components of the medial layer—particularly type I collagen—become exposed to the circulating blood. Marked platelet activation typically occurs, with release of adenosine diphosphate, thromboxane $A_2$, serotonin, and other substances from intracytoplasmic granules, potentiating platelet aggregation and thrombus formation. Vascular damage of this magnitude also stimulates thrombin synthesis through both the intrinsic (surface-activated) and extrinsic (tissue factor-dependent) coagulation pathways, in which the platelet membrane interacts with clotting factors. Thrombin promotes the polymerization of fibrin, which is responsible for stabilizing the expanding thrombotic mass, resisting dislodgement by arterial blood flow (2, 3).

Similar to collagen, thrombin is a powerful activator of platelet aggregation, and the interactions of platelets and thrombin form the basis for emerging approaches to the management of thrombosis in a variety of cardiovascular disease states.

Delivery of platelets to the site of vascular injury and their local activation depend on the severity of vessel wall injury and on shear rate, a measure of the gradient in blood flow velocity between the center and the periphery of the vascular lumen (4). In areas of stenosis, high shear rate promotes contact between blood elements and the vessel wall (5), favoring platelet activation. The relationship between the severity of vascular injury and thrombus formation has been shown in perfusion chamber experiments in which different tissue substrates were exposed to blood at various shear rates (6). With superficial injury, platelet deposition and thrombus formation are transient; with deep injury, however, platelet deposition is more extensive, leading to thrombus fixation and vascular occlusion. Where shear rate is relatively high (e.g., in the region of a stenotic, irregularly shaped, or disrupted atherosclerotic plaque), thrombus composed predominantly of platelets and fibrin extends distally in the lumen; in regions where shear rate is low, the proportion of fibrin and erythrocytes in the thrombus is greater.

These concepts are important in the pathogenesis of acute coronary syndromes such as unstable angina pectoris, in which plaque disruption is associated with transient thrombotic vessel occlusion, and myocardial infarction, in which coronary occlusion is more persistent. After lysis of thrombus in patients with acute myocardial infarction, angiographic studies have demonstrated that the risk of subsequent reocclusion is related to residual stenosis, even in the presence of anticoagulation with heparin (7). Stenosis increases local shear rate, facilitating platelet deposition and activation, and is a powerful stimulus to platelet aggregation and fibrin formation. Residual thrombus after thrombolysis is an important component of the material narrowing the coronary lumen and is a highly thrombogenic substrate (8).

## Cardiac Chambers

Intracavitary mural thrombi often develop in patients with acute myocardial infarction, chronic left ventricular aneurysm, dilated cardiomyopathy, and atrial fibrillation (AF). The pathogenesis of thrombosis may follow the approach established more than a century ago by Rudolph Virchow, who defined a triad of precipitating factors: endothelial injury, a zone of circulatory stasis, and a hypercoagulable state (9). The clinical significance of these mural thrombi derives from their potential for systemic embolism and, hence, depends on dynamic forces of the circulation and other factors responsible for migration into the arterial tree.

### *Endocardial Injury*

In the first few days after acute myocardial infarction, leukocytic infiltration separates endothelial cells from their basal lamina (10). The resulting exposure of subendothelial tissue to intracavitary blood serves as the nidus for thrombus development. Specific endocardial abnormalities have been identified histologically in surgical and postmortem specimens from patients with left ventricular aneurysms (11) and at necropsy in patients with idiopathic dilated cardiomyopathy (12). Endocardial disruption by surgical sutures may contribute to the increased risk of thromboembolism in the first 3 months after prosthetic heart valve replacement.

### *Blood Stasis*

Both experimental (13) and clinical studies (14, 15) emphasize the importance of wall motion abnormalities in the development of left ventricular mural thrombi, and stasis of blood in akinetic or dyskinetic regions appears to be an essential factor. Similarly, stasis is important in the development of atrial thrombi (16) when effective mechanical atrial activity is impaired by atrial fibrillation (AF), chamber dilatation, mitral stenosis, or cardiac failure. Stasis is analogous to a condition of low shear rate, in which activation of the coagulation system, rather than platelets, leads to fibrin formation, thus constituting the predominant pathogenetic mechanism in the development of intracavitary thrombi.

### *Hypercoagulable State*

One study of patients with acute myocardial infarction found a significantly greater incidence of thromboembolism in cases of elevated serum fibrinogen (17), and recent reports cite similar changes in subsets of patients with AF (18), suggesting that there are hypercoagulable tendencies in these conditions. Although this limb of Virchow's triad is controversial, a systemic procoagulant tendency conceivably arises during the acute stage of myocardial infarction or in cases of AF associated with intraatrial stasis, predisposing the patient to thromboembolic events. Moreover, the surface of fresh thrombus is itself highly thrombogenic, producing a local if not a systemic hypercoagulable state (19).

### *Dynamic Circulatory Forces*

The problems of thromboembolism originating from the cardiac chambers prompt consideration of the balance between the effects of regional injury, stasis, and procoagulant factors, which favor thrombus formation, and dynamic forces of the circulation, which are responsible for the migration of thrombotic material into the systemic circulation. Although stasis favors thrombus formation within the cavity of a ventricular aneurysm, isolation from dynamic circulatory forces protects against embolic migration (20, 21). In diffusely dilated cardiomyopathy, however, mural thrombus is not isolated from the circulation, and the risk of embolism is greater. Thus, factors leading to thrombus formation are not the same as those that produce systemic embolism, and this paradox must not be neglected in the consideration of therapeutic options.

## Prosthetic Valves

### *Mechanical Prostheses*

Platelet deposition begins almost immediately once circulation is restored after implantation of a prosthetic cardiac valve, both on the prosthetic surface itself—particularly on the endocardium-suture-prosthesis interfaces—and on damaged perivalvular tissues (22). The exposed prosthetic surface area is the major factor leading to platelet deposition and to activation of factor XII, thus initiating the coagulation cascade (23). Flow stasis and abnormal hemodynamic characteristics of prosthetic devices promote fibrin generation and, to a lesser degree, platelet activation.

**Biologic Prostheses.** Bioprosthetic valves are considerably less thrombogenic than mechanical devices, at least before fibrocalcific degeneration occurs (24), mainly because of the natural properties of the material used in their construction and the characteristics of axial flow profile, leaflet pliability, and cyclic sinusoidal washout.

In contrast to arterial thrombosis, the pathogenesis of which involves damage to the vessel wall and exposure of a thrombogenic substrate leading to platelet activation and fibrin formation, intracavitary thrombosis develops mainly in situations of blood stasis, which favor activation of the coagulation system and generation of thrombin. Endocardial injury and the presence of a hypercoagulable stimulus may contribute to thrombus formation on the surfaces of the cardiac chambers. Mechanical prosthetic surfaces promote activation of the coagulation system in relation to localized areas of deranged flow, and platelet aggregation plays an additional role in thromboembolism associated with these devices. Biologic prostheses are significantly less thrombogenic than their mechanical counterparts, because of characteristics of materials used and flow dynamics when these valves function normally.

## RISK STRATIFICATION AND IMPLICATIONS FOR ANTITHROMBOTIC THERAPY

The various clinical heart disease syndromes may be classified according to absolute and relative risks of thromboembolic events. Three general risk categories will be considered in this chapter: the highest involving more than 6% per year, a medium risk range of 2–6% annually, and a low risk rate less of than 2% per year (Table 10.1) (25). Individuals without overt heart disease

**Table 10.1**
**Thromboembolism in Cardiac Disease Based on Pathogenesis and Risk**

| | Thromboembolic Risk | | |
|---|---|---|---|
| Pathogenesis | High (>6% per year) | Medium (2–6% per year) | Low (<2% per year) |
| Arterial system Platelets and fibrin | Unstable angina<br>Acute MI<br>After thrombolysis<br>PTCA early phase<br>SVBG early phase | Chronic stable angina<br>Chronic phase after MI<br>PTCA chronic phase<br>SVBG chronic phase | Primary prevention of coronary artery disease |
| Cardiac chambers Fibrin | AF, prior embolism<br>AF, mitral stenosis<br>AF, other risk factors | NVAF with heart disease<br>Early phase after anterior MI<br>Dilated cardiomyopathy | Lone AF<br>Chronic LV aneurysm |
| Prosthetic valves Fibrin and platelets | Old mechanical prostheses<br>Mechanical prostheses, prior embolism | Recent mechanical prostheses<br>Bioprostheses, AF | Bioprostheses, NSR |

AF = atrial fibrillation; LV = left ventricular; MI = myocaradial infarction; NSR = normal sinus rhythm; NVAF = nonvalvular atrial fibrillation; PTCA = percutaneous transluminal coronary angioplasty; SVBG = saphenous vein bypass graft.

have a comparable annual event rate well below 1%. For patients at high risk, aggressive antithrombotic management is recommended, whereas less intensive strategies are required for those at medium risk, and antithrombotic therapy may be avoided altogether for those at the lowest risk (Table 10.2).

## Coronary Arteries

During the early phase of unstable angina and acute myocardial infarction, the risk of developing thrombotic occlusion (or reocclusion after vessel reperfusion) varies from 5–20%. (26) Patients with stable angina and survivors of myocardial infarction are at intermediate risk of coronary thrombosis. According to the Framingham Heart Study (27), patients with stable angina followed for 10 years develop myocardial infarction or suspected cardiac death at averaged annual rates of 5% for men and 2.5% for women. In survivors of myocardial infarction the annual rate of recurrent coronary events is just over 5% regardless of gender. Patients in the stable phase after coronary angioplasty and saphenous vein bypass surgery are also at continuous risk of developing thrombotic coronary events. Individuals without clinical evidence of coronary disease, however, have a risk of thrombotic arterial events of less than 1% annually (28).

### *Unstable Angina Pectoris*

Although disruption of an atherosclerotic plaque, with or without superimposed thrombus, is a frequent finding in patients with unstable

**Table 10.2**
**Antithrombotic Therapy Based on Pathogenesis and Risk**

| | Thromboembolic Risk | | |
|---|---|---|---|
| Location | High (>6% per year) | Medium (2–6% per year) | Low (<2% per year) |
| Arterial system | Platelet inhibitor; addition of heparin in acute setting may be beneficial | Platelet inhibitor; anticoagulant also effective but has increased bleeding risk | Platelet inhibitor in patients at higher risk for coronary disease |
| Cardiac chambers | Anticoagulant (PT 1.5–2.0 × control; INR 3.0–4.5) | Anticoagulant (PT 1.3–1.5 × control; INR 2.0–3.0) | Usually no need for therapy |
| Prosthetic valves | Anticoagulant (PT 1.5–2.0 × control; INR 3.0–4.5) *plus* platelet inhibitor | Anticoagulant (INR 3.0–4.5 or 2.0–3.0) | Usually no need for therapy |

INR = international normalized ratio; PT = prothrombin time.

angina as shown by angiography (29), angioscopy (30), and histologic studies (31), thrombosis may be evanescent and occur without appreciable myocardial necrosis. Vasospasm and changes in myocardial oxygen balance also may be important; however, the high risk of subsequent myocardial infarction when thrombotic coronary occlusion occurs makes antithrombotic therapy advisable for most patients with unstable angina.

The results of several randomized trials support administration of aspirin as a platelet inhibitor in patients with unstable angina. In particular, a Veterans Administration cooperative study (32) found a 51% collective reduction in mortality and nonfatal myocardial infarction with a daily aspirin dose of 324 mg during a period of 12 weeks, and benefit was detectable even after 1 year. A Canadian multicenter trial (33) corroborated these findings using higher aspirin dosage (1300 mg daily) over a mean of 18 months and found an identical (51%) reduction in myocardial infarction and death. Sulfinpyrazone conferred no additional benefit. Aspirin and heparin, alone and in combination, were compared in a short-term (6-day) randomized trial; aspirin (325 mg twice daily) reduced the combined rate of fatal and nonfatal myocardial infarction by 72% compared with placebo (34). Patients treated with heparin, with or without aspirin, had 89% fewer infarcts than those given placebo, but the sample size was insufficient to allow statistical comparisons among the three treatment arms. In another trial, intravenous heparin reduced the incidence of myocardial infarction in patients with unstable angina by as much as 80%; however, there was an increase in the rate of infarction after cessation of heparin therapy, implying rebound coagulation phenomena (35).

Evidence supporting the use of heparin, aspirin, or both in patients with unstable angina is strong, and treatment should be initiated promptly after the onset of the unstable syndrome. Because a substantial proportion of patients develop myocardial infarction despite treatment with one agent or the other, combinations of low-dose aspirin and heparin are currently under investigation in large clinical trials. The combination may be superior to either agent alone for prevention of infarction in the acute phase (36). Beyond this phase, aspirin alone is recommended in a dose of 160–325 mg daily, although ongoing trials are addressing maintenance therapy with low-dose combinations of warfarin and aspirin.

### *Acute Myocardial Infarction*

As in unstable angina, rupture of an atherosclerotic plaque and superimposed thrombotic occlusion play major roles in the development of acute myocardial infarction. In some patients, particularly those with nonQ-wave infarction, spontaneous early vessel reperfusion occurs because of thrombolysis or resolution of vasospasm, limiting myocardial necrosis but setting the stage for subsequent ischemic events. Extensive necrosis that occurs in Q-wave infarction probably results from persistent thrombotic coronary occlusion and inadequate collateral flow. Because spontaneous vessel recanalization seems to occur in both types of infarction, an aggressive antithrombotic approach to these patients is emerging for prevention of thrombotic reocclusion.

In the large Second International Study of Infarct Survival (ISIS-2), patients with suspected myocardial infarction treated with aspirin within 24 hours of onset had a 23% reduction in 5-week vascular mortality compared with those given placebo (37). This dramatic benefit may have been related to prevention of reinfarction in patients with spontaneous vessel recanalization. Aspirin reduced the rate of nonfatal reinfarction by almost 50%. Short-term anticoagulation, aimed at reducing the incidence of death, infarct extension, or reinfarction, is still not settled for patients with acute myocardial infarction in the absence of thrombolytic therapy. Despite several studies published during more than 40 years, only three randomized controlled trials were of sufficient scope to establish a significant reduction in mortality with anticoagulants. Of these, only one (38) found a statistically significant decrease in mortality; others (39, 40) showed a trend toward lower reinfarction rate. When the results of six published randomized trials are pooled (41), a significant 21% reduction in mortality in treated patients emerges. Despite the limitation inherent in retrospective metaanalysis of heterogeneous trials, short-term anticoagulation in acute myocardial infarction appears to provide a modest reduction in early mortality. Because of the high risk of reinfarction and death in the first weeks after acute infarction, however, the combination of aspirin and an anticoagulant may prove beneficial and is currently under investigation.

Patients with acute myocardial infarction treated with thrombolytic agents are at high risk of early coronary reocclusion (5–20%) (42, 43). The importance of concomitant platelet inhibitor therapy in patients undergoing thrombolysis was emphasized by the results of the ISIS-2 trial, in which streptokinase alone decreased early cardiovascular mortality by 25%, whereas the combination of aspirin and streptokinase decreased mortality by 42% compared with placebo (37). The benefits of these agents appeared independent of one another, and the addition of aspirin to streptokinase reduced the clinical reinfarction rate by 50%. Aspirin (160–325 mg daily) is advocated as early as possible in the treatment of acute myocardial infarction, irrespective of whether thrombolytic agents are given. Given the marked thrombogenicity of the residual thrombus following vessel recanalization, and supported by the results of the Gruppo Italiano per lo Studio della Sopravvivenza nell'Infarto Miocardico-II (GISSI-II) trial (44), heparin therapy is recommended for a period of 3–7 days after thrombolysis with alteplase. Aspirin should be continued daily beyond discharge. The lower incidence of reocclusion in some thrombolytic trials may be related to the use of combined therapy with aspirin plus heparin. The use of low-dose combinations of aspirin plus an anticoagulant is now being compared with aspirin alone for prevention of reinfarction and related coronary occlusive events in the Coumadin Aspirin Reinfarction Study (CARS) and Combination Hemotherapy and Mortality Prevention Study (CHAMP) studies in North America, and simultaneously in several European investigations (45).

### *Chronic Phase after Myocardial Infarction*

Survivors of acute myocardial infarction are at persisting risk of recurrent infarction or cardiac death that falls into the intermediate risk category. Because cardiac morbidity and mortality within 2 years of infarction may be related to several factors, including left ventricular dysfunction, ventricular arrhythmias, and recurrent myocardial infarction, the advantage of antithrombotic therapy has remained controversial for decades and difficult to prove. Since 1974, no fewer than 10 randomized trials involving platelet inhibitors in patients with prior myocardial infarction have been reported and subjected to metaanalysis (Fig. 10.1) (46). From these data, it appears that among survivors of myocardial infarction, platelet inhibitors reduced vascular mortality by 13%, nonfatal reinfarction by 31%, nonfatal stroke by 42%, and other important vascular events by 25%. Aspirin alone was at least as effective as the combination of aspirin and dipyridamole and more effective than sulfinpyrazone. Available data do not justify the additional cost, frequency of administration, and occasional side effects of drugs other than aspirin for this group of patients.

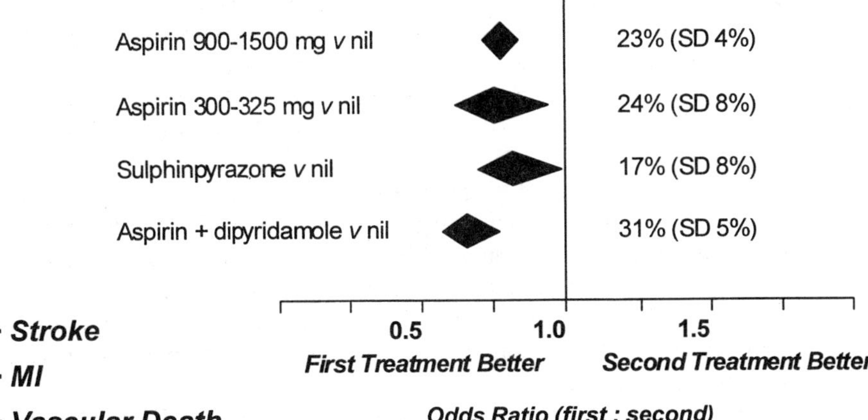


Figure 10.1 Platelet inhibitor therapy in cardiovascular trials. MI = myocardial infarction; SD = standard deviation. Reproduced with permission from Antiplatelet Trialists' Collaboration. Secondary prevention of vascular disease by prolonged antiplatelet treatment. Br Med J 1988;296: 320.

Despite numerous trials of long-term anticoagulation conducted since 1950, few have been adequately designed to show a salutary effect in late postinfarction patients. A British study (47) showed a trend toward lower case fatality rate, and the Veterans Cooperative trial suggested a reduction in reinfarction of 25–50% (48), but only the Norwegian Warfarin Re-Infarction Study (WARIS) trial has convincingly demonstrated significant reductions in rates of reinfarction and mortality over several years after acute myocardial infarction (49).

Thus, evidence supporting the use of aspirin for secondary prevention of cardiovascular morbidity and mortality beyond the acute phase of myocardial infarction is almost as strong as that supporting anticoagulation. At a daily dose of 325 mg, aspirin offers several advantages over long-term anticoagulants in cost, ease of administration, and safety. Ongoing trials are investigating the relative safety and efficacy of fixed combination doses of warfarin and aspirin for survivors of myocardial infarction, and results are expected to accumulate over the next 1–4 years.

### *Chronic Stable Coronary Artery Disease*

Patients with a remote history of myocardial infarction (beyond 2 years) and those with chronic stable angina pectoris are at medium risk of ischemic events, varying between 2.5–5% per year. Recurrent coronary thrombotic events are probably the main cause of mortality. Most studies of platelet inhibitors in survivors of myocardial infarction have shown a beneficial trend toward lower mortality and reinfarction, which became significant only when the data derived from all available trials were pooled

(45). With regard to anticoagulant therapy, in the Sixty-Plus Reinfarction Study (50), patients treated for an average of 6 years with warfarin after myocardial infarction were randomly assigned to continue anticoagulant or substitute placebo for 2 more years. Mortality was 26% lower ($P = 0.071$) and the rate of reinfarction was 55% lower ($P = 0.0005$) among the anticoagulated group.

Safe use of sustained anticoagulant medication was obviously favored in this group of patients by their toleration of warfarin for an extended period before randomization. It appears that aspirin or anticoagulation each represent an effective strategy for prevention of reinfarction and mortality in asymptomatic patients late after myocardial infarction; although the two alternatives have not been directly compared, aspirin is associated with lower cost and toxicity.

Although no randomized trials of antithrombotic therapy in chronic stable angina have been published, the sustained benefits of aspirin after initial treatment of patients with unstable angina suggests a role for platelet inhibitor therapy in patients with stable coronary disease. Aspirin doses of 325 mg daily or less are associated with minimal gastrointestinal toxicity and should be considered in these patients. Evidence from an angiographic study in patients with stable coronary disease suggests that platelet inhibitors reduce the incidence of myocardial infarction and new lesion formation, but do not prevent progression of disease in those with preexisting lesions (51). Such therapy also appears appropriate for patients with documented atherosclerotic disease involving other vascular beds, including those with intermittent claudication or carotid stenosis.

### *Primary Prevention of Coronary Events*

Although platelet inhibitor therapy decreases the incidence of vascular events by 25% in patients with cardiovascular or cerebrovascular disease (46), such benefit is less apparent when aspirin is used for primary prevention in apparently healthy individuals. In the US Physicians' Health Study (52) of 22,071 male physicians followed 4.8 years, aspirin (325 mg every other day) significantly reduced the incidence of nonfatal myocardial infarction by 44%, from about 0.4–0.2% per year. The incidence of cardiovascular death was identical in the aspirin and placebo groups, but aspirin was associated with a slight increase in the number of severe hemorrhagic strokes (13 versus 6, not significant). In a British primary prevention trial (53) of 5139 male physicians in which the control group was not given a placebo, there was no difference in the incidence of myocardial infarction or cardiovascular mortality in those given aspirin (500 mg daily) for 6 years. Although the number of enrolled subjects was smaller than that in the American trial, cardiovascular event rates were 5–10 times higher. When both studies are considered together, there appears to be reduction in coronary events with aspirin but at the price of a small increase in the risk of cerebral hemorrhage. Before aspirin is recommended to every adult, therefore, the risks of therapy must be weighed against potential benefits. Patients with risk factors for coronary atherosclerotic disease (54), particularly those aged above 50 years, and those with cerebral or peripheral arterial disease are among the best candidates for aspirin prophylaxis.

## Coronary Intervention

### *Coronary Angioplasty*

Coronary angioplasty is associated with endothelial denudation and exposure of thrombogenic elements of the disrupted atherosclerotic plaque and vessel wall, which may lead to mural thrombosis and acute occlusion. Experimentally, when angioplasty results in mild arterial injury, only minimal deposition of platelets occurs (55). On the other hand, severe damage or dissection of the arterial wall leads to exposure of collagen, smooth muscle cells, and other components of the atherosclerotic lesion and to the release of tissue thromboplastin. Contact with these substances results in activation of platelet and coagulation processes, predisposing to acute thrombotic occlusion. Thrombus formation at the site of angioplasty is not only important in acute occlusion but may also contribute to later restenosis.

Several studies have shown that pretreatment of patients with aspirin alone, aspirin and dipyridamole, or ticlopidine significantly reduces the rate of acute thrombotic complications after angioplasty (56, 57). Experimental evidence suggests an inverse relationship between the dose of heparin and both platelet deposition and the extent of mural thrombosis (58), and clinical observations also indicate that treatment with heparin reduces the incidence of acute thrombotic complications during and after angioplasty (59). High-dose heparin is generally used during such interventional procedures in catheterization laboratories and, because of the substantial risk of acute thrombotic complications associated with angioplasty, pretreatment with aspirin combined with adequate heparinization throughout the procedure is widely recommended. The angiographic appearance of intraluminal thrombus or vessel dissection usually dictates the duration of anticoagulant therapy on completion of the procedure, although detailed investigations are needed to establish appropriate guidelines.

New interventional methods such as intraluminal stenting are typically employed when the risk of reocclusion is higher than that with conventional balloon angioplasty. More aggressive antithrombotic strategies may be required in these circumstances. The problem of late restenosis after angioplasty is beyond the scope of this chapter, but data from clinical trials regarding the use of antithrombotic agents to prevent restenosis have been inconsistent. Although one group of investigators found no difference in the number of patients with restenosis 4–7 months after angioplasty among those treated with aspirin plus dipyridamole compared with placebo (55), the antithrombotic regimen reduced the severity of restenosis. Based on favorable experience in chronic coronary artery disease, long-term aspirin therapy has been recommended for secondary prevention of ischemic complications.

### *Saphenous Vein Bypass Grafts*

Saphenous vein graft disease is the most important factor leading to recurrent myocardial ischemia after coronary artery bypass surgery. The risk of graft occlusion is greatest during the first postoperative year: occlusion rates are 8–18% per distal anastomosis at 1 month and 16–26% by 12 months (60). Early occlusion appears to be related to endothelial disruption caused by surgical manipulation and exposure of the graft to high rates of arterial flow. This process is mainly of thrombotic origin, and platelets play a major pathogenetic role. The etiology of late vein graft disease is multifactorial, involving a hyperplastic intimal proliferative response to chronic injury and a superimposed thrombotic tendency. Several months after surgery, vein grafts develop an accelerated form of atherosclerosis, similar to that seen in the native coronary circulation (61).

Antithrombotic therapy is most effective in reducing the rate of early postoperative thrombotic occlusion. Several trials (62, 63) document that aspirin, with or without dipyridamole, reduces the incidence of early vein graft occlusion. Antiplatelet therapy should be instituted preoperatively or in the immediate postoperative period, because benefit is reduced if therapy is initiated after platelet deposition has occurred. Administration of aspirin before surgery increases the risk of postoperative bleeding; it is not clear, however, whether addition of dipyridamole preoperatively offers any value over postoperative aspirin alone. Because extracorporeal circulation activates the coagulation system and platelets, the routine use of heparin intraoperatively is also important for prevention of thrombus formation and early graft occlusion.

Two studies have addressed the effect of anticoagulation on vein graft patency. In one (64), there was a trend toward higher graft patency with warfarin (begun 3–4 days postoperatively), but in the other (65), this drug offered no avantage over placebo. These studies were compromised by incomplete angiographic documentation, small sample size, or late initiation of antithrombotic therapy. Although no comparative studies have been published, it is difficult to advocate the use of anticoagulants because of the impressive success of aspirin after saphenous vein graft surgery. It should also be emphasized that the results cited here do not apply to internal mammary arterial grafts, in which the long-term patency rate is substantially higher than that with saphenous vein grafts. Beyond the first year after coronary bypass surgery, patients are at intermediate risk of recurrent ischemic events associated with either native coronary thrombosis or vein graft closure; in such cases long-term aspirin therapy appears to be appropriate.

In summary, thrombosis within the arterial system involves both platelet and clotting mechanisms. Therefore, in patients at high risk, a combination of a platelet inhibitor and an anticoagulant can be implemented. In those at medium risk, either a platelet inhibitor or an anticoagulant should be considered, and in those at low risk, a platelet inhibitor can be recommended to selected patients.

## Cardiac Chambers

### *AF with Valvular Heart Disease*

Systemic embolism is a common and potentially devastating complication of AF associated with both mitral valve disease and certain other forms of organic heart disease. Blood stasis appears to play a predominant pathogenetic role in thrombus formation in patients with AF. Patients at highest risk are those with a history of systemic embolism in the previous 2 years. In this group, the embolic risk approaches 10–20% in the first 1 or 2 years (66). Recent prospective randomized trials found anticoagulation with warfarin more effective than anticoagulation with aspirin for secondary prevention after ischemic stroke in patients with nonvalvular AF, and statistical analysis suggests that the optimum intensity may fall in the range of 2–5 international normalized ratio (INR) units (Table 10.2) (67).

Patients with AF associated with mitral stenosis are also at substantial risk of embolism (approximately 6% per year). Data from uncontrolled studies suggest that anticoagulation reduces the rates of embolism and death in patients with rheumatic valvular disease by 25%. Based on known embolic risk and clinical observations, chronic anticoagulation to maintain INR in the range of 2.0–4.0 is recommended for these patients. In addition, patients with uncontrolled hyperthyroidism and heart failure appear to be at increased risk of embolism (68–70).

Although anticoagulation for this patient group has not been evaluated by prospective randomized trials, warfarin therapy is recommended at least until the patient becomes euthyroid or for several weeks after reversion to sinus rhythm has occurred (71).

### *Lone Atrial Fibrillation*

Young patients with AF without associated organic heart disease have a low embolic risk. The natural history of lone AF was addressed by the Framingham investigators (72), but the inclusion of older patients and those with hypertension make the relatively high event rate inapplicable to a population in which lone AF is more rigorously defined. In an observational study from the Mayo Clinic (73), 97 normotensive patients aged 60 years or less with lone AF were followed a mean of 17 years, mostly without anticoagulants. Only eight ischemic events were identified, an overall incidence well under 1% per year. In the Stroke Prevention in Atrial Fibrillation Study (SPAF-I) randomized trial of aspirin versus placebo, no ischemic events occurred among 51 patients with lone AF who were followed for an average of 1.3 years. These data suggest that for patients aged less than 60 years with rigidly defined lone AF but without organic heart disease, chronic anticoagulation is not required, and even aspirin prophylaxis may be unnecessary.

### *Nonvalvular Atrial Fibrillation in Patients with Cardiovascular Disease*

Between the two poles of lone AF and AF associated with rheumatic heart disease, prosthetic heart valves, or prior thromboembolism exists a large group of patients with an intermediate but incompletely defined risk of embolism: those with nonvalvular AF associated with other forms of cardiovascular disease (66). Six recent randomized trials and several other studies have confirmed the magnitude of the problem: AF raises the risk of stroke in more than 1.5 million Americans to a degree matching that which follows transient ischemic attack. Because the absolute rate of stroke varies with coexistent cardiovascular disease, stratification of AF patients into those at high and low risk of thromboembolism has become a crucial determinant of optimal antithrombotic prophylaxis. AF increases in prevalence and risk with age, and about half of AF-associated strokes occur in patients over the age of 75 years; AF is the most frequent cause of disabling stroke in elderly women. Special consideration of these older patients is therefore a critical aspect of an effective stroke prevention strategy (74).

Most ischemic strokes associated with AF are probably caused by embolism of stasis-induced thrombi forming in the left atrium and its appendage. Transesophageal echocardiography shows left atrial thrombi more frequently in AF patients with ischemic stroke than AF patients without stroke (75, 76). Nevertheless, approximately 25% of AF-associated strokes are due to intrinsic cerebrovascular diseases, other cardiac sources of embolism, or atheromatous pathology in the proximal aorta (77). About 50% of elderly AF patients have chronic hypertension (a major risk factor for cerebrovascular disease) and about 12% harbor cervical carotid artery stenosis. The frequency of carotid stenosis, however, is not substantially greater in AF patients with stroke and is probably a minor contributing factor (78). Although atherosclerotic carotid lesions may contribute to stroke risk through thromboembolic mechanisms unrelated to the severity of luminal stenosis, the available data do not support routine screening of AF patients without symptoms of brain ischemia for cervical carotid stenosis.

Identification of AF subpopulations with relatively high or low absolute rates of stroke determines which patients will benefit most from chronic anticoagulation with warfarin, offsetting its risk, expense, and inconvenience. Because clinical classification of ischemic strokes according to etiologic subtypes is imperfect and not adequately validated (79), risk stratification is presently based on combined analysis of all ischemic strokes. Schemes for stratification of risk in AF patients have been pursued using clinical and echocardiographic parameters; two prospective studies encompass sufficient numbers of patients and stroke events for meaningful multivariate analysis, providing the most reliable basis for risk stratification available (Table 10.3) (80–82). Intermittent (or paroxysmal) AF does not appear to be an independent predictor of thromboembolic risk. Stroke in AF patients is directly related to coexistent heart disease, hypertension, age, and perhaps, female gender. The five clinical variables listed in Table 10.3 are independently predictive of thromboembolic risk and clinically useful to characterize AF patients at high or low risk for stroke.

Echocardiographic correlates of thromboembolic risk in patients with AF are enlargement of the left atrium (mitigated by mitral regurgitation) and impairment of left ventricular systolic function, which may promote stasis of blood within the left atrium in the presence of AF. Precordial echocardiographic findings can be combined with clinical risk stratifiers to identify AF patients without risk factors, who are at low inherent risk of thromboembolism. Transesophageal echocardiography offers better visualization of the left atrium and its appendage than precordial echocardiography, and more often identifies atrial thrombi and spontaneous echogenic contrast ("smoke" probably indicative of stasis) in AF patients with thromboembolism than in those without thromboembolism (83). The predictive value of these findings for subsequent stroke has yet to be validated by adequate clinical studies, however, and current data are insufficient to justify routine transesophageal echocardiography to stratify thromboembolic potential.

**Table 10.3**
**Risk Stratification in Atrial Fibrillation: Independent Predictors of Thromboembolic Risk[a]**

| | SPAF-I Placebo | AFI Pooled Analysis |
|---|---|---|
| Number of patients | 568 | 1236 |
| Number of events | 46 | 81 |
| High risk variables | History of hypertension<br>Prior stroke/TIA<br>Diabetes<br>Recent heart failure | History of hypertension<br>Prior stroke/TIA<br>Diabetes<br>Age > 65 years |
| Thromboembolic rate (95% CI) | | |
| Low risk | 1.4% annually (0.05–3.7) | 1.0% annually (0.3–3.1) |
| High risk | > 7% annually | > 5% annually |
| Percent at low risk | 38% | 15% |

[a] Prospectively acquired data analyzed by multivariable techniques. The SPAF-I placebo data set (80) was included in the pooled analysis of clinical trials by the Atrial Fibrillation Investigators (79).
AFI = Atrial Fibrillation Investigators; CI = confidence interval; SPAF = Stroke Prevention in Atrial Fibrillation study; TIA = transient ischemic attack.

Anticoagulation with warfarin is highly effective for reducing ischemic stroke in AF patients. Five recent randomized clinical trials using prothrombin time INR ranges between approximately 1.8 and 4.2 showed a mean reduction in ischemic stroke of nearly 70% in patients assigned anticoagulation; on therapy analysis indicated an even greater benefit (80). The incremental risk of severe bleeding was less than 1% annually among anticoagulated patients, a selected group followed carefully according to clinical trial protocols. Whether such low bleeding risks can be achieved in general clinical practice is an important, unresolved issue (84). Safe anticoagulation monitoring requires use of the INR, which corrects for variable thromboplastin sensitivities. Low-intensity anticoagulation (INR 2–3) clearly confers benefit (80, 85), and it is clear that warfarin is highly effective in subgroups of AF patients who carry a high inherent risk of thromboembolism (Table10.3) (80, 86, 87).

The safety and tolerability of chronic anticoagulation to conventional levels has not been well defined in patients aged more than 75 years, who account for nearly half of AF-associated strokes. All but one of the anticoagulation trials enrolled AF patients about 10 years younger. The single placebo-controlled trial involving AF patients with a mean age of 75 years reported an overall withdrawal rate from anticoagulation of 38% after 1 year, and the attrition rate among the oldest patients may have been even higher. The risk of major hemorrhage during anticoagulation (INR range 2.0–4.5, mean 2.7) in another trial was substantially greater among older AF patients (more than 75 years of age) than among their younger counterparts anticoagulated to similar intensities. Although the elderly have a greater risk of AF-associated stroke, the benefit of anticoagulation is offset somewhat by this greater toxicity, and the inability of the very elderly to sustain chronic anticoagulation is a noteworthy finding of several trials. Until ongoing trials are completed, a lower intensity of anticoagulation (INR approximately 2) may be more appropriate in older AF patients who have risk factors for thromboembolism.

The efficacy of aspirin, a platelet inhibitory agent, for stroke prevention in AF patients is less clear and more controversial (80, 88). The effect of aspirin in doses of 75–325 mg/day has been assessed in three placebo-controlled trials with a statistically significant pooled risk reduction of about 25% (range, 14–44%) in aspirin-treated patients (86, 89, 90). Aspirin was less effective than warfarin in two of these trials analyzed on intention-to-treat paradigms (86, 90) and according to on-treatment (efficacy) analysis of the third (87). There is no compelling evidence that the specific dose of aspirin between 75 and 325 mg/day confers more or less benefit, although the individual trial results suggest greater efficacy at the higher dosage. Aspirin thus appears active for preventing stroke in AF patients, but is less uniformly effective than warfarin.

Platelet inhibitors and anticoagulants may influence cardioembolic and noncardioembolic sources of stroke differently. Aspirin could have a greater prophylactic impact on noncardioembolic mechanisms than on strokes of presumed cardioembolic origin. Aspirin is particularly effective in younger AF patients with a history of diastolic hypertension (79). Most AF-related stroke, particularly in women, seems attributable to cardiogenic embolism; this type of stroke may be more effectively prevented by anticoagulation (79). AF patients with high rates of stroke during aspirin therapy are typically older women and those with impaired left ventricular function, in which cardiogenic embolism is the predominant mechanism of cerebral infarction (74, 79). These pathophysiologic constructs, however, require further study before they can be confidently applied to patient management.

The risk of thromboembolism in AF patients aged 75 years or less given aspirin is relatively low, less than 3% annually (74). These younger AF patients, if prospectively identified as at low risk based on clinical criteria, have an extremely low rate of thromboembolism averaging 0.5% annually (95% confidence interval, 0.1–1.9% per year; Table 10.4) when treated with aspirin (74). Pending the results of ongoing confirmatory studies, low-risk AF patients can be treated with aspirin, 325 mg/day, to prevent stroke, but they must be observed carefully for the development of risk factors for thromboembolism (including systolic hypertension over 160 mm Hg, episodes of minor cerebral ischemia, and changes in ventricular function). "High-risk" patients deemed safe candidates for anticoagulation should be treated with warfarin. For "high-risk" AF patients aged 75 years or less, an INR range of 2–3 is effective and fairly safe; for those patients aged more than 75 years, a lower target INR of 2 seems more sensible. AF patients who cannot safely take warfarin should be given aspirin; the value of other antiplatelet agents has not been assessed in this situation.

Conventional wisdom holds that most ischemic strokes in AF patients are large and disabling, but it is now clear that minor stroke and transient ischemic attack (TIA) are frequent accompaniments of AF. AF-related

**Table 10.4**
**Rates of Thromboembolism During Aspirin Therapy in High-Risk and Low-Risk Patients: Results of the SPAF-II Study**

| | Clinical Risk Factors for Thromboembolism | |
|---|---|---|
| | Yes | No |
| Patients ≤ 75 years old | | |
| % of cohort | 57% | 43% |
| Aspirin event rate[a] (95% CI) | 2.9% (1.9–4.6) | 0.5% (0.1–1.9) |
| Patients > 75 years old | | |
| % of cohort | 61% | 39% |
| Aspirin event rate[a] (95% CI) | 7.2% (4.3–11.9) | 1.8 (0.6–5.5) |

[a] One or more of the following: a history of hypertension, prior thromboembolism, or recent (within 3 months) congestive heart failure (81).
CI = confidence interval; SPAF = Stroke Prevention in Atrial Fibrillation study.

stroke carries a high mortality rate, related to advanced patient age and associated heart disease. Previously unrecognized AF discovered in a patient with acute stroke might be a consequence of brain infarction mediated by other processes. A large randomized trial found warfarin (INR 2.5–4.0) highly effective, superior to aspirin, and comparatively safe (86); secondary analysis suggested that a target INR value of 3 may be optimal for preventing stroke in AF patients with previous cerebral ischemia (91).

### *Acute Myocardial Infarction*

Clinicopathologic studies have shown that left ventricular mural thrombi occur in approximately one third of patients in the first 2 weeks after anterior myocardial infarction, and the incidence is greater in those with large infarcts involving the left ventricular apex (92–95) Recent trials examining the impact of thrombolytic therapy suggest a lower incidence of left ventricular thrombus formation (96–101), but this is controversial (102). Systemic embolism occurs in about 10% of patients with left ventricular thrombi within the first month, and in up to 35% of patients within the first 3 months when anticoagulant medication is not given (92, 93), (103–106). Clinically evident cerebral infarction occurs in approximately 10% of patients with left ventricular thrombi in the absence of anticoagulant therapy (107, 108).

Serial studies of acute myocardial infarction spanning the past decade are fairly consistent with respect to the incidence of ventricular thrombi. Left ventricular thrombus occurs in approximately one third of patients with anterior infarctions; the incidence is much lower with inferior infarction (Table 10.5) (92, 95, 102, 105), (109–112). In patients with large infarcts, up to two thirds of thrombi are visible by echocardiography within 48 hours of hospital presentation (106, 113–116) and the vast majority form within the first 2 weeks (111, 116). Thrombi are most prevalent on precordial echocardiographic examinations performed 6–14 days after infarction (92–94, 103, 105, 111, 113, 116–118). Echocardiography is useful to characterize thrombus size, shape, mobility, site of attachment, and adjacent regional left ventricular wall thickness and function (108, 119–121)—features related to the risk of thromboembolic events including ischemic stroke. The sensitivity and specificity of echocardiography for the detection of left ventricular thrombi range from 77–95% and 86–94%, respectively (117, 118, 121, 122). Despite the availability of alternative methods, echocardiography performed serially at selected intervals in the postinfarction period is considered the best available means of detecting left ventricular thrombi.

Heparin is commonly given parenterally from the time of diagnosis of anterior infarction until the presence or absence of thrombus is investigated by two-dimensional echocardiography. An oral antithrombotic medication regimen is then substituted (for about 3 months) based upon the

**Table 10.5**
**Incidence of Left Ventricular Thrombis (LVT) after Q-wave Myocardial Infarction**

| | Total | Anterior Infarction | | | Inferior Infarction | | |
|---|---|---|---|---|---|---|---|
| | N | N | LVT (No.) | LVT (%) | N | LVT (No.) | LVT (%) |
| Asinger, 1981 (14) | 70 | 35 | 12 | 34 | 35 | 0 | 0 |
| Friedman, 1982 (106) | 52 | 21 | 8 | 38 | 13 | 2 | 15 |
| Weinreich, 1984 (95) | 261 | 130 | 44 | 34 | 131 | 2 | 2 |
| Visser, 1984 (103) | 96 | 65 | 21 | 32 | 31 | 1 | 3 |
| Johannessen, 1984 (109) | 90 | 53 | 15 | 28 | 28 | 0 | 0 |
| Gueret, 1986 (110) | 90 | 46 | 21 | 46 | 44 | 0 | 0 |
| Nihoyannopoulos, 1989 (111) | 87 | 53 | 21 | 40 | 34 | 0 | 0 |
| Keren, 1990 (112) | 198 | 124 | 38 | 31 | 74 | 0 | 0 |
| Aggregate | 944 | 527 | 180 | 34 | 390 | 5 | 1 |

results of the ultrasound examination and other clinical circumstances. Two randomized trials (123, 124) have documented that therapeutic anticoagulation reduces the incidence of left ventricular thrombi complicating anterior myocardial infarction within the initial hospital period (1–2 weeks postinfarction) by about 50%, and several studies suggest acceleration of thrombus resolution with anticoagulation (94,116, 125, 126). Furthermore, anticoagulant therapy reduces the incidence of systemic and cerebral embolism in patients with left ventricular thrombi in the early phase after myocardial infarction (93, 127–128).

The use of platelet inhibitors to reduce the incidence of left ventricular thrombi has not been studied extensively. Clinical investigation using indium-111 platelet imaging to assess the effect of aspirin on the hematologic activity of left ventricular thrombi has yielded conflicting results (129, 130). One trial involving a small number of patients found aspirin superior to no treatment in achieving regression of left ventricular thrombi (126), and a second, nonrandomized trial showed that aspirin is effective in reducing thromboembolic events in patients with dilated cardiomyopathy (131). Other studies, however, found no influence of aspirin on the incidence of left ventricular thrombi (132–134). A study comparing aspirin, anticoagulants, and placebo in patients with echocardiographically documented left ventricular thrombi found anticoagulants and aspirin associated with equal rates of thrombus resolution (126).

Based upon available clinical trial results, the American College of Chest Physicians and National Heart, Lung and Blood Institute have promulgated class I recommendations that oral anticoagulant therapy be given to patients with echocardiographically detected left ventricular thrombi after anterior myocardial infarction, but no consensus has been reached regarding the duration of anticoagulant treatment (135). The persistence of stroke risk for several months after infarction in these patients can be surmised from aggregate results of several studies (Table 10.6), but alternative antithrombotic regimens were not systematically evaluated in these investigations. The risk of thromboembolism appears to decrease beyond the first 1–3 months, and in patients with chronic ventricular aneurysm the risk of embolism is comparatively low, even though intracavitary thrombi occur frequently in this condition.

Two studies addressing the echocardiographic detection of thrombi after hospital discharge seem concordant in finding left ventricular thrombi in approximately 10% of patients with anterior Q-wave infarcts not on anticoagulant therapy (112, 116). Although the number of anticoagulated patients was small, none developed thrombi. In patients without echocardiographic evidence of thrombi at the time of hospital discharge, the most

**Table 10.6**
**Myocardial Infarction, Left Ventricular Thrombi (LVT), and Embolism Beyond the First Month**

| Author | Time to Thrombus Detection | Follow-up (months) | No. with LVT | No. with Emboli | % with Emboli |
|---|---|---|---|---|---|
| Tramarin et al (104) | 4 weeks | 11 | | | |
| No anticoagulation | | | 17 | 0 | 0% |
| Anticoagulation | | | 17 | 0 | 0% |
| Keating et al (94) | 2 weeks | 11 | | | |
| No anticoagulation | | | 5 | 3 | 60% |
| Anticoagulation | | | 9 | 0 | 0% |
| Weinreich et al (95) | 1–3 weeks | 15 | | | |
| No anticoagulation | | | 14 | 3 | 22% |
| Anticoagulation | | | 25 | 0 | 0% |
| Asinger et al (14) | 7 days | 9 | | | |
| No anticoagulation | | | 2 | 0 | 0% |
| Anticoagulation | | | 7 | 0 | 0% |
| Turpie et al (123) | 10 days | 6 | | | |
| No anticoagulation | | | 8 | 0 | 0% |
| Anticoagulation | | | 30 | 0 | 0% |
| Visser et al (103) | 2–3 days | 12 | | | |
| No anticoagulation | | | 10 | 1 | 10% |
| Anticoagulation | | | 11 | 1 | 9% |
| Domenicucci et al (116) | 12 days | 14 | | | |
| No anticoagulation | | | 59 | 5 | 8% |
| Nihoyannopoulos et al (111) | 6 days | 39 | | | |
| No anticoagulation | | | 21 | 0 | 0% |
| Keren et al (112) | 10 months | 29 | | | |
| No anticoagulation | | | 26 | 6 | 23% |
| Anticoagulation | | | 22 | 0 | 0% |
| Aggregate | | | | | |
| No anticoagulation | | | 162 | 18 | 11% |
| Anticoagulation | | | 121 | 1 | 1% |

pressing clinical question is whether anticoagulation, administration of a platelet inhibitor, or some combination of both approaches is most effective for preventing the development of thrombosis and embolism.

### *Chronic Left Ventricular Aneurysm*

In contrast to the prevalence of thromboembolism in acute myocardial infarction, the incidence of embolism in chronic left ventricular aneurysm is significantly lower (approximately 0.3% per year) (21). Two possible explanations exist for this difference. First, thrombi formed after acute infarction are usually mobile, friable, and protrude into the ventricular cavity, whereas thrombi in the cavity of a chronic aneurysm are laminated and more adherent to the endocardium. Second, thrombi within an aneurysmal sac devoid of contractile fibers are less prone to propulsion into the ventricular outflow tract (133). Although some investigators have found a persistent risk of embolism in postinfarction patients (136), it was not the presence of an aneurysm but rather the mobility and protrusion of thrombus that predicted embolic events. Patients with remote infarction and chronic left ventricular aneurysm are at low risk of embolism and do not need anticoagulant therapy. Whether warfarin should be given selectively to patients with echocardiographically mobile or protruding thrombi, however, remains to be determined.

### *Dilated Cardiomyopathy*

When left ventricular systolic function is more diffusely reduced, as with dilated cardiomyopathy, most studies suggest that the risk of cerebral embolism is between 3 and 4% per year (137). The echocardiographic findings of protrusion and mobility of the thrombotic mass in the ventricular chamber are, again, associated with greater embolic potential (138).

Surface pathology of endocardial tissue, including myxomatous or fibrotic changes in mitral or aortic valve leaflets, annular dilatation or calcification, damaged chordae tendineae, or other lesions may stimulate platelet aggregation and the coagulation system, influencing the mechanism and clinical features of thromboembolism (30, 139). Alterations in hemostatic function have also been identified in patients with dilated cardiomyopathy associated with AF, including higher plasma concentrations of von Willebrand factor, coagulation factor VIIc, fibrinogen, the fibrinolytic product D-dimer, β-thromboglobulin, and platelet factor 4, the platelet component released upon platelet adhesion (140). These biochemical changes may be either a cause or effect of ongoing thrombosis, however, and correlation with clinical thrombus formation and occurrence in dilated cardiomyopathy without AF has not been established.

Beyond these primary thrombotic mechanisms, coexisting atherosclerotic lesions in the aorta or extracranial or intracranial arteries may reduce cerebral perfusion by direct obstruction or as a result of thrombus formation provoked by exposure of lipid material and subintimal vascular collagen (21). Patients with chronic left ventricular dysfunction often have a history of atherosclerosis, hypertension, or other disorders associated independently with disease of the cerebral vasculature, which may be direct causes of ischemic stroke of noncardioembolic origin.

The sensitivity and specificity of transthoracic two-dimensional echocardiography have not been as clearly established in patients with dilated cardiomyopathy as in those with mural thrombi developing after myocardial infarction. A consensus is emerging regarding echocardiographic criteria for diagnosis of left ventricular thrombi, more applicable to the type that form after acute myocardial infarction than the laminar thrombi prevalent in patients with chronic dilated cardiomyopathy (141). Spontaneous echo-contrast, seen most often in dilated cardiac chambers with reduced blood flow, appears to reflect rouleaux formation, platelet aggregation, and fibrin within areas of blood stasis in the ventricular cavity adjacent to a thrombogenic mural surface, and may be a precursor of thrombus development (142). Left ventricular spatial flow patterns identified by Doppler echocardiography exhibit little predictive capacity for thrombus formation (143). Transesophageal echocardiography more frequently identifies potential sources of cerebral embolism in patients with acute brain infarction than does transthoracic echocardiography (144). Atherosclerotic lesions of the proximal aorta are relatively frequently discovered by transesophageal ultrasound imaging, sometimes accompanied by mobile echodensities protruding into the aortic lumen representing potentially additional sources of atheroembolism and thromboembolism. Although transesophageal echocardiography is superior to transthoracic imaging for the detection of left atrial thrombi, this technique has not been validated for the diagnosis of left ventricular thrombi.

Contrast ventriculography appears to have lower sensitivity and specificity than echocardiography for detection of left ventricular mural thrombi, and carries the risk of inducing embolism of dislodged of thrombotic material. $^{111}$Indium-labeled platelet scintigraphy requires a latency of 48–72 hours for detection of intracardiac thrombi and, similar to "ultra-fast" gated cardiac computed tomography and magnetic resonance imaging, this technique has been investigated in a relatively small number of cases (117). False-positive results may occur less frequently than with echocardiographic imaging and it has been hypothesized that the former method may identify thrombotically active masses prone to embolism (145). The diagnostic accuracy and clinical usefulness of computed tomography and magnetic resonance imaging for detection of ventricular thrombi have not been superior to those of echocardiography, and none of these methods has been validated for identification of patients who require more intensive antithrombotic therapy. In one study involving more than 1000 echocardiograms of 126 patients with dilated cardiomyopathy followed over a 3-year period, echocardiography revealed left ventricular thrombi in 11% of patients, half localized to the apex and a nearly equal proportion of the mural type. Anticoagulant treatment resulted in a thromboembolism rate of 1.4% per year, but there was no correlation between identification of intracavitary thrombi and clinical thromboembolic events (14).

Postmortem (146) and echocardiographic (147) studies have found a high prevalence of right and left ventricular mural thrombi in patients with idiopathic dilated cardiomyopathy (more than 50% and 36%, respectively). Blood stasis and low shear rate present in a dilated, hypocontractile ventricle lead to activation of coagulation processes. Since the mural thrombus is not mechanically isolated, as occurs in a ventricular aneurysm, embolism of thrombotic material is more likely. In one retrospective study, patients treated with anticoagulants had no evidence of systemic embolism, whereas those not on anticoagulation therapy had an embolic rate of 3.5% per year (148). The only independent predictor of thromboembolism, however, was AF.

Within the poorly contracting left ventricle, blood stasis causes coagulation to predominate over platelet activation as the principal mechanism of thrombus formation, and anticoagulant therapy alone seems most appropriate in the management of these patients. At high risk are patients with AF and prior embolism and those with thrombogenic abnormalities of the endocardial surface; at highest risk are those who also have prosthetic heart valves. Dilated cardiomyopathy associated with clinical congestive heart failure is another high-risk situation, and there is sufficient evidence to favor chronic anticoagulation in such cases.

For most patients with long-standing ventricular dysfunction related to dilated cardiomyopathy, the optimum type and dosage of antithrombotic medication has not been established by prospective clinical trials. In the absence of such a trial, available evidence supports chronic warfarin administration for patients with idiopathic dilated cardiomyopathy, particularly those with overt heart failure or AF. For patients with chronic dilated cardiomyopathy associated with advanced coronary atherosclerotic heart disease remote from acute myocardial infarction, there are no studies upon which to base a decision regarding the use of either anticoagulant medication or a platelet inhibitor such as aspirin for preventing either systemic embolism or ischemia-related mortality. In the Vasodilator-Heart Failure Trial (V-HeFT), rates of ischemic stroke and systemic embolism were lower with platelet inhibitor treatment; however, these results should be treated with caution because antithrombotic therapy was not randomized (149).

The best approach to prevention of embolism in patients with dilated cardiomyopathy in patients with chronic ischemic heart disease is currently under investigation. Among the many issues that need to be addressed are the following: (1) should echocardiography be performed routinely to detect left ventricular thrombi, (2) what is the minimum effective intensity of anticoagulant medication, and (3) does the addition of a platelet inhibitor such as aspirin, ticlopidine, or clopidogrel add significantly to efficacy or toxicity? Less intense regimens of anticoagulant therapy have shown promise for prevention of venous thrombosis in patients at risk following gynecologic surgery or with malignancy treated with indwelling catheters (150, 151). Several trials of low-dose combinations of warfarin and aspirin are in progress for patients with prior myocardial infarction, coronary bypass graft surgery, and AF. A similar study is also called for in patients with dilated cardiomyopathy.

In summary, because thrombosis within the cardiac chambers is related to activation of the coagulation system, anticoagulation (of variable intensity) is recommended in patients at high and medium risk for thromboembolism. In contrast, patients at low risk need not be subjected to the risk, expense, and disutility of chronic warfarin therapy.

## Prosthetic Valves

### *Mechanical Prostheses*

Prosthetic surfaces are thrombogenic by virtue of activation of both the intrinsic coagulation system and platelets. Increased shear rate, blood stasis (particularly in high-profile prosthetic devices), and associated abnormalities of the cardiac chambers related to chronic valvular pathology predispose to thromboembolism. Patients with a history of embolism and those with valves manufactured before the mid-1970s are at highest risk, exceeding 6% per year. AF and left atrial thrombi contribute additional risk (23).

Warfarin, at a dose sufficient to prolong the INR to 3.0–4.5, is the most important agent for prevention of thromboembolism. Studies in patients with mechanical prostheses have consistently shown that anticoagulation significantly reduces the incidence of valvular thrombosis and embolism (23). Platelet inhibitors alone cannot be expected to reduce the incidence of embolic events in this high-risk group, but addition of a platelet inhibitor such as dipyridamole (300–400 mg daily) to warfarin may reduce the thromboembolic risk to less than that of warfarin alone (23). The antithrombotic effects of dipyridamole may be more evident on prosthetic materials such as artificial heart valves than on biologic surfaces (152, 153). In patients with mechanical prostheses, the combination of warfarin and aspirin appears more effective than anticoagulation alone, although the risk of bleeding, particularly in the gastrointestinal tract, is increased (154). Supplementation of warfarin with a platelet inhibitor might be considered for patients with mechanical prostheses who have sustained prior embolism and in those with older prosthetic devices, in whom the increased risk of hemorrhage may be offset by improved antithrombotic efficacy.

Patients with mechanical prostheses of more modern design have a risk of thromboembolism between 1 and 5% per year despite anticoagulants: the risk is higher for those with prosthetic valves in the mitral position, multiple prostheses, and Starr-Edwards models. Inadequate anticoagulation increases the thromboembolic risk, whereas excessive anticoagulation increases the risk of bleeding complications (154). Platelet inhibitors alone do not confer protection against embolism in patients with mechanical prostheses. Studies of aspirin and dipyridamole in these patients have shown an incidence of thromboembolism as high as 10% per year (155). Patients with mechanical prostheses treated with warfarin had significantly fewer thromboembolic events compared with those treated with aspirin combined with either dipyridamole or pentoxifylline (156). It seems clear, therefore, that patients with mechanical prostheses should receive anticoagulant therapy indefinitely, aimed at an INR of 3.0–4.5.

In patients with prosthetic heart valves on anticoagulant therapy, the incidence of ischemic thromboembolism is about 2.5% for the Starr-Edwards and Omniscience prostheses, 2% for the Medtronic Hall prosthesis, and 1.5% for the St. Jude Medical prosthesis, compared with about 1% for the pericardial and porcine bioprostheses (157, 158). These values are about half the rate among nonanticoagulated patients. The risk persists over years postoperatively, but it is highest in the first month for both bioprosthetic and mechanical prosthetic valve devices (159, 160). Recurrent embolism is frequent among those with prior (even preoperative) embolic events. In a series from the Mayo Clinic, 20% of patients with mitral prostheses and 27% of those with aortic prostheses had recurrent embolism (160).

The optimal anticoagulant regimen may be defined as that intensity of anticoagulation that leads to the lowest incidence of valve thrombosis or systemic embolism, with the minimum number of bleeding episodes. It appears from retrospective studies of late postoperative thromboembolic and bleeding complications that the generally recommended INR of 3.0–4.5 may not be necessary after aortic or mitral valve replacement with mechanical prostheses (161, 162). Thus, for mechanical prostheses, an INR of 2.5–3.5 may be adequate; a lower level of anticoagulation with an INR of 2.0–3.0 may suffice in bioprosthetic valves in patients with AF or no anticoagulation at all (sinus rhythm) in bioprosthetic valves on sinus rhythm. A large scale, prospective, randomized trial (German Experience with Low Intensity Anticoagulation, GELIA) has begun, therefore, to provide conclusive evidence regarding the optimum level of anticoagulation after valve replacement with the St. Jude Medical prosthesis.

No randomized placebo-controlled clinical trials have tested the use of platelet inhibitors alone as an antithrombotic regimen in mechanical heart valve replacement. However, combination antiplatelet therapy with dipyridamole and aspirin, or pentoxifylline and aspirin, was associated with a significantly higher incidence of thromboembolism over a 2-year follow-up period (13.6 and 10.5%, respectively) when compared with warfarin (4.1%) in an open prospective randomized trial of patients with mitral or aortic Starr-Edwards valves (163). In other nonrandomized series, aspirin or dipyridamole alone or in combination has not shown significant protective effects.

Although consistent and optimal anticoagulant therapy is critical for patients with mechanical heart valve prostheses, there is still a relatively high residual risk of systemic thromboembolism. The pathophysiologic importance of platelet activation and the demonstration of increased platelet consumption in such patients, as reflected by a measured decrease in platelet survival, has led to the clinical evaluation of combination therapy with oral anticoagulants and platelet inhibitors. The platelet inhibitor dipyridamole has been tested in several trials, because at a dose of 400 mg/day the agent normalized platelet survival in patients with prosthetic intracardiac surfaces. Five randomized controlled trials have therefore been conducted comparing the antithrombotic efficacy of warfarin plus dipyridamole (5–6 mg/kg/day) with warfarin alone in recipients of mechanical ball or tilting disc valves. In three trials, combination therapy was significantly better than warfarin alone, resulting in a 70–92% reduction in embolic events. In the other two trials, the addition of dipyridamole to warfarin resulted in statistically insignificant differences, perhaps because event rates in both groups were relatively low. In three studies, high-dose aspirin (500–1000 mg/day) combined with warfarin reduced systemic embolism compared with warfarin alone. In each instance, this combination led to a significant increase in serious hemorrhage requiring blood transfusion; therefore, this dosage combination is not recommended.

In a more recent study by Turpie and colleagues (164), warfarin (INR 3.0–4.5) was given in combination with aspirin (100 mg/day) to 370 patients with prosthetic heart valves implanted between 1987 and 1991 (75% mechanical). The combination of warfarin and aspirin reduced event rates for the composite end point of major systemic embolism and vascular death from 8.5% to 1.9% over warfarin anticoagulation alone ($P < 0.01$). The risk of hemorrhagic events was higher in the combination therapy group than in patients given warfarin alone (35 versus 22% per year, $P = 0.02$), mainly because of minor bleeding. The rates of major hemorrhagic events were not significantly different. In fact, when the end points of major systemic embolism, vascular death, hemorrhagic death, and nonfatal intracranial hemorrhage were combined, there was a significant risk reduction in the combination therapy group (3.9% per year) compared with the group receiving warfarin alone (9.9% per year, $P = 0.005$). One explanation is that aspirin decreased the rate of myocardial infarction in a population at risk of coronary events. Furthermore, the rate of major systemic embolism or death in the warfarin group was higher than that generally reported in other series. Although the intended INR range was 3.0–4.5, the INR actually achieved was 3.1 in the warfarin group and 3.0 in the combination group, which may have contributed to the higher thromboembolism rates observed in patients not receiving platelet inhibitor therapy. Additional studies are necessary to clarify whether the combination of aspirin and a low-intensity anticoagulant is safe while preserving antithrombotic efficacy in patients with mechanical valve prostheses.

*Biologic Prostheses*

Although bioprosthetic valves are less thrombogenic than mechanical devices, thromboembolism may occur in two to three per 100 patients per year, particularly in the first 3 months after surgery, and more often in those patients with mitral rather than aortic prostheses and in those with AF or prior embolism (23, 24). Patients with mitral bioprostheses should receive warfarin postoperatively, aimed at an INR of 2–3 for 1–3 months, unless AF persists, in which case warfarin should be used indefinitely. Although aortic bioprostheses are associated with a lower incidence of embolism, concomitant AF also may warrant chronic warfarin therapy in these patients.

Patients maintaining sinus rhythm postoperatively who do not have left ventricular dysfunction or prior embolism are at lower risk and may not need sustained anticoagulant therapy. This is particularly true for patients with aortic bioprostheses in whom even platelet inhibitors may be unnecessary (24). No randomized, controlled studies of platelet inhibitors in patients with bioprostheses have been reported, although in an uncontrolled series (165), long-term aspirin use was associated with a low incidence of embolism.

In summary, activation primarily of the coagulation system and secondarily of platelets occurs in patients with prosthetic valves. For patients at highest risk, the combination of an anticoagulant and a platelet inhibitor is suggested, although precise dosing regimens have yet to be established. Patients at intermediate risk should be treated with anticoagulant medication alone, and those at low risk may be treated with aspirin, or they may not require antithrombotic therapy at all.

## CONCLUSIONS

Rooted in ideas about thrombosis and embolism planted more than a century ago, an approach to antithrombotic therapy in various cardiovascular disease states has emerged based on current knowledge of pathophysiology and an understanding of differential clinical features determining morbid risk. The essential parameters of this approach form the framework of Tables 10.1 and 10.2. In Table 10.1, the numerical values corresponding to the relatively high-, medium-, and low-risk clinical situations, defined at the top of the columns, should be considered approximate and even flexible, because distinguishing variables in individual patients avoid rigidly defined categories. In Table 10.2, a therapeutic approach is formulated based on anatomic location and pathogenesis (horizontal rows) and relative risk (columns).

In the arterial circulation, vessel wall injury leads to both platelet activation and production of thrombin and fibrin, suggesting a combined therapeutic approach with a platelet inhibitor and an anticoagulant. The propensity to thrombosis determines the intensity of antithrombotic therapy. High-risk patients with unstable angina or evolving acute myocardial infarction may be treated aggressively, perhaps with a combination of a platelet inhibitor and an anticoagulant, although final recommendations await the results of ongoing clinical trials. Patients undergoing coronary angioplasty or saphenous vein bypass surgery should receive platelet inhibitors and adequate anticoagulation during the procedure. Coronary disease patients at moderate risk in the chronic phase of stable angina or post-myocardial infarction, angioplasty, or bypass surgery are best managed with a platelet inhibitor rather than an anticoagulant for reasons of convenience, safety, and economy. In low-risk patients in whom prevention of complications of atherosclerosis is desired, aspirin may be prescribed to those with certain risk factors such as diabetes, familial history, tobacco exposure, and hypercholesterolemia. However, long-term aspirin therapy may be associated with an escalated risk of intracerebral hemorrhage; therefore this agent should be used discriminately.

Within the cardiac chambers, stasis of blood flow causes coagulation to predominate over platelet activation as the principal mechanism of thrombus formation, and anticoagulant therapy alone seems most appropriate in management of these patients. At highest risk are patients with AF and prior embolism and those with mitral stenosis and uncontrolled hyperthyroidism. Patients at medium risk are those who have just had large anterior myocardial infarction and dilated cardiomyopathy associated with congestive heart failure. For these patients, there is sufficient evidence to indicate chronic anticoagulation. Many patients with nonvalvulopathic AF associated with hypertension, heart failure, or prior thromboembolism benefit from long-term warfarin therapy, but other subgroups in this population are at substantially lower risk and require only aspirin prophylaxis. At lowest risk are patients with lone AF without overt heart disease and patients in sinus rhythm with chronic left ventricular aneurysm, who do not require anticoagulant therapy.

The thrombogenicity of prosthetic heart valves involves both fibrin formation and, to a lesser degree, platelet activation, and is considerably greater for mechanical than biologic devices. Patients with older mechanical prostheses or prior embolism are at highest risk and should be treated with a combination of an anticoagulant and a platelet inhibitor. Although dipyridamole and aspirin have proven beneficial, their relative efficacy has not been compared; dipyridamole has the advantage of not potentiating bleeding. At medium risk are patients with modern mechanical valvular prostheses and those in AF with bioprostheses; they should be treated with anticoagulant medication alone. When bioprostheses are in place along with sinus rhythm, the embolic risk is low enough that antithrombotic therapy is not needed, although a platelet inhibitor is frequently employed.

Coronary atherosclerotic disease, AF, cardiomyopathy and valvular heart disease can be regarded not only as markers of thromboembolic risk but also as valuable opportunities for effective clinical intervention. Even so, many issues remain unresolved. Lower intensity regimens of anticoagulation, which should cause less bleeding, and combinations of anticoagulants and platelet inhibitory agents are under study to establish safety and efficacy. These efforts are particularly important for elderly patients, for whom conventional anticoagulation carries substantial toxicity. Better characterization of the role of aspirin and of "low-risk" patients awaits clarification of mechanisms of thromboembolism in cardiovascular disease.

## REFERENCES

1. Dalen JE, Hirsh J, eds. Third ACCP Consensus Conference on Antithrombotic Therapy. Chest 1992; 102(Suppl):303S–549S.
2. Fuster V, Badimon L, Badimon JJ, et al. The pathogenesis of coronary artery disease and the acute coronary syndromes (I). N Engl J Med 1992;226:242–250.
3. Fuster V, Badimon L, Badimon JJ, et al. The pathogenesis of coronary artery disease and the acute coronary syndromes (II). N Engl J Med 1992;326:310–318.
4. Goldsmith HL, Turitto VT. Rheological aspects of thrombosis and hemostasis: basic principals and applications. Thromb Haemost 1986;55:415–435.
5. Badimon L, Badimon JJ, Turitto VT, et al. Mechanism of arterial thrombosis: platelet thrombus deposition in areas of stenosis. Circulation 1987;76:IV-102.
6. Badimon L, Badimon JJ, Galvez A, et al. Influence of arterial wall damage and wall shear rate on platelet deposition: ex vivo study in a swine model. Arteriosclerosis 1986;6:312–320.
7. Chesebro JH, Knatterud G, Roberts R, et al. Thrombolysis in myocardial infarction (TIMI) trial, phase I: a comparison between intravenous tissue plasminogen activator and intravenous streptokinase. Circulation 1992;86:III-100–III-110.
8. Lierde JV, DeGeest H, Verstraete M, et al: Angiographic assessment of the infarct-related residual coronary stenosis after spontaneous or therapeutic thrombolysis. J Am Coll Cardiol 1990;16:1545–1549.
9. Virchow R: Gesammelte Abhandlungen zur Wissenschaftlichen Medicine. Frankfurt: Meidinger Sohn & Co, 1856;219–732.
10. Johnson RC, Crissman RS, Didio LJA. Endocardial alterations in myocardial infarction. Lab Invest 1979;40:183–193.
11. Hochman JS, Platia EB, Bulkley BH. Endocardial abnormalities in left ventricular aneurysms: a clinicopathological study. Ann Intern Med 1984;100:29–35.
12. Roberts WC, Siegel RJ, McManus BM. Idiopathic dilated cardiomyopathy: analysis of 152 necropsy patients. Am J Cardiol 1987;60:1340–1355.
13. Mikell FL, Asinger RW, Elsperger KJ, et al. Regional stasis of blood in the dysfunctional left ventricle: echocardiographic detection and differentiation from early thrombosis. Circulation 1982;66:755–763.
14. Asinger RW, Mikell FL, Elsperger J, et al. Incidence of left ventricular thrombosis after acute transmural myocardial infarction: serial evaluation by two-dimensional echocardiography. N Engl J Med 1981;305:297–302.
15. Weinrich DJ, Burke JF, Pauletto FJ. Left ventricular mural thrombi complicating acute myocardial infarction: long-term follow-up with serial echocardiography. Ann Intern Med 1984;100:789–94.
16. Shresta NK, Moreno FL, Narcisco FV, et al. Two-dimensional echocardiographic diagnosis of left atrial thrombus in rheumatic heart disease: a clinicopathologic study. Circulation 1983;67:341–347.

17. Fulton RM, Duckett L: Plasma-fibrinogen and thromboemboli after myocardial infarction. Lancet 1976;2:1161–1164.
18. Fatkin D Herbert E, Feneley MP. Hematologic correlates of spontaneous echo contrast in patients with atrial fibrillation and implications for thromboembolic risk. Am J Cardiol 1994;73:672–676.
19. Fuster V, Badimon L, Cohen M, et al. Insights into the pathogenesis of acute ischemic syndromes. Circulation 1988;77:1213–1220.
20. Cabin HS, Roberts WC. Left ventricular aneurysm, intra-aneurysmal thrombus and systemic embolus in coronary heart disease. Chest 1980;77:586–590.
21. Fuster V, Halperin JL. Left ventricular thrombi and cerebral embolism: an emerging approach. N Engl J Med 1989;320:392–394.
22. Dewanjee MK, Fuster V, Rao SA, et al. Noninvasive radioisotopic technique for detection of platelet deposition in mitral valve prostheses and quantification of visceral microembolism in dogs. Mayo Clin Proc 1983;58:307–314.
23. Chesebro JH, Adams PC, Fuster V. Antithrombotic therapy in patients with valvular heart disease and prosthetic heart valves. J Am Coll Cardiol 1986;8:41B–56B.
24. Edmunds LH. Thrombotic and bleeding complications of prosthetic heart valves. Ann Thorac Surg 1987;44:430–445.
25. Stein B, Fuster V, Halperin JL, et al. Antithrombotic therapy in cardiac disease: an emerging approach based upon pathogenesis and risk. Circulation 1989;80: 1501–1513.
26. Resnekov L, Chediak J, Hirsch J, et al. Antithrombotic agents in coronary artery disease. Chest 1989;95:52S–72S.
27. Kannel WB, Wolf PA, Garrison RJ. Survival following initial cardiac events: Framingham study. Section 35. (Publication No. PB 88–204029.) Washington, DC: US Department of Health and Human Services, National Institutes of Health, US Department of Commerce, National Technical Information Center, 1988.
28. Fuster V, Cohen M, Halperin JL. Aspirin in the prevention of coronary disease. N Engl J Med 1989;321:183–185.
29. Ambrose JA, Winters SL, Arora RH, et al. Angiographic evolution of coronary artery morphology in unstable angina. J Am Coll Cardiol 1986;7:472–478.
30. Sherman CT, Litvak F, Grundfest W, et al. Coronary angioscopy in patients with unstable angina. N Engl J Med 1986;315:913–919.
31. Falk E. Unstable angina with fatal outcome, dynamic coronary thrombosis leading to infarction and/or sudden death: autopsy evidence of recurrent mural thrombosis with peripheral embolization culminating in total vascular occlusion. Circulation 1985;71:699–708.
32. Lewis HD, Davis JW, Archibald DG, et al. Protective effects of aspirin against acute myocardial infarction and death in men with unstable angina: results of a Veterans Administration Cooperative Study. N Engl J Med 1983;309:396–403.
33. Cairns JA, Gent M, Singer J, et al. Aspirin, sulfinpyrazone, or both in unstable angina. N Engl J Med 1985;313:1369–1375.
34. Theroux P, Ouimet H, McCans J, et al. Aspirin, heparin or both to treat acute unstable angina. N Engl J Med 1988;319:1105–1111.
35. Telford AM, Wilson C. Trial of heparin versus atenolol in prevention of acute myocardial infarction in intermediate coronary syndrome. Lancet 1981;1:1225–1228.
36. Cohen M, Adams PC, Parry G, et al. Combination antithrombotic therapy in unstable rest angina and non-Q-wave infarction in nonprior aspirin users. Circulation 1994;89:81–88.
37. ISIS-2 (Second International Study of Infarct Survival) Collaborative Group. Randomized trial of intravenous streptokinase, oral aspirin, both, or neither among 17,187 cases of suspected acute myocardial infarction. Lancet 1988;2:349–360.
38. Drapkin A, Merskey C. Anticoagulation therapy after acute myocardial infarction: relation of therapeutic benefit to patient's age, sex and severity of infarction. JAMA 1972;222:541–548.
39. Working Party on Anticoagulant Therapy in Coronary Thrombosis. Report to the Medical Research Council. Assessment of short-term anticoagulant administration after cardiac infarction. Br Med J 1969;1:335–342.

40. Veterans Administration Cooperative Study Group. Anticoagulants in acute myocardial infarction: results of a cooperative clinical trial. JAMA 1973;225:541–548.
41. Chalmers TC, Matta RJ, Smith JH, et al. Evidence favoring the use of anticoagulants in the hospital phase of acute myocardial infarction. N Engl J Med 1977;297: 1091–1096.
42. GUSTO Agiographic Investigators. The effects of tissue plasminogen activator, streptokinase, or both on coronary artery patency, ventricular function, and survival after acute myocardial infarction. N Engl J Med 1993;329:1615–1622.
43. Roux S, Christeller S, Ludin E. Effects of aspirin on coronary reocclusion and recurrent ischemia after thrombolysis: a meta-analysis. J Am Coll Cardiol 1992; 19:671–677.
44. Gruppo Italiano per lo Studio della Sopravvivenza nell'infarto Miocardico: GISSI-2: a factorial randomized trial of alteplase and heparin versus no heparin among 12,490 patients with acute myocardial infarction. Lancet 1990;336:65–71.
45. Cairns JA, Markham BA. Economics and efficacy in choosing oral anticoagulants or aspirin after myocardial infarction. JAMA 1995;273:965–967.
46. Antiplatelet Trialists' Collaboration. Secondary prevention of vascular disease by prolonged antiplatelet treatment. Br Med J 1988;296:320–331.
47. Working Party on Anticoagulant Therapy in Coronary Thrombosis. Second Report to the Medical Research Council. An assessment of long-term anticoagulant administration after cardiac infarction. Br Med J 1964;2:837–843.
48. Ebert RV, Borden CW, Hipp HR, et al. Long-term anticoagulation therapy after myocardial infarction: final report of the Veterans Administration Cooperative Study. JAMA 1969;207:2263–2267.
49. Smith P, Arnesen H, Holme I. The effect of warfarin on mortality and reinfarction after myocardial infarction. N Engl J Med 1990;323:147–152.
50. Sixty-Plus Reinfarction Research Group. A double-blind trial to assess long-term oral anticoagulant therapy in elderly patients after myocardial infarction. Lancet 1980;2:989–993.
51. Chesebro JH, Webster MWI, Zolhelyi P, et al. Antithrombotic therapy and progression of coronary artery disease. Circulation 1992;86(Suppl III):III-100–III-111.
52. Steering Committee of the US Physicians' Health Study Research Group. Final report on the aspirin component of the ongoing Physicians' Health Study. N Engl J Med 1989;321:129–135.
53. Peto R, Gray R, Collins R, et al. A randomized trial of the effects of prophylactic daily aspirin among male British doctors. Br Med J 1988;296:313–316.
54. Fuster V, Cohen M, Halperin JL. Aspirin in the prevention of coronary disease. N Engl J Med 1989;321:183–185.
55. Steele PM, Chesebro JH, et al. Balloon angioplasty: natural history of the pathophysiological response to injury in a pig model. Circ Res 1985;57:1005–1012.
56. Barnathan ES, Schwartz JS, Taylor L, et al. Aspirin and dipyridamole in the prevention of acute coronary thrombosis complicating coronary angioplasty. Circulation 1987;76:125–134.
57. Schwartz L, Bourassa MG, Lesperance J, et al. Aspirin and dipyridamole in the prevention of restenosis after percutaneous transluminal coronary angioplasty. N Engl J Med 1988;318:1714–1719.
58. Heras M, Chesebro JH, Penny WJ, et al. Importance of adequate heparin dosage in arterial angioplasty in a porcine model. Circulation 1988;78:654–660.
59. Gabliani G, Deligonul U, Kern MJ, et al. Acute coronary occlusion occurring after successful percutaneous transluminal coronary angioplasty: temporal relationship to discontinuation of anticoagulation. Am Heart J 1988;116:696–700.
60. Fuster V, Chesebro JH. Role of platelets and platelet inhibitors in aortocoronary artery vein-graft disease. Circulation 1986;73:227–232.
61. Bulkley BH, Hutchins GM. Accelerated "atherosclerosis": a morphologic study of 97 saphenous vein coronary artery bypass grafts. Circulation 1977;55:163–169.
62. Chesebro JH, Clements IP, Fuster V, et al. A platelet-inhibitor drug trial in coronary-artery bypass operations: benefit of perioperative dipyridamole and aspirin therapy on early postoperative vein-graft patency. N Engl J Med 1982;307:73–78.

63. Goldman S, Copeland J, Moritz T, et al. Improvement in early saphenous vein graft patency after coronary artery bypass surgery with antiplatelet therapy: results of a Veterans Administration Cooperative Study. Circulation 1988;77:1324–1332.
64. McEnany MT, Salzman EW, Mundth ED, et al. The effect of antithrombotic therapy on patency rates of saphenous vein coronary artery bypass graft. J Thorac Cardiovasc Surg 1982;83:81–89.
65. Pantely GA, Goodnight SH, Rahimtoola SH, et al. Failure of antiplatelet and anticoagulant therapy to improve patency of grafts after coronary-artery bypass: a controlled randomized study. N Engl J Med 1979;301:962–966.
66. Halperin JL, Hart RG. Atrial fibrillation and stroke: new ideas, persisting dilemmas. Stroke 1988;19:937–941.
67. European Atrial Fibrillation Trial Study Group. Optimal oral anticoagulant therapy in patients with nonrheumatic atrial fibrillation and recent cerebral ischemia. N Engl J Med 1995;333:5–10.
68. Bar-Sela S, Ehrenfeld M, Eliakim M. Arterial embolism in thyrotoxicosis with atrial fibrillation. Arch Intern Med 1981;141:1191–1192.
69. Yuen RWM, Gutteridge DH, Thompson PL, et al. Embolism in thyrotoxic atrial fibrillation. Med J Austr 1979;1:630–631.
70. Staffurth JS, Gibberd MC, Tang Fui SN. Arterial embolism in thyrotoxicosis and atrial fibrillation. Br Med J 1977;2:688–690.
71. Laupacis A, Albers G, Dalen J, et al. Antithrombotic therapy in atrial fibrillation. Chest 1995;108(Suppl 4):352S–359S.
72. Brand FN, Abbott RD, Kannel WB, et al. Characteristics and prognosis of lone atrial fibrillation: 30-year follow-up in the Framingham study. JAMA 1985;254:3449–3453.
73. Kopecky SL, Gersh BJ, McGoon MD, et al. The natural history of lone atrial fibrillation: a population-based study over three decades. N Engl J Med 1987;317:669–674.
74. Hart RG, Halperin JL. Atrial fibrillation and stroke: revisiting the dilemmas. Stroke 1994;25:1337–1334.
75. Daniel WG, Grote J, Freedberg RS, et al. Assessment of left atrial thrombi by transesophageal echo in non-valvular atrial fibrillation: a multicenter study. Eur Heart J 1993; 14(Suppl):355.
76. Mugge A, Kuhn H, Nikutta P, et al. Assessment of left atrial appendage function by biplane transesophageal echocardiography in patients with nonrheumatic atrial fibrillation: identification of a subgroup of patients at increased embolic risk. J Am Coll Cardiol 1994;23:599–607.
77. Amarenco P, Duyckaerts C, Tzourio C, et al. The prevalence of ulcerated plaques in the aortic arch in patients with stroke. N Engl J Med 1992;326:221–225.
78. Kanter MC, Tegeler CH, Pearce LA, et al. on behalf of the SPAF investigators. Carotid stenosis in patients with atrial fibrillation: prevalence, risk factors and relationship to stroke. Arch Intern Med 1994;154:1372–1377.
79. Miller VT, Rothrock JF, Pearce LA, et al. Ischemic stroke in patients with atrial fibrillation: effect of aspirin according to stroke mechanism. Neurology 1993;43:32–36.
80. Atrial Fibrillation Investigators. Risk factors for stroke and efficacy of antithrombotic therapy in atrial fibrillation: analysis of pooled data from five randomized controlled trials. Arch Intern Med 1994;154:1449–1457.
81. Stroke Prevention in Atrial Fibrillation Investigators. Predictors of thromboembolism in atrial fibrillation: I. Clinical features of patients at risk. The Stroke Prevention in Atrial Fibrillation Study. Ann Intern Med 1992;116:1–5.
82. Stroke Prevention in Atrial Fibrillation Investigators. Predictors of thromboembolism in atrial fibrillation: II. Echocardiographic features of patients at risk. The Stroke Prevention in Atrial Fibrillation Study. Ann Intern Med 1992;116:6–12.
83. Chimowitz MI, DeGeorgia MA, Poole RM, et al. Left atrial spontaneous echo contrast is highly associated with previous stroke in patients with atrial fibrillation. Stroke 1993;24:1015–1019.
84. Lundstrom T, Ryden L. Haemorrhagic and thromboembolic complications in patients with atrial fibrillation on anticoagulant prophylaxis. J Intern Med 1989;226:137–142.
85. Veterans Affairs Stroke Prevention in Nonrheumatic Atrial Fibrillation Investigators. Warfarin in the prevention of stroke associated with nonrheumatic atrial fibrillation. N Engl J Med 1992;327:1406–1412.

86. EAFT Study Group. European Atrial Fibrillation Trial: secondary prevention of vascular events in patients with nonrheumatic atrial fibrillation and recent transient ischemic attack or minor ischemic stroke. Lancet 1993;342:1255–1262.
87. Stroke Prevention in Atrial Fibrillation Investigators. Warfarin compared to aspirin for prevention of thromboembolism in atrial fibrillation: results of the Stroke Prevention in Atrial Fibrillation II study. Lancet 1994;343:687–691.
88. Singer DE. Aspirin and prevention of stroke. Lancet 1994;343:233–234 (letter).
89. Stroke Prevention in Atrial Fibrillation Study Investigators. Stroke Prevention in Atrial Fibrillation Study: final results. Circulation 1991;84:527–539.
90. Petersen P, Boysen G. Prevention of stroke in atrial fibrillation. N Engl J Med 1990:323:482 (letter).
91. The European Atrial Fibrillation Trial Study Group. Optimal oral anticoagulant therapy in patients with nonrheumatic atrial fibrillation and recent cerebral ischemia. N Engl J Med 1995;333:5–10.
92. Asinger RW, Mikell FL, Elsperger J, et al. Incidence of left ventricular thrombosis after acute transmural myocardial infarction: serial evaluation by two-dimensional echocardiography. N Engl J Med 1981;305:297–302.
93. Mikell F, Asinger R, Elsperger J, et al. Long term prospective evaluation of left ventricular thrombus in acute myocardial infarction. Circulation 1981; 64(Suppl 4):93.
94. Keating EC, Gross SA, Schlamowitz RA, et al. Mural thrombi in myocardial infarction: prospective evaluation by two-dimensional echocardiography. Am J Med 1983; 74:989–995.
95. Weinreich DJ, Burke JF, Pauletto FJ. Left ventricular mural thrombus complicating acute myocardial infarction: long-term follow-up with serial echocardiography. Ann Intern Med 1984;100:789–794.
96. Nataarajan D, Hotchandani RK, Nigam PD. Reduced incidence of left ventricular thrombi with intravenous streptokinase in acute anterior myocardial infarction: prospective evaluation by cross-sectional echocardiography. Int J Cardiol 1988; 20:201–207.
97. Bhatnagar SK, Al-Yusuf AR. Effects of intravenous recombinant tissue-type plasminogen activator therapy on the incidence and associations of left ventricular thrombus in patients with a first acute Q-wave anterior myocardial infarction. Am Heart J 1991;122:1251–1256.
98. Eigler NN, Maurer G, Shah PK. Effect of early thrombolytic therapy on left ventricular mural thrombus formation in acute anterior myocardial infarction. Am J Cardiol 1984;54:261–263.
99. Karatasakis G, Kalkandi H, Handanis H, et al. Thrombolysis and intraventricular thrombus formation: an echocardiographic study. Eur Heart J 1990; 11 (Suppl):147 (Abstract).
100. Lupi G, Domenicucci S, Chiarella F, et al. Influence of thrombolytic therapy followed by full dose anticoagulation on the frequency of left ventricular thrombi in acute myocardial infarction. Am J Cardiol 1989; 64:588–590.
101. Motro M, Barbash GI, Hod H, et al. Incidence of left ventricular thrombi formation after thrombolytic therapy with recombinant tissue plasminogen activator, heparin and aspirin in patients with acute myocardial infarction. Am Heart J 1991; 122:23–26.
102. Visser C, Roelandt J. Left ventricular thrombus. Echocardiography 1985;2:245–255.
103. Visser CA, Kan G, Meltzer RS, et al. Long-term follow-up of left ventricular thrombus after acute myocardial infarction: a two-dimensional echocardiographic study in 96 patients. Chest 1984;86:532–536.
104. Tramarin R, Pozzolli M, Febo O, et al. Echocardiographic assessment of therapy efficacy in left ventricular thrombosis post myocardial infarction. Circulation 1983;68 (Suppl 3):331 (Abstract).
105. McEntee CW, VanReet RE, Winters WL, et al. Incidence and natural history of mural thrombi in acute myocardial infarction by two-dimensional echocardiography. Circulation 1981;64(Suppl 4):93 (Abstract).
106. Friedman MJ, Carlson K, Marcus FI, et al. Clinical correlations in patients with acute myocardial infarction and left ventricular thrombus detected by two-dimensional echocardiography. Am J Med 1982;72:894–898.

107. Chesebro JH, Fuster V. Antithrombotic therapy for acute myocardial infarction: mechanisms and prevention of deep venous, left ventricular, and coronary artery thromboembolism. Circulation 1986; 4 (Suppl III):1–10.
108. Meltzer RS, Visser CA, Fuster V. Intracardiac thrombi and systemic embolization. Ann Intern Med 1986;104:689–698.
109. Johannessen KA, Nordehaug JE, von der Lippe G. Left ventricular thrombosis and cerebrovascular accident in acute myocardial infarction. Br Heart J 1984;51: 553–556.
110. Gueret P, Dubourg O, Ferrier A, et al. Effects of full-dose heparin anticoagulation on the development of left ventricular thrombosis in acute transmural myocardial infarction. J Am Coll Cardiol 1986;8:419–426.
111. Nihoyannopoulos P, Smith GC, Maseri A, et al. The natural history of left ventricular thrombus in myocardial infarction: a rationale in support of masterly inactivity. J Am Coll Cardiol 1989;14:903–911.
112. Keren A, Goldberg S, Gottlieg S, et al. Natural history of left ventricular thrombi: their appearance and resolution in the posthospitalization period of acute myocardial infarction. J Am Coll Cardiol 1990;15:790–800.
113. Spirito P, Bellotti P, Chiarella F, et al. Prognostic significance and natural history of left ventricular thrombi in patients with acute myocardial infarction: a two-dimensional echocardiographic study. Circulation 1985;72;774–780.
114. Visser CA, Kan G, Lie KI, et al. Left ventricular thrombus following acute myocardial infarction: a prospective serial echocardiographic study of 96 patients. Eur Heart J 1983;4:333–337.
115. Vecchio C, Chiarella F, Lupi G, et al. Left ventricular thrombus in acute myocardial infarction after thrombolysis: a GISSI-2 connected study. Circulation 1991;84: 512–519.
116. Domenicucci S, Bellotti P, Chiarella F, et al. Spontaneous morphologic changes in left ventricular thrombi: a prospective two-dimensional echocardiographic study. Circulation 1987;75:737–743.
117. Ezekowitz MD, Wilson DA, Smith EO, et al. Comparison of indium-111 platelet scintigraphy and two-dimensional echocardiography in the diagnosis of left ventricular thrombi. N Engl J Med 1982;306:1509–1513.
118. DeMaria AN, Bommer W, Neumann A, et al. Left ventricular thrombi identified by cross-sectional echocardiography. Ann Intern Med 1979;90:14.
119. Judgutt BI, Sivaram CA, Wortman C, et al. Prospective two-dimensional echocardiographic evaluation of left ventricular thrombus and embolism after acute myocardial infarction. J Am Coll Cardiol 1989;13:554–564.
120. Johannessen KA, Nordrehaug JE, von der Lippe G, et al. Risk factors for embolisation in patients with left ventricular thrombi and acute myocardial infarction. Br Heart J 1988;60:104–110.
121. Visser CA, Kan G, Meltzer RS, et al. Embolic potential of left ventricular thrombus after myocardial infarction: a two-dimensional echocardiographic study of 119 patients. J Am Coll Cardiol 1985;1276–1280.
122. Stratton JR, Lighty GW, Pearlman AS, et al. Detection of left ventricular thrombus by two-dimensional echocardiography: sensitivity, specificity, and causes of uncertainty. Circulation 1982;66:156–166.
123. Turpie AGG, Robinson JG, Doyle DJ, et al. Comparison of high-dose with low-dose subcutaneous heparin to prevent left ventricular mural thrombosis in patients with acute transmural anterior myocardial infarction. N Engl J Med 1989;320:352–357.
124. The SCATI (Studio sulla Calciparin nell'Angina e nella Thrombosi Ventriculare nell'Infarto) group. Randomized controlled trial of subcutaneous calcium-heparin in acute myocardial infarction. Lancet 1989;2:182–186.
125. Tramarin R, Pozzoli M, Febo O, et al. Two-dimensional echocardiographic assessment of anticoagulant therapy in left ventricular thrombosis early after acute myocardial infarction. Eur Heart J 1986;7:482–492.
126. Kouvras G, Chronopoulus G, Soufras G, et al. The effects of long-term antithrombotic treatment on left ventricular thrombi in patients after an acute myocardial infarction. Am Heart J 1990;119:73–78.

127. Arnott WM, Biggs R, Gilchrist AR, et al. for the Working Party on Anticoagulant Therapy in Coronary Thrombosis. Assessment of short term anticoagulant administration after cardiac infarction. Br Med J 1969;1:335–342.
128. Veterans Administration Cooperative Study. Anticoagulants in acute myocardial infarction: results of a cooperative clinical trial. JAMA 1973;225:724–729.
129. Stratton JR, Ritchie JL. The effects of antithrombotic drugs in patients with left ventricular thrombi: assessment with indium-111 platelet imaging and two-dimensional echocardiography. Circulation 1984;69:561–568.
130. Ezekowitz MD, Smith EO, Cox AC, et al. Failure of aspirin to prevent incorporation of indium-111 labelled platelets into cardiac thrombi in man. Lancet 1981;1: 440–443.
131. Dunkman WB, Johnson GR, Carson PE, et al. Incidence of thromboembolic events in congestive heart failure. Circulation 1993;87(Suppl VI):94–101.
132. Funke Kupper AJ, Verheugt FWA, Peels, CH, et al. Left ventricular thrombus incidence and behavior studied by serial two-dimensional echocardiography in acute anterior myocardial infarction: left ventricular wall motion, systemic embolism and oral anticoagulation. J Am Coll Cardiol 1989;13:1514–1520.
133. Johanessen KA, Stratton JR, Taulow E, et al. Usefulness of aspirin plus dipyridamole in reducing left ventricular thrombus formation in anterior wall acute myocardial infarction. Am J Cardiol 1989;63:101–102.
134. Funke Kupper AJ, Verheugt FWA, Peels CH, et al. Effect of low dose acetylsalicylic acid on the frequency and hematologic activity of left ventricular thrombus in anterior wall acute myocardial infarction. Am J Cardiol 1989;63:917–920.
135. American College of Cardiology and American Heart Association. Guidelines for the early management of patients with acute myocardial infarction. Circulation 1990;82:664–707.
136. Stratton JR, Nemanich JW, Johannessen KA, et al. Fate of left ventricular thrombi in patients with remote myocardial infarction or idiopathic cardiomyopathy. Circulation 1988;78:1388–1393.
137. Cerebral Embolism Task Force. Cardiogenic brain embolism. Arch Neurol 1986;43: 71–84.
138. Cerebral Embolism Task Force. Cardiogenic brain embolism: the second report of the Cerebral Embolism Task Force. Arch Neurol 1989;46:727–743.
139. Hochman JS, Platia EB, Bulkley BH. Endocardial abnormalities in left ventricular aneurysms: a clinicopathologic study. Ann Intern Med 1984;100: 29–35.
140. Sherman DG, Dyken ML, Fisher M, et al. Cerebral embolism. Chest 1986;89 (Suppl):82S–98S.
141. Dolara A, Cecchi F, Ciaccheri M. Cardiomyopathy in Italy today: extent of the problem. G Ital Cardiol 1989;19:1074–1079.
142. Mikell FL, Asinger RW, Elsperger KJ, et al. Regional stasis of blood in the dysfunctional left ventricle: echocardiographic detection and differentiation from early thrombosis. Circulation 1982;66:755–763.
143. Johnson RC, Crissman RS, Didio LJA. Endocardial alterations in myocardial infarction. Lab Invest 1979;40:183–193.
144. Lee RJ, Bartzokis T, Yeoh TK, et al. Enhanced detection of intracardiac sources of cerebral emboli by transesophageal echocardiography. Stroke 1991;22:734–739.
145. Sechtem U, Theissen P, Heindel W, et al. Diagnosis of left ventricular thrombi by magnetic resonance imaging and comparison with angiocardiography, computerized tomography and echocardiography. Am J Cardiol 1989;64:1195–1199.
146. Shresta NK, Moreno FL, Narciso FV, et al. Two-dimensional echocardiographic diagnosis of left atrial thrombus in rheumatic heart disease: a clinicopathologic study. Circulation 1983;67:341–347.
147. Fulton RM, Duckett K. Plasma-fibrinogen and thromboemboli after myocardial infarction. Lancet 1976;2:1161–1164.
148. Kumagai K, Fukunami M, Ohmori M, et al. Increased intravascular clotting in patients with chronic atrial fibrillation. J Am Coll Cardiol 1990;16:377–380.
149. Dunkman WB, Johnson GR, Carson PE, et al. Incidence of thromboembolic events in congestive heart failure. Circulation 1993;87 (Suppl VI) 94–101.

150. Poller L, McKernan A, Thomson JM, et al. Fixed minidose warfarin: a new approach to prophylaxis against venous thrombosis after major surgery. Br Med J 1987;295:1309–1312.
151. Bern MM, Lokich JJ, Wallach SR, et al. Very low doses of warfarin can prevent thrombosis in central venous catheters. Ann Intern Med 1990;112:423–428.
152. Sullivan JM, Harken DE, Gorlin R. Pharmacologic control of thromboembolic complications of cardiac-value replacement. N Engl J Med 1971;284:1391–1394.
153. Chesebro JH, Fuster V, Elveback LR, et al. Trial of combined warfarin plus dipyridamole or aspirin therapy in prosthetic heart valve replacement: danger of aspirin compared with dipyridamole. Am J Cardiol 1983;51:1537–1541.
154. Cannegieter SC, Rosedaal FR, Wintzen AR, et al. Optimal oral anticoagulant therapy in patients with mechanical heart valves. N Engl J Med 1995;333:11–17.
155. Myers ML, Lawrie GM, Crawford ES, et al. The St. Jude valve prosthesis: analysis of the clinical results in 815 implants the need for systemic anticoagulation. J Am Coll Cardiol 1989;13:57–62.
156. Mok CY, Boey J, Wang R, et al. Warfarin versus dipyridamole-aspirin and pentoxifylline-aspirin for the prevention of prosthetic heart valve thromboembolism: a prospective randomized clinical trial. Circulation 1985;72:1059–1063.
157. Fuster V, Badimon L, Badimon JJ, et al. Prevention of thromboembolism induced by prosthetic heart valves. Semin Thromb Hemost 1988;14:50–58.
158. Israel DH, Sharma SK, Fuster V. Antithrombotic therapy in prosthetic heart valve replacement. Am Heart J 1994;127:400–411.
159. Heras M, Chesebro JH, Fuster V, et al. High risk of thromboembolic events early after bioprosthetic cardiac valve replacement. J Am Coll Cardiol 1995;25: 1111–1119.
160. Butchart EG. Thrombogenicity, thrombosis and embolism. In: Butchart EG, Bodnar E, eds. Current issues in heart valve disease: thrombosis, embolism and bleeding. London: ICR Publishers, 1992:172–205.
161. Piper C, Schulte HD, Horstkotte D. Optimization of oral anticoagulation for patients with mechanical heart valve prostheses. J Heart Valve Dis 1995;4:127–137.
162. Butchart EG. Rationalizing antithrombotic management for patients with prosthetic heart valves. J Heart Valve Dis 1995;4:106–113.
163. Mok DC, Boey J, Wang R, et al. Warfarin versus dipyridamole-aspirin and pentoxifylline-aspirin for the prevention of prosthetic heart valve thromboembolism: a prospective randomized clinical trial. Circulation 1985;72:1059–1063.
164. Turpie AGG, Gent M, Laupacis A, et al. A comparison of aspirin with placebo in patients treated with warfarin after heart valve replacement. N Engl J Med 1993;329: 524–529.
165. Nunez L, Gil Aguado M, Larrea JL, et al. Prevention of thromboembolism using aspirin after mitral valve replacement with porcine bioprostheses. Ann Thorac Surg 1984;37:84–87.

# PART V

# Therapy of Congestive Heart Failure

# CHAPTER 11

## Pharmacologic Intervention for the Treatment of Congestive Heart Failure

Thierry H. LeJemtel, MD, Laura A. Demopoulos, MD, and Edmund H. Sonnenblick, MD

Optimal pharmacologic management of congestive heart failure (CHF) requires an in-depth understanding of the pathophysiology of the syndrome. Clinical manifestations of CHF can result from either left ventricular systolic or diastolic dysfunction. Left ventricular diastolic dysfunction is characterized by reduced ventricular compliance (most commonly resulting from hypertrophy, with or without fibrosis) and by increased ventricular filling pressures that can produce pulmonary congestion. Systolic function is maintained with a normal ejection fraction. Left ventricular systolic dysfunction, which is identified by a reduced ejection fraction, can be associated with a variable degree of diastolic dysfunction. Although CHF cannot always be attributed exclusively to either left ventricular systolic or diastolic dysfunction, left ventricular systolic dysfunction is most often assumed to play a preponderant role when the left ventricular ejection fraction is lower than 35% (1).

This chapter focuses on the pharmacologic management of CHF caused by left ventricular systolic dysfunction. However, most of the pharmacologic interventions that are discussed in the framework of managing CHF owing to left ventricular systolic dysfunction also apply to the management of CHF caused by left ventricular diastolic dysfunction, with one exception: positive inotropic therapy is specific for patients with left ventricular systolic dysfunction and detrimental in patients with left ventricular diastolic dysfunction. The latter may also be worsened by tachycardia that reduces time to ventricular filling and thus leads to augmented filling pressures.

### PATHOPHYSIOLOGY OF CHF

Independently from the nature of the initial cardiac insult, the left ventricle undergoes remodeling that eventually leads to the clinical picture of CHF (2). The phase of left ventricular remodeling is most often asymptomatic. It is associated with ventricular dilatation, myocyte loss, and slippage (see Chapter 12 for a detailed discussion). As the left ventricle dilates to maintain an adequate stroke volume, left ventricular wall stress increases, and functional mitral regurgitation develops. These factors promote further myocyte loss with elongation and slippage in the remaining myocytes. In addition, myocyte hypertrophy is promoted by the persistent activation of the local renin-angiotensin system with increased levels of angiotensin II and the sympathetic nervous system with increased levels of norepinephrine(3).

The symptomatic phase of CHF is also associated with the development and progression of abnormalities of the skeletal muscle vasculature, metabolism, and mass (4). The abnormalities of the peripheral circulation are characterized by impaired endothelium-mediated vasodilation (5, 6), whereas those of the skeletal muscle are characterized by a loss of oxidative metabolic capacity. From a therapeutic viewpoint, it is important to emphasize that the symptoms of CHF mainly result from impaired end organ perfusion and the peripheral abnormalities in the circulation and skeletal muscles.

## ANGIOTENSIN-CONVERTING ENZYME INHIBITORS

The pharmacologic characteristics of angiotensin-converting enzyme (ACE) inhibitors are shown in Table 11.1.

### Rationale

The activation of the renin-angiotensin-aldosterone system, which characterizes CHF, results from reduced effective vessel perfusion and possibly the use of diuretics. Angiotensin II produces arterial vasoconstriction and stimulation of aldosterone secretion from the adrenal cortex, which enhances sodium accumulation and potassium loss. ACE inhibitors also inactivate bradykinin, a vasodilating peptide. ACE inhibitors inhibit the conversion of angiotensin I to angiotensin II and also the breakdown of bradykinin.

### Clinical Trials

Large randomized, double-blind trials have demonstrated the beneficial clinical effects of long-term ACE inhibition throughout the course of CHF caused by left ventricular systolic dysfunction (7). In asymptomatic patients with left ventricular systolic dysfunction because of a recent myocardial infarction, captopril improves survival, delays the progression to overt heart failure, and reduces the incidence of recurrent myocardial infarction (8). In patients who developed clinical evidence of heart failure early in the course of an acute myocardial infarction, ramipril demonstrated similar benefits (9). In the late phase of left ventricular remodeling and the symptomatic phase of CHF, enalapril has been shown to improve survival and morbidity (10, 11). In the end stage of CHF, enalapril clearly improved survival of patients who had severe but stable symptoms of CHF compatible with functional class IV of the New York Heart Association (NYHA) (12).

**Table 11.1**
**Pharmacologic Characteristics of Angiotensin-Converting Enzyme Inhibitors**

| | Onset of Action (h) | Peak Effect (h) | Duration of Action (h) | Plasma Half-life (h) | Bioavailability (%) | Renal Excretion (%) | Protein Binding (%) | Dose L/R (mg) | Schedule |
|---|---|---|---|---|---|---|---|---|---|
| Captopril | 0.5 | 1–2 | 6–12 | <3 | 70 | 40 | 25 | 6.25/50 | t.i.d. |
| Enalapril[a] | 1–2 | 4–6 | >24 | 11 | 40 | 100 | 50 | 2.5/20 | b.i.d. |
| Fosinopril[a] | 1 | 2–6 | 24 | 11.5 | 25 | 50 | 95 | 10/20 | q.d. |
| Lisinopril | 1 | 6 | >24 | 12.6 | 25 | 100 | 0 | 5/20 | q.d. |
| Quinapril[a] | <1 | 2–4 | 12–14 | 1–2 | 30 | 100 | 97 | 5/40 | q.d. |

[a]Enalapril, fosinopril and quinapril are prodrugs with hepatic conversion to enalaprilat, fosinoprilat and quinaprilat, respectively.
b.i.d. = twice daily; h = hour; L/R = low/recommended dose; q.d. = once daily; t.i.d. = three times daily.

Based on these concordant results and the early experience of the Captopril Multicenter Research Group, long-term ACE inhibition has become the central pharmacologic intervention for the treatment of left ventricular systolic dysfunction and CHF (13, 14). The results of the large trials and published experience with smaller studies clearly indicate that the majority of patients with left ventricular systolic dysfunction and CHF are clinically improved by ACE inhibition (15–17).

## Practical Considerations

In view of their clear benefits, therapy with ACE inhibitors should be initiated in all patients with left ventricular systolic dysfunction and CHF. A few exceptions exist, however; these include patients with known bilateral renal artery stenosis, pregnant women, patients with previously documented hypersensitivity to ACE inhibitors, and patients on hemodialysis who may develop anaphylactoid reactions when treated with ACE inhibition. In addition, ACE inhibition is clearly contraindicated when CHF is caused by critical aortic or mitral stenosis or severe left ventricular outflow tract obstruction.

Therapy with ACE inhibitors can be safely initiated in most patients with CHF provided a few precautions are taken (18). Baseline determination of renal function and electrolytes should be obtained. Overt intravascular depletion or hyperkalemia should be corrected before ACE inhibition is initiated. Because symptomatic hypotension is an early potentially adverse effect of ACE inhibition, the first two doses should be taken at bedtime on subsequent days (19). If well tolerated despite decreases in blood pressure (i.e., absence of dizziness, fainting or headache), the frequency of administration can be increased according to the schedule recommended for the ACE inhibitor chosen. Determination of renal function and electrolytes should be repeated within 4–7 days of initiation of ACE therapy. In the absence of change or only modest change in renal function and potassium concentration, the ACE inhibitor should be gradually titrated up to the highest recommended dose and renal function and electrolytes should be reevaluated.

Patients with systolic blood pressure less than 100 mm Hg, creatinine level more than 2.5 mg/dL, diabetes mellitus, or evidence of diffuse atherosclerosis should be monitored closely during initiation of ACE inhibition. Renal function and electrolytes should be frequently monitored, particularly after each dose increase. Moreover, the dose of most ACE inhibitors should be adjusted in patients with chronic renal insufficiency according to creatinine level. Modest but stable increases in creatinine are acceptable. The rise in creatinine does not indicate renal damage, but rather is secondary to decrease in glomerular filtration to efferent glomerular arterial dilation. Finally, patients who are already treated with loop diuretics or thiazides require special attention because they are the most likely to develop symptomatic hypotension after receiving an ACE inhibitor. When feasible, diuretics should be withheld for 48 hours before ACE inhibition. If diuretics cannot be withheld for 48 hours, because of the severity of symptoms, their dose should be reduced by half in order to minimize the likelihood of inducing symptomatic hypotension. Potassium-sparing diuretics and potassium supplements should be withheld in all patients before ACE inhibition. Similarly, nonsteroidal antiinflammatory agents should be discontinued as much as possible in patients with CHF because they may increase the risk of worsening renal function.

ACE inhibition is extremely well tolerated in patients with left ventricular systolic dysfunction and CHF, but some adverse effects may occur. Cough, which is probably related to increased levels of kinins, may occur in up to 30% of patients and may be severe enough to prevent use of the drug in 5% of patients. Angioedema is extremely rare but mandates discontinuation of ACE inhibition. In these circumstances, angiotensin II receptor antagonists, such as losartan, may be useful (20).

Patients who cannot tolerate ACE inhibitors because of hyperkalemia or worsening of renal function may benefit from combined administration of hydralazine and nitrates. Such combined therapy has been shown to improve survival in patients with CHF when compared with placebo (21). Hydralazine should be started at a dose of 25 mg administered four times daily and increased up to 75 mg if tolerated. Nitrate therapy with isosorbide dinitrate can be initiated at 20 mg, which can be increased to 40 mg administered three times daily.

## β-ADRENERGIC BLOCKADE

### Rationale

CHF is associated with stimulation of the sympathetic nervous system, resulting in high levels of plasma norepinephrine. The potential detrimental effects of elevated circulatory catecholamines include proarrhythmic effects, direct toxicity on the myocardium, and down-regulation of myocyte $\beta_1$ receptors. Therapy with β-adrenergic blocking agents may then result in improved survival and morbidity by preventing or reversing these effects.

### Clinical Trials

The beneficial effects of short-term β-adrenergic blockade on mortality have been well documented in patients with acute myocardial infarction (22). Moreover, the benefits of prolonging β-adrenergic blockade for 1–2 years after the acute event have also been well established, because mortality and reinfarction are reduced by 25% (23). The larger the myocardial infarct and the greater the reduction in ejection fraction, the greater is the potential benefit. The presence of heart failure does not contraindicate careful use of β-adrenergic blockade.

The clinical benefits of β-adrenergic blockade in patients with symptomatic CHF have been increasingly documented at later stages of CHF over the past 20 years (24, 25). Despite the growing number of favorable reports about the use of β-adrenergic agents in patients with CHF, however, this pharmacologic approach has not been widely embraced by clinicians (26–28). The lack of enthusiasm may, in part, result from the close and extensive follow-up required during the progressive up-titration of β-blockade at initiation of therapy and the lack of an impressive response in terms of functional capacity and peak exercise performance. The lack of improvement in peak exercise performance is more apparent with nonselective than selective $\beta_1$-adrenergic blockade. The issue of selectivity versus nonselectivity may also play a role in the mechanisms by which β-adrenergic blockade reduces mortality in CHF. Selective β-adrenergic blockers apparently fail to prevent sudden death, whereas nonselective agents do appear to prevent sudden death (24). In addition, long-term administration of bucindolol, a nonselective agent, lowers norepinephrine levels, whereas metoprolol, a $\beta_1$-selective agent, does not (24). The effects of β-adrenergic blockers on β-receptor density appear to be variable. In contrast to ACE inhibitors, all of which seem to produce comparable clinical benefits, β-adrenergic blockers appear to differ in their action. Although the initial experience in CHF was acquired mostly with selective β-blockade, current data indicate that nonselective β-adrenergic blockers with direct vasodilating properties, such as bucindolol and carvedilol, appear to be the most promising agents for the treatment of CHF (29, 30).

### Practical Considerations

Of the many β-blocking agents currently in use, none has been approved by the Food and Drug Administration for the treatment of CHF, although several of them are approved for use after myocardial infarction. As previously mentioned, β-adrenergic agents with vasodilating properties are currently undergoing clinical investigation for the treatment of CHF. Their approval by the Food and Drug Administration for this use will depend on their overall effect on mortality.

## DIURETICS

The pharmacologic characteristics of oral loop diuretics and thiazide diuretics are shown in Tables 11.2 and 11.3.

### Rationale

CHF caused by left ventricular systolic dysfunction is characterized by a steadily progressive state of avid renal salt and water retention (31). When inhibition of the renin-angiotensin system and a low-sodium diet are no longer sufficient to prevent salt and water retention, the addition of loop

**Table 11.2**
**Pharmacologic Characteristics of Oral Loop Diuretics**

| | Onset of Action (h) | Peak Effect (h) | Duration of Action (h) | Plasma Half-life (h) | Bioavailability (%) | Renal Excretion (%) | Protein Binding (%) | Dose L/H (mg) | Metabolism |
|---|---|---|---|---|---|---|---|---|---|
| Bumetanide | 0.5 | 1–2 | 4–6 | 1.5 | 80 | 81 | 95 | 0.5/4 | Hepatic |
| Ethacrynic acid | 0.5 | 2 | 6–8 | 1.0 | 100 | 67 | 80–90 | 50/400 | Hepatic/renal |
| Furosemide | 0.3 | 1–2 | 6–8 | Variable | 60 | 88 | 96 | 20/360 | Hepatic |
| Torsemide | 1.0 | 1–2 | 6 | 2.4 | 80 | 100 | 99 | 10/200 | Hepatic |

h = hour; L/H = low/high dose.

**Table 11.3**
**Pharmacologic Characteristics of Thiazide Diuretics**

| | Onset of Action (h) | Peak Effect (h) | Duration of Action (h) | Plasma Half-life (h) | Bioavailability (%) | Renal Excretion (%) | Protein Binding (%) | Dose L/H (mg) |
|---|---|---|---|---|---|---|---|---|
| Hydrochlorothiazide | 2 | 4 | 6–12 | 6–14 | 70 | 100 | 60 | 25/200 |
| Metolazone | 1 | 4–24 | 24–28 | 8 | 60 | 80 | 60 | 2.5/10 |

h = hour; L/H = low/high dose.

diuretics is indicated (32). Loop diuretics such as bumetanide, ethacrynic acid, furosemide, and torsemide are more potent than thiazide diuretics in treating the sodium and water retention of moderate to severe CHF. Furosemide is the most frequently prescribed loop diuretic in patients with CHF.

## Pharmacology

Furosemide is secreted into the lumen of the proximal tubule via the organic anion exchanger (33). Similar to all loop diuretics, furosemide inhibits the sodium-chloride cotransport system located in the apical membrane of the cells in the medullary thick ascending limb of Henle, resulting in inhibition of sodium and chloride reabsorption (34, 35). In addition, part of the natriuretic effect of loop diuretics has been attributed to increased renal prostaglandin (PG) synthesis, particularly of $PGE_2$, which is natriuretic (36). It is therefore essential to discontinue or avoid administration of nonsteroidal agents in patients with CHF (37). Suppression of renal prostaglandin biosynthesis by nonsteroidal agents exposes patients with CHF to renal complications. This effect is compounded by concomitant administration of potent diuretics.

Thiazides and thiazide-like diuretics such as hydrochlorothiazide and metolazone, act on the early distal tubule where approximately 5–10% of the filtered load of sodium is ordinarily reabsorbed. They inhibit sodium and chloride reabsorption by competing for the chloride site on the apical sodium-chloride cotransporter.

As cardiac function deteriorates and renal perfusion is reduced, less filtrate is delivered to the distal tubule, rendering the thiazide diuretic less effective. Proximal tubular reabsorption of sodium increased from 67% in normal subjects to as much as 80% in patients with CHF (32). A decrease in renal plasma flow and glomerular filtration rate tends to further reduce filtrate delivery to the distal tubule.

## Practical Considerations

The diuretic dosage should be individualized in each patient according to daily and cumulative net negative fluid balance, which can be estimated from accurate daily weights taken at the same time each day. The dose of a loop diuretic such as furosemide should be adjusted for renal impairment. A good estimate can be obtained by multiplying 40 mg by the serum creatinine level. When the response to a diuretic is insufficient, the dosing frequency may be increased to twice daily. If the desirable diuretic effect is not obtained, the dose may be increased up to 160 mg. Above this dose the addition of a distal-acting diuretic such as metolazone (2.5 to 10 mg) before administration of furosemide should be considered (38–41). Because the combination of furosemide and metolazone can induce massive diuresis, the potassium level should be assessed before the next dose of metolazone is administered. The oral administration of high-dose furosemide (more than 500 mg daily) may be indicated in an outpatient setting, particularly when severe renal impairment exists.

When immediate diuresis is necessary, furosemide should be administered intravenously. The natriuretic effect of intravenous furosemide is brief, ranging from 1–2 hours, and initiation of oral therapy shortly after the intravenous administration may ensure a sustained natriuretic response. When the combination of metolazone and an intravenous bolus of furosemide fail to produce the desired diuretic effect, continuous intravenous administration of furosemide is indicated. The loading dose of intravenous furosemide should be adjusted to renal function and followed by continuous intravenous administration at a rate of 3 mg/hour. Blood pressure, serum potassium, magnesium, and renal function should be closely monitored during intensive diuretic therapy to avoid, for example, the proarrhythmic effect of potassium levels of less than 4 mEq/dL in patients with dilated left ventricles treated with digitalis. In that regard, long-term administration of spironolactone, an aldosterone receptor antagonist, is currently under investigation to determine if it will prevent loop diuretic-induced hypokalemia and improve survival in patients with CHF (42).

## CARDIAC GLYCOSIDES

The pharmacologic characteristics of oral digitalic agents are shown in Table 11.4.

### Rationale

The aim of positive inotropic therapy with cardiac glycosides in patients with CHF is to enhance global left ventricular function and thereby increase cardiac output at rest and during exercise. In addition, acute administration of digitalis has been shown to result in profound sympathoinhibition and peripheral vasodilation in animal models (43). Acute administration of digitalis has also been shown to normalize the baroreceptor-mediated reflexes in patients with CHF (44). The relative contributions of the positive inotropic action and the neuroinhibitory effect of digitalis in mediating long-term clinical benefits in patients with CHF are at present unknown.

### Clinical Trials

The clinical benefits of long-term administration of digitalis in patients in sinus rhythm have been demonstrated recently by randomized double-blind studies of the withdrawal of digoxin (45). In the Prospective Randomized Study of Ventricular Failure and the Efficacy of Digoxin (PROVED) trial, functional capacity deteriorated in patients who received placebo when compared with patients who continued to receive digoxin (46). The Randomized Assessment of the Effect of Digoxin on Inhibitors of the

**Table 11.4**
**Pharmacologic Characteristics of Oral Digitalic Agents**

| | Onset of Action (h) | Peak Effect (h) | Duration of Action (h) | Plasma Half-life (h) | Bioavailability (%) | Renal Excretion (%) | Protein Binding (%) | Hepatic Metabolism |
|---|---|---|---|---|---|---|---|---|
| Digitoxin | 1–4 | 8–14 | 14 | 120–216 | 100 | Yes | >90 | Yes |
| Digoxin | 1–2 | 1–4 | 6 | 32–48 | 70 | 60% | 20 | No |

h = hours.

Angiotensin-Converting Enzyme (RADIANCE) trial demonstrated similar findings after double-blind randomized withdrawal of study drug in patients in sinus rhythm who were already treated with ACE inhibitors (47). Of interest, confirmation of the therapeutic efficacy of digitalis for CHF was shown at a plasma level of 1.2 mg/mL, which used to be considered at the low end of digitalization (46).

### Practical Considerations

The precise plasma level of digoxin that should be achieved during long-term therapy has not been determined as yet. Thus, from an efficacy standpoint, monitoring the plasma level of digoxin is not helpful. It is, however, clearly beneficial from a safety standpoint, because the incidence of digitalis intoxication has considerably decreased since the advent of a convenient radioimmunoassay and the use of lower digoxin doses. Such monitoring is especially indicated when function of the cardiac and renal systems is fluctuating (48). Two oral preparations of digitalis are available for administration—digoxin and digitoxin. Digoxin is the most frequently used.

Thus, the clinical efficacy of long-term administration of digoxin has been well documented with regard to symptom relief and improved exercise tolerance in selected patients with CHF, e.g., patients with atrial fibrillation and CHF and patients with $S_3$ gallop. Whether long-term therapy with digoxin prolongs, shortens, or does not alter survival of all patients with CHF will soon be determined by the results of a large double-blind randomized trial (49).

## POSITIVE INOTROPIC AGENTS

The pharmacologic characteristics of intravenous positive inotropic agents are shown in Table 11.5.

### Rationale

The use of intravenous positive inotropic therapy is limited to patients with acute CHF in whom systemic hypotension and severely depressed

**Table 11.5**
**Pharmacologic Characteristics of Intravenous Positive Inotropic Agents**

| | Onset of Action (min) | Peak Effect (min) | Duration of Action (min) | Plasma Half-life (min) | Bioavailability (%) | Renal Excretion | Protein Binding (%) |
|---|---|---|---|---|---|---|---|
| Milrinone | 1–2 | 10 | 180–240 | 150 | 100 | 80% | 70 |
| Dobutamine | 1–2 | 10 | <5–10 | 2 | 100 | Partial | Unknown |

min = minute.

cardiac output preclude the administration of vasodilator and β-adrenergic blockers, respectively. Additionally, decompensation of chronic CHF secondary to a coexisting illness or excessive sodium intake, leading to a low output state, can be reversed by short-term administration of intravenous positive inotropic agents.

## Pharmacology

Two intravenous inotropes are currently approved by the Food and Drug Administration: they are dobutamine, a synthetic-catecholamine that acts through β-adrenergic stimulation, and milrinone, a second-generation specific phosphodiesterase inhibitor devoid of the thrombocytopenic side effect of amrinone. Both β-adrenergic stimulation and specific phosphodiesterase inhibition share a common final pathway—an increase in intracellular cyclic adenosine monophosphate (cAMP) (50–52). In turn, increased cAMP levels with subsequent phosphorylation of several proteins augment intracellular concentration of calcium, thereby enhancing myocardial contractility. β-adrenergic agonists such as dobutamine activate the stimulatory guanine nucleotide-binding regulatory protein, which stimulates adenyl cyclase and enhances production of cAMP (53). In contrast, specific phosphodiesterase inhibitors such as milrinone do not affect production of cAMP, but they prevent its degradation, thereby increasing cAMP levels (54). In addition to their positive inotropic effects, both dobutamine and milrinone have vasodilatory effects.

## Practical Considerations

Patients should be observed in an intensive care environment with continuous electrocardiographic (ECG) monitoring during intravenous administration of positive inotropic agents. Treatment with inotropic agents should be initiated at the lowest recommended dose and titrated up according to the clinical response of the patient. When available, hemodynamic parameters obtained by right heart catheterization are helpful in guiding therapy. The hemodynamic goals of positive inotropic therapy are to increase cardiac output by 20–30% while reducing left ventricular filling pressure. When clinical or hemodynamic benefits are obtained with intravenous positive inotropic agents, administration should be continued for at least 48 hours, then the patient should be gradually weaned from this therapy over 24–36 hours.

Dobutamine is the preferred agent for patients with borderline hypotension, whereas milrinone is more suitable for patients at risk for myocardial ischemia caused by a critical coronary lesion. Concurrent use of dobutamine and milrinone may be indicated when dobutamine alone, at a dose of 5 μg/kg/minute, fails to produce clinical or hemodynamic improvement (55). The increases in heart rate and myocardial oxygen consumption that accompany inotropic support may precipitate ischemia. Increased intracellular calcium levels may predispose patients to ventricular arrhythmias. Dobutamine may result in excessive tachycardia because of β-adrenergic stimulation of the sinus node, and milrinone may cause hypotension as a result of cAMP-mediated vascular smooth muscle relaxation.

## ANTICOAGULATION

### Rationale

Patients with CHF are at risk for systemic and cerebral embolic events because poor left ventricular function predisposes them to intracavitary flow stasis and clot formation. The reported annual risk of systemic embolization varies widely from less than 1% to 12% (56–59). Evidence of left ventricular thrombus is present in a substantial proportion of patients with CHF. One autopsy study reported mural thrombi in more than 50% of patients with idiopathic dilated cardiomyopathy (60), and echocardiographic studies have reported an incidence in selected patients ranging from 36–50% (61, 62). A significant relationship between the presence of left ventricular thrombus and subsequent embolic events has not been well established, with some studies reporting (58, 59) and some refuting (63) a correlation. Established risk factors for systemic or cerebral embolization in patients with CHF include severe left ventricular dysfunction, chronic or paroxysmal atrial fibrillation, a prior history of thromboembolic disease, hypertension, and diabetes mellitus.

### Clinical Trials

A retrospective analysis of the Veterans Administration Heart Failure Trials (VHeFT) I and II databases suggests that the incidence of thromboembolic events is not reduced in patients treated with warfarin (58). Similarly, five of nine cerebral embolic events in a group of prospectively followed patients with CHF occurred in those receiving warfarin treatment (62). Neither of these studies, however, was primarily designed to evaluate the efficacy of anticoagulant therapy in the prevention of embolic events. Other studies have suggested a benefit from treatment with warfarin in preventing thromboembolic disease in patients with CHF (57, 64). The duration of follow-up may not have been adequate, however, to fully evaluate long-term embolic risk.

### Practical Considerations

Despite the lack of conclusive data, anticoagulant therapy is likely to be beneficial in selected patients from the time of initial myocardial injury, through asymptomatic left ventricular dysfunction, and finally, in symptomatic CHF. Patients are at increased risk for thromboembolic events following acute myocardial infarction, and several studies suggest efficacy of warfarin therapy in stroke prevention after myocardial infarction (65–67) but report a high complication rate when the prothrombin time is prolonged to an international normalized ratio (INR) of 2.5–4.8 (67).

It is important to recognize that warfarin is used empirically in patients with advanced CHF. Until a prospective trial to determine the risk:benefit ratio of anticoagulant therapy in unselected patients with CHF is performed, the use of this treatment must be determined on an individual basis, and patients who are at high risk for events and low risk for treatment should receive warfarin. An appropriate dose of warfarin has, similarly, not been established. To maximize therapeutic benefit while minimizing bleeding risk, however, the warfarin dose should probably be adjusted to maintain a prothrombin time prolonged to an INR of 2–3.

## SUMMARY

Early in the course of CHF, pharmacologic interventions are aimed at preventing, delaying, or even reversing the process of left ventricular remodeling and at improving survival. Long-term ACE inhibition is currently the only proven therapy to achieve these goals. The clinical benefits of intervening at an early stage of CHF, when patients are asymptomatic, are difficult to demonstrate because trials require large numbers of patients. However, these benefits are likely to be much more substantial than those observed at late stages of the syndrome. Current experience suggests that long-term β-adrenergic blockade may exert additive benefits on left ventricular remodeling over those produced by ACE inhibition in asymptomatic patients. When symptoms develop despite long-term ACE inhibition, and possibly β-adrenergic blockade, loop diuretics and digoxin should be added to the medical regimen for symptom relief. The effects of loop diuretics and digoxin on the course of CHF and survival are presently unknown. In the late stages of the syndrome of CHF, when patients are refractory to standard medical management, however, therapy is aimed primarily at relieving symptoms without having a negative impact on life expectancy.

---

## REFERENCES

1. Factor SM, Sonnenblick EH. The pathogenesis of clinical and experimental congestive cardiomyopathies: recent concepts. Prog Cardiovas Dis 1985;27:395–420.
2. Pfeffer MA, Braunwald E. Ventricular remodeling after myocardial infarction: experimental observations and clinical implications. Circulation 1990;81:1161–1172.
3. Schunkert H, Lorell BH. Role of angiotensin II in the transition of left ventricular hypertrophy to cardiac failure. Heart Failure 1994;10:142–149.
4. Mancini D, LeJemtel TH, Factor S, et al. The central and peripheral components of heart failure. Am J Med 1986;80 (Suppl 2B):2–13.
5. Kubo SH, Rector TS, Bank AJ, et al. Endothelium-dependent vasodilation is attenuated in patients with heart failure. Circulation 1991;84:1589–1596.
6. Katz SD, Biasucci L, Sabba C, et al. Impaired endothelium-mediated vasodilation in the peripheral vasculature of patients with congestive heart failure. J Am Coll Cardiol 1992;19:918–925.

7. Lonn EM, Yusuf S, Jha P, et al. Emerging role of angiotensin-converting enzyme inhibitors in cardiac and vascular protection. Circulation 1994;90:2056–2069.
8. Pfeffer MA, Braunwald E, Moye LA, et al. Effect of captopril on mortality and morbidity in patients with left ventricular dysfunction after myocardial infarction. N Engl J Med 1992;327:669–677.
9. Acute Infarction Ramipril Efficacy (AIRE) Study Investigators. Effect of ramipril on mortality and morbidity of survivors of acute myocardial infarction with clinical evidence of heart failure. Lancet 1993;342:821–828.
10. SOLVD Investigators. Effect of enalapril on survival in patients with reduced left ventricular ejection fraction and congestive heart failure. N Engl J Med 1991;325: 293–302.
11. SOLVD Investigators. Effect of enalapril on mortality and the development of heart failure in asymptomatic patients with reduced left ventricular ejection fractions. N Engl J Med 1992;327:685–691.
12. CONSENSUS Trial Study Group. Effects of enalapril on mortality in severe congestive heart failure. Results of the Cooperative North Scandinavian Enalapril Survival Study (CONSENSUS). N Engl J Med 1987;316:1429–1435.
13. Captopril Multicenter Research Group. A cooperative multi-center study of captopril in congestive heart failure: hemodynamic effects and long-term response. Am Heart J 1985;110:439–447.
14. Captopril Multicenter Research Group. A placebo-controlled trial of captopril in refractory chronic congestive heart failure. J Am Coll Cardiol 1983;2:755–763.
15. TD, Katz R, Sullivan JM, et al. Short- and long-acting angiotensin converting enzyme inhibitors: a randomized trial of lisinopril versus captopril in the treatment of congestive heart failure. J Am Coll Cardiol 1989;13:1240–1247.
16. Fonarow GC, Chelimsky-Fallick C, Warner Stevenson L, et al. Effect of direct vasodilation with hydralazine versus angiotensin converting enzyme inhibition with captopril on mortality in advanced heart failure: the Hy-C trial. J Am Coll Cardiol 1992;19:842–850.
17. Pflugfelder PW, Baird MG, Tonkon MJ, et al. for the Quinipril Heart Failure Trial Investigators. Clinical consequences of angiotensin-converting enzyme inhibitor withdrawal in chronic heart failure: a double-blind, placebo-controlled study of quinapril. J Am Coll Cardiol 1993;22:1557–1563.
18. LeJemtel TH, Gentilucci M, Testa M, et al. Practical aspects of ACE inhibition for the treatment of left ventricular systolic dysfunction and congestive heart failure. Congestive Heart Failure 1994;1:32–36.
19. Hood WB Jr., Youngblood M, Ghali JK, et al. Initial blood pressure response to enalapril in hospitalized patients (Studies of Left Ventricular Dysfunction [SOLVD]). Am J Cardiol 1991;68:1465–1468.
20. Crozier I, Ikram H, Awan N, et al. Losartan in heart failure: hemodynamic effects and tolerability. Circulation 1995;91:691–697.
21. Cohn JN, Johnson G, Ziesche S, et al. A comparison of enalapril with hydralazine-isosorbide dinitrate in the treatment of chronic congestive heart failure. N Engl J Med 1991;325:303–310.
22. Yusuf S, Sleight P, Held P, et al. Routine medical management of acute myocardial infarction: lessons from overviews of recent randomized controlled trials. Circulation 1990;82(Suppl II):II-117–II-134.
23. Yusuf S, Peto R, Lewis J, et al. Beta blockade during and after myocardial infarction: an overview of the randomized trials. Prog Cardiovasc Dis 1985;35:335–371.
24. Eichhorn EJ, Hjalmarson A. β-Blocker treatment for chronic heart failure. The frog prince. Circulation 1994;90:2153–2156.
25. Waagstein F, Hjalmarson A, Varnauskas E, et al. Effect of chronic beta-adrenergic blockade in congestive cardiomyopathy. Br Heart J 1975;37:1022–1036.
26. Waagstein F, Caidahl K, Wallentin I, et al. Long-term β-blockade in dilated cardiomyopathy. Effects of short- and long-term metoprolol treatment followed by withdrawal and readministration of metoprolol. Circulation 1989;80:551–563.
27. Eichhorn EJ, Bedotto JB, Malloy CR, et al. Effect of β-adrenergic blockade on myocardial function and energetics in congestive heart failure. Improvements in

hemodynamic, contractile, and diastolic performance with bucindolol. Circulation 1990; 82:473–483.
28. Waagstein F, Bristow MR, Swedberg K, et al. Beneficial effects of metoprolol in idiopathic dilated cardiomyopathy. Lancet 1993;342:1441–1446.
29. Eichhorn EJ, Heesch CM, Barnett JH, et al. Effect of metoprolol on myocardial function and energetics in patients with nonischemic dilated cardiomyopathy: a randomized, double-blind, placebo-controlled study. J Am Coll Cardiol 1994;24: 1310–1320.
30. Metra M, Nardi M, Giubbini R, et al. Effects of short-and long-term carvedilol administration on rest and exercise hemodynamic variables, exercise capacity and clinical conditions in patients with idiopathic dilated cardiomyopathy. J Am Coll Cardiol 1994;24:1678–1687.
31. Schrier RW. Pathogenesis of sodium and water retention in high output and low output cardiac failure: nephrotic syndrome, cirrhosis and pregnancy. N Engl J Med 1988;319:1065–1072.
32. Mokrzycki MH. Diuretic treatment of heart failure. Heart Failure 1994;10:181–191.
33. Boles Ponto LL, Schoenwald RD. A pharmacokinetic/pharmaco-dynamic review. Clin Pharmacokinet 1990;18:381–408.
34. Haas M, McManus TJ. Bumetidine inhibits (Na-K-Cl) co-transporters. Am J Physiol 1983;245:C235–C240.
35. Brater DC, Day B, Burdette A, et al. Bumetidine and furosemide in heart failure. Kidney Int 1984;26:183–189.
36. Patak RV, Fadem SZ, Rosenblatt SG, et al. Diuretic-induced changes in renal blood flow and prostaglandin E excretion in the dog. Am J Physiol 1979;236:F494–F500.
37. Clive DM, Stoff JS. Renal syndromes associated with nonsteroidal antiinflammatory drugs. N Engl J Med 1984;310:563–572.
38. Epstein M, Lepp BA, Hoffman DS, et al. Potential of furosemide by metolazone in refractory edema. Curr Ther Res 1977;21:656–667.
39. Olesen KH, Siguard B. The supra-additive natriuretic effect addition of quinethazone or bendroflumethiazide during long-term treatment with furosemide and spironolactone. Acta Med Scand 1971;190:233–240.
40. Ram CV, Reichgott MJ. Treatment of loop diuretic resistant edema by the addition of metolazone. Curr Ther Res 1977;22:686–691.
41. Channer KS, McLean KA, Lawson-Matthew P, et al. Combination diuretic treatment in severe heart failure: a randomised-controlled trial. Br Heart J 1994;71 146–150.
42. Pitt B. "Escape" of aldosterone production in patients with left ventricular dysfunction treated with an angiotensin converting enzyme inhibitor: implications for therapy. Cardiovasc Drug Ther 1995;9:145–149.
43. Ferguson DW. Digitalis and neurohormonal abnormalities in heart failure and implications for therapy. Am J Cardiol 1992;69:24G–33G.
44. Ferguson DW, Berg WJ, Sanders JS, et al. Sympathoinhibitory responses to digitalis glycosides in heart failure patients. Direct evidence from sympathetic neural recordings. Circulation 1989;80:65–77.
45. Gheorghiade M, Zarowitz BJ: Review of randomized trials of digoxin therapy in patients with chronic heart failure. Am J Cardiol 1992; 69:48G–63G.
46. Uretsky BF, Young JB, Shahidi FE, et al. Randomized study assessing the effect of digoxin withdrawal in patients with mild to moderate chronic congestive heart failure: results of the PROVED trial. J Am Coll Cardiol 1993;22:955–962.
47. Packer M, Gheorghiade M, Young JB, et al. Withdrawal of digoxin from patients with chronic heart failure treated with angiotensin-converting-enzyme inhibitors. N Engl J Med 1993;329:1–7.
48. Lewis RP. Clinical use of serum digoxin concentrations. Am J Cardiol 1992; 69:97G–107G.
49. Yusuf S, Garg R, Held P, et al. Need for a large randomized trial to evaluate the effects of digitalis on morbidity and mortality in congestive heart failure. Am J Cardiol 1992;69:64G–70G.
50. Colucci WS, Wright RF, Braunwald E. New positive inotropic agents in the treatment of congestive heart failure. N Engl J Med 1986;314:349–358.

51. Sonnenblick EH, Frishman WH, LeJemtel TH. Dobutamine: a new synthetic cardioactive sympathetic amine. N Engl J Med 1979;300:17–22.
52. Anderson JL, Baim DS, Fein SA, et al. Efficacy and safety of sustained (48 hour) intravenous infusions of milrinone in patients with severe congestive heart failure: a multicenter study. J Am Coll Cardiol 1987;9:711–722.
53. Feldman AM. Classification of positive inotropic agents. J Am Coll Cardiol 1993; 22:1223–1227.
54. Bohm M, Morano I, Pieske B, et al. Contribution of cAMP-phosphodiesterase inhibition and sensitization of the contractile proteins for calcium to the inotropic effect of pimobendan in the failing human myocardium. Circ Res 1991;68:689–701.
55. Gage J, Rutman H, Lucido D, et al. Additive effects of dobutamine and amrinone on myocardial contractility and ventricular performance in patients with severe heart failure. Circulation 1986;74:367–373.
56. Diaz RA, Obasohan A, Oakley CM. Prediction of outcome in dilated cardiomyopathy. Br Heart J 1987;58:393–399.
57. Fuster V, Gersh BJ, Giuliani ER, et al. The natural history of idiopathic dilated cardiomyopathy. Am J Cardiol 1981;47:525–531.
58. Dunkman WB, Johnson GR, Carson PE, et al. Incidence of thromboembolic events in congestive heart failure. Circulation 1993;87(Suppl VI):VI-94–VI-101.
59. Falk RH, Foster E, Coats MH. Ventricular thrombi and thromboembolism in dilated cardiomyopathy: a prospective follow-up study. Am Heart J 1992;123:136–142.
60. Roberts EC, Ferrans VJ. Pathologic aspects of certain cardiomyopathies. Circ Res 1974;34/35(Suppl II):II-128–II-144.
61. Gottdiener JS, Gay JA, Van Voorhees L, et al. Frequency and embolic potential of left ventricular thrombus in dilated cardiomyopathy: assessment by two-dimensional echocardiography. Am J Cardiol 1983;52:1281–1285.
62. Katz SD, Marantz PR, Biasucci L, et al. Low incidence of stroke in ambulatory patients with heart failure: a prospective study. Am Heart J 1993;126:141–146.
63. Ciaccheri M, Castelli G, Cecci F, et al. Lack of correlation between intracavitary thrombosis detected by cross sectional echocardiography and systemic emboli in patients with dilated cardiomyopathy. Br Heart J 1989;62:26–29.
64. Kyrle PA, Korninger C, Gossinger H, et al. Prevention of arterial and pulmonary embolism by oral anticoagulants in patients with dilated cardiomyopathy. Thromb Haemost 1985;54:521–523.
65. The Sixty Plus Reinfarction Study Research Group. A double-blind trial to assess long-term oral anticoagulant therapy in elderly patients after myocardial infarction. Lancet 1980;2:989–994.
66. Smith P, Arnesen H, Holme I. The effect of warfarin on mortality and reinfarction after myocardial infarction. N Engl J Med 1990;323:147–152.
67. The Sixty Plus Reinfarction Study Research Group. Risks of long-term oral anticoagulant therapy in elderly patients after myocardial infarction. Lancet 1982;1: 64–68.

CHAPTER 12

# Drug Therapy to Prevent Congestive Heart Failure and Left Ventricular Remodeling

Evan Loh, MD, and Marc A. Pfeffer, MD, PhD

Congestive heart failure has grown in scope and importance as the United States population continues to grow and age (1). With an estimated 3–4 million Americans affected (2) and 600,000 new cases diagnosed annually (3), heart failure is the leading hospital admission diagnostic-related group (DRG); 4), costing the American health care system 5.5 billion dollars annually (2). Despite the fact that clinical trials have demonstrated improved survival in patients with symptomatic heart failure treated with enalapril (5, 6) or hydralazine plus isosorbide dinitrate (7) in addition to therapy with digoxin and diuretics, more than 40% of patients enrolled in these trials in the 1990s died during 4 years of follow-up. Furthermore, patients who present with symptomatic heart failure, regardless of pharmacologic therapy, have a poor prognosis, with a median survival of 1.7 years for men and 3.5 years for women (8).

Thus, therapeutic interventions in patients with left ventricular dysfunction are now being aimed at preventive strategies. After the index event that results in myocardial damage, there is often obvious evidence of left ventricular dysfunction without clinical evidence of cardiac insufficiency, circulatory congestion, or edema. Nevertheless, these patients remain at risk of developing overt congestive heart failure. Physiologic data support the concept that progression to the symptomatic phase of the clinical heart failure syndrome is gradual, and once myocardial damage is present, proceeds independently of further myocardial injury.

Symptomatic heart failure is the end result of a lengthy sequence of the "maladaption" of initially appropriate "adaptive" processes, including neuroendocrine activation (9–11), cardiac myocyte hypertrophy (12), myocardial collagen synthesis (13), and progressive ventricular enlargement (Fig. 12.1) (14). After myocardial damage such as that from myocardial infarction, the excessive workload necessary to maintain stroke volume results in initial configurational changes. If left unchecked, these "adaptive" responses to myocardial injury result in the damaged left ventricle further enlarging with changes in morphology and shape in a process referred to as *remodeling* (15). Such remodeling involves left ventricular hypertrophy to preserve wall stress (see Glossary) as the end-diastolic volume rises to

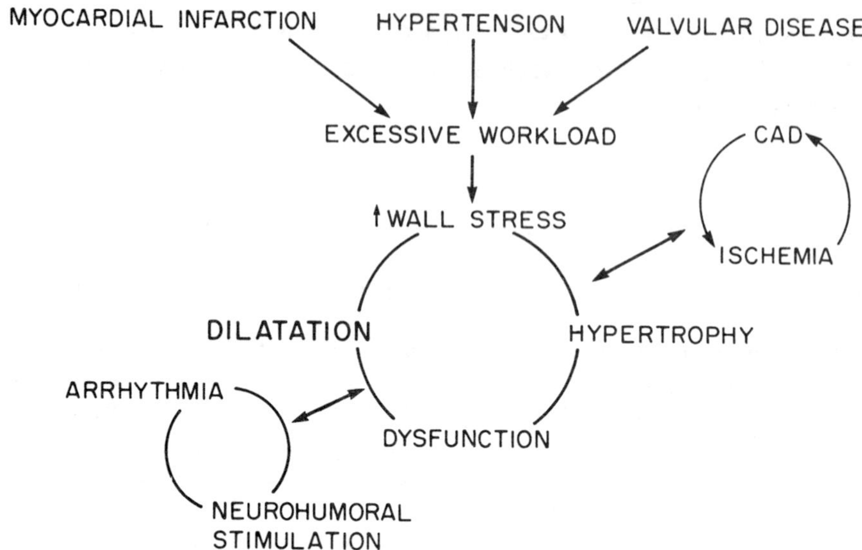


**Figure 12.1** Hyperfunction-remodeling-failure hypothesis. In this model, a hyperfunctional state exists when an excessive workload is placed on the heart, leading to an increase in wall stress that, if chronic, may lead to detrimental changes in ventricular architecture. Depending on the relative contributions of myocardial hypertrophy and cavitary dilation, wall stress may not be restored to normal and may increase even further, leading to a state of dysfunction, and thereby setting up a positive feedback cycle. There are other potential interacting factors, such as the presence of progressive coronary artery disease (CAD) and ischemia, that would exacerbate the vicious circle. Another potentially adverse influence is the relationship of dysfunction to neurohumoral stimulation, arrhythmias, and, indeed, dilation. Reproduced with permission from Pfeffer MA, Pfeffer JM. Ventricular enlargement following a myocardial infarction. J Cardiovasc Pharmacol 1987;9:S21–S23.

restore an adequate stroke volume. However, if hypertrophy does not occur in concert with ventricular dilatation, especially in infarcted areas of the left ventricle that can vasodilate only with a hypertrophy response, wall stress increases, which leads to further decreases in contractile reserve and decreased stroke volume. Once the framework for this pathophysiologic construct is established, it is easy to understand how neurohormonal stimulation can further exacerbate the process, leading to the development of the chronic, symptomatic heart failure syndrome. This chronic neurohormonal stimulation exacerbates the compensatory, excessive hypertrophy with deposition of fibrosis (15). Myocyte hypertrophy (16) may be the central event around which the remodeling process pivots. This chapter presents a paradigm of how external signals are transduced within the myocyte (17), leading to left ventricular hypertrophy and remodeling. These data provide a rational basis for therapeutic and preventive strategies for patients with asymptomatic left ventricular dysfunction designed to slow or impede this apparently inexorable progression to the chronic heart failure syndrome.

## DEFINITION OF SYMPTOMATIC LEFT VENTRICULAR DYSFUNCTION

Heart failure has been defined traditionally and most simply as a syndrome in which the heart fails to pump adequate quantities of blood to supply the metabolic needs of the peripheral organs. For the purposes of this chapter, heart failure is described pathophysiologically in terms of left ventricular systolic dysfunction (depressed left ventricular ejection fraction; see Glossary) with a focus on the accompanying hemodynamic abnormalities such as decreased renal blood flow with subsequent sodium retention leading to pulmonary and peripheral congestion or edema (18). Current clinical practice has confirmed that considerable left ventricular dysfunction may exist in the absence of clinical symptoms of heart failure. Studies have demonstrated that the correlation between left ventricular ejection fraction and maximal exercise tolerance ($VO_2$) remains poor (19). In fact, it is not uncommon for patients with depressed left ventricular ejection fraction to have near normal exercise capacity. Therefore, although the quantitative establishment of a reduced left ventricular ejection fraction is necessary, it remains inadequate to fully define the chronic heart failure syndrome.

The principle clinical manifestation of heart failure is reduced exercise capacity (20) as a result of dyspnea or fatigue. Although there is a substantial cohort of patients with reduced ejection fraction and normal exercise capacities, the chronic heart failure syndrome develops when the compensatory hemodynamic, peripheral, and neurohormonal processes are overwhelmed or exhausted, resulting in progressive exercise intolerance and pump failure.

The chain of events following myocardial injury that occur before the onset of the chronic heart failure syndrome are discussed, and a schema is then proposed for the early initiation of drug therapy to delay the onset of symptomatic left ventricular dysfunction.

## COMPENSATORY PATHOPHYSIOLOGY OF ASYMPTOMATIC LEFT VENTRICULAR DYSFUNCTION

### Index Event

The index event leading to heart failure often involves the loss of a critical quantity of functioning myocardial cells after an injury to the heart. This injury may be secondary to prolonged cardiovascular load stresses (hypertension, valvular disease), acute myocardial infarction, toxins (alcohol, anthracyclines), or inflammation (viral myocarditis, Chagas' disease). In many cases, the cause of the injury remains unknown (idiopathic cardiomyopathy). Nevertheless, myocardial infarction continues to be the leading cause of left ventricular dysfunction in patients who present with symptomatic congestive heart failure (21).

## Compensatory Mechanisms

After cardiac injury, both hemodynamic and neurohormonal mechanisms become activated to enhance the contractile force of the noninjured myocardium to preserve forward cardiac output. Because of decreased emptying during systole and increased ventricular preload, the impaired ventricle compensates to augment its contractile force by the Frank-Starling principle (22, 23). The sympathetic nervous system is activated simultaneously to increase the inotropic state of the myocardium (24). Enhanced adrenergic receptor stimulation increases both the force and frequency of the contractile response of the noninjured myocardium, thereby providing inotropic support for the impaired ventricle. This compensated phase after myocardial injury is also characterized by neurohormonal activation, including progressive increases in atrial natriuretic factor (9) and arginine vasopressin (9), and activation of the renin-angiotensin-aldosterone system (25–28). The potential physiologic effects of this neuroendocrine profile result in an increase in vascular resistance and a decrease in vascular compliance, primarily caused by the effects of norepinephrine, angiotensin II and arginine vasopressin. Other potent vasoconstrictors, such as endothelin (29), are also increased in the circulation of patients with heart failure, contributing to increased vascular resistance (30). Although this increase in vascular tone raises impedance to left ventricular ejection, recent studies have suggested that elevations in plasma endothelin levels are associated with poor prognosis in patients after myocardial infarction (31).

Initially after myocardial injury, ventricular "distension" occurs, i.e., left ventricular filling pressures and size increase without structural changes in the ventricle. Over the next weeks to months, "adaptive" processes in response to neurohormonal activation evolve, which include cardiac myocyte hypertrophy and progressive ventricular enlargement, or remodeling (Fig. 12.2). The hypertrophy of myocytes facilitates adaptation to the loss of contractile strength and unfavorably altered loading conditions of the left ventricle (i.e., increased preload and afterload) to maintain wall stress (hypertrophy) and preserve stroke volume, albeit at a greater end-diastolic volume (ventricular "dilatation") (Fig. 12.3) (32).

These increases in diastolic wall stress induce the expression of specific proto-oncogenes (c-myc, c-fos, c-jun) (33–35) that promote synthesis of fetal isoforms of β-myosin heavy chain, α-actin and atrial natriuretic factor by ventricular myocytes (36–41). Angiotensin II and arginine vasopressin also stimulate the hypertrophic response in myocytes (42, 43). In fact, elevations of angiotensin II may link increased ventricular wall stress to increased gene expression as shown in an in vitro model examining the effect of physical stretch on myocytes (44). The increased wall thickness seen with this myocyte hypertrophic response is initially important as a mechanism to reduce wall stress (LaPlace). In addition, new collagen is synthesized by fibroblasts to strengthen the infrastructure of the damaged myocardium and

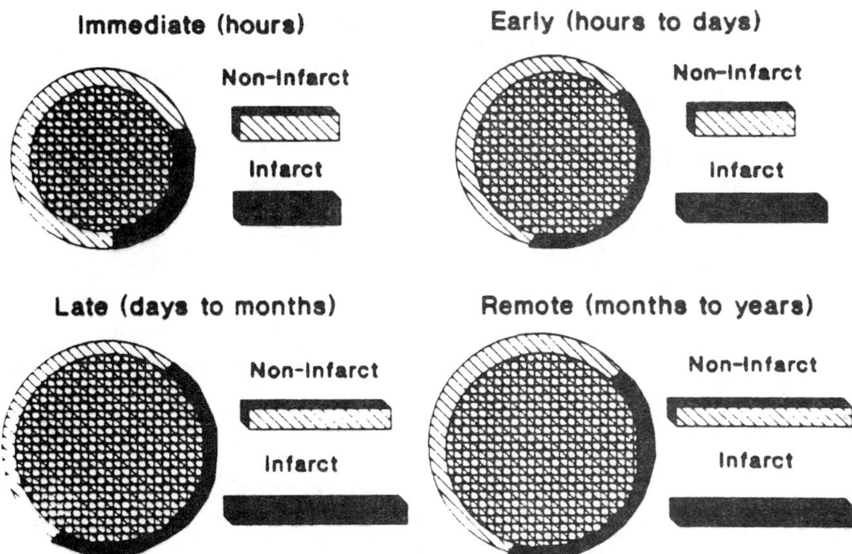


Figure 12.2 Schematic depiction of the serial (early and late) cavity remodeling/dilatation adaptations of both the infarcted (black) and noninfarcted (hatched) regions after myocardial infarction. It is important to note that these changes occur throughout the ventricle, with the greatest increases in wall stress seen at the border zones between infarcted and noninfarcted zones. Reproduced with permission from Rumberger JA. Ventricular dilatation and remodeling after myocardial infarction. Mayo Clin Proc 1994;69:664–674.

to compensate for the disruption of collagen by injury-activated collagenase (13). As a result, these processes are designed to limit left ventricular enlargement and wall stress, thus maintaining compensated ventricular function and preserved stroke volume.

The stimulation of the sympathetic nervous system, observed when the initial myocardial injury occurs, is counterbalanced by the effects of the increased diastolic wall stress (secondary to increased preload) on atrial stretch receptors. These receptors inhibit sympathetic outflow from the vasomotor center in the central nervous system (19). For example, atrial stretch leads to production of atrial natriuretic factor that inhibits secretion of norepinephrine and results in peripheral vasodilation. In addition, in an experimental model of myocardial infarction, the size of the infarct was the primary determinant of the extent of activation and production of atrial natriuretic factor activity (45). Atrial natriuretic factor also exerts direct vasodilator (46) and natiuretic effects on the kidney, which reduces ventricular preload via sodium excretion (47). The renin-angiotensin-aldosterone system is also activated early after myocyte injury (i.e., after myocardial infarction), even in patients without overt symptoms of heart failure (48). This activation results in increased production of angiotensin II, which is well known to induce hypertrophy of isolated smooth muscle

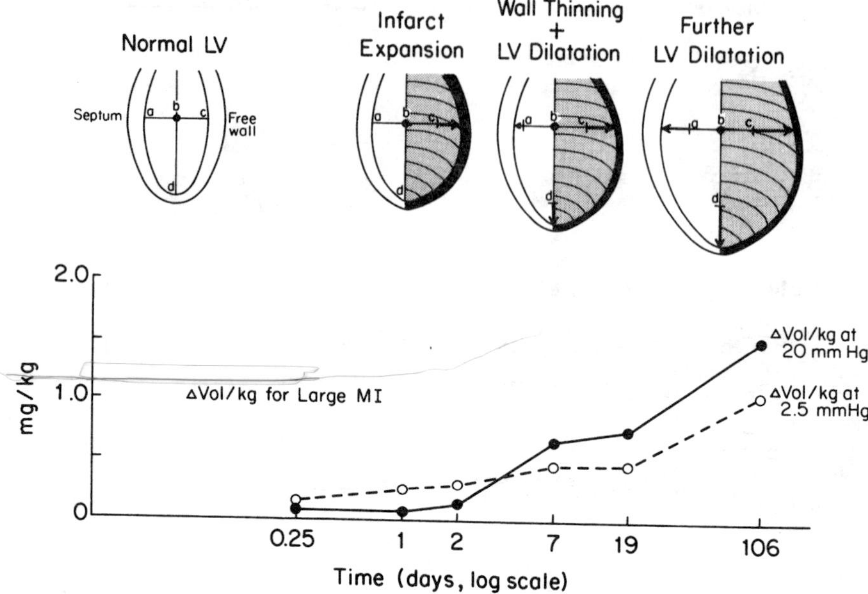


Figure 12.3 Schema of volume changes occurring in the left ventricle (LV) during the early and late postinfarction phases in an experimental myocardial infarction animal model. In the normal left ventricle the lengths *ba* and *bc* represent the distance (minor radius) from the midpoint of the left ventricle to the septum and free wall, respectively; the length *bd* represents the distance (major radius) from the midpoint to the apex. These distances are presented in the infarcted left ventricle as a frame of reference. The directional arrows attached to the normal radii illustrate the extent of the regions involved in volume changes during the various postinfarction phases. The shaded area represents an infarction comprising 50% of the surface area of the left ventricle. The graph in the lower portion of the figure depicts the net increase in absolute volume per kilogram for ventricles with large-sized infarcts compared with ventricles without infarcts. MI = myocardial infarct. Reproduced with permission from Pfeffer JM. Progressive ventricular dilation in experimental myocardial infarction and its attenuation by angiotensin-converting enzyme inhibition. Am J Cardiol 1991;68:17D–25D.

cells in vitro (49), increase left ventricular mass (13), induce myocyte necrosis (50), and stimulate collagen deposition with myocardial fibrosis (13).

All of these data are compelling in support of the importance of circulating neurohormones in the remodeling process. The results of the Survival and Ventricular Enlargement (SAVE) trial (48, 51), however, suggest that the circulating neurohormonal profile of patients after significant myocardial injury is variable, at best, compared with patients who have overt, symptomatic heart failure (Fig. 12.4) (51). Furthermore, recent data have suggested that myocardial tissue expression of the angiotensin converting enzyme (ACE) gene may be an important companion marker of the remodeling process (52). Therefore, the activity of circulating neurohormones may not accurately reflect the extent of tissue activity of the ACE gene. The unique role of ACE inhibition in stabilizing the remodeling process remains speculative.

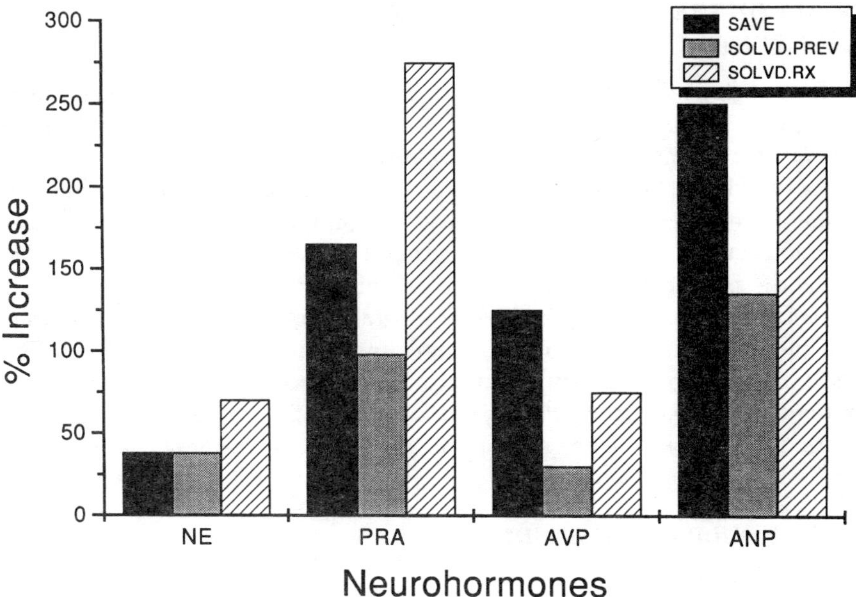


Figure 12.4 Neurohormonal profile of asymptomatic versus symptomatic patients with left ventricular dysfunction. Depicted are the mean serum levels of various neurohormones in two trials with asymptomatic patients (SAVE trial, SOLVD prevention trial) compared with symptomatic patients (SOLVD treatment trial). These results suggest that these levels do differ between the two groups and cannot be used to reliably predict symptomatic versus asymptomatic clinical status in patients with left ventricular dysfunction. ANP=atrial natriuretic peptide; AVP=arginine vasopressin; NE=norepinephrine; PRA=plasma renin activity; SAVE=SAVE trial; SOLVD.PREV=SOLVD prevention trial; SOLVD.RX=SOLVD treatment trial.

In summary, the combination of ventricular dilatation and hypertrophy, balanced activation of vasoconstrictor and vasodilator peptides, and neuroendocrine activation results in a delicate balance composed of preserved cardiac function with a more energy-efficient protein matrix. Patients at this stage of compensated, preclinical heart failure must be identified for early pharmacologic intervention because they are at increased risk for the development of symptomatic heart failure. The goal is to prevent the further loss of these favorable physiologic effects because, although ventricular remodeling may be useful in preserving stroke volume in the early weeks after injury to the myocardium, sustained hemodynamic stress and neurohormonal activation lead to progressive deterioration of left ventricular function with necrosis of myocardial cells in previously noninjured segments of the heart and further deterioration of ventricular function with the onset of chronic, symptomatic heart failure (15). This group of patients, albeit asymptomatic, remains at high risk for developing overt congestive heart failure.

## GOALS OF THERAPY FOR ASYMPTOMATIC LEFT VENTRICULAR DYSFUNCTION

Recent clinical trials have elucidated the goals of early pharmacologic intervention in patients with asymptomatic left ventricular dysfunction (53–56). The primary goal is to prevent progression to symptomatic, chronic congestive heart failure. This end point is paramount to the secondary goal of improving survival. Individuals with asymptomatic left ventricular dysfunction have a median expected survival of more than 5 years (54). Because the prognosis of patients who present with symptomatic heart failure continues to remain poor (1-year mortality, is 50%) (6, 8, 57), therapies designed to keep these individuals asymptomatic should be the focus (Fig. 12.5). A third goal of early pharmacologic intervention is to improve that patient's quality of life by preventing the onset of exercise intolerance, congestion, and edema. This end point is more difficult to define, yet it is integrally linked to a comprehensive therapeutic approach for all patients.

## WHO SHOULD BE TREATED?

### Hypertension

Epidemiologic studies have established that hypertension remains the most important risk factor associated with the development of clinical congestive heart failure (58). The Framingham Study has noted a sixfold-increase in the likelihood of heart failure in patients with hypertension

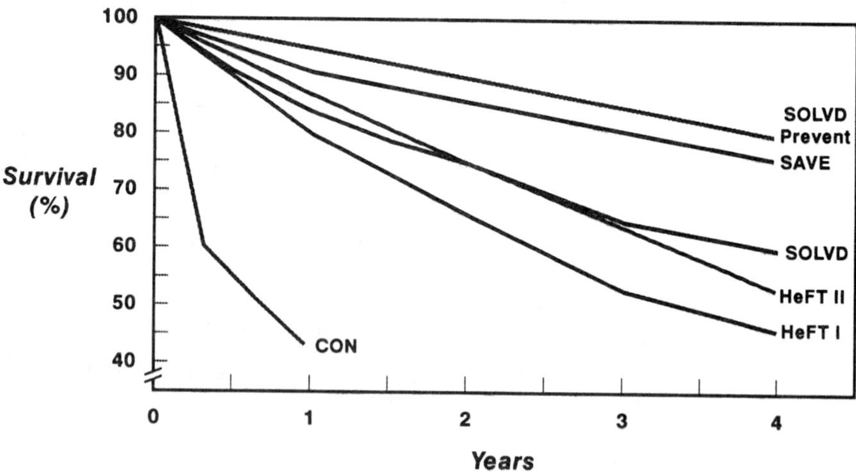


Figure 12.5 Actuarial survival of patients with asymptomatic versus that of patients with symptomatic left ventricular (LV) dysfunction. Survival rates differ significantly based upon the presence or absence of symptoms of congestive heart failure (CHF), as illustrated in this composite figure. This difference emphasizes the importance of the early identification and treatment of patients with asymptomatic left ventricular dysfunction. CON=CONSENSUS trial; HeFT=Vasodilator-Heart Failure Trial; SOLVD prevent=SOLVD prevention trial.

(59–61). Furthermore, a direct relationship exists between hypertension and an increased prevalence of left ventricular hypertrophy . The presence of left ventricular hypertrophy alone has also been associated with a higher incidence of clinical cardiovascular events, including myocardial infarction, stroke, heart failure, and cardiac death (62–64). Hypertrophy appears to be the final chronic adaptation to any myocardial injury whether it is from coronary artery disease, valvular heart disease, or essential hypertension (Fig. 12.1).

Further adaptive responses have been demonstrated in patients with mild hypertension. Alderman and colleagues (65) have demonstrated that activation of the renin-angiotensin-aldosterone system is an independent risk factor for myocardial infarction (the overall most common etiology of heart failure) (21). Therefore, chronic load stresses on the ventricle and exposure to trophic growth factors (i.e., angiotensin II) lead to ventricular remodeling, with changes in ventricular shape and myocyte hypertrophy (66), increased fibrosis (66), and abnormal coronary flow reserve (67). These observations have led to the concept that ACE inhibition may exert beneficial effects through direct actions and not only secondarily through the effects of blood pressure reduction. The goal of therapy is to diminish ventricular dilatation, which has been associated with increased risk for cardiovascular morbidity and mortality (67), thus supporting early and aggressive pharmacologic therapy for hypertension.

Drug therapy recommendations for mild or moderate hypertension remain beyond the scope of this chapter. Nevertheless, findings from several trials support the hypothesis that treatment of these individuals results in substantial reductions in cardiovascular morbidity and mortality, regardless of class of agents used (68–70). Regarding the specific choice of class of agent, several trials (71–73) have demonstrated that β-blockers should be considered first-line therapy to reduce coronary events and total cardiovascular mortality in hypertensive patients. Diuretics used as first-line therapy are also effective in patients who have mild hypertension, with demonstrated reductions in cardiovascular mortality (74, 75). Comparison trials are needed, however, to determine which class of agents is preferred as first-line monotherapy.

### Valvular Heart Disease

Major advances in the diagnosis, evaluation, and surgical therapy of patients with valvular heart disease have resulted in significant improvements in maintenance of systolic function and long-term survival. However, the role of medical therapy in either delaying the timing of valve replacement or in preservation of left ventricular function remains controversial. Regurgitant valvular lesions, such as aortic or mitral insufficiency, share many of the morphologic and clinical features of acutely injured hearts (i.e.,those after myocardial infarction) that have undergone a remodeling process, with cavity dilation and reduced systolic performance. For example, in aortic insufficiency, the regurgitant flow of blood contributes to a chronic increase in left ventricular end-diastolic volume. This increase in ventricular volume is associated with increased wall stress. The adaptive changes of eccentric hypertrophy, replication of sarcomeres in series, elongation of fibers, and increased wall thickness return left ventricular wall stress to normal (76). If this process is left untreated, significant left ventricular hypertrophy with increased wall stress and increased left ventricular end-diastolic dimensions evolve with loss of forward left ventricular stroke volume (77). The final common pathway is the extent of ventricular enlargement.

Several studies have recently defined the role of vasodilator agents in patients with asymptomatic aortic regurgitation. Greenberg and colleagues (78) studied 80 patients with minimally symptomatic aortic insufficiency randomized to hydralazine versus placebo. Enlargement of left ventricular end-diastolic and end-systolic volumes and reductions in left ventricular ejection fractions were significantly smaller in the cohort randomized to hydralazine. In 143 patients with asymptomatic aortic regurgitation, Scognamiglio and colleagues (56) demonstrated that nifedipine therapy (20 mg twice daily) reduced the need for aortic valve replacement for the indications of progressive left ventricular dysfunction, increased left ventricular end-diastolic and end-systolic volume indices and mass, with overall preserved left ventricular ejection fraction when compared with therapy with digoxin alone (0.25 mg daily). Lin and colleagues (79) studied 76 patients with asymptomatic aortic regurgitation and showed that enalapril (mean dose, 31 mg daily) reduced left ventricular end-diastolic and end-systolic dimensions, and left ventricular mass index and significantly reduced activation of the renin-angiotensin-aldosterone system during 1-year of follow-up. Finally, recent studies examining the effect of ACE inhibition on the transition to heart failure and survival in a rat model of ascending aortic stenosis have suggested that histologic left ventricular hypertrophy, systolic performance, and survival were all enhanced with ACE inhibitor therapy (80). This suggests that ACE inhibition of cardiac tissue has direct beneficial effects on myocyte hypertrophy in addition to improving the systemic hemodynamic stimulus for hypertrophy. Clinical studies to address this hypothesis have yet to be designed.

Nevertheless, current clinical data indicate that blood pressure reduction is important in delaying progression to symptomatic heart failure in patients with aortic insufficiency. The use of nifedipine in patients with asymptomatic aortic regurgitation with normal systolic function appears to be beneficial in delaying the onset of symptomatic heart failure. Preliminary data also suggest that ACE inhibitors may also play a role in preventing progression to symptomatic heart failure. Other calcium channel blocking agents with more negative inotropic effects cannot be recommended currently, and these agents cannot be used routinely in patients with systolic dysfunction. Finally, there are no data available that allow routine recommendation of vasodilating agents in asymptomatic patients with other regurgitant or stenotic valve abnormalities.

## Postmyocardial Infarction

Myocardial infarction continues to be the leading cause of symptomatic heart failure (2, 21). Depending upon the residual left ventricular ejection fraction after myocardial infarction, the onset of the clinical manifestations of heart failure often may not appear until many years later (2, 81, 82). Accordingly, modalities directed at limiting initial infarct size during the acute phase of infarction include the early use of aspirin (83) and thrombolytic therapy (84). Both approaches are vital to these patients and have both short-term and long-term benefits on survival in patients after myocardial infarction.

As discussed previously, myocyte necrosis from infarction can result in elongation of the infarcted segment (expansion) (85), followed by ventricular dilatation and associated hypertrophy of the border zone myocardium. Myocardial cell hypertrophy and chamber dilatation facilitate adaptation of the injured myocardium to loss of contractile strength and unfavorably alter loading conditions by maintaining stroke volume, albeit from a greater end-diastolic volume. Both eccentric (sarcomeres in series) and concentric (increased cell diameter) hypertrophy occur. This remodeling process results in increased left ventricular cavitary dilatation in excess of mass (increased wall stress) leading to further depression of left ventricular ejection fraction (15, 86). The increase in wall stress then leads to further cavity dilatation via eccentric hypertrophy, elongation of myocytes, myocyte "slippage" and cell drop-out, and further deposition of collagen, which begets further deterioration in ventricular mechanics. Finally, it is important to understand that the remodeling process is not only limited to the infarct zone, but also involves the border zones of the infarct where wall stress remains high. Hypertrophy, elongation and ventricular dilatation occur in these areas, and contribute significantly to the ventricular enlargement seen after myocardial infarction (Fig. 12.3) (87, 88).

Recent clinical trials have now helped focus attention on the need to identify the postmyocardial infarction patient with preclinical left ventricular dysfunction and to design pharmacologic interventions directed at minimizing subsequent left ventricular enlargement or remodeling to delay the onset of symptomatic heart failure. These patients clearly differ from those with symptomatic heart failure in both natural history (Fig. 12.5) and clinical features, as identified by left ventricular function. Furthermore, this patient group possesses a unique neurohormonal profile at the time of myocardial infarction (Fig. 12.4). Plasma norepinephrine, renin activity, arginine vasopressin and atrial natriuretic peptide levels are intermediate between age-matched normal subjects and patients with symptomatic heart failure (42, 43, 51, 89). In fact, in the SAVE trial (48), plasma renin activity, atrial natriuretic factor, and arginine vasopressin levels were independently predictive of the development of severe heart failure and total cardiovascular mortality. Finally, although currently still a research tool, pro-atrial natriuretic factor levels (90) provide an independent and potentially more sensitive prediction of prognosis than atrial natriuretic factor, norepinephrine, plasma renin activity, or arginine vasopressin levels, with respect to cardiovascular mortality and the development of heart failure after myocardial infarction.

For the prevention of chronic heart failure after myocardial infarction, a small body of literature supports the use of β-blocker therapy. Although symptomatic heart failure presentations remained equal with control rates in β-Blocker in Heart Atack Trial (BHAT; a prospectively, randomized, placebo-controlled trial), mortality rates continued to decrease in patients with and without heart failure over 25 months of follow-up (91), suggesting at least a stabilizing effect of β-blocker therapy on left ventricular function. Further, in a retrospective analysis of the the Multicenter Diltiazem Post-Infarction Research Group (MDPIT) study, although β-blocker therapy was not specifically controlled, in all postmyocardial infarction left ventricular ejection fraction groups, patients on β-blocker therapy were at a significantly reduced risk of developing clinical heart failure symptoms at 2.5 years of follow-up (82).

The most dramatic evolution in the drug therapy of patients with asymptomatic left ventricular dysfunction after myocardial infarction is the use of ACE inhibitors to maintain left ventricular ejection fraction and delay progression to clinical congestive heart failure symptoms. From a clinical efficacy perspective, Sharpe and colleagues (91–94) have demonstrated that initiation of ACE inhibitor therapy within 1 week of Q-wave myocardial infarction in patients without symptoms of heart failure reduced ventricular enlargement, improved left ventricular ejection fraction, and decreased the rate of development of symptomatic heart failure (left ventricular ejection fraction 45% or less). Pfeffer (95) and Lamas (96) and their colleagues demonstrated that in patients with first anterior infarction and left ventricular ejection fractions of 40% or less, those who received ACE inhibitor therapy developed less ventricular enlargement (Fig. 12.6) and fewer clinical symptoms of heart failure than patients given placebo. Finally, other studies have demonstrated consistent improvement in left ventricular ejection fraction at 3 months after uncomplicated myocardial infarction (97) and similar reductions in both mortality and the onset of progressive heart failure (98).

These mechanistic studies suggesting that ACE inhibition preserved ventricular function after myocardial infarction provided the basis for a large clinical trial. The SAVE trial (54) had 2231 patients with left ven-

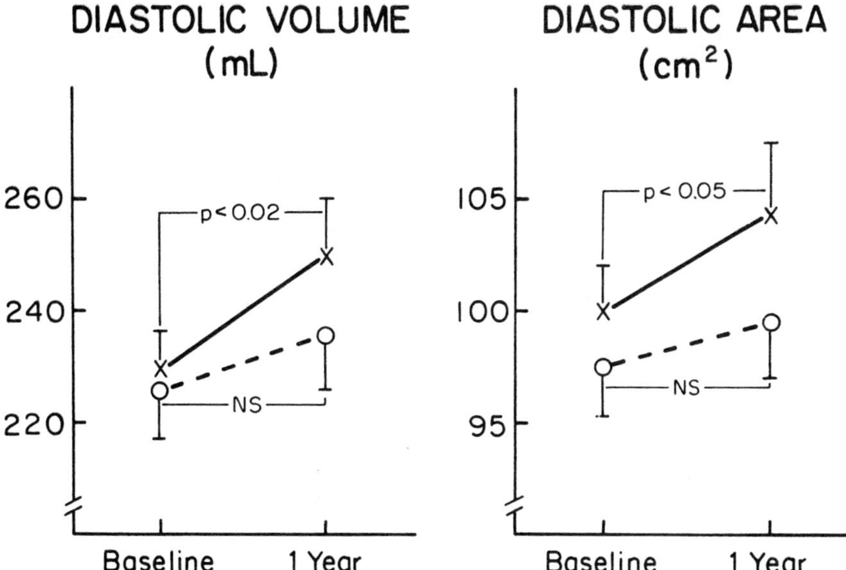


**Figure 12.6** Increases over a 1-year period of follow-up in left ventricular end-diastolic volume and area as assessed by quantitative ventriculography in patients after anterior myocardial infarction treated with captopril (o) versus placebo (x). Captopril therapy decreased the degree of ventricular dilatation over this one period of follow-up. NS=not significant. Reproduced with permission from Pfeffer MA, Lamas GA, Vaughan DE, et al. Effect of captopril on progressive ventricular dilatation after anterior myocardial infarction. N Engl J Med 1988;319:80–86.

tricular ejection fractions of 40% or less after myocardial infarction without symptoms of heart failure and randomized them to captopril treatment (maximum of 150 mg daily) or placebo. Active therapy reduced the following: the incidence of severe heart failure by 37% ($P < 0.001$), the development of heart failure requiring hospitalization by 22% ($P = 0.019$), and all-cause mortality by 19% ($P = 0.019$; Figure 12.7). In the Survival of Patients with Left Ventricular Dysfunction (SOLVD)-prevention trial (55), 4228 patients with left ventricular ejection fractions of 35% or less (83% with ischemic heart disease 30 days or more from myocardial infarction) without symptoms of heart failure were randomized to enalapril treatment (maximum of 20 mg daily) or placebo. Active therapy reduced the incidence of symptomatic heart failure by 29% ($P < 0.001$). In both trials, patients who survived 1 year but manifested symptomatic heart failure had greater ventricular enlargement and lower ejection fractions than those without heart failure symptoms. Both of these trials had mechanistic substudies that supported the prestudy rationale that preventing left ventricular enlargement would be protective from both a prevention of heart failure and mortality standpoint. Both Konstam and colleagues (99) and St. John Sutton and colleagues (100) have demonstrated that therapy that minimizes

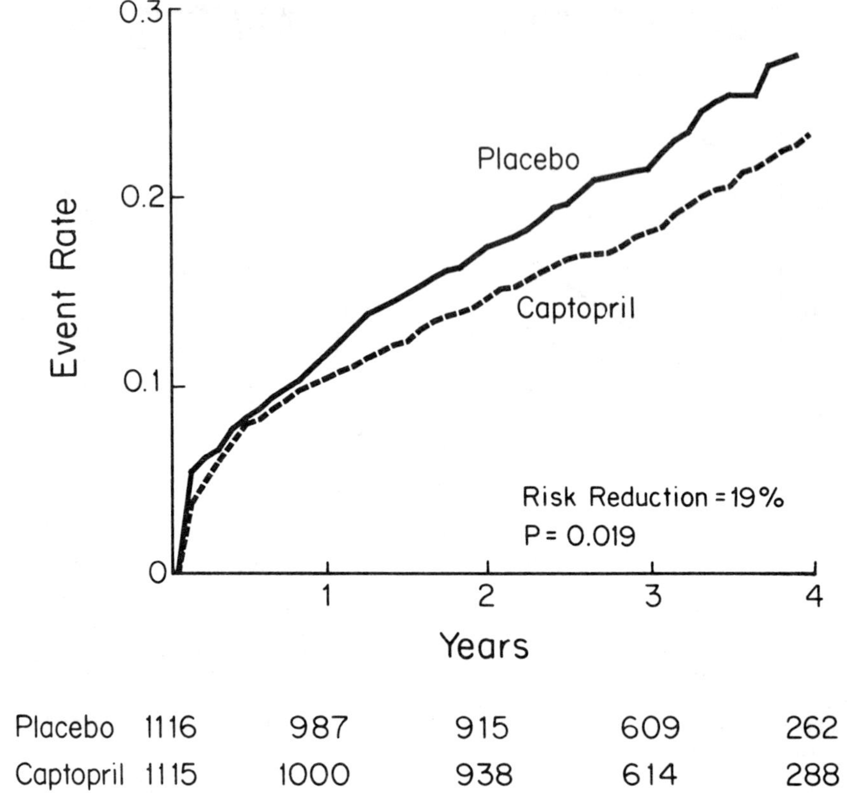


Figure 12.7 SAVE trial results illustrating the 19% reduction in overall mortality in patients with asymptomatic left ventricular (LV) dysfunction (LV ejection fraction 40%) treated with captopril versus those receiving placebo after myocardial infarction. Note that the mortality advantage was not observed until after 1 year of follow-up, emphasizing that the goals of this therapy are long term. Reproduced with permission from Pfeffer MA, Braunwald E, Moye LA, et al. Effect of captopril on mortality and morbidity in patients with left ventricular dysfunction after myocardial infarction: results of the survival and ventricular enlargement trial. N Engl J Med 1992;327:669–677

left ventricular dilatation results in improved survival and a reduced incidence of symptomatic heart failure. Finally, mortality from progressive heart failure was also significantly reduced in patients treated with ACE inhibition in both the SAVE and SOLVD-prevention trials. Taken together, these results strongly support a role for ACE inhibitor therapy in the asymptomatic patient with left ventricular dysfunction after myocardial infarction.

Currently, few data exist to support the routine use of digoxin in patients with asymptomatic left ventricular dysfunction for prevention of the onset of symptomatic heart failure. In fact, 52 patients with anterior infarction (left ventricular ejection fraction less than 40%) were randomized to captopril (50 mg three times daily) or digoxin (0.125–0.375 mg daily) treatment and followed for 1 year (101). The clinical end points were left ventricular end-diastolic and end-systolic volumes, ejection fraction, and global wall motion index. Captopril prevented ventricular dilatation whereas digoxin therapy did not, again supporting early therapy with ACE inhibition. The clinical role of nitrate preparations, calcium channel antagonists, or other vasodilator agents such as hydralazine or prazosin to prevent or delay progression of asymptomatic left ventricular dysfunction to symptomatic congestive heart failure in patients after myocardial infarction remains unclear.

### Idiopathic Dilated Cardiomyopathy

No large-scale prospective clinical trials have been conducted to address the role of drug therapy in asymptomatic patients with idiopathic cardiomyopathy. Potential extrapolations for preventive indications for ACE inhibitor therapy may be gleaned from trials in which idiopathic cardiomyopathy as a cause of left ventricular dysfunction was included, i.e. the SOLVD-prevention trial. Another trial with 170 patients with New York Heart Association (NYHA) class I to III heart failure (75% class I–II; 20% idiopathic dilated cardiomyopathy) demonstrated that ACE inhibition significantly decreased the rate of progression to class IV heart failure over 2.7 years of follow-up (102). Together, these data suggest that for asymptomatic patients with idiopathic dilated cardiomyopathy, ACE inhibition is probably indicated to delay progression to symptomatic heart failure. A definitive recommendation, however, awaits results from a prospective clinical trial.

## RECOMMENDATIONS FOR THE ASYMPTOMATIC PATIENT

This chapter has attempted to emphasize the concept that once the index event has occurred that results in myocardial damage, a process of ventricular remodeling begins with regional and global ventricular dilatation. The progression of this remodeling process is clearly delayed by the early initiation of ACE inhibition, as is the incidence and onset of symptomatic heart failure. Accordingly, pharmacologic therapy designed to prevent or minimize damage to the left ventricle by an "index" event is the foremost recommendation that can be made. These recommendations include therapy for mild essential hypertension, cholesterol lowering, smoking cessation, and limitation of alcohol consumption. If myocardial infarction occurs, the data support the role of aggressive therapy to restore patency of the infarct-related vessel with thrombolytics. Once left ventricular dysfunction is present, recommendations for pharmacologic therapy to prevent progression to symptomatic heart failure include ACE inhibitors, digoxin, β-blockers, calcium channel blockers, diuretics, and nitrates.

## ACE Inhibitors

The most compelling data exist for use of ACE inhibitors in asymptomatic patients with left ventricular dysfunction to prevent the onset of symptoms of chronic congestive heart failure. As mentioned above, ACE inhibition alone in patients with minimally symptomatic left ventricular dysfunction improves exercise tolerance and ejection fraction (53). Furthermore, ACE inhibition prevents progression to symptomatic heart failure and presentations of severe heart failure and cardiovascular death because of pump failure (54, 55, 102). The data are mostly derived from patients with ischemic heart disease, but the extrapolation to patients with other forms of dilated cardiomyopathy seems logical, especially since two trials (Captopril-Digoxin and SOLVD-prevention) specifically enrolled these patient groups.

The left ventricular ejection fraction to use as a criterion for initiation of ACE inhibitor therapy is less clear, especially because preliminary data with ACE inhibition in patients with normal left ventricular function and aortic insufficiency may demonstrate less progression to symptomatic heart failure (79). For patients with minimally symptomatic left ventricular dysfunction, the Munich trial used a left ventricular ejection fraction of 45% or less as an inclusion criterion to prevent progression to more symptomatic heart failure class. We support this as a minimum amount of left ventricular dysfunction for which initiation of therapy with ACE inhibitors is warranted. Specifically, for postmyocardial infarction patients, a left ventricular ejection fraction of 40% or less should be used to initiate therapy with ACE inhibitors. Other clinical measures of increased risk to develop heart failure such as anterior infarction (Survival of Myocardial Infarction Long-Term Evaluations; SMILE) (98) and advanced Killip class (Acute Infarction Ramipril Efficacy; AIRE) (103) should also be integrated into the decision-making process to initiate ACE inhibitor therapy. The dosages should approach the goals used in the SAVE (captopril, 50 mg three times a day) and SOLVD-prevention (enalapril, 10 mg twice daily) trials. These agents should be administered at low doses and increased every 1–2 weeks until maximal doses are achieved, or patients are limited by symptomatic orthostasis or progressive azotemia. Diuretic therapy should be reduced to minimize these symptoms to allow for achievement of these dosages.

## Digoxin

Digoxin therapy in the asymptomatic patient with left ventricular dysfunction is questionable. Despite studies by Arnold (104) and Lee (105) and their colleagues that suggest digitalis may be useful improving hemodynamic and ejection fraction end points in patients with symptomatic heart failure, this benefit was apparent only in patients with symptomatic heart failure (i.e., NYHA class III or higher). Compared with ACE inhibition (101), digoxin did not prevent ventricular enlargement. Furthermore, in a multicenter trial of ACE inhibitor versus digoxin versus placebo in patients with "mild" heart failure (87% NYHA class II or less; both ischemic and idiopathic dilated left ventricular dysfunction), digoxin therapy improved ejection fraction and overall functional class without increasing exercise duration (53). The recent digoxin withdrawal trials (106, 107) have also suggested that this agent is important for at least the maintenance of functional class in patients with symptomatic heart failure. However, the routine use of digitalis in patients with left ventricular dysfunction who are truly asymptomatic from a heart failure perspective remains unaddressed.

## β-Blockers

Although almost every parameter of functional status (108), ejection fraction (109), and neurohormonal profile (110) is improved in symptomatic patients with heart failure, no trial has specifically examined a preventive role of early β-blockade therapy in patients with left ventricular dysfunction who are totally asymptomatic from a heart failure perspective, especially postmyocardial infarction (BHAT) and hypertensive patients. Accordingly, the prophylactic use of β-blockers cannot be recommended at this time for patients with asymptomatic left ventricular dysfunction.

## Calcium Channel Blockers

Specific indications for use of this class of drug cannot be made at this time except for patients with aortic insufficiency and normal left ventricular function (56, 79). Patients in this category should be given either nifedipine at 20 mg twice daily or enalapril at 15 mg twice daily. For patients with left ventricular dysfunction postmyocardial infarction, diltiazem was associated with an increased incidence of clinical heart failure. For all other patient groups with asymptomatic left ventricular dysfunction, these agents await the results of the Veterans Administration Vasodilator-Heart Failure Trial (VHeFT-III) (felodipine) and Prospective Randomized Trial of Amlodipine in Symptomatic Heart Failure (PRAISE) (amlodipine) trials.

## Diuretics

Diuretic therapy remains important for the management of patients with symptomatic heart failure. The role of diuretics in the prevention of progression to symptomatic heart failure has not been examined. Most physicians prescribe a low sodium diet and diuretics to patients with congestive symptoms of heart failure. This practice, although effective and pivotal in relieving symptoms, has never been shown to either prolong life or reduce the likelihood of progression to more advanced heart failure.

### Nitrates

Although nitrates have been shown to improve both rest and exercise functional capacity and pulmonary hemodynamics in patients with NYHA III and IV heart failure (111), no controlled trial has addressed the issue of their use as agents to prevent progression to symptomatic heart failure in patients with asymptomatic left ventricular dysfunction.

## FUTURE DIRECTIONS

Despite the recommendations made in this chapter, the best definition of the truly asymptomatic patient with left ventricular dysfunction remains unclear. Left ventricular ejection fraction has been the operative tool used to date. However, improved characterization of these patients with ventricular volumes (112), neurohormonal profiles, endothelial function, or skeletal muscle function (113) may help in the understanding of their true natural history and in the design of clinical trials with more end points than the gold standard of survival.

Exploration of new classes of drugs for patients with asymptomatic left ventricular dysfunction may yet prove fruitful. Current possibilities include angiotensin II-receptor antagonists (114), synthetic atrial natriuretic factor analogues (115, 116), $\alpha$1-receptor antagonists (117), and endopeptidase inhibitors (118). Each of these agents appears to have beneficial hemodynamic and neurohormonal effects in heart failure patients (114–116, 118), and they have been found to delay or prevent ventricular remodeling in an animal model of heart failure following direct current (DC) shock therapy (117). These agents should be considered for inclusion in future clinical trials.

## CONCLUSION

The understanding of the progression of compensated left ventricular dysfunction to decompensated, chronic heart failure has grown enormously. Clearly, the accurate identification of these patients by clinical or neurohormonal parameters remains paramount because initial studies have now demonstrated that early intervention with ACE inhibition therapy is beneficial. Better characterization of these patients is increasingly important because the design of therapy for heart failure is shifting from initiating therapy only when symptoms exist to identifying patients with asymptomatic left ventricular dysfunction who are at risk for developing heart failure. The implications of these observations are that trials that prospectively test the protective effects of new drugs in these patients would require greater screening and larger patient numbers. Nevertheless, if such trials were carried out, the results would have greater public health implications.

Finally, the understanding of the mechanical and molecular forces that are responsible for the maintenance of asymptomatic left ventricular dysfunction and the processes leading to terminal heart failure will assist in the rational design of drug therapy approaches that will substantively change the natural history of these asymptomatic patients with left ventricular dysfunction. New drug development, neurohormonal modulation, and cytokine research remain exciting areas of future research in the prevention of progressive heart failure. It is clear that we have the opportunity to intervene in this process, to reduce the deterioration in ventricular function, decrease the incidence of heart failure, and improve long-term survival.

---

## REFERENCES

1. Rice DP, Feldman JJ. Living longer in the United States: demographic changes and health needs of the elderly. Milbank Q 1983;61:362–396.
2. Smith WM. Epidemiology of congestive heart failure. Am J Cardiol 1985;55:3A–8A.
3. Graves EJ. 1989 summary: National Hospital Discharge Survey. Adv Data Vital Health Stat 1991;199:1–11
4. Ghali JK, Cooper R, Ford E. Trends in hospitalization rates for heart failure in the United States. 1973–1986: evidence for increasing population prevalence. Arch Intern Med 1990;150:769–773.
5. The SOLVD Investigators. Effect of enalapril on survival in patients with reduced left ventricular ejection fractions and congestive heart failure. N Engl J Med 1991;325: 293–302.
6. The CONSENSUS Trial Study Group. Effects of enalapril on mortality in severe congestive heart failure: results of the Cooperative North Scandinavia Enalapril Survival Study (CONSENSUS). N Engl J Med 1987;316:1429–1435.
7. Cohn JN, Archibald DG, Ziesche S, et al. Effect of vasodilator therapy on mortality in chronic congestive heart failure: results of a Veterans Administration Cooperative Study. N Engl J Med 1986;314:1547–1552.
8. Ho KL, Anderson KM, Kannel WB, et al. Survival after the onset of congestive heart failure in Framingham Heart Study subjects. Circulation 1993;88:107–151.
9. Francis GS, Goldsmith SR, Levine TB, et al. The neurohumoral axis in congestive heart failure. Ann Intern Med 1984;101:370–377.
10. Dzau VJ. Renal and circulatory mechanisms in congestive heart failure. Kidney Int 1987;31:1402–1415.
11. Benedict CR, Johnstone DE, Weiner DH, et al. Relation of neurohumoral activation to clinical variables and degree of ventricular dysfunction: a report from the registry of studies of left ventricular dysfunction. J Am Coll Cardiol 1994;23:1410–1420.
12. Sabbah HN, Goldstein S. Ventricular remodeling: consequences and therapy. Eur Heart J 1993;14(Suppl C):24–29.
13. Weber KT, Sun Y, Guarda E. Structural remodeling in hypertensive heart disease and the role of hormones. Hypertension 1994;23:869–877.
14. Sabbah HN, Kono T, Stein PD, et al. Left ventricular shape changes during the course of evolving heart failure. Am J Physiol 1992;263:H266–H270.
15. Pfeffer MA, Braunwald E. Ventricular remodeling after myocardial infarction: experimental observations and clinical implications. Circulation 1990;81:1161–1172.
16. Morgan HE, Baker KM. Cardiac hypertrophy: mechanical, neural, and endocrine dependence. Circulation 1991;83:13–25.
17. Weber KT, Brilla CG. Pathological hypertrophy and cardiac insterstitium. Circulation 1991;83:1849–1865.
18. Packer M. Pathophysiology of chronic heart failure. Lancet 1992;340:88–92.
19. Cohn JN, Johnson GR, Shabetai R, Loeb H, et al. Ejection fraction, peak exercise oxygen consumption, cardiothoracic ratio, ventricular arrhythmias, and plasma norepinephrine as determinants of prognosis in heart failure. Circulation 1993;87(suppl VI):VI-5–VI-16.

20. Liang CS, Stewart DK, LeJemtel TH, et al. Characteristics of peak aerobic capacity in symptomatic and asymptomatic subjects with left ventricular dysfunction. Am J Cardiol 1992;69:1207–1211.
21. Teerlink JR, Goldhaber SZ, Pfeffer MA. An overview of contemporary etiologies of congestive heart failure. Am Heart J 1991;121:1852–1853.
22. Frank O. On the dynamics of cardiac muscle. (Translated by Chapman CB, Waserman E). Am Heart J 1959;58:282, 467.
23. Starling EH. Linacre lecture on the law of the heart (1915). London: Longmans, Green and Co., 1918.
24. Cohn JN, Levien TB, Olivaro MT, et al. Plasma norepinephrine as a guide to prognosis in patients with chronic congestive heart failure. N Engl J Med 1984;311: 819–823.
25. Schunkert H, Ingelfinger JR, Hirsch AT, et al. Evidence for tissue-specific activation of renal angiotensinogen mRNA expression in chronic stable experimental heart failure. J Clin Invest 1992;90:1523–1529.
26. Hirsch AT, Pinto YM, Schunkert H, et al. Potential role of the tissue renin-angiotensin system in the pathophysiology of congestive heart failure. Am J Cardiol 1990;66:22D–30D.
27. Grinstead WC, Young JB. The myocardial renin-angiotensin system: existence, importance, and clinical implications. Am Heart J 1992;123:1039–1045.
28. Urata H, Healy B, Stewart RW, et al. Angiotensin II-forming pathways in normal and failing human hearts. Circ Res 1990;66:883–890.
29. Cody RJ, Haas GJ, Binkley PF, et al. Plasma endothelin correlates with the extent of pulmonary hypertension in patients with congestive heart failure. Circulation 1992;85:504–509.
30. Wei C-M, Lerman A, Rodeheffer RJ, et al. Endothelin in human heart failure. Circulation 1994;89:1580–1586.
31. Omland T, Lie RT, Aakvaag A, et al. Plasma endothelin determination as a prognostic indicator of 1-year mortality after acute myocardial infarction. Circulation 1994;89:1573–1579.
32. Gaudron P, Eilles C, Ertl G, et al. Adaptation to cardiac dysfunction after myocardial infarction. Circulation 1993;89(Suppl IV):IV-83–IV-89.
33. Naftilan AJ, Pratt RE, Eldrige CS, et al. Angiotensin II induces c-fos expression in smooth muscle via transcriptional control. Hypertension 1989;13:706–711.
34. Naftilan AJ, Gilliland GK, Eldrige CS, et al. Induction of the proto-oncogene c-jun by angiotensin II. Mol Cell Biol 1990;10:5536–5540.
35. Yazaki Y, Tsuchimochi H, Kurabayashi M, et al. Molecular adaptation to pressure overload in human and rat hearts. J Mol Cell Cardiol 1989;21(Suppl V): 91–101.
36. Feldman AM, Ray PE, Bristow MR. Expression of a-subunits of G proteins in failing human heart: a reappraisal utilizing quantitative polymerase chain reaction. J Mol Coll Cardiol 1991;23:1355–1358.
37. Feldman AM, Ray PE, Silan CM, et al. Selective gene expression in failing human heart: quantification of steady-state levels of messenger RNA in endomyocardial biopsies using the polymerase chain reaction. Circulation 1991;83:1866–1872.
38. Tsuchimochi H, Sugi M, Kuro-o M, et al. Isozymic changes in myosin of human atrial myocardium induced by overload: immunohistochemical study using monoclonal antibodies. J Clin Invest 1984;74:662–665.
39. Mercadier JJ, de la Bastie D, Menasche P, et al. Alpha-myosin heavy chain isoform and atrial size in patients with various types of mitral valve dysfunction: a quantitative study. J Am Coll Cardiol 1987;9:1024–1030.
40. Cummins P. Transitions in human atrial and ventricular myosin light-chain isoenzymes in response to cardiac-pressure-overload-induced hypertrophy. Biochem J 1982;205:195–204.
41. Kurabayashi M, Komuro I, Tsuchimochi H, et al. Molecular cloning and characterization of human atrial and ventricular myosin alkali light chain cDNA clones. J Biol Chem 1988;263:13930–13936.
42. Geisterfer A, Owens GK. Arginine vasopression-induced hypertrophy of cultured rat aortic smooth muscle cells. Hypertension 1989;14:413–420.

43. Geisterfer A, Peach MJ, Owens GK. Angiotensin II induces hypertrophy, not hyperplasia, of cultured rat aortic smooth muscle cells. Circ Res 1988;62:749–756.
44. Sadoshima J, Xu J, Slayter HS, et al. Autocrine release of antiotensin II mediates stretch-induced hypertrophy of cardiac myocytes in vitro. Cell 1993;75:977–984.
45. Mendez RE, Pfeffer JM, Ortola FV, et al. Atrial natriuretic peptide transcription, storage, and release in rats with myocardial infarction. Am J Physiol 1987;253: H1449–H1455
46. Wei CM, Heublein DM, Perrella MA, et al. Natriuretic peptide system in human heart failure. Circulation 1993;88:1004–1009.
47. Kinnunen P, Vuolteenaho O, Ruskoaho H. Mechanisms of atrial and brain natriuretic peptide release from rat ventricular myocardium: effect of stretching. Endocrinology 1993;132:1961–1970.
48. Rouleau JL, Packer M, Moye L, et al. Prognostic value of neurohumoral activation in patients with an acute myocardial infarction: effect of captopril. J Am Coll Cardiol 1994;24:583–591.
49. Simpson P, McGrath A. Norepinephrine-stimulated hypertrophy of cultured rat myocardial cells is an alpha1-adrenergic response. J Clin Invest 1983;72:732–738.
50. Tan LB, Jalil JE, Pick R, et al. Cardiac myocyte necrosis induced by angiotensin II. Circ Res 1991;69:1185–1195.
51. Rouleau JL, Moye LA, de Champlain J, et al. Activation of neurohumoral systems following acute myocardial infarction. Am J Cardiol 1991;68:80D–86D.
52. Schunkert H, Jackson B, Tang SS, et al. Distribution and functional significance of cardiac angiotensin converting enzyme in hypertrophied rat hearts. Circulation 1993;87:1328–1339.
53. The Captopril-Digoxin Multicenter Research Group. Comparative effects of therapy with captopril and digoxin in patients with mild to moderate heart failure. JAMA 1988;259:539–544.
54. Pfeffer MA, Braunwald E, Moye LA, et al. Effect of captopril on mortality and morbidity in patients with left ventricular dysfunction after myocardial infarction: results of the survival and ventricular enlargement trial. N Engl J Med 1992;327:669–677.
55. The SOLVD Investigators. Effect of enalapril on mortality and the development of heart failure in asymptomatic patients with reduced left ventricular ejection fractions. N Engl J Med 1992;327:685–691.
56. Scognamiglio R, Rahimtoola SH, Fasoli G, et al. Nifedipine in asymptomatic patients with severe aortic regurgitation and normal left ventricular function. N Engl J Med 1994;331:689–694.
57. Rodeheffer RJ, Jacobson SJ, Gersch BJ, et al. The incidence and prevalence of congestive heart failure in Rochester, Minnesota. Mayo Clinic Proc 1993;68:1143–1150.
58. Schwartzkopff B, Motz W, Vogt M, et al. Heart failure on the basis of hypertension. Circulation 1993;87(Suppl IV):IV-66–IV-72.
59. McKee PA, Castelli WP, McNamara PM, et al. The natural history of congestive heart failure: the Framingham Study. N Engl J Med 1971;285:1441–1446.
60. Kannel WB, Castelli WP, McNamara PM, et al. Role of blood pressure in the development of congestive heart failure: the Framingham Study. N Engl J Med 1972;287: 781–787.
61. Kannel WB. Role of blood pressure in cardiovascular morbidity and mortality. Prog Cardiovasc Dis 1974;17:5–24.
62. Koren MJ, Devereux RB, Casale PN, et al. Relation of left ventricular mass and geometry to morbidity and mortality in uncomplicated essential hypertension. Ann Intern Med 1991;114:345–352.
63. Levy D, Garrison RJ, Savage DD, et al. Prognostic implications of echocardiographically determined left ventricular mass in the Framingham Heart Study. N Engl J Med 1990;322:1561–1566.
64. Levy D, Garrison RJ, Savage DD, et al. Left ventricular mass and incidence of coronary heart disease in an elderly cohort: the Framingham Heart Study. Ann Intern Med 1989;110:101–107.
65. Alderman MH, Madhavan S, Oot WL, et al. Association of the renin-sodium profile with the risk of myocardial infarction in patients with hypertension. N Engl J Med 1991;324:1098–1104.

66. Katz AM. Cardiomyopathy of overload: a major determinant of prognosis in congestive heart failure. N Engl J Med 1990;322:100–110.
67. Frohlich ED, Apstein C, Chobanian AV, et al. The heart in hypertension. N Engl J Med 1992;327:998–1008.
68. Wikstrand J, Warnold I, Olsson G, et al. Primary prevention with metoprolol in patients with hypertension. JAMA 1988;259:1976–1982.
69. SHEP Cooperative Research Group. Prevention of stroke by antihypertensive drug treatment in older persons with isolated systolic hypertension. JAMA 1991;265:3255–3264.
70. Dahlof B, Lindholm LH, Hansson L, et al. Morbidity and mortality in the Swedish Trial in Old Patients with Hypertension (STOP-Hypertension). Lancet 1991;338:1281–1285.
71. Medical Research Council Working Party on Mild Hypertension: Coronary heart disease in the Medical Research Council trial of treatment of mild hypertension. Br Heart J 1988;59:364–378.
72. The IPPPSH Collaborative Group. Cardiovascular risk and risk factors in a randomized trial of treatment based on the beta-blocker oxprenolol: the International Prospective Primary Prevention Study in Hypertension (IPPPSH). J Hypertens 1985;3:379–392.
73. Wikstrand J, Warnold I, Tuomilehto J, et al. Metoprolol versus thiazide diuretics in hypertension: morbidity results from the MAPHY study. Hypertension 1991;17:579–588.
74. Siscovick DS, Rachunathan TE, Psaty BM, et al. Diuretic therapy for hypertension and the risk of primary cardiac arrest. N Engl J Med 1994;330:1852–1857.
75. Cutler JA, Psaty BM, MacMahon S, et al. Public health issues in hypertension control: what has been learned from clinical trials. In: Laragh JH, Brenner BM, eds. Hypertension: pathophysiology, diagnosis and management. 2nd ed. New York: Raven Press, 1995.
76. Grossman W, Jones D, McLaurin LP. Wall stress and patterns of hypertrophy in the human left ventricle. J Clin Invest 1975;56:56–64.
77. Bonow RO, Rosing DR, McIntosh CL, et al. The natural history of asymptomatic patients with aortic regurgitation and normal left ventricular function. Circulation 1983;68:509–517.
78. Greenberg B, Massie B, Bristow JD, et al. Long-term vasodilator therapy of chronic aortic insufficiency. A randomized double-blind, placebo-controlled clinical trial. Circulation 1988;78:92–103, 150, 168.
79. Lin M, Chiang H-T, Lin S-L, et al. Vasodilator therapy in chronic asymptomatic aortic regurgitation: enalapril versus hydralazine therapy. J Am Coll Cardiol 1994;24:1046–1053.
80. Weinberg EO, Schoen FJ, George D. Angiotensin-converting enzyme inhibition prolongs survival and modifies the transition to heart failure in rats with pressure overload hypertrophy due to ascending aortic stenosis. Circulation 1994;90:1410–1422.
81. Greene HL, Richardson DW, Hallstrom AP, et al. Congestive heart failure after acute myocardial infarction in patients receiving antiarrhythmic agents for ventricular premature complexes (Cardiac Arrhythmia Pilot Study). Am J Cardiol 1989;63:393–398.
82. Lichstein E, Hager WD, Gregory JJ, et al. Relation between beta-adrenergic blocker use, various correlates of left ventricular function and the chance of developing congestive heart failure. The Multicenter Diltiazem Post-Infarction Research Group. J Am Coll Cardiol 1990;16:1327–1332.
83. ISIS-3 (Third International Study of Infarct Survival) Collaborative Group. ISIS-3: a randomized comparison of streptokinase vs. tissue plasminogen activator vs. anistreplase and of aspirin plus heparin vs. aspirin alone among 41, 299 cases of suspected acute myocardial infarction. Lancet 1992;339:753–770.
84. Shammas NW, Zeitler R, Fitzpatrick P. Intravenous thrombolytic therapy in myocardial infarction: an analytical review. Clin Cardiol 1993;16:283–292.
85. Weisman HF, Healy B. Myocardial infarct expansion, infarct extension, and reinfarction: pathophysiologic concepts. Prog Cardiovasc Dis 1987;30:73–110.

86. Pfeffer MA, Pfeffer JM, Lamas GA. Development and prevention of congestive heart failure following myocardial infarction. Circulation 1993;87(Suppl IV): IV-120–IV-125.
87. Pfeffer JM, Pfeffer MA, Fletcher PJ, et al. Progressive ventricular remodeling in rat with myocardial infarction. Am J Physiol 1991;260:H1406–1414.
88. Mitchell GF, Lamas GA, Vaughan DE, et al. Left ventricular remodeling in the year after first anterior myocardial infarction: a quantitative analysis of contractile segment lengths and ventricular shape. J Am Coll Cardiol 1992;19:1136–1144.
89. Francis GS, Benedict C, Johnstone DE, et al. Comparison of neuroendocrine activation in patients with left ventricular dysfunction with and without congestive heart failure: a substudy of the studies of left ventricular dysfunction. Circulation 1990;82:1724–1729.
90. Hall C, Rouleau JL, Moye L, et al. N-terminal proatrial natriuretic factor. An independent predictor of long-term prognosis after myocardial infarction. Circulation 1994;89:1934–1942.
91. Chadda K, Goldsmith S, Byington R, et al. Effect of propranolol after acute myocardial infarction in patients with congestive heart failure. Circulation 1986;73: 503–510.
92. Sharpe N, Smith H, Murphy J, et al. Treatment of patients with symptomless left ventricular dysfunction after myocardial infarction. Lancet 1988;1:255–259.
93. Sharpe N, Smith H, Murphy J, et al. Early prevention of left ventricular dysfunction after myocardial infarction with angiotensin-converting-enzyme inhibition. Lancet 1991;337:872–876.
94. Sharpe N, Murphy J, Smith H, et al. Preventive treatment of asymptomatic left ventricular dysfunction following myocardial infarction. Eur Heart J 1990:11 (Suppl B);147–156.
95. Pfeffer MA, Lamas GA, Vaughan DE, et al. Effect of captopril on progressive ventricular dilatation after anterior myocardial infarction. N Engl J Med 1988;319:80–86.
96. Lamas GA, Vaughan DE, Parisi AF, et al. Effects of left ventricular shape and captopril therapy on exercise capacity after anterior wall acute myocardial infarction. Am J Cardiol 1989;63:1167–1173.
97. Foy SG, Crozier IG, Turner JG, et al. Comparison of enalapril versus captopril on left ventricular function and survival three months after acute myocardial infarction (the "PRACTICAL" study). Am J Cardiol 1994;73:1180–1186.
98. Ambrosioni E, Borghi C, Magnani B for the Survival of Myocardial Infarction Long-Term Evaluation (SMILE) study investigators. The effect of the angiotensin-converting-enzyme inhibitor zofenopril on mortality and morbidity after anterior myocardial infarction. N Engl J Med 1995;332:80–85
99. Konstam MA, Rousseau MF, Kronenberg MW, et al. Effects of the angiotensin converting enzyme inhibitor enalapril on the long-term progression of left ventricular dysfunction in patients with heart failure. Circulation 1992;86:431–438.
100. St. John Sutton MG, Pfeffer MA, Plappert T, et al. Quantitative two-dimensional echocardiographic measurements are major predictors of adverse cardiovascular events after acute myocardial infarction. The protective effects of captopril. Circulation 1994;89:68–75.
101. Bonaduce D, Petretta M, Arrichiello P, et al. Effects of captopril treatment on left ventricular remodeling and function after anterior myocardial infarction: comparison with digitalis. J Am Coll Cardiol 1992;19:858–863.
102. Kleber FX, Niemoller L, Doering W. Impact of converting enzyme inhibition on progression of chronic heart failure: results of the Munich Mild Heart Failure Trial. Br Heart J 1992;67:289–296.
103. AIRE Investigators. Effect of ramipril on mortality and morbidity of survivors of acute myocardial infarction with clinical evidence of heart failure. The Acute Infarction Ramipril Efficacy (AIRE) study investigators. Lancet 1993;342:821–828.
104. Arnold SB, Byrd RC, Meister W, et al. Long-term digitalis therapy improves left ventricular function in heart failure. N Engl J Med 1980;303:1443–1448.
105. Lee DC, Johnson RA, Bingham JB, et al. Heart failure in outpatients: a randomized trial of digoxin versus placebo. N Engl J Med 1982;306:699–705.

106. Uretsky BF, Young JB, Shahidi FE, et al., for the PROVED investigative group. Randomized study assessing the effect of digoxin withdrawal in patients with mild to moderate chronic congestive heart failure: results of the PROVED trial. J Am Coll Cardiol 1993;22:955–962.
107. Packer M, Gheorghiade M, Young JB, et al. Withdrawal of digoxin from patients with chronic heart failure treated with angiotensin-converting-enzyme inhibitors. N Engl J Med 1993;329:1–7.
108. Andersson B, Hamm C, Persson S, et al. Improved exercise hemodynamic status in dilated cardiomyopathy after beta-adrenergic blockade treatment. J Am Coll Cardiol 1994;23:1397–1404.
109. Eichhorn EJ, Bedotto JB, Malloy CR, et al. Effect of beta-adrenergic blockade on myocardial function and energetics in congestive heart failure: improvements in hemodynamic, contractile, and diastolic performance with bucindolol. Circulation 1990;82:473–483.
110. Eichhorn EJ, McGhie AL, Bedotto JB, et al. Effects of bucindolol on neurohormonal activation in congestive heart failure. Am J Cardiol 1991;67:67–73.
111. Leier CV, Huss P, Magorien RD, et al. Improved exercise capacity and differing arterial and venous tolerance during chronic isosorbide dinitrate therapy for congestive heart failure. Circulation 1983;67:817–822.
112. White HD, Norris RM, Brown MA, et al. Left ventricular end-systolic volume as the major determinant of survival after recovery from myocardial infarction. Circulation 1987;76:44–51.
113. Mancini DM, Wilson JR, Bolinger L, et al. In vivo magnetic resonance spectroscopy measurement of deoxymyoglobin during exercise in patients with heart failure: demonstration of abnormal muscle metabolism despite adequate oxygenation. Circulation 1994;90:500–508.
114. Gottlieb SS, Dickstein K, Fleck E, et al. Hemodynamic and neurohormonal effects of the angiotensin II antagonist losartan in patients with congestive heart failure. Circulation 1993;88(part I):1602–1609.
115. Fifer MA, Molina CR, Quiroz AC, et al. Hemodynamic and renal effects of atrial natriuretic peptide in congestive heart failure. Am J Cardiol 1990;65:211–215.
116. Cody RJ, Atlas SA, Laragh JH, et al. Atrial natriuretic factor in normal subjects and heart failure patients: plasma levels and renal, hormonal, and hemodynamic responses to peptide infusion. J Clin Invest 1986;78:1362–1374.
117. McDonald KM, Garr M, Carlyle PF, et al. Relative effects of α1-adrenoceptor blockade, converting enzyme inhibitor therapy, and angiotensin II subtype 1 receptor blockade on ventricular remodeling in the dog. Circulation 1994;90:3034–3046.
118. Elsner D, Muntze A, Kromer KP, et al. Effectiveness of endopeptidase inhibition (candoxatril) in congestive heart failure. Am J Cardiol 1992;70:494–498.

---

## GLOSSARY

**Clinical Trials**

***CONSENSUS (Cooperative North Scandinavian Enalapril Survival Study) trial (6):*** In this study, 253 patients with NYHA class IV heart failure symptoms were randomized to receive either enalapril treatment or placebo. There was a significant 1-year reduction (31%) in mortality in the enalapril arm.

***SAVE (Survival and Ventricular Enlargement) trial (54):*** This trial enlisted 2231 patients with left ventricular ejection fractions of 40% or less without symptoms of heart failure after myocardial infarction and randomized them to receive either captopril treatment or placebo. There was a significant (19%) reduction in 4-year mortality in the captopril arm.

***SMILE (Survival of Myocardial Infarction Long-Term Evaluations) trial (98):*** In this trial, 1556 patients after anterior myocardial infarction were randomized within the first 24 hours to zofenopril treatment versus placebo. There was a significant (34%) reduction in the risk of death or severe congestive heart failure at 1 year of follow-up.

***SOLVD (Survival of Patients with Left Ventricular Dysfunction) prevention trial (55):*** In this trial, 4228 patients with left ventricular ejection fractions of 35% or less without symptoms of heart failure were randomized to receive either enalapril treatment or placebo. There was a significant (29%) reduction in the combined end point of mortality and placebo, and a significant (29%) reduction in the combined end point of mortality and new-onset congestive heart failure at 4 years.

***SOLVD treatment trial (5):*** In this study, 2569 patients with left ventricular ejection fraction of 35% or less with NYHA class II or III heart failure symptoms were randomized to receive either enalapril treatment or placebo. There was a significant 16% overall reduction in mortality.

***VHeFT (Veterans Administration Vasodilator-Heart Failure Trial) I (7):*** In this trial, 642 men with NYHA class II and III heart failure symptoms were randomized to placebo, prazosin, or hydralazine/isosorbide dinitrate. A significant (34%) reduction in 2-year mortality was noted in the patients randomized to hydralazine/isosorbide dinitrate compared with placebo. No beneficial effect of prazosin was seen.

**Other Terms**

***Ejection fraction:*** This is a common measurement used clinically to represent the contractile performance of the left ventricle. This is a dimensionless parameter because it is a percent and it represents the fraction of blood ejected from the heart during systole as expressed in the following equation:

$$\mathrm{EF} = \frac{EDV - \mathrm{ESV}}{\mathrm{EDV}} = \frac{SV}{\mathrm{EDV}}$$

where EF = ejection fraction, EDV = end-diastolic volume, ESV = end-systolic volume, and SV = stroke volume.

***Wall stress:*** Wall stress ($\sigma$) in this chapter refers specifically to the left ventricle. Wall stress is the force normalized to the cross-sectional area to which the force is applied. In the ellipsoid left ventricle, there is circumferential ($\sigma$c), meridional ($\sigma$m), and radial ($\sigma$r) stress. The wall stress formula makes possible the calculation of the magnitude of ventricular myocardial loading normalized to the amount of myocardium that is supporting the load. Summated wall stress of the left ventricle can be expressed in the equation:

$$\sigma = \mathrm{PR_i} / (2\mathrm{h}(1 + \mathrm{h}/2\mathrm{R_i}))$$

where P = cavity pressure, $R_i$ = cavity radius, and h = wall thickness.

Therefore, total wall stress of the ventricle is proportional to the magnitude of intracavitary pressure and radius and inversely proportional to the wall thickness. In this chapter, increased wall stress most typically occurs when the left ventricle dilates or remodels (increased $R_i$) without compensatory hypertrophy (increased h).

CHAPTER 13

# Treatment of Advanced Congestive Heart Failure

Robert J. Cody, MD

Heart failure is not a disease. It is a clinical expression of left ventricular dysfunction, occurring as the result of various causes. More than 400,000 new patients are diagnosed with congestive heart failure (CHF) annually in the United States (1), and the number will probably increase as more patients survive acute myocardial infarction with progressive left ventricular dysfunction. The estimated number of patients with heart failure may currently be approaching 800,000 new patients. Treatment of advanced heart failure begins with the assumption that heart failure has progressed from an asymptomatic stage to one of significant symptoms (such as New York Heart Association [NYHA] functional class III or IV), and limited exercise or functional capacity. At this advanced stage of the disease, therapeutic management is intensified, and transplantation is often suggested. Practitioners who treat heart failure find that many patients initially thought to require transplantation because of their symptoms at presentation actually can be managed with current medical therapy. This is illustrated by the fact that many patients who have been cleared for a transplant waiting list can be stabilized for periods of 1–2 years while awaiting a donor heart. Given the limited availability of heart transplantation as a treatment modality, a vigorous effort must be made in the medical management of advanced heart failure (2). This chapter focuses on the medical treatment of advanced heart failure, providing information for management of complex cases of this disorder.

Many factors contribute to progression of heart failure from mild forms to advanced or refractory conditions (Table 13.1). However, the precise characteristics that govern the rate of progression are not fully understood. As a result, the onset of decompensation or refractory presentation is difficult to predict and may be abrupt. Evidence of deterioration therefore must be monitored carefully. Some features that define advanced heart failure, or are a prelude to decompensation, are listed in Table 13.2. In some individuals, particularly those with combined systolic and diastolic dysfunction or coronary artery disease, there may be no warning, and these patients present with pulmonary edema.

**Table 13.1**
**Mechanisms Contributing to the Progression of Heart Failure From Mild to Advanced Forms**

Progression of the primary disease process
- Coronary artery disease
- Myocarditis

Persistent or progressive comorbid disorders
- Coronary artery disease (if not demonstrably the primary disease process)
- Hypertension
- Diabetes mellitus
- Hyperlipidemia
- Renal dysfunction

Progressive geometric ventricular remodeling with increase of end-systolic and end-diastolic volume

Neurohormonal activation
- Autonomic/baroreceptor abnormalities
- Renin-angiotensin-aldosterone system
- Arginine vasopressin
- Reduced responsiveness to natriuretic peptides
- Endothelin

**Table 13.2**
**Clinical Situations that Define "Advanced" Heart Failure**

Progressive or persistent severe sodium retention
Fatigue or weakness with minimal exertion or rest
Frequent nocturnal decompensation/dyspnea
New or recurrent angina
Progressive unexplained weight loss
Loss of independent function
Progressive renal failure
Decompensation resulting from associated medical problems:
- Chronic obstructive lung disease
- Hypertension
- Infections
- Renal failure of independent disorders (diabetes mellitus, hypertension)
- Cerebrovascular disorders
- Anemia
- Gastrointestinal disorders

## GOALS OF TREATMENT

There are several goals of treatment for CHF. These include identification of correctable causes and cofactors, prevention of disease progression, maintenance of physical activity, and prevention of sodium retention through sensible dietary sodium intake. Obviously, some of these factors can be achieved or optimized only through medical therapy for heart failure, particularly as the disorder reaches advanced stages. Treatment of advanced heart failure can be divided into oral therapy and acute parenteral therapy. Oral therapy for advanced heart failure recognizes the need for aggressive management, which includes digoxin, a diuretic, and angiotensin-converting enzyme (ACE) inhibitor therapy. If an ACE inhibitor is not tolerated, combined therapy with hydralazine and isosorbide dinitrate is an acceptable alternative. ACE inhibitors have a more established pattern of benefit for clinical and survival outcome and are therefore preferred. Patient acceptance and benefit can be achieved in most patients when adequate dosage and attention to dose titration are established. It may be necessary to combine drugs with vasodilator properties to achieve desired end points, such as blood pressure reduction, or clinical attenuation of mitral regurgitation. This is discussed in greater detail later in this chapter. Additional issues include control of rhythm disturbances when possible, anticoagulation or antiplatelet therapy when indicated, electrolyte balance, and continued patient adherence to lifestyle factors such as controlled dietary sodium intake (2–3 g) and smoking cessation.

Parenteral therapy typically is used for abrupt decompensation of new or chronic failure, or as a means to stabilize a patient who has gradual progressive deterioration. In addition to parenteral treatment, a patient's oral regimen should be augmented or modified during parenteral therapy (see discussion on management of clinical deterioration).

## DRUG THERAPY

A rational, step-wise approach to therapy can be discussed, but this is often a luxury rather than a realistic option. When a patient has gradual progression to advanced heart failure, the progressive addition of drug treatment may be considered (Table 13.3). In many cases. however, this is not an option and several classes of therapy must be initiated simultaneously. Current evidence supports the use of digoxin, even in patients with normal sinus rhythm. Diuretics are typically required in advanced heart failure, except for patients with advanced cachexia and no edema. Because ACE inhibitors are recommended for all stages of heart failure, they certainly are the mainstay of treatment for the most advanced stages of the disease, and additional therapy is added as clinically indicated. Each of the specific drug classes is discussed below, with emphasis on their use in advanced stages of heart failure.

### Digoxin

New information has indicated that there is a role for digoxin therapy in patients with significant heart failure (3, 4). This was largely supported by specific directed studies, as well as large multicenter studies demonstrating a favorable effect of digoxin therapy. Furthermore, digoxin has additional therapeutic mechanisms including suppression of the renin-angiotensin system (5) and favorable resetting of autonomic tone. (6) In determining whether digoxin therapy is optimal for a given patient, the

**Table 13.3**
**Drugs for Long-term Treatment of Advanced Heart Failure**

| |
|---|
| Digoxin |
| Diuretics |
| Loop |
| Thiazide[a] |
| K sparing[a] |
| Ace inhibitors[b] |
| Captopril |
| Enalapril |
| Lisinopril |
| Quinapril |
| Vasodilators |
| Hydralazine/isosorbide |
| Rhythm management[c] |
| Atrial |
| Ventricular |
| Anticoagulation |
| Warfarin |
| Aspirin |
| Electrolyte management |
| Potassium replacement |
| Magnesium replacement |

[a]Diuretics in these groups are usually used in combination with a loop diuretic.
[b]Others may be approved in the near future.
[c]Treatment is complex and must be individualized.

factors to be considered include institution of standard dosage, indexing this to a serum digoxin level when appropriate. Another important consideration is adequate absorption. A patient may be stable on digoxin for months or even years; with progressive decompensation and advanced status, however, absorption can be adversely affected.

Based on recent clinical trials, the standard digoxin dosage is 0.125 or 0.25 mg daily. Reduction of the dose to an every other day regimen is recommended for patients with significant renal disease (serum creatinine more than 2.5–3.0 mg/dL), the elderly, or patients receiving other drugs that interfere with the metabolism of digoxin. When digoxin is administered for the first time, a loading dose given either orally or intravenously is still required, irrespective of the ultimate oral dose. In patients with atrial fibrillation or advanced heart failure, digoxin dosage may be increased to 0.375 mg daily. Routine surveillance of digoxin levels is generally not required when routine doses are used. If a patient requires dose reduction for the concomitant conditions discussed earlier, or the dosage is increased in problematic patients, routine surveillance of serum levels may then be required. In the latter situation, attention must be given to the timing of serum sampling to avoid erroneous or spurious recording of serum levels. Serum levels are of less clinical importance in patients with atrial fibrillation, in whom the end point of treatment is control of the ventricular response rather than a specific drug level. Digitoxin is a more desirable preparation in heart failure patients because of its hepatic metabolism; thus, concerns regarding renal dysfunction are less important. However, because digoxin is used by most physicians, introduction of digitoxin in a random fashion will increase the risk of error in drug prescription and dosage. When acute decompensation occurs or when oral intake is otherwise compromised, patients should be given the drug intravenously. Withholding therapy for a short period of time (2–3 days) is generally without consequence in patients with normal sinus rhythm. In patients with atrial fibrillation, an increase of ventricular response can be seen even with limited withdrawal. In addition, data from the Randomized Assessment of (the effect of) Digoxin on Inhibitors of the Angiotensin-Converting Enzyme (RADIANCE) and Prospective Randomized Study of Ventricular Failure and the Efficacy of Digoxin (PROVED) trials clearly demonstrate clinical deterioration when digoxin is withheld (7, 8). The trials were similar in design and purpose; both tested the hypothesis that withdrawal of digoxin would result in clinical and functional deterioration. In each trial, patients receiving long-term digoxin therapy, in addition to an ACE inhibitor and diuretic as needed, were randomized in double-blind fashion to continue digoxin or receive placebo. Clinical status and exercise tolerance were prospectively assessed. In each study, withdrawal of digoxin (placebo group) was associated with deterioration of exercise tolerance and worsening of NYHA functional class, compared with patients who continued on digoxin therapy. The mechanism for deterioration is not known. However, in view of the effects of digoxin on ventricular contractile performance, baroreceptor function, and the renin-angiotensin system, the mechanism may be multifactorial. Because exercise performance deteriorated as early as 1 month after digoxin withdrawal, structural cardiovascular changes are less likely than functional or neurohormonal causes. In current heart failure trials, improved survival has become a primary end point of evaluation. A clinical trial currently in progress (digoxin investigator's group, DIG) is assessing whether digoxin therapy has an adverse effect on survival during long-term use.

## Other Inotropic Agents

There are no alternative oral inotropic agents available for the treatment of heart failure, and the use of these agents is currently limited to parenteral intravenous administration. In patients with advanced heart failure oral milrinone was associated with a higher mortality rate than placebo in the Prospective Randomized Milrinone Survival Evaluation (PROMISE) trial; therefore, it was withdrawn from development. Pimobendan, an inotrope with calcium-sensitizing properties, was also withdrawn from development because of the PROMISE trial, but it may re-enter developmental studies. Vesnarinone, a positive inotropic agent, demonstrated initial benefit in clinical trials; however, concerns regarding dosage and clinical outcome persist, and it remains in development. Vesnarinone also can produce neutropenia, and cases of agranulocytosis have been reported.

## Diuretics

Although the appropriateness of diuretics in patients with asymptomatic or mild left ventricular dysfunction is currently debated (10, 11), their use in patients with advanced or refractory heart failure is accepted (12). Patients with advanced heart failure will require diuretics, with few exceptions (Table 13.4). Renal insufficiency and aging may influence a patient with CHF to become resistant to diuretics (13, 14). Furthermore, concomitant therapy with noncardiac drugs that affect renal function such as nonsalicylate antiinflammatory drugs and indomethacin can also attenuate the response to diuretics. Because renal dysfunction progresses gradually, a diuretic response may become progressively attenuated. Edema of the gastrointestinal tract can also reduce drug absorption, thereby limiting efficacy. Different classes of diuretic agents may act at different locations within the nephron, so that combination therapy may be appropriate in the patient with developing refractory heart failure. A patient should not be considered refractory to diuretic therapy if only moderate doses of an oral loop diuretic are being given. There are several approaches to the management of resistance to diuretics that can aid in the optimization of diuretic therapy for the refractory heart failure patient (15, 16). A single large bolus of intravenous diuretics may substantially improve urinary flow and natriuresis. An alternative approach is frequent administration of smaller, effective intravenous doses to achieve a cumulative effect. Although not typically used in practice, continuous intravenous infusion of a loop diuretic also may be efficacious (17, 18).

Perhaps the most versatile and effective approach is the combination of a loop diuretic with a thiazide diuretic (15, 16, 19, 20). Long-standing

**Table 13.4**
**Diuretic Therapy for Advanced Heart Failure**

Restrict sodium to a normal 2–3 g intake (80–120 mEq)
*plus*
Loop diuretic, adjusting for renal function if necessary

*If Unsatisfactory Response, Progress To:*
Loop diuretic combined with an intermittent thiazide diuretic
*or*
Loop diuretic combined with a thiazide or potassium-sparing diuretic

*Treatment Measures for Refractory Sodium Retention*
Intermittent intravenous loop diuretic
Continous intravenous infusion of a loop diuretic
Intensified combination therapy
Ultrafiltration or dialysis

treatment with a loop diuretic can result in hypertrophy of the distal segment of the nephron (21, 22), producing enhanced sodium reabsorption. This can often attenuate the previous favorable response to a loop diuretic. Coadministration of a thiazide diuretic that acts at the distal nephron can therefore result in a substantial increase of net sodium and water excretion. Intermittent outpatient intravenous loop diuretic therapy should also be considered because not all patients with severe sodium retention require hospitalization. If the patient can be brought to an outpatient area where an intravenous loop diuretic can be administered, sufficient diuresis may be achieved without hospitalization. This would also be particularly effective in the holding area of an emergency room.

Continued moderate sodium intake is important to prevent or manage advanced CHF. The "normal" sodium requirement in humans is defined as 2–3 g of sodium (80–120 mEq), which is quite palatable. Data from experimental animal models and humans demonstrate that the response to a loop diuretic can be overcome with ad lib sodium intake (21, 23) compared with animals in whom sodium intake is restricted (19). Insistence that a patient ingest a normal sodium diet, as defined above, enables the patient to participate in the therapeutic process. Other clinical studies have shown that functional impairment and ability to excrete sodium in response to a saline challenge also correlate best with hemodynamic and neurohormonal indices of heart failure severity (24). If the patient remains resistant to diuretics, additional factors such as intensification of combined therapy can be considered. Combination therapy may include adding up to three diuretics that potentially act at different sites of the nephron such as a loop diuretic, thiazide diuretic, and amiloride or spironolactone. Although typically not required for refractory heart failure, ultrafiltration, hemofiltration, hemodialysis, or peritoneal dialysis can be used for rapid removal of fluid (25–27). These modalities are obviously important for CHF that accompanies chronic renal failure.

The site of action of diuretics and their specific pharmacokinetic and cellular actions have been summarized elsewhere (15, 16, 28, 29). Although each diuretic may have altered pharmacokinetics and pharmacodynamics in heart failure, furosemide is highlighted to show the changes that occur in the heart failure process. It should be noted that the renal tubular urine concentration of a diuretic is the actual amount of the drug delivered to its primary site of action, rather than simply a measure of drug excretion. Consequently, route of administration and blood concentration affect diuretic effectiveness only to the extent that they influence the delivery of effective concentrations of the diuretic to the site of action within the tubular lumen. Compared with normal subjects, the rate of sodium excretion in heart failure patients is reduced at any given renal tubular furosemide concentration (30). In view of these changes, the ceiling dose of a loop diuretic in heart failure should be considered twice that of normal subjects.

Hypertrophy of the distal tubule occurs, whereby the sodium that was inhibited at the thick ascending limb of the loop of Henle is ultimately reabsorbed at the distal portion of the tubule. Changes in both of these properties have been demonstrated with furosemide and bumetanide. The pharmacokinetics of thiazide diuretics can also be abnormal in CHF. As with loop diuretics, the changes include a prolonged absorption phase and a time delay to peak concentration in the urine after oral administration (15, 16), resulting in a slower onset and a longer duration of action. For instance, metolazone absorption can be substantially reduced, requiring several days to achieve adequate urinary concentration.

Increases in both plasma renin activity and plasma norepinephrine have been demonstrated with acute intravenous administration (31, 32) and short-term oral treatment (10, 11, 31) with diuretics. Aldosterone responses parallel those of renin. Increased renin release may be related to a direct effect on the macula densa, activation of baroreceptor control of renin release, and diuretic-induced volume contraction. Important consequences of neurohormonal stimulation include increased secretion of renin, which also leads to increased aldosterone secretion. Augmentation of sympathetic activity, reflected by increased plasma catecholamines, is observed in some, but not all, studies of diuretics. Whether this reflects a true adverse effect of diuretics has not been adequately evaluated. It should also be remembered that the neurohormonal abnormalities reported with diuretics preceded the more widespread use of ACE inhibitors. Reduction of diuretic dosage in this setting should reduce the extent of neurohormonal activation, but this requires prospective evaluation.

Electrolyte disorders are the most common adverse effect of all diuretics (15, 16, 28, 29). Long-term diuretic use may produce hypokalemia, hyponatremia, hypocalcemia, hypomagnesemia, hyperuricemia, and metabolic alkalosis (15, 16, 33). Electrolyte abnormalities have diverse clinical presentations. For example, hypokalemia and hypomagnesemia may be associated with myalgias, leg cramps, and an increase in ventricular arrhythmias. The increase in ventricular arrhythmias may be associated with an increase in the incidence of sudden arrhythmic death, particularly in patients treated with digoxin (34, 35).

The predisposition for electrolyte abnormalities in CHF is the result of both the underlying pathophysiology and the concurrent administration of diuretic therapy. The pathologic factors predisposing to electrolyte abnormalities include abnormal neurohormonal activation and marked reduction of renal blood flow and function. Although hyponatremia, a hallmark of CHF, is well correlated with activation of the renin system, it is also stimulated as a result of enhanced vasopressin activity, which reduces free water clearance and, in conjunction with uncontrolled sodium intake, results in hyponatremia. Diuretic therapy intensifies these electrolyte abnormalities. First, diuretic therapy can result in further activation of the renin angiotensin system. Second, by increasing the renal tubular load of electrolytes, through electrolyte transport inhibition, diuretics produce an indiscriminate wasting of electrolytes. The use of potassium-sparing diuretics in combination with loop or thiazide diuretics limits the excessive potassium and magnesium. Few controlled studies, however, have evaluated the efficacy of addition of potassium-sparing diuretics in this setting.

The most common electrolyte abnormality is hypokalemia (16). Usually, diuretic-induced hypokalemia is associated with a metabolic alkalosis and a coexisting chloride deficit. Therefore, chloride is the preferred salt of potassium over the gluconate or bicarbonate for supplementation in this setting (36). Intravenous administration of potassium is recommended to correct moderate to severe potassium deficits, with or without the occurrence of cardiac arrhythmias. This route is also useful when oral replacement is not feasible or not tolerated because of a decrease in gastrointestinal motility. Oral, slow-release potassium chloride preparations are employed in the long-term management of diuretic-induced hypokalemia. Patient preference and cost should be considered in product selection. The dosage of potassium chloride is adjusted on an individual basis and depends on the use of other medications, such as ACE inhibitors or concomitant diuretics. Generally, patients require between 40–120 mEq/day to maintain potassium homeostasis.

Long-term diuretic therapy with loop and thiazide diuretics also leads to hypomagnesemia (16, 37). Magnesium, primarily an intracellular ion, plays a pivotal role in mitochondrial functions, oxidation-phosphorylation reaction, and neuromuscular transmission (16). Potassium and magnesium have a interrelationship whereas magnesium is a cofactor in the appropriate function of the sodium-potassium ATPase pump. Therefore, hypokalemia may persist until the magnesium deficiency is corrected (38). Although normal serum magnesium concentrations range from 1.6–2.0 mEq/L, only 1% of the ion is found in the extracellular space, with the remainder occurring in bone, muscle, and other soft tissues (39). Consequently, serum and urinary concentrations do not accurately reflect the total body content (40). Intravenous supplementation is essential in the presence of cardiac arrhythmias. Administration of 2–5 g (equal to 16–40 mEq) of magnesium sulfate by slow intravenous infusion, at 1 g/hour, to be repeated in 12 hours if needed, should yield a better end result. Oral dosing of magnesium poses a problem because all of the salt forms are poorly absorbed and frequently associated with diarrhea when administered in large amounts. Maintenance regimens frequently used are 14 mEq of magnesium administered 4 times a day based on patients with normal gastrointestinal and renal function (39, 40).

Intravenous diuretic therapy may be used acutely in several clinical situations. In pulmonary edema, acute intravenous diuretic therapy results in the rapid clearance of pulmonary congestion. Because subacute decompensation is a prelude to pulmonary edema, the goals of intravenous diuretic therapy are similar to those of treatment of pulmonary edema. Acute intravenous diuretic therapy may also be used to supplement chronic oral therapy for sodium retention, to augment outpatient. For acute reversal of sodium retention and fluid overload, therapy with a loop diuretic is indicated. It should be administered intravenously, to a ceiling dose that is twice the normal dose (e.g., furosemide 80 mg; bumetanide 2 mg) and increased as necessary, in combination with other agents. A thiazide diuretic combined with a loop diuretic is often very effective. However, an oral thiazide-type diuretic, particularly metolazone, may require several days to achieve its maximal favorable response, because of delayed absorption. The ability to use intravenous chlorothiazide (Diuril; Merck and Company, West Point, Pennsylvania) is often overlooked. Unlike hydrochlorothiazide, chlorothiazide can be administered intravenously in a dose of 250–500 mg, which is equivalent to oral hydrochlorothiazide dosage of 25–50 mg; when combined with a loop diuretic, it produces greater diuresis than that caused by the loop diuretic alone.

In view of the results of several clinical trials of heart failure, there is clear evidence for the use of ACE inhibitors at all stages of heart failure. Although ACE inhibitors block the secretion of aldosterone, they should not be considered "diuretics." Clinical studies demonstrate the lack of efficacy of ACE inhibitors as primary diuretic therapy. The clinical response to ACE inhibitors may be inadequate when it is administered as single therapy (41–43), and the coadministration of diuretics is required. For relief of edema and congestive symptoms, diuretic therapy alone is more effective than an ACE inhibitor (41).

## ACE Inhibitors

Recent insights into the mechanisms underlying progressive myocardial dysfunction (44) support a beneficial role for ACE inhibitors in attenuating the neurohormonal abnormalities that characterize CHF (45–47). Large-scale survival studies provide practical evidence that the addition of enalapril or captopril to conventional therapy with diuretics and digoxin can significantly reduce the number of hospitalizations and risk of death attributable to progressive CHF. The clinical and hemodynamic benefits of ACE inhibitors in CHF and hypertension have been firmly established (48–51). ACE inhibitors reduce systemic vascular resistance and blood pressure, lower left ventricular filling pressure, and improve ventricular function. They also improve clinical signs and symptoms, exercise tolerance, and NYHA functional class in patients with moderate to severe CHF treated with diuretics or digitalis. ACE inhibitors also slow the onset of symptomatic CHF and clinical progression in those patients with mild CHF. ACE inhibitors have been shown to prolong survival in CHF patients, including asymptomatic and symptomatic left ventricular function in acute myocardial infarction. In many patients, coronary artery disease or previous myocardial infarction is the primary etiology of CHF. For this reason, ACE inhibitors have also been utilized to prevent the progression of left ventricular enlargement and dysfunction after myocardial infarction. This discussion of ACE inhibitors is limited to the context of moderate to severe CHF.

The biochemical pathway of ACE inhibitors has been summarized previously (45, 52). Angiotensinogen is the substrate for the rate-limiting enzyme renin. Renin cleaves angiotensinogen, resulting in production of the decapeptide, angiotensin I. Two additional amino acids are subsequently cleaved from this decapeptide by converting enzyme, a carboxypeptidase that was originally identified in the pulmonary circulation but subsequently has also been identified in blood vessel walls. In addition, this enzyme inhibited the degradation of bradykinin, with implications also for prostaglandin biosynthetic pathways. Recently, the key elements of the renin system have been identified in several tissues, suggesting the importance of local tissue regulation of the pathway. Newer, potent, specific, angiotensin II antagonists have been developed, and their use in heart failure is under investigation.

Angiotensin II is one of the most potent endogenous vasoconstrictors. In a situation in which an inappropriate increase of vascular tone may accompany severe reduction of left ventricular function, the elaboration of angiotensin II would result in further impedance to forward flow, thereby further reducing cardiac output and regional flow. In addition to intense vasoconstriction, angiotensin II directly stimulates release of aldosterone from the adrenal gland, resulting in sodium and water retention. Aldosterone release also directly stimulates potassium excretion by the kidney. Activation of the paracrine and autocrine functions of this system contribute to the progressive cellular dysfunction in CHF. Increased wall tension in the ventricle is associated with induced ACE gene expression. Studies in isolated myocardial preparations demonstrate that ACE inhibitors normalize isomyosin patterns and prevent myointimal proliferation induced by injury to the endothelium. Long-term ACE inhibition increases oxidative metabolism in biopsied skeletal muscle, indicating reversal of adverse regional flow and skeletal muscle abnormalities in CHF. This effect on peripheral oxygen use may be involved in the overall beneficial effect of long-term treatment with ACE inhibitors. It is interesting to note, therefore, that genetic overexpression of ACE has been identified as a potent independent risk factor for myocardial infarction (53). The effects of ACE inhibitors on heart rate have been variable, with heart rate remaining unchanged or demonstrating an overall reduction, thus suggesting a direct effect on autonomic activity. This effect may have many mechanisms, but autonomic and baroreceptor normalization and improved parasympathetic tone predominate (54, 55). Treatment with ACE inhibitors restores the reflex response; receptor density and the level of G-protein transducing this receptor signal are increased (56), and baroreceptor function is improved after treatment (54). However, plasma norepinephrine and adrenaline levels are not themselves consistently affected by ACE inhibitor treatment (57, 58).

The pharmacology of ACE inhibitors has been typically published in small patient populations, often with acute dosing. Many of these studies have been previously summarized (59, 60). The difficulty with the pragmatic aspects of these studies is that the clinical benefit of ACE inhibitors does not parallel plasma drug concentration, as is seen with other drug classes, such as antiarrhythmic agents.

A review of existing pharmacokinetic studies for all ACE inhibitors identifies two factors that are germane to the use of this class of agents in heart failure, and helps to explain observations from clinical trials. First, aging produces a measurable and significant increase in serum levels of ACE inhibitors. Despite the background, abnormalities produced by heart failure, cross-sectional studies reveal persistence of an aging profile that parallels normal subjects (61, 62). Because the elderly constitute the majority of heart failure patients, the effect of aging on the pharmacokinetics and pharmacodynamics of ACE inhibitors must be considered. Although this "aging effect" is evident at many physiologic levels, the reduction of renal function in the elderly heart failure patient is an important factor (61). Second, pharmacokinetic studies of all of the ACE inhibitors repeatedly demonstrate that renal insufficiency is associated with increased serum drug concentration (60). Because all ACE inhibitors are primarily excreted by the kidneys, this relationship is readily apparent. Less apparent, however, is whether the clinical use of ACE inhibitors in CHF takes this relationship into consideration. In general, the renal insufficiency of ambulatory heart failure does not approach severe chronic renal insufficiency (creatinine clearance less than 20 mL/minute). Nonetheless, many heart failure patients have a creatinine clearance in the range of 40–70 mL/minute, particularly within the elderly group (61). The clinical concern for these pharmacodynamic effects is the occurrence of hypotension or progressive renal deterioration.

The acute hemodynamic effects are sustained during long-term ACE inhibition, unlike the tolerance that develops to nonspecific vasodilators. Although the acute hemodynamic response to ACE inhibitors is well correlated with plasma renin activity, long-term hemodynamic and clinical responses to ACE inhibitors are weakly correlated to pretreatment plasma renin activity. This is because of multiple adaptations of hemodynamics, renal function, and neurohormonal activity that occur during long-term therapy. The response may be greater when dependence on plasma renin activity is induced by sodium restriction or diuretic administration. The effect of ACE inhibitors on the tissue renin system may be an important aspect of long-term response, but this remains speculative because it cannot be clinically quantified.

Because the extensive experience of ACE inhibitors in CHF has been summarized recently (50, 51), only the response in patients with moderate to advanced heart failure will be discussed in this chapter. The Cooperative North Scandinavian Enalapril Survival Study (CONSENSUS) was the first prospectively designed mortality trial of an ACE inhibitor in severe CHF (63). At enrollment, patients were NYHA functional class IV despite background digoxin and diuretic therapy. Many patients were also receiving traditional vasodilators, such as nitrates. It is important to note that the mean age of patients in this trial was 70 years, thus the effect of ACE inhibitors in elderly CHF patients was observed. This study was designed to evaluate the effect of enalapril treatment (mean dose 18.4 mg/day) versus placebo in 253 patients with severe (NYHA class IV) CHF. Conventional therapy was continued in all patients. The study was terminated early; results after 20 months showed a 27% reduction in deaths in the group treated with enalapril. Deaths attributable to progressive heart failure were decreased by 50% in the group treated with enalapril, but there was no difference between enalapril and placebo with respect to sudden cardiac deaths.

In the treatment arm of the Survival of Patients with Left Ventricular Dysfunction (SOLVD) trial, enalapril therapy and placebo were compared with regard to their influence on mortality and hospitalization in 2569 patients with NYHA class II or III CHF (64). In addition to conventional therapy, patients were randomly assigned to either treatment with enalapril (mean dose 11.2 mg/day) or placebo and followed for an average of 41.4 months. Enalapril treatment was associated with a reduction in mortality and fewer hospitalizations for decompensated CHF. The largest reduction of mortality was seen in deaths owing to progressive heart failure (22% reduction in risk); no significant effect was apparent in the subgroup where death was because of presumed arrhythmias in the absence of pump failure. The effects of enalapril were consistent across most patient subgroups such as functional class and baseline ejection fraction.

Most of the large clinical trials of ACE inhibitors involved upward titration of dosage to maximal toleration, targeting doses of captopril of 50 mg three times daily, and enalapril, 20 mg twice daily, or lisinopril, 20 mg daily. Even higher doses were used in many of the earlier trials, such as captopril, 100 mg three times daily. An advantage of new prospective trials, particularly in mild heart failure, is that ACE inhibition can be initiated before development of severe heart failure or before coadministration of a high dose of diuretic. Even within the severe CHF group, careful titration can limit adverse outcome, while permitting administration of an ACE inhibitor at a dose that would achieve levels compatible with those prescribed in large clinical trials. This is exemplified by the CONSENSUS trial (63) in which, in the early stages, unacceptable hypotension with enalapril treatment was observed with the initial planned dosage of 20 mg twice a day. This resulted in a downward titration of the dose to 20 mg a day. In fact, because the majority of the patients in this trial were elderly, it was subsequently recognized that approximately 20% of patients had clinical improvement with a dose of 5 mg a day. Overall, the mean dose of enalapril in CONSENSUS was just under 20 mg daily.

Several guidelines can be given therefore for all ACE inhibitors. First, the baseline renal function and extent of diuretic-induced prerenal azotemia should be assessed, particularly in the elderly patient. Second, ACE inhibitor therapy should be initiated in relatively small doses. Third, the ACE inhibitor dose should be progressively increased toward the dosage levels used in the clinical trials that have established long term benefit. For captopril, this is 6.25 mg three times a day, increasing to 50 mg three times a day as tolerated; some investigators have advocated 75–100 mg three times a day in the most refractory patients. For enalapril, the dose is 2.5 mg twice a day, increasing to 20 mg twice a day as tolerated. These considerations apply equally to lisinopril (65) and quinapril, which have been approved by the Food and Drug Administration for the treatment of CHF. Lisinopril should be started at a dose of 2.5 or 5 mg daily and can be increased to 20 mg daily. It is a once-daily drug with prolonged half-life, which is increased in the elderly and in the presence of renal dysfunction or CHF. Lisinopril has not been as extensively studied in CHF as captopril and enalapril have been. Quinapril has also shown clinical benefit in heart failure patients. Dosage recommendations suggest initiation of therapy at 5 mg twice a day, increasing to 40 mg twice a day, although the latter dose has been used primarily for the treatment of hypertension. The lack of more experience with dosing identifies the problem of new ACE inhibitors. As with the Zestril (Stuart Pharmaceuticals, Wilmington, Delaware) formulation of lisinopril, Accupril (Parke-Davis, Morris Plains, New Jersey) is being tested in a high-dose versus low-dose strategy to define a drug response range to better define treatment outcomes. These recommendations are summarized in Table 13.5.

The adverse effect profile of ACE inhibitors is well characterized (50, 51, 65–67). Experience with CHF patients indicates that hypotension remains the most common reason for treatment withdrawal. When ACE inhibitor therapy is initiated for CHF, particularly a long-acting ACE inhibitor, upward titration from a low starting dose is recommended. Diuretic dosage should be reduced if hypotension still remains during maintenance treatment. Symptomatic hypotension, or reduction of systolic blood pressure below physiologic lower limits of 80–85 mm Hg, would prevent the use of ACE inhibitor therapy until diuretics are further decreased or the cause of hypotension is clarified. However, reduction of blood pressure to

**Table 13.5**
**ACE Inhibitors: Range of Doses for Heart Failure Therapy**

| ACE Inhibitor | Dose |
|---|---|
| Captopril[a] | |
| Capoten (Bristol-Myers Squibb, Princeton, NJ) | 6.25–75 mg t.i.d. |
| Enalapril[a] | |
| Vasotec (Merck and Company, West Point, PA) | 2.5–20 mg b.i.d. |
| Lisinopril[a] | |
| Prinivil (Merck and Company, West Point, PA) | 5–20 mg daily |
| Zestril (Stuart Pharmaceuticals, Wilmington, DE) | 5–20 mg daily |
| Quinapril[a] | |
| Accupril (Parke-Davis, Morris Plains, NJ) | 5–20 mg b.i.d. (40 mg in some reports) |
| Ramipril[b] | |
| Altace (Hoechst-Roussel Pharmaceuticals, Somerville, NJ) | 1.25–10 mg b.i.d. |
| Benazapril[b] | |
| Lotensin (CIBA Consumer Pharmaceuticals, Woodbridge, NJ) | 10–20 mg b.i.d. |
| Fosinopril[b] | |
| Monopril (Bristol-Myers Squibb, Princeton, NJ) | 10–20 mg b.i.d. |

[a] Approved in the United States (dosage varies in published reports).
[b] Reported in the literature: heart failure indication and dosage not established.
ACE = angiotensin-converting enzyme; b.i.d. = twice a day; t.i.d. = three times a day.

90–100 mm Hg should not be considered an adverse effect; it is evidence of achieving therapeutic end point. In patients with CHF, maintenance of renal function is dependent on the renin-angiotensin system. ACE inhibitors reduce perfusion pressure by decreasing systemic vascular resistance and reduce intraglomerular pressure and therefore glomerular filtration. Although this may occur because of decreasing vasoconstrictor tone of the efferent arteriole, careful physiologic studies demonstrate that the increased renal resistance and decreased glomerular filtration rate in CHF are primarily because of afferent vasoconstriction. Because of the known underlying renal impairment of CHF, however, small increases after the addition of an ACE inhibitor should not discourage continued use of the drug because these increases may actually revert toward baseline with prolonged treatment. Reducing diuretic dosage and avoiding prostaglandin synthesis inhibitors such as indomethacin, which interfere with renal perfusion autoregulation, are important to minimize the impact of ACE inhibitors. Other class effects of ACE inhibitors include hyperkalemia, nonproductive cough, skin rash, altered taste, and rarely, angioedema (65–67).

## Other Oral Vasodilators

Although ACE inhibitors have become standard therapy for advanced heart failure, patient intolerance does exist, and alternative therapy should be considered. In view of the favorable outcome with hydralazine and isosorbide dinitrate therapy in the Veterans Administration Heart Failure Trials (VHeFT), this combination should be considered a viable alternative for long-term management of advanced heart failure (68). Despite intense study of vasodilators, there are currently no additional compounds that can be given unequivocal consideration. Vasodilators that are effective in hypertension, such as α-blockers and minoxidil, are not effective for long-term management of CHF. The calcium channel antagonists have also remained a paradoxical group of agents for heart failure management, complicated by their diverse pharmacologic properties. Specific aspects of this treatment class are discussed below.

Because hydralazine and isosorbide dinitrate are currently long-standing generic preparations, there has not been a strong impetus to pursue detailed studies in heart failure that would otherwise be valuable because of the VHeFT trials. For example, the relative contribution of each of these compounds to the aggregate effect that is produced in heart failure remains speculative. It is unclear whether hydralazine or the nitrate preparations account for the long-term mortality benefit and clinical efficacy in these trials. Furthermore, precise information regarding dose of the individual compounds or the combined dosage is difficult to obtain. The best guidance, therefore, is to titrate the dosage indicated in the VHeFT trials. Finally, the effect of this combination on the mortality of advanced heart failure has not been established.

Calcium channel antagonists have not been successful as primary or early therapy for the management of heart failure (69). Because this has been attributed to the putative "negative inotropic" effects of these compounds, the issue is clearly more complex. First, these agents are not pharmacologically uniform. Second, the direct negative inotropic effect of the prototype compound verapamil has not been substantiated in clinical trials of the new dihydropyridines. Third, these compounds have differing effects on electrical conduction within the myocardium. Despite the limited applicability of these compounds as primary therapy for systolic ventricular dysfunction, they are effective for the treatment of hypertension and angina. Thus, when persistent hypertension or angina accompany advanced heart failure, calcium channel antagonists can be added to the standard combination of digoxin, a diuretic, and an ACE inhibitor. Studies in progress are examining the efficacy and survival impact of calcium channel antagonists when added to background therapy consisting of digoxin, a diuretic, and an ACE inhibitor. Preliminary results from large-scale clinical trials suggest that calcium channel antagonists do not adversely affect survival in patients with moderate to severe CHF. In fact, survival may improve in some subsets of patients. These results are preliminary, and therefore recommendations for clinical use cannot be made at this time. The use of new calcium channel antagonists for the treatment of hypertension or active angina in patients with left ventricular dysfunction is appropriate, however, but the decision should be made on an individual patient basis.

### β-Adrenergic Blockade

At the current time, β-adrenergic blockers cannot be recommended for routine use, particularly in patients with severe heart failure. Nonetheless, broad guidelines can be given. β-Blockade is certainly appropriate in patients with acute myocardial infarction and, if clinically tolerated, can also be used in patients with left ventricular dysfunction after an acute infarction. Ironically, in large-scale clinical trials of β-blockade in chronic heart failure, the mortality benefit was greater when the cause was nonischemic, whereas heart failure of ischemic origin does not always show improvement. Additional issues regarding use of this therapy include severity of heart failure, gradual dose titration, and maintenance dosage. These issues remain empiric at the current time.

A unique β-blocker is carvedilol. Although predominantly a β-blocker, it also has α-blocking properties and is associated with mild vasodilator effects. In addition, it has antioxidant and antiinflammatory effects in experimental models. In initial trials and recent survival studies, clinical and survival benefit has been shown in patients who were already receiving standard therapy, including mandatory ACE inhibitor utilization. Similar to other β-blockers, slow titration is required, with vasodilation and heart rate reduction occurring even at relatively low doses. At the time of this writing, the compound is under evaluation but has not yet been approved for a heart failure indication.

## MANAGEMENT OF CLINICAL DETERIORATION IN HEART FAILURE

CHF is considered refractory in a patient with advanced heart failure (NYHA functional class III or IV heart failure) in whom symptoms of CHF have not improved, or have worsened, despite recently escalated therapy (2). Typically, this patient population presents with evidence of substantial fluid retention or reduction in cardiac output ("low-flow state"). CHF should not be considered "refractory" unless optimal therapy with digoxin, a diuretic, and an ACE inhibitor (or alternative vasodilator regimen) has already been initiated.

That such patients are common is evident by patient enrollment in new drug therapy trials for heart failure, which require patients to have functional class III or IV heart failure at baseline, despite background therapy with digoxin, a diuretic, and an ACE inhibitor. This implies that the standard "triple therapy" of heart failure is not sufficient to maintain patients in a symptom-free state indefinitely.

The approach to the patient with refractory CHF, therefore, includes three components: (1) assessment of changing clinical status and pathophysiology of the underlying disorder that is producing heart failure, (2) adjustment of current oral medical therapy to provide optimal standard treatment, and (3) temporary parenteral therapeutic support and hospitalization for management of the underlying disorder and to determine prospective treatment options.

## Changing Clinical Status and Pathophysiology

The appearance of refractory CHF should immediately raise questions regarding changes in clinical status and pathophysiology (Table 13.6). The first major issue is ongoing myocardial ischemia or infarction. In the United States, coronary artery disease is the main cause of CHF. When clinical management dictates close attention to advanced heart failure, a remote history of coronary artery disease or myocardial infarction can be overlooked in the absence of clinically overt ischemia such as chest pain, or new electrocardiographic changes. However, progressive transmural or endocardial ischemia can produce abrupt decompensation in a previously stable patient with heart failure. A new myocardial infarction is an obvious cause of decompensation. Deterioration of systolic or diastolic function, increased mitral regurgitation, and rhythm disorders are less overt reasons for progressive or abrupt deterioration of otherwise stable heart failure.

Mitral regurgitation of any origin produces an adverse effect on myocardial function in an otherwise stable heart failure patient, particularly because the severity of mitral regurgitation is not correlated with the acoustic properties of the accompanying murmur. In addition, the appearance of a new rhythm disorder, most commonly atrial fibrillation, will produce decompensation.

Similar to myocardial ischemia, coexistent hypertension also may be overshadowed by advanced heart failure. In fact, the presence of a systolic arterial pressure of 140–150 mm Hg may be erroneously interpreted as evidence of good ventricular function. However, a systolic blood pressure of 130–140 mm Hg or a diastolic blood pressure of 85–100 mm Hg, requires greater blood pressure control in an individual with abnormal systolic function and heart failure. In a patient with coexistent heart failure and hypertension, as the ventricle fails to the extent that excessive systolic blood pressure is not generated (despite increased diastolic blood pressure), continued attention to blood pressure regulation is required. Systolic blood pressure ideally should be maintained in the range of 100–120 mm Hg, but it may be difficult to achieve reduction to this level in the elderly patient with isolated systolic hypertension.

**Table 13.6**
**Factors Altering the Underlying Clinical Status and Pathophysiology of Refractory Heart Failure**

New myocardial ischemia/infarction
New or progressive myocardial mechanical defect: mitral regurgitation
New rhythm disorder (most commonly atrial fibrillation)
Inadequately controlled hypertension
Diabetes mellitus (particularly insulin-dependent)
Dietary sodium indiscretion
Progressive renal failure
Pulmonary disorders
  Thromboembolic disease
  Secondary pulmonary hypertension
  Progressive obstructive lung disease
Infectious processes
  Pneumonia
  Upper respiratory infection
  Urosepsis
Errors in drug consumption

The importance of controlled dietary sodium intake has already been discussed. A low-sodium diet (2–3 g) is important in all stages of heart failure, even when diuretic therapy is used.

Other coexistent medical disorders may trigger decompensation. Insulin-dependent diabetes mellitus, progressive renal dysfunction, and pulmonary disease can adversely influence outcome. Pulmonary embolic events and chronic lung disease are not unusual in the patient with heart failure. Pulmonary and upper respiratory infections are common in patients with stable heart failure, particularly in the fall and winter. Likewise, urinary tract infections are not uncommon in the elderly patient with heart failure. All of these disorders are difficult to differentiate from progressive heart failure and may trigger left ventricular decompensation.

## Optimizing Current Oral Therapy

All patients with severe heart failure should be treated with the combination of digoxin, a diuretic, and an ACE inhibitor. If an ACE inhibitor is not tolerated, an alternate vasodilator regimen such as hydralazine and isosorbide dinitrate must be given (Table 13.3). Rhythm management and anticoagulation must be individualized, however. Atrial arrhythmias, particularly atrial fibrillation, limit ventricular filling and performance. Electrical or pharmaceutical cardioversion should be attempted, and if it is unsuccessful, ventricular response should be controlled to a moderate range. Management of asymptomatic ventricular ectopy is more problematic, although most investigators and clinicians use amiodarone therapy. Clinical trials of amiodarone suggest this agent is beneficial, but they have not been uniformly successful. When amiodarone is unsuccessful, particularly with symptomatic ventricular ectopy, an implantable defibrillator may be required.

Anticoagulation may take two forms. In the "ischemic" cardiomyopathy population, antiplatelet therapy with aspirin is common: dosage is maintained at 80 mg daily to minimize the known compromise of ACE inhibitor benefit that occurs during coadministration of high-dose aspirin. Warfarin therapy is recommended in most patients with abnormal ventricular function, particularly when the ejection fraction is less than 20%. Recently, some experts have questioned routine use of warfarin; however, if not contraindicated, most recommend its use.

The standard dosage of digoxin should be 0.25 mg daily. Upward adjustment to 0.375 mg is typical in patients with atrial fibrillation. Downward titration to 0.125 mg is often necessary in elderly patients in whom renal function is impaired. Digoxin therapy is often used in substandard doses because of concern about toxicity. It would be unusual for a patient to be in an adequate therapeutic range at a dose of 0.125 mg every other day, unless profound renal impairment exists (e.g., creatinine clearance less than 20 mL/minute). Likewise, it would be unusual for toxicity to occur at doses of 0.125 or 0.25 mg daily. As noted previously, digoxin levels do not correlate with clinical outcome or therapeutic effect. They are useful, however, if patient compliance or toxicity is questioned.

"Optimal" therapeutic management of diuretics remains a clinical decision, based on the clinical assessment of edema. Use of more objective criteria to document the presence of sodium retention on physical examination may provide a guideline for edema, but there is no single laboratory test to demonstrate an optimal therapy (70). Typically, diuretics are escalated until prerenal azotemia occurs. This is a vague and potentially dangerous end point. For refractory CHF, a combination of diuretics is normally required. Although combined diuretics are beneficial, additional attention should be directed to their clinical and biochemical side effects, as outlined previously, so that metolazone is not used excessively.

Several ACE inhibitors have been approved for the treatment of heart failure, and approval of additional agents may be forthcoming (Table 13.5). This should not be construed as endorsement for particular agents or encouragement to use ACE inhibitors not officially approved for treatment of heart failure. The common feature for all of these agents is to provide therapy in doses consistent with those in large clinical trials. Typically, these are at the high end of the dosage range. Several studies are underway to compare the efficacy of high-dose versus low-dose therapy.

Currently, hydralazine and isosorbide dinitrate is the only other drug combination with vasodilator properties that has approval for treatment of heart failure. Efficacy versus placebo was not established in severe end stage heart failure, but rather, in moderate disease. For this and other reasons, an ACE inhibitor should be the initial agent to be considered. If it is not tolerated, the hydralazine and isosorbide dinitrate regimen is an alternative approach. Many experienced heart failure investigators use one of the following regimens, although they have not been tested formally in combination: (1) an ACE inhibitor and isosorbide dinitrate for patients with ongoing angina or those in whom additional preload reduction is desired or (2) an ACE inhibitor and hydralazine for the management of severe heart failure. Hydralazine does not typically induce greater blood pressure reduction than the ACE inhibitor alone, but this varies from patient to patient. This combination is particularly useful when mitral or tricuspid regurgitation exists. In all combinations, excess hypotension should be avoided. Typically systolic blood pressure must be maintained in the range of 85–90 mm Hg, or more. If a patient has symptomatic hypotension, reduction of vasodilator therapy is warranted, irrespective of the absolute blood pressure level.

At the current time there is no established role of calcium channel antagonists for the treatment of heart failure, particularly in patients with advanced disease. Studies are currently underway to assess this issue. Particular subsets of patients who theoretically could benefit from the addition of a calcium channel antagonist to standard "triple" therapy include those with persistent angina or hypertension. There are no major studies underway that test the efficacy of a calcium channel antagonist against an ACE inhibitor or in place of an ACE inhibitor, and the calcium antagonists should not be used in this manner for the treatment of heart failure.

Finally, patient-related drug therapy issues must be considered. Noncompliance with therapy is important. In a symptomatic heart failure patient, the incidence of noncompliance may be less than it is in disorders such as hypertension, because the perception of illness is greater in heart failure. Other factors may also limit the persistence of therapy. Treatment of heart failure requires several drugs to be taken throughout the day. A patient may misunderstand the use of the medications and inadvertently alter drug therapy. Confusion, memory deficit, and other central neurologic disorders are common in heart failure, particularly in the elderly patient, and may lead to inaccurate drug consumption.

## Admission for Diagnostic Studies and Parenteral Therapy

A patient should be hospitalized when he or she can no longer be managed on an outpatient basis for persistent severe edema, weakness, fatigue, or dyspnea. To maximize outcome, and limit the length of hospitalization, the plan of admission should be developed to address relevant diagnostic and treatment approaches (Table 13.7). Refractory heart failure can occur because of altered underlying pathophysiology or intercurrent clinical disorders. In a patient with known coronary disease, a coronary lesion with potential reversible ischemia should be managed by appropriate

**Table 13.7**
**Management of Acutely Decompensated Heart Failure**

Step 1: Assessment for hospitalization
- Refractory sodium retention
- Progressive fatigue/weakness
- Mental status obtundation
- Marked renal dysfunction
- Infection (usually pneumonia)
- Restructuring of a complex medical regimen

Step 2: Initial urgent treatment
- Intravenous diuretics
- Oxygen
- Temporizing treatment (nitrates)

Step 3: Acute therapy
- Parenteral diuretic
- Dobutamine or milrinone
- Blood pressure management
  - Reduce: parenteral or oral vasodilators
- Support: dopamine or phenylephrine

Step 4: Transition therapy
- Convert parenteral to oral therapy
- Reassess previous oral regimen
- Treat associated medical disorders
- Establish cardiac rehabilitation
- Give intruction about dietary sodium
- Counsel about/discuss prognosis

intervention. Hyperglycemia in the diabetic patient and hypertension should be controlled. Evidence of infection should be aggressively pursued. New onset or suspicion of progressive mitral regurgitation should be evaluated. Intermediate diagnostic studies, such as assessing change in ejection fraction, are not beneficial in most patients.

Parenteral therapy (including intravenous diuretics and electrolyte replacement) should be initiated from the moment of admission, while diagnostic studies are pending (Table 13.8). As soon as feasible, intravenous inotropic support (usually with dobutamine) can be initiated to support the heart while other oral medications are being optimized or changed (71). In many centers, low dose intravenous dobutamine can be given in a step-down unit, which obviates the need for coronary or intensive care unit admission. When dobutamine is given in doses of 2–5 μg/kg/minute, excessive tachycardia and/or ventricular ectopy are usually avoided, but telemetry provides important monitoring of the clinical response. The final dose required for stabilization varies, but many patients show almost immediate clinical improvement by the time that the infusion is titrated to 5 μg/kg/minute. Higher administration rates can be given, but the need for more than 10 μg/kg/minute is of concern, suggesting severe morbidity. In acute decompensation, when oral vasodilator therapy cannot be implemented or precise

**Table 13.8**
**Therapy for Advanced Heart Failure: Acute Decompensation**

| |
|---|
| Initial Supportive therapy |
| Intravenous loop diuretics |
| Oxygen |
| Nitrates |
| Morphine for pulmonary edema |
| Parenteral diuretics |
| Loop diuretic |
| Intravenous chlorothiazide |
| Dobutamine |
| Standard short-term inotropic support |
| Can be given at low infusion rates in a step-down unit |
| Nitroprusside |
| Permits afterload reduction by a peripheral route |
| Milrinone |
| Combined inotropic and vasodilator properties |
| Can be given in combination with dobutamine |
| Electrolyte replacement |
| Intravenous or oral potassium and magnesium supplementation |
| Rhythm control |
| Urgent management if contributing to the acute decompensation (e.g., atrial Fibrillation) |

dose adjustment is required, intravenous nitroprusside can be used; however, this often requires an arterial catheter to monitor rapid changes of blood pressure. Infusion is efficacious when vasodilator therapy is the primary therapy or is combined with inotropic agents such as dobutamine. Although intravenous nitroglycerin is frequently used to treat acute decompensation of heart failure, most patients demonstrate hemodynamic tachyphylaxis within the first 24 hours of administration. The hemodynamics then return toward baseline and are not significantly different from those seen with placebo. An alternative approach to therapy is the use of intravenous milrinone, which has both inotropic and direct vasodilator properties (72). The direct vasodilator response to milrinone is mediated by an increase of cyclic adenosine monophosphate (AMP). The degree of vasodilation produced by milrinone is less than that of nitroprusside, when the two are compared on an equimolar basis. Experience with intravenous milrinone for the treatment of heart failure is more limited; for this reason, it should be administered in a coronary or intensive care unit. Milrinone requires a loading dose to reach effective drug levels. Tachycardia and ventricular ectopy are also observed with milrinone, but direct comparisons to dobutamine are limited. Because milrinone has vasodilator properties, it is more likely to lower systemic blood pressure than is dobutamine.

Inotropic support of the decompensated patient should continue for 2–4 days. Many patients demonstrate substantial improvement with short-term dobutamine administration. In some cases this benefit is maintained during long-term follow-up. However, this outcome does not occur in all patients. The requirement for short-term inotropic administration at gradually shortening intervals is evidence of progressive ventricular deterioration. The observed benefit with short-term inotropic support has resulted in an industry of outpatient and home dobutamine programs. When dobutamine is administered at intervals mandated by patient deterioration, this is an appropriate management approach. However, the concepts that dobutamine administered for 4–8 hours weekly is beneficial and that continuous home dobutamine improves clinical outcome or survival have never been substantiated. Limited data suggest that the latter approach actually may decrease survival.

Discharge planning should include an optimized oral treatment program, dietary instruction for sodium intake, and a plan for cardiac rehabilitation, if clinically feasible. Prognosis should also be discussed with the patient and family members. The issue of cardiac transplantation is often raised when the patient reaches the point of advanced heart failure, particularly with progressive deterioration. This remains a complex approach to heart failure management and is available to only approximately 2200 patients per year. A detailed discussion of this approach is beyond the context of this chapter, but the topic has recently been summarized (73).

## SUMMARY

Despite advances in the therapy for CHF, many patients still present with refractory symptoms and findings. If a logical approach is taken to the management of such patients, heroic and less available forms of therapy such as cardiac transplantation can often be avoided or delayed. Such a logical approach would include that all patients with functional NYHA class III to IV CHF, particularly those who continue to manifest symptoms, receive digoxin, a diuretic, and an ACE inhibitor (or alternative vasodilator therapy) on a long-term basis. If a patient experiences decompensation despite this approach, the patient should be assessed for changing clinical status or pathophysiologic conditions. Should these two steps prove to be insufficient, hospital-based parenteral therapy with diuretics and inotropic agents should be considered to permit restructuring of a subsequent oral regimen.

---

## REFERENCES

1. McFate Smith W. Epidemiology of congestive heart failure. Am J Cardiol 1985;55:3A.
2. Cody RJ. Management of the patient with refractory congestive heart failure. Am J Cardiol 1992;69:141G–149G.
3. Gheorghiade M, Zarowitz BJ. Review of randomized trials of digoxin therapy in patients with chronic heart failure. Am J Cardiol 1992;69:48Q–63Q.
4. Kulick DL, Rahimtoola SH. Current role of digitalis therapy in patients with congestive heart failure. JAMA 1991;265:2995–2997.

5. Covit AB, Schaer GL, Sealey JE, et al. Suppression of the renin-angiotensin system by intravenous digoxin in chronic congestive heart failure. Am J Med 1983;75: 445–447.
6. Gheorghiade M, Ferguson D. Digoxin: a neurohormonal modulator? Circulation 1991;84:2181–2186.
7. Uretsky BF, Young JB, Shahidi E, et al. Randomized study assessing the effect of digoxin withdrawal in patients with mild to moderate chronic congestive heart failure: results of the PROVED Trial. J Am Coll Cardiol 1993;22:955–967.
8. Packer M, Gheorghiade M, Young JB, et al. [On behalf of the RADIANCE Study. Effects of digoxin withdrawal in patients with chronic heart failure treated with converting-enzyme inhibitors. N Engl J Med 1993;329:1–7
9. Packer M, Carver JR, Rodeheffer RJ, et al. for the PROMISE Study Research Group. Effect of oral milrinone or mortality in severe chronic heart failure. N Engl J Med 1991;325:1468–1475.
10. Bayliss J, Norell M, Canepa-Anson R, et al. Untreated heart failure: clinical and neuroendocrine effects of introducing diuresis. Br Heart J 1987;57:17–22.
11. Kubo SH, Clark M, Laragh JH, et al. Identification of normal neurohormonal activity in mild congestive heart failure and the stimulating effect of upright posture and diuretics. Am J Cardiol 1987;60:1322–1328.
12. Gerlag PG, Meijel J. High-dose furosemide in the treatment of refractory congestive heart failure. Arch Intern Med 1988;148:286–291.
13. Brater DC. Resistance to diuretics: emphasis on a pharmacological perspective. Drugs 1981;22:477–494.
14. Brater DC. Resistance to loop diuretics: why it happens and what to do about it. Drugs 1985;30:427–443.
15. Cody RJ, Kubo SH, Pickworth KK. Diuretic utilization for the sodium retention of congestive heart failure. Arch Intern Med 1905;154:1905–1914.
16. Cody RJ, Pickworth KK. Approaches to diuretic therapy and electrolyte imbalance in congestive heart failure. Cardiol Clin 1994;12:37–50.
17. Rudy DW, Voelker JR, Greene PK, et al. Loop diuretics for chronic renal insufficiency: a continuous infusion is more efficacious than bolus therapy. Ann Intern Med 1991;115:360–366.
18. Krasna MJ, Scoot GE, Scholz PM, et al. Postoperative enhancement of urinary output in patients with acute renal failure using continuous furosemide therapy. Chest 1986;89:294–295.
19. Oster JR, Epstein M, Smoller S. Combined therapy with thiazide-type and loop diuretic agents for resistant sodium retention. Ann Intern Med 1983;99:405–406.
20. Wollam GL, Tarazi RC, Bravo EL, et al. Diuretic potency of combined hydrochlorothiazide and furosemide therapy in patients with azotemia. Am J Med 1982;72:929–938.
21. Ellison D, Velazquez H, Wright FS. Adaptation of the distal convoluted tubule of the rat: structural and functional effects of dietary salt intake and chronic diuretic infusion. J Clin Invest 1989;83:113–126.
22. Ellison DH. The physiologic basis of diuretic synergism: its role in treating diuretic resistance. Ann Intern Med 1991;114:886–894.
23. Wilcox CS, Mitch WE, Kelly RA, et al. Response to furosemide. I. Effect of salt intake and renal compensation. J Lab Clin Med 1983;102:450–458.
24. Cody RJ, Covit AB, Schaer GL, et al. Sodium and water balance in chronic congestive heart failure. J Clin Invest 1986;77:1441–1452.
25. Agostoni PG, Marenzi GC, Pepi M, et al. Isolated ultrafiltration in moderate congestive heart failure. J Am Coll Cardiol 1993;21:424–431.
26. Rimondini A, Cipolla CM, Bella PD, et al. Hemofiltration as short-term treatment for refractory congestive heart failure. Am J Med 1987;83:43–48.
27. Rubin J, Ball R. Continuous ambulatory peritoneal dialysis as treatment of severe congestive heart failure in the face of chronic renal failure: report of eight cases. Arch Intern Med 1986;146:1533–1535.
28. Lant A. Diuretics: clinical pharmacology and therapeutic use (part 1). Drugs 1985; 29:57–87.
29. Lant A. Diuretics: clinical pharmacology and therapeutic use (part 2). Drugs 1985;29:162–188.

30. Brater DC, Chennavasin P, Seiwell R. Furosemide in patients with heart failure: shift in dose-response curves. Clin Pharmacol Ther 1980;28:182–186.
31. Ikram H, Chan W, Espiner EA, et al. Hemodynamic and hormone responses to acute and chronic furosemide therapy in congestive heart failure. Clin Sci 1980;59: 443–449.
32. Francis GS, Siegel RM, Goldsmith SR, et al. Acute vasoconstrictor response to intravenous furosemide in patients with chronic congestive heart failure. Ann Intern Med 1985;103:1–6.
33. Dyckner T, Wester PO. Plasma and skeletal muscle electrolytes in patients on long-term diuretic therapy for arterial hypertension and/or congestive heart failure. Acta Med Scand 1987;222:231–236.
34. Gradman A, Deedwania P, Cody R, et al. Predictors of total mortality and sudden death in mild to moderate heart failure. J Am Coll Cardiol 1989;14:564–570.
35. Holmes J, Kubo SH, Cody RJ, et al. Arrhythmias in ischemic and nonischemic dilated cardiomyopathy: prediction of mortality by ambulatory electrocardiography. Am J Cardiol 1985;55:146–151.
36. Morgan T, Myers J. Potassium maintenance, potassium supplements or potassium sparing agents. Acta Med Scand 1981;657(Suppl):117–123.
37. Massery SG, Seelig MS. Hypomagnesemia and hypermagnesemia. Clin Nephrol 1977;7:147–153.
38. Reinhart RA. Magnesium metabolism: a review with special reference to the relationship between intracellular content and serum levels. Arch Intern Med 1988; 148:2415–2420.
39. Juan D. Clinical review. The importance of hypomagnesemia. Surgery 1982;91: 510–517.
40. Rude RK, Singer FR. Magnesium deficiency and excess. Annu Rev Med 1981; 32:245–259.
41. Anand IS, Kabra GS, Ferrari R, et al. Enalapril as initial and sole therapy in severe chronic heart failure with sodium retention. Int J Cardiol 1990;28:341–346.
42. Kelly RA, Wilcox CS, Mitch WE, et al. Response of the kidney to furosemide. II Effect of captopril on sodium balance. Kidney Int 1983;24:233–239.
43. Odemuyiwa of, Gilmartin J, Kenny D, et al. Captopril and the diuretic requirements in moderate and severe chronic heart failure. Eur Heart J 1989; 10:586–590.
44. Pfeffer MA, Braunwald E, Moy LA, et al. on behalf of the SAVE Investigators. Effect of captopril on mortality and morbidity in patients with left ventricular dysfunction after myocardial infarction: results of the Survival and Ventricular Enlargement Trial. N Engl J Med 1992;327:669–677.
45. Cody RJ, Laragh JH. The renin-angiotensin-aldosterone system in chronic congestive heart failure: pathophysiology and implications for treatment. In: Cohn J, ed. Drug treatment of heart failure. Secaucus: Advanced Therapeutics Communications International, 1988;79–104.
46. Francis GS, Goldsmith SR, Levine TB, et al. The neurohormonal axis in congestive heart failure. Ann Intern Med 1984;101:370–377.
47. Cody RJ. Neurohormonal influences in the pathogenesis of congestive heart failure. Cardiol Clin 1989;7:73–86.
48. Cody RJ. Hemodynamic responses to specific renin angiotensin inhibitors in hypertension and heart failure: a review. Drugs 1984;28:144–169.
49. Kubo SH, Cody RJ. Clinical and hemodynamic aspects of angiotensin inhibition for the management of congestive heart failure. In: Ferguson R, Vlasses P, eds. The clinical applications of angiotensin converting enzyme inhibitors. Mt. Kisco, NY: Futura Publications, 1987: 87–106.
50. Cody RJ. ACE inhibitors: mechanisms, pharmacodynamics, and clinical trials in heart failure. Cardiol Rev 1994;3:145–156.
51. Cody RJ. Comparing angiotensin-converting enzyme inhibitor trial results in patients with acute myocardial infarction. Arch Intern Med 1994;154:2029–2036.
52. Cody RJ. The clinical potential of renin inhibitors and angiotensin antagonists. Drugs 1994;47:586–598.
53. Alderman MH, Madhavan S, Ooi WL, et al. Association of the renin-sodium profile with the risk of myocardial infarction in patients with hypertension. N Engl J Med 1991;324:1098–1104.

54. Cody RJ, Franklin KW, Kluger J, et al. Mechanisms governing the postural response, and baroreceptor abnormalities in chronic congestive heart failure: effects of acute and long-term converting enzyme inhibition. Circulation 1982;66:135–141.
55. Binkley PF, Haas GJ, Starling RC, et al. Sustained augmentation of parasympathetic tone with angiotensin converting enzyme inhibition in patients with congestive heart failure. J Am Coll Cardiol 1993;21:655–661.
56. Horn EH, Orwin SJ, Steinberg SF, et al. Reduced lymphocyte stimulatory guanine nucleotide regulatory protein and adrenergic receptors in congestive heart failure and reversal with angiotensin converting enzyme inhibitor therapy. Circulation 1989;78:1373–1379.
57. Cody RJ, Franklin KW, Kluger J, et al. Sympathetic responsiveness and plasma norepinephrine during therapy of chronic congestive heart failure with captopril. Am J Med 1982;72:791–797.
58. Kubo S. Neurohormonal activation and the response to converting enzyme inhibition in congestive heart failure. Circulation 1990;81(Suppl III):107–114.
59. Kubo SH, Cody RJ. Clinical pharmacokinetics of angiotensin converting enzyme inhibitors: a review. Clin Pharmacokinet 1985;10:377–391.
60. Cody RJ. Optimizing ACE inhibitor therapy of congestive heart failure: Insights from pharmacodynamic studies. Clin Pharmacokinet 1993;22:59–70.
61. Cody RJ, Ljungman S, Covit AB, et al. Regulation of glomerular filtration rate in chronic congestive heart failure patients. Kidney Int 1988;34:361–367.
62. Cody RJ, Torre S, Clark M, et al. Age related hemodynamic, renal, and hormonal differences in patients with congestive heart failure. Arch Intern Med 1989;149: 1023–1028.
63. CONSENSUS Trial Study Group. Effects of enalapril on mortality in severe congestive heart failure. N Engl J Med 1987;316:1425–1435.
64. The SOLVD Investigators. Effect of enalapril on survival in patients with reduced left ventricular ejection fractions and congestive heart failure. N Engl J Med 1991;325:293–302.
65. Lancaster SG, Todd PA. Lisinopril: a preliminary review of its pharmacodynamic and pharmacokinetic properties, and therapeutic use in hypertension and congestive heart failure. Drugs 1988;35:646–669.
66. Brogden RN, Todd PA, Sorkin EM. Captopril: An update of its pharmacodynamic and pharmacokinetic properties, and therapeutic use in hypertension and congestive heart failure. Drugs 1988;36:540–562.
67. Todd PA, Heel RC. Enalapril: a review of its pharmacodynamic and pharmacokinetic properties and therapeutic use in hypertension and congestive heart failure. Drugs 1986;31:198–248.
68. Cohn JN, Johnson G, Ziesche S, et al. A comparison of enalapril with hydralazine-isosorbide dinitrate in the treatment of chronic congestive heart failure. N Engl J Med 1991;35:303–310.
69. Cody RJ. Vascular and myocardial responses to calcium channel antagonists: Implications for hypertension and congestive heart failure. In: Epstein M, ed. Calcium antagonists in clinical medicine. Philadelphia: Hanley and Belfus, 1992;105–112.
70. Cody RJ. The need for a sodium retention score in clinical trials of heart failure. Clinical Pharmacol Ther 1993;54:7–10.
71. Leier CV, ed. Cardiotonic drugs. New York: Marcell Dekker, 1991.
72. Konstam MA, Cody RJ. Short term use of intravenous milrinone for heart failure. Am J Cardiol 1995;75:822–826.
73. Twenty-Fourth Bethesda Conference. Cardiac transplantation. J Am Coll Cardiol 1993;22:1–64.

# PART VI

# Antiarrhythmic Therapy

CHAPTER 14

# Antiarrhythmic Drugs

Joel Kupersmith, MD

This chapter reviews the pharmacology of the commonly used antiarrhythmic drugs. Because the bridge between basic principles and the clinic is very short in this area, we will first briefly review the generalities of arrhythmia mechanisms and how drugs interfere with them. Subsequently we will address testing in patients with arrhythmia and proarrhythmic effects of drugs, then describe each antiarrhythmic drug currently in use.

## BASIC ELECTROPHYSIOLOGY

The fundamental recording of electrophysiologic activity of the heart is the action potential. Figure 14.1*A* shows the two main types of cardiac action potentials, fast and slow responses. The fast response occurs in atrial, ventricular, and His-Purkinje tissue whereas the slow response occurs in the sinus and atrioventricular (AV) nodes. The upstroke of the fast response, which is mediated by a rapid inward movement of sodium ions, is blocked by the "local anesthetic" class I drugs (see below). The upstroke of the slow response is mediated mainly by a slow inward movement of calcium ions and is blocked by the β-blockers and calcium channel blockers (classes II and IV, respectively) (1–3).

Certain action potential parameters are important in respect to antiarrhythmic drugs. The rate of rise of the upstroke is related to conduction (i.e., a slowed upstroke is associated with depression of conduction) and therefore to effects on reentrant arrhythmias (see below) and adverse effects (heart block). Action potential duration and refractory period (i.e., the time from the onset of the action potential to the earliest new action potential that can be initiated) are also relevant to reentry. In addition, certain tissues in the heart (sinus, AV nodes, and His-Purkinje system) are capable of automaticity, i.e., firing on their own (Fig. 14.1*A*). This property of the sinus node initiates the recurrent electrical activity of each heart beat while lower automatic centers (AV node and His-Purkinje system) assume control when the sinus node fails. Under certain circumstances automaticity may be enhanced or develop in certain tissue to cause tachyarrhythmia.

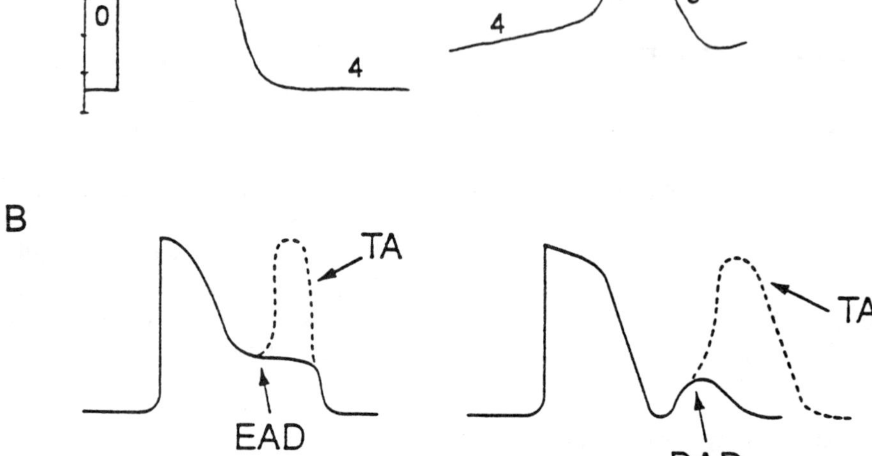


Figure 14.1. Action potentials recorded from the heart under normal and abnormal circumstances. *A,* Normal action potentials. On the left is a "fast response," which exists in normal myocardium and the His-Purkinje system. It is mediated by a rapid inward movement of sodium ions. On the right is an example of a "slow response" action potential, which occurs in the sinus (shown here) and atrioventricular (AV) nodes. Upstroke in these tissues is slower and smaller than the fast response and is mediated by a slow inward movement of mainly Ca++. Note that the sinus node action potential also displays automaticity (phase 4 depolarization). Numbers refer to the various phases of the action potential. *B,* Action potentials recorded under certain abnormal conditions. On the left are early afterdepolarizations (EADs), which are prolonged depolarizations interrupting the repolarization phase of the action potential. On the right are delayed afterdepolarizations (DADs), which are depolarizations occurring after the end of the action potential. Both EADs and DADs may lead to triggered activations (TA), which are new action potentials that may become repetitive to cause tachycardia. EADs occur in congenital prolonged QT syndrome and as a result of toxicity with a number of drugs that prolong action potential duration. DADs may occur in digitalis toxicity.

## MECHANISMS OF ARRHYTHMIAS

The two major categories of arrhythmia mechanisms are reentry (4–8) and automaticity. Most arrhythmias occur because of reentry. Figure 14.2*A* shows a zone of depressed conduction displaying unidirectional block. Impulses are blocked at this junction in an antegrade direction, but they proceed in retrograde direction to complete a reentrant circuit that may then become repetitive to cause tachycardia. Antiarrhythmic drugs either prolong refractoriness or depress conduction further at the abnormal segment to convert one-way block to two-way block and thus prevent reentry (Fig 14.2*B*). However, depression of conduction in other instances

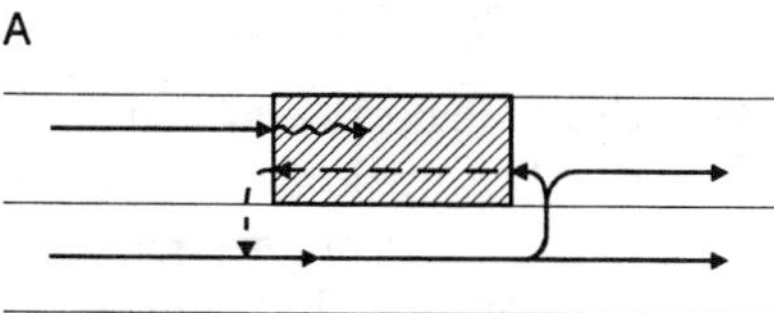


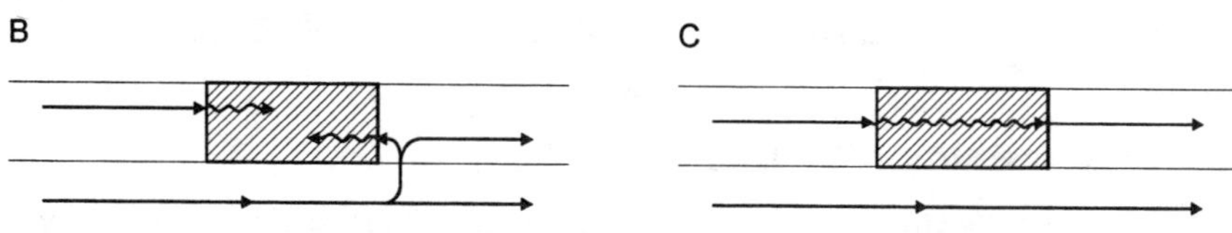


Figure 14.2 Schematic depiction of reentry. *A,* Shows reentry in myocardium. Here, there are two contiguous strips of ventricular muscle. The upper strip has a depressed segment that displays one-way block. An impulse (*arrow*) proceeds into this zone and is blocked in an antegrade direction. The corresponding impulse proceeds in a contiguous strip and then reenters in a retrograde direction through the zone of one-way block to complete a reentrant cycle, which may become repetitive to cause a reentrant tachycardia. *B,* Shows the usual effects of antiarrhythmic drugs, i.e., further depression of conduction and/or prolongation of refractoriness in the depressed segment. Here the impulse again proceeds in an antegrade direction, slows, and is blocked as in *A;* however, in this case the retrograde impulse is also blocked. *C,* Shows a more favorable and probably less common effect of antiarrhythmic drugs. Here the impulse, rather than being blocked in an antegrade direction, passes on through, making reentry impossible. Adapted with permission from Kupersmith J. Antiarrhythmic drugs: general principles. In: Singer I, Kupersmith J, eds. Clinical manual of electrophysiology. Baltimore: Williams & Wilkins, 1993.

may actually promote reentry and cause arrhythmias, a fundamental paradox in antiarrhythmic therapy.

Automaticity, the other mechanism of arrhythmias, can be subdivided into enhanced automaticity and triggered activity. Enhanced automaticity relates to a cell or groups of cells developing rapid automatic activity, (i.e., rapid firing). It is believed to be the cause of atrial and ventricular tachyarrhythmias during catecholamine excess, e.g., pheochromocytoma, (enhanced normal automaticity) (9) or accelerated idioventricular rhythm (abnormal automaticity) (10–11).

Triggered activity is a type of abnormal automaticity in which undriven action potentials arise from early or late afterdepolarizations (Fig. 14.1*B*). Mechanisms related to early afterdepolarizations are believed to be the cause of torsades de pointes ventricular arrhythmias (a dangerous arrhythmia characterized by bursts of rapid polymorphic ventricular tachycardia that occur in the congenital and acquired—i.e., usually drug related—long QT syndrome) (12). Delayed afterdepolarizations are responsible for certain digitalis-induced arrhythmias (13).

## EVALUATION OF ANTIARRHYTHMIC DRUGS

The goals of antiarrhythmic drug therapy are (1) prevention of sudden cardiac or other death; (2) diminution of symptoms; (3) diminution of complications secondary to arrhythmias such as emboli, syncope, and hypotension; and (4) suppression of arrhythmic events in patients with implantable cardioverter defibrillators to prevent excessive firing of the device (14). The major methods of evaluating antiarrhythmic drugs are electrophysiologic (EP) testing, ambulatory and other electrocardiographic (ECG) monitoring, drug level monitoring, and observation of symptoms.

### Electrophysiologic Testing

Clinical EP testing is an invasive approach most frequently used in ventricular arrhythmias and certain of the supraventricular arrhythmias. The basic premises of EP testing are: arrhythmias that occur spontaneously may be induced and reenacted in the catheterization laboratory via electrical stimulation; and treatments that successfully prevent induction of arrhythmias in the laboratory are likely to be successful in long-term therapy (Fig. 14.3) (15).

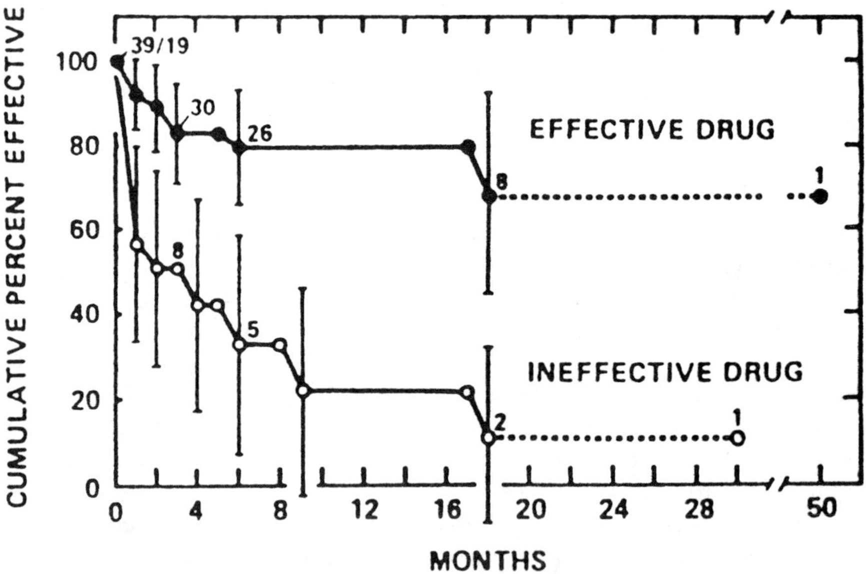


**Figure 14.3** Electrophysiologic (EP) testing used to determine efficacy of antiarrhythmic drugs. Cumulative percentage of efficacy, i.e., freedom from arrhythmia events, is shown on the vertical axis. *Solid circles* represent patients in whom drug efficacy has been shown by EP testing and *open circles* represent patients in whom drugs were ineffective. Data were from a nonrandomized study. Reproduced with permission from Mason JW, Winkle RA. Accuracy of the ventricular tachycardia-induction study for predicting long-term efficacy and inefficacy of antiarrhythmic drugs. N Engl J Med 1980;303:1073–1077.

It is beyond the scope of this chapter to discuss the particulars and pitfalls of EP testing (15–20). However, the ability of EP testing to predict events has been questioned. For example, one study found a limited predictive ability of the test: if ventricular arrhythmias continued to be inducible in the EP laboratory despite drug treatment, prognosis was worse than if the arrhythmia was suppressed by drugs. However, empiric treatment with the β-blocker metoprolol in another group had an outcome similar to that of EP-guided therapy (21). Doubts about EP testing have also been expressed in the case of amiodarone therapy (22).

In spite of the questions that have been raised, the test has numerous uses and is still widely used to evaluate drugs and pacing devices for ventricular arrhythmias and in Wolff-Parkinson-White syndrome mainly as a prelude to catheter ablation but also to test drugs. EP testing is not useful in atrial fibrillation.

## Ambulatory ECG Monitoring

Ambulatory ECG (or Holter) monitoring is an important technique in evaluating arrhythmias and the effects of antiarrhythmic drugs. Here the arrhythmia is analyzed during a baseline evaluation or monitoring period, and the evaluation is repeated after drug administration. Ambulatory ECG monitoring is also useful for correlating symptoms with arrhythmias because there may be surprises, e.g., the occurrence of sinus tachycardia rather than paroxysmal supraventricular tachycardia during symptomatic episodes in patients with the Wolff-Parkinson-White syndrome (23). Monitoring periods usually last 24 hours but may vary from 8–72 hours.

Although it is easy to use and interpret, ambulatory ECG monitoring has many pitfalls. First, it is costly and there is a limit to the frequency of its use, an issue in establishing drug dosages or changing therapy. Second, arrhythmias have to occur frequently. For example, it is not uncommon in patients with paroxysmal atrial fibrillation or ventricular tachycardia for arrhythmias not to occur during the particular monitoring period chosen. On the other hand, event monitors of various kinds, particularly transtelephonic devices (which are worn for several weeks), are useful for infrequently occurring arrhythmias. Third, there is significant spontaneous variation in frequently occurring arrhythmias. Ventricular premature complexes, for example, have a 23% day-to-day and 48% hourly variation (24). Finally, use of one arrhythmia as a proxy for another poses problems. These problems were manifest acutely in the Cardiac Arrhythmias Suppression Trial (CAST) when ventricular premature complexes were used as proxy for more life-threatening arrhythmias. On the other hand results of the Electrophysiologic Study Versus Electrodiographic Monitoring (ESVEM) trial in patients with inducible ventricular tachycardia or fibrillation and frequent ventricular premature complexes (admittedly a rather small universe) were different. In the ESVEM study, suppression of ventricular premature complexes on monitoring and electrophysiologic testing had similar predictive capacity for serious ventricular events and similar costs (25–27).

### Standard ECGs

Standard ECGs are useful more for monitoring drug toxicity, e.g., prolongation of PR, QRS, or $QT_c$ intervals, and they may also detect arrhythmias.

### Signal-Averaged ECGs

Although signal-averaged ECGs (SA-ECGs) yield prognostic information and certain antiarrhythmic drugs may influence the SA-ECG, there are no SA-ECG parameters that predict drug efficacy. Thus, the SA-ECG cannot be used to guide antiarrhythmic drug therapy (28).

### Drug Levels

Drug levels may be monitored as outlined in Chapter 1.

### Symptoms

For non–life-threatening arrhythmias (and those not associated with emboli) the goal of therapy is to control symptoms. This should be kept in mind during the evaluating of aggressive therapy for arrhythmia suppression.

## PROARRHYTHMIA AND OTHER POTENTIALLY LETHAL EFFECTS

The paradox of antiarrhythmic therapy is the ability of drugs to both cause and suppress arrhythmias. This two-edged sword can be explained by the depressive electrophysiologic properties of drugs described above (e.g., Fig. 14.2*B*) and the ability of drugs to induce triggered activity (early and delayed afterdepolarizations) (Fig. 14.1*B*). It may also be related to direct depression of myocardial pump function.

Primary evidence of proarrhythmia is an increase in arrhythmias on ambulatory or other ECG monitoring or on EP testing (29, 30). In the case of ventricular premature complexes (31) and EP testing for ventricular tachycardia or fibrillation (22), criteria have been established for proarrhythmia. Atrial proarrhythmia has been less clearly characterized, although it occurs, e.g., increased atrial arrhythmia with class IC agents (32) and increased atrial fibrillation with digoxin (33) and calcium channel blockers (34, 35).

Certain ventricular arrhythmias have been characterized as specifically related to drug-induced proarrhythmia, i.e., torsades de pointes (12, 36, 37) and incessant ventricular tachycardia. Torsades de pointes (Fig. 14.4) is associated with drugs that lengthen action potential duration and $QT_c$ interval, e.g., quinidine (36, 38) (although $QT_c$ may not be prolonged in all patients with the arrhythmia); the effect is fostered by hypokalemia and

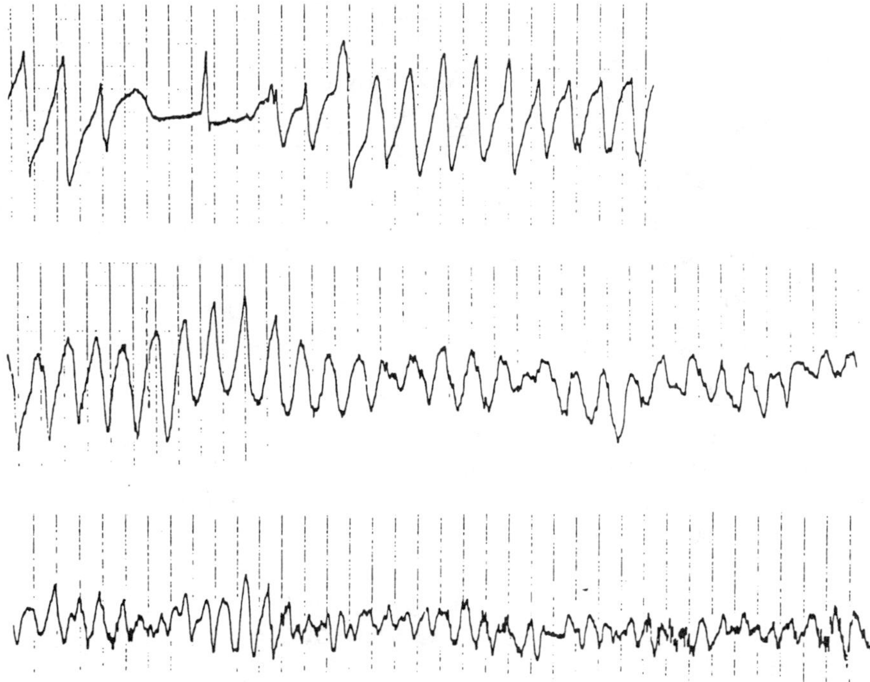

Figure 14.4 Torsades de pointes (polymorphic ventricular tachycardia) progressing to ventricular fibrillation. Reproduced with permission from Roden DM. The long Q-T syndrome and torsades de pointes: basic and clinical aspects. In: El-Sherif N, Samet P, eds. Cardiac pacing and electrophysiology. Philadelphia: WB Saunders, 1991; 265–284.

bradycardia and can occur even at low drug levels. Recent data suggest that $QT_c$ dispersion on ECG leads is particularly associated with torsades de pointes (39). Incessant ventricular tachycardia is a toxic manifestation of drugs that block the sodium channel, especially the class IC agent flecainide (40) (and now unavailable encainide) as well as quinidine.

Besides proarrhythmia per se, the increased mortality observed in certain antiarrhythmic drug trials is also disturbing. Although these results may be due to proarrhythmia, they may also result from myocardial failure and other factors. The most widely known study is CAST (41), which showed that patients with ventricular arrhythmia given encainide or flecainide postmyocardial infarction had a higher mortality rate (and rate of myocardial pump failure) than those on placebo; the increased mortality occurred in those with mild as well as in those with severe disease features. A similar but less conclusive trend was later shown for morcizine (42) and for mexiletine in another study (43). Figure 14.5*A* shows an overview of mortality risk after myocardial infarction (MI) from drugs in all classes (44). Mortality is significantly increased with class I and significantly decreased with class II agents (β-blockers) and amiodarone.

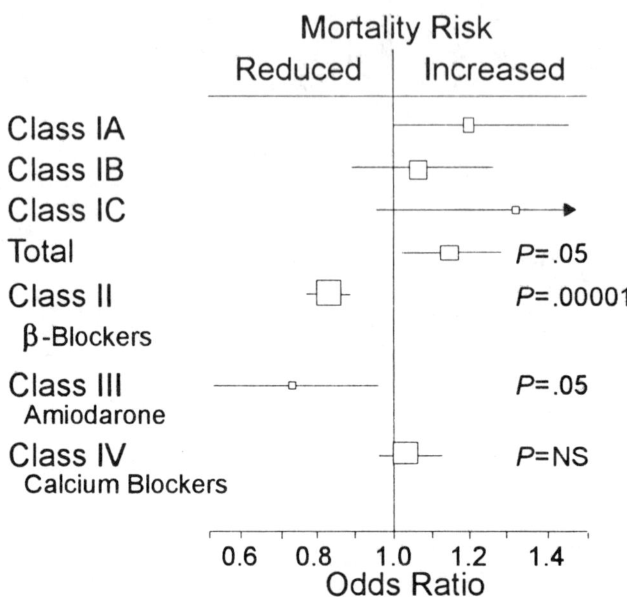
Post MI Trials
Mortality Risk
Reduced
Increased
Class IA
Class IB
Class IC
Total
P=.05
Class II
β-Blockers
P=.00001
Class III
Amiodarone
P=.05
Class IV
Calcium Blockers
P=NS
0.6
0.8
1.0
1.2
1.4
Odds Ratio

A

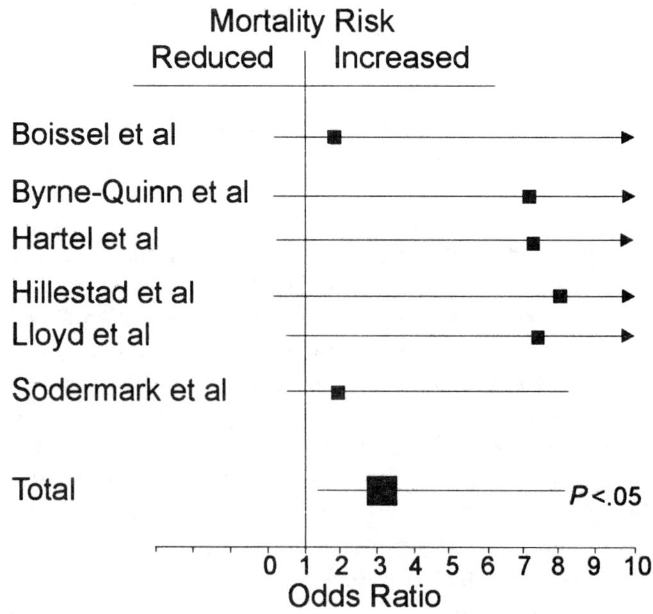
Quinidine: AF Post Cardioversion
Mortality Risk
Reduced
Increased
Boissel et al
Byrne-Quinn et al
Hartel et al
Hillestad et al
Lloyd et al
Sodermark et al
Total
P<.05
0 1 2 3 4 5 6 7 8 9 10
Odds Ratio

B

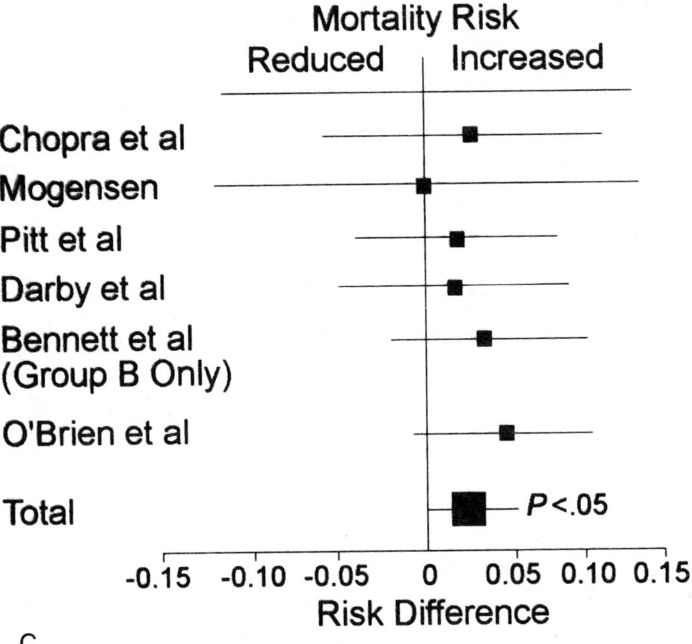


**Figure 14.5** Antiarrhythmic drug effects on mortality under various circumstances. *A,* Odds ratio of mortality risk for various classes of drugs after myocardial infarction (MI). *B,* Odds ratio for quinidine in atrial fibrillation (AF) patients after cardioversion. *C,* Risk difference for lidocaine during the treatment period of MI. Horizontal lines show 95% confidence intervals. In *A, P* values are shown on the right. Total patient numbers and percent mortality drug/placebo for these studies are as follows: Class IA: N = 6582, 7.7/6.6%; Class IB: N = 14,013, 4.3/4.0%; Class IC: N = 2538, 7.4/6.0%. Totals, all Class I drugs: N = 23,229, 5.6/5.0%; Class II (β-blockers): N = 53,268, 5.4/6.6%; Class III (amiodarone only): N = 1557, 9.9/13.0%; Class IV calcium channel blockers: N = 20,342, 9.7/9.3%. Note statistically significant results in favor of drug therapy for the β-blockers and amiodarone and in favor of the placebo (i.e., higher mortality on drug) for the Class IC drugs as a group. In the case of the Class IC drugs, however, the results of the CAST trial on flecainide-encainide were statistically significant on their own (41). For the Class III drugs, only studies on amiodarone were analyzed. A recent study on d-sotalol (Survival with oral d-sotalol; SWORD) in patients with left ventricular dysfunction revealed an increased mortality on drug (44). In *B,* results were for 12 months after electroconversion, during which time the AF patients remaining in sinus rhythm at 3, 6, and 12 months in the quinidine group were 45%, 33%, and 25%, respectively, versus 24%, 23%, and 24%, respectively, for placebo. Mortality/total patient numbers were: quinidine 12/413, control 3/387 (2.9% versus 0.8%) ($P < .05$). Thus, in spite of a modest but beneficial effect on the arrhythmia, albeit for a relatively short period of time, there was a statistically significant increased mortality with quinidine (45). In *C,* analysis of 6 studies (54–59) was for the period of lidocaine treatment only (24–48 hours). Mortality/total numbers were 37/705 for lidocaine and 21/702 for control (5.2% versus 3.0%) ($P < .05$). There was no statistically significant difference in mortality between lidocaine and placebo when the prehospital phase or when the total hospitalization was taken into account (not shown). Reproduced with permission from Hine LK, Laird N, Hewitt P, et al. Meta-analytic evidence against prophylactic use of lidocaine in acute myocardial infarction. Arch Intern Med 1989;149:2694–2698.

Disturbing information has also come from metaanalyses of drug trials in other situations. For example, a metaanalysis of six studies of quinidine administered to patients with atrial fibrillation during the first year after cardioversion showed that mortality was increased as arrhythmia was suppressed (2.9 versus 0.8%, odds ratio 2.98, $P < 0.05$) (44–50) (Fig. 14.5*B*) A retrospective review of the Stroke Prevention in Atrial Fibrillation (SPAF) trial also revealed an increased mortality in congestive heart failure patients taking antiarrhythmics (nonrandomized data) (51). In hospitalized patients with myocardial infarction, lidocaine reduced primary VF but also increased mortality (52–58) (Fig. 14.5*C*).

## CLASSIFICATION OF ANTIARRHYTHMIC DRUGS

Classification of antiarrhythmic drugs has always been problematic. Although classifications of other drug types usually devolve around structure (e.g., tricyclic antidepressants) with variances of function expected, attempts to classify antiarrhythmic drugs focus mainly on electrophysiologic properties and specifically on ion channel blockade. The approach creates excessive expectations that cannot be realized, e.g., that drugs in a certain class will be interchangeable as to their antiarrhythmic effect in a specific patient. This goal is unachievable because an absolute pharmacologic specificity of a drug does not exist. In addition, differences in kinetics, local tissue concentration (especially in abnormal tissue) (59) and other similar factors play important roles in antiarrhythmic properties. Thus, the effects of drugs in the clinic are not entirely predictable based on ionic or receptor effects (60).

The most widely used antiarrhythmic drug classification is the Vaughan-Williams classification with the Harrison modification (1–3, 61) based mainly on electrophysiologic properties (Table 14.1). There are five classes of drugs. Class I are sodium channel blockers that influence mainly atrial, His-Purkinje, and ventricular cardiac tissue. This class is divided into subclasses A, B, and C based on the degree of sodium channel blockade and the rate of binding and unbinding (association and dissociation) of drugs from the sodium channel (i.e., use dependent block; see Table 14.1). Class II drugs are β-blockers. Class III drugs prolong action potential and either block the potassium channel or enhance slow inward sodium current (a subclassification has been suggested for different types of potassium channel blockade, but it is not currently used) (62). Class IV drugs are calcium channel blockers and class V consists of miscellaneous drugs.

Recently, the Vaughan-Williams classification has been attacked by a group of concepts called the "Sicilian gambit" (61–64) ("Sicilian" because it was discussed at a meeting housed in Taormina, Sicily; "gambit" because it is an opening strategy rather than a fully developed concept). In the Sicilian gambit, all antiarrhythmic drugs are listed according to their channel and receptor blocking (i.e., βα, or parasympathetic) properties and in

**Table 14.1**
**Classification of Antiarrhythmic Drugs**

| | |
|---|---|
| Class I: | Local anesthetic agents |
| Class IA: | Intermediate suppression of sodium current and UDB with intermediate rate kinetics[a,b] |
| Class IB: | Modest suppression of sodium ions and UDB with rapid kinetics[a,c] |
| Class IC: | Considerable suppression of sodium ions and UDB with slow kinetics[a,d] |
| Class II: | β-Adrenergic blocking agents |
| Class III: | Drugs that primarily prolong action potential duration |
| Class IV: | Calcium channel blockers |
| Class V: | Miscellaneous (e.g., adenosine) |

[a]All drugs that block the sodium channel have greater affinity to the channel and thus greater effects during rapid rates. This phenomenon is referred to as use-dependent block (UDB). Drugs with rapid UDB kinetics bind and unbind to the channel quickly and thus have a substantially greater enhancement of effect during tachycardias. For reasons related to the electrophysiologic properties of damaged tissue, they also have greater effects on conduction in abnormal than in normal tissue (e.g., they exhibit "ischemic zone selectivity") (83, 84).
[b]Class IA agents also prolong action protential duration.
[c]Class IB agents also shorten action potential duration.
[d]Class IC agents also have no effect on action potential duration.
Data from Harrison DC. Antiarrhythmic drug classification: new science and practical applications. Am J Cardiol 1985;56:185–187; Kupersmith J. Antiarrhythmic drugs: specific agents. In: Singer I, Kupersmith J, eds. Clinical manual of electrophysiology. Baltimore: Williams & Wilkins, 1993;186–207; Vaughan-Williams EM. A classification of antiarrhythmic actions re-assessed after a decade of new drugs. J Clin Pharmacol 1984;24:129–147; Vaughan-Williams EM. Classification of the antiarrhythmic action of moricizine. J Clin Pharmacol 1991;31:216–221.

one case enzymatic (sodium-potassium adenosine triphosphatase) effect. The thrust of the gambit is to match electrophysiologic properties of drugs with what are termed *vulnerable parameters* of arrhythmias, i.e., those electrophysiologic properties that may be associated with termination of arrhythmia such as block of reentry. For example, drugs that block sodium channel are thought to be better for certain reentrant arrhythmias (e.g., type I atrial flutter) and those that prolong action potential duration and refractoriness for others (e.g., atrial fibrillation).

The Sicilian gambit at present is not a classification but a framework and departure point for discussions by experts regarding drug properties in relation to arrhythmias. One's choice of drug is still ordinarily based mainly on clinical experience and empiricism and only somewhat on knowledge of electrophysiologic properties. This chapter follows the Vaughan-Williams classification with the realization, however, that it does not offer complete predictability in regard to antiarrhythmic effect within a class and that its days may be numbered.

## SPECIFIC AGENTS

Table 14.2 shows dosages, Table 14.3 various pharmacologic attributes of each antiarrhythmic drug, and Table 14.4 important pharmacokinetic drug interactions.

**Table 14.2**
**Dosage of Antiarrhythmic Drugs**

| | Intravenous Dosage | | Oral Dosage | | |
|---|---|---|---|---|---|
| | Loading[a] | Maintenance | Initial | Loading (mg)[a,b] | Maintenance (mg/day) |
| Class IA | | | | | |
| Quinidine | 6–10 mg/kg at 0.3–0.5 mg/kg/min[c] | | 200 mg q 6 h (sulfate) | 600–1000 (sulfate) | 648–1944 (gluconate) 800–1600 (sulfate) |
| Procainamide | 6–15 mg/kg at 0.2–0.5 mg/kg/min[d] | 2–6 mg/min | 500 mg q 6 h (SR) | 500–1000 | 2000–6000 (SR) (50 mg/kg) |
| Disopyramide | | | 100 mg q 6 h | | 300–800 |
| Class IB | | | | | |
| Lidocaine | —[e] | —[e] | — | — | — |
| Mexiletine | — | — | 200 mg q 8 h | initial dose of 400 mg, then 200 mg q 8 h | 200–400 q 8 h or 450 q 12 h |
| Class IC | | | | | |
| Flecainide | — | — | 50 mg q 12 h[f] | | 200–400[g] |
| Propafenone | — | — | 150 mg q 8 h | | 300–900 |
| Class III | | | | | |
| Amiodarone | —[e] | —[e] | —[e] | —[e] | —[e] |
| Sotalol | | | 80 mg bid | | 160–640 |
| Bretylium | 5–10 mg/kg, over <8 min[i] | 0.5–2 mg/min | | | |
| Ibutilide | 1 mg over 10 min ×2 if necessary[i,j] | — | — | — | — |
| Class IV | | | | | |
| Verapamil | 5–10 mg over 2–3 min × 2 q 30 min[g] 0.25 mg/kg over 2 | 0.125 μg/min | 80–120 mg | — | 240–1600 SR or tablet |

**Table 14.2—*continued***
**Dosage of Antiarrhythmic Drugs**

| | Intravenous Dosage | | Oral Dosage | | |
|---|---|---|---|---|---|
| | Loading[a] | Maintenance | Initial | Loading mg[a,b] | Maintenance (mg/day) |
| Diltiazem | min, 2nd dose:0.35 mg/kg/over 2 min, 15 min later[g] | 5–15 mg/h | 120–240 mg/day | | 180–480 (SR or CD) |
| Class V | | | | | |
| Adenosine | 6–12 mg × 2 q 1–2 min[g,k] | | | | |
| Digoxin | 0.75–1 mg | 0.125–0.375 mg/day | 0.25–0.50 mg | 1–1.5 mg | 0.125–0.5 mg |

[a] *Loading dosages are highly individual and depend on response, observation of toxicity, and presence of renal, hepatic, or congestive heart failure.*
[b] Oral loading must be done with caution and careful observation.
[c] Now uncommonly used. Intramuscular quinidine gluconate can also be used at a dose of 400 mg initially and up to 200 mg Q2H.
[d] Alternative dosing regimen for acute arrhythmias: 100 mg every 5 minutes until arrhythmia terminates, toxicity (hypotension), or a total dose of 1000 mg is administered.
[e] See text for dosage regimens.
[f] For supraventricular tachycardia. Start at 100 mg every 12 hours for ventricular tachycardia. Maximum dose: 300 mg for supraventricular tachycardia, 400 mg for ventricular tachycardia.
[g] Second dose only if necessary.
[h] Repeat if necessary at 10 mg in cardiac arrests or at 1–2 hours in other situations.
[i] For patients weighing less than 60 kg, dose is: 01 mg/kg.
[j] Second dose can be administered if arrhythmia does not convert within 10 minutes.
[k] Drug must be administered rapidly; it is less effective when given slowly.
CD = ; IV = intravenous; h = hour; mg = milligram; min = minutes; ng = nanograms; po = oral; q = every; SR = sustained release.
Data Antiarrhythmic drugs. Medical Lett Drug Ther 1991;33:55–60; Beaufils P, Leenhardt A, Denjoy E, et al. Antiarrhythmic drugs in the adult population. In: Rosen MR, Janse MJ, Wit AL, eds. Cardiac electrophysiology. Mt. Kisco, NY: 1990:1175–1187; Frishman WH, Sonnenblick EH. Calcium channel blockers. In: Hurst JW, Schlant RC, eds. The heart. New York: McGraw-Hill, 1990:1731–1748; Funck-Brentano C, Woosley RL. Current antiarrhythmic agents: clinical pharmacology. In: El-Sherif N, Samet P, eds. Cardiac pacing and electrophysiology. Philadelphia: WB Saunders, 1991:409–435; Kupersmith J. Antiarrhythmic drugs: specific agents. In: Singer I, Kupersmith J, eds. Clinical manual of electrophysiology. Baltimore: Williams & Wilkins, 1993:186–207; Marcus FI, Huang SK. Digitalis. In: Hurst JW, Schlant RC, eds. The heart. 7th ed. New York: McGraw-Hill, 1990:1748–1761; Scheiner LB, Tozer TN. Clinical pharmacokinetics. The use of plasma concentrations of drugs. In: Melmon KL, Morrelli HF, eds. Clinical pharmacology. New York: MacMillan, 1978:71–109; Woosley RLJ. Antiarrhythmic agents. In: Hurst JW, Schlant RC, eds. The heart. New York: McGraw-Hill, 1990:1682–1711; Zipes DP: Management of cardiac arrhythmias: pharmacological, electrical, and surgical techniques. In: Braunwald E, ed. Heart disease. Philadelphia: WB Saunders, 1988:621–657.

**Table 14.3**
**Pharmacology of Antiarrhythmic Drugs**

| | Time to Peak Level ($t_{max}$) (po) (h) | Bioavailability (%) | Volume of Distribution ($V_D$) (L/kg) | Protein Binding (%) | Beta $T_{1/2}$ (h) | Therapeutic Levels[a] (mg/L) | Route(s) of Elimination | Active Metabolites |
|---|---|---|---|---|---|---|---|---|
| Class IA | | | | | | | | |
| Quinidine | 1.5–3 | 60–80 | 2.5 | 80–90 | 5–9 | 2–5 | Liver | 3-OH quinidine[i] 2'Oxoquinidinone[i] O-Desmethyl quinidine[i] |
| Procainamide | 1 (tab) 2–3 (SR) | 80–100 | 2 | 15 | 3–5[b] | 4–10[c] | Liver and kidneys[d] | N-acetylprocainamide |
| Disopyramide | 1–2 | 80–90 | 1.5 | 20–50[e] | 4–10 | 2–5 | Kidneys | N-Diisopropyl disopyramide |
| Class IB | | | | | | | | |
| Lidocaine | —[f] | 35[f] | 2 | 40–70 | 1.5–2.5 | 1.5–5.0 | Liver (first pass)[g] | Monoethlyglycine xylidine Glycine xylidine |
| Mexiletine | 2–4 | 70–90 | 5.5–9.5 | 70 | 8–17 | 0.5–2.0 | Liver and kidneys | — |
| Class IC | | | | | | | | |
| Flecainide | 2–4 | 90–95 | 7–10 | 40 | 12–27 | 0.2–1.0 | Liver and kidneys | — |
| Propafenone | 1–3 | —[h] | 3–4 | 90 | 2–32[b] | 0.5–3.0[c] | Liver and kidneys[d] | 3-OH propafenone N-dealkyl propafenone |
| Class III | | | | | | | | |
| Amiodarone | 3–5 | 35–65 | 20–200 | 95 | 14–53[i] days | 1–2.5.0[c] | Liver | Desethyl amiodarone |
| Sotalol | 2.5–3.5 | 95–100 | 1.5–1.8 | 20–40 | 10–18 | 1.5–4.0 | Kidneys | — |
| Bretylium | —[f] | 10–35[f] | 3–4 | Low | 7–8 | 0.5–1.5 | Kidneys | — |
| Ibutilide | —[f] | —[f] | 11 | 40 | 2–12 | — | Liver and kidneys[d] | ω Hydroxy ibutilide[j] |

**Table 14.3—*continued***
**Pharmacology of Antiarrhythmic Drugs**

| | Time to Peak Level ($t_{max}$) (po) (h) | Bioavailability (%) | Volume of Distribution ($V_D$) (L/kg) | Protein Binding (%) | Beta $T_{1/2}$ (h) | Therapeutic Levels[a] (mg/L) | Route(s) of Elimination | Active Metabolites |
|---|---|---|---|---|---|---|---|---|
| Class IV | | | | | | | | |
| Verapamil | 1–2 | 10–35 | 4–5 | 90 | 6–10 | 0.05–0.4[c] | Liver (first pass)[g] | Norverapamil |
| Diltiazem | 1.5 (tablets) (3–4 SR or CD) | 30–40 | 5 | 80–90 | 2–11 | 0.05–.03[3] | Liver (first pass)[g] | *N*-monodemthyl diltiazem Deacetyl diltiazem |
| Class V | | | | | | | | |
| Adenosine | | | | | 1–7 sec | | | — |
| Digoxin | 1–2 | 50–80 (tablet) 80–100 (caplet) | 4–8 | 25 | 1.1–1.9 days | 1.2–2.0 ng/mL | Liver and kidneys | — |

[a]Therapeutic levels are an approximate range; they may vary considerably among individuals as well as among conditions for which the drug is used.
[b]Genetic variation in metabolism (see text).
[c]Active metabolite(s) may play an important role (see text).
[d]Parent compound and active metabolites are eliminated by the kidneys.
[e]Protein binding is concentration dependent.
[f]Not used as an oral agent for arrhythmias.
[g]Requires dosage modification in congestive heart failure.
[h]Saturable hepatic first-pass metabolism (see text).
[i]Highly variable
[j]Minor role.
CD = ; h = hour; po =by mouth; SR = sustained-release form.
Data from Beaufils P, Leenhardt A, Denjoy E, *et al.* Antiarrhythmic drugs in the adult population. In: Rosen MR, Janse MJ, Wit AL, eds. Cardiac electrophysiology. Mt. Kisco, NY. Futura, 1990. 1175–1187; Frishman WH, Sonnenblick EH. Calcium channel blockers. In: Hurst JW, Schlant RC, eds. The heart. 7th ed. New York: McGraw-Hill, 1990:1731–1748; Funck-Bretano C, Woosley RL. Current antiarrhythmic agents: clinical pharmacology. In: El-Sherif N, Samet P, eds. Cardiac pacing and electrophysiology. Philadelphia: WB Saunders, 1991:409–435; Marcus FI, Huang SK. Digitalis. In: Hurst JW, Schlant RC, eds. The heart. 7th ed. New York: McGraw-Hill, 1990:1748–1761; Medical Lett Drug Ther Drugs for cardiac arrhythmias. 1991;33:55–60; Slama R. Antiarrhythmic drugs in the adult population. In: Rosen MR, Janse MJ, Wit AL, eds. Cardiac electrophysiology. Mt. Kisco, NY: Futura, 1990:1175–1187; Woosley RL. Antiarrhythmic agents. In: Hurst JW, Schlant RC, eds. The heart. 7th ed. New York: McGraw-Hill, 1990:1682–1711; Zipes DP: Management of cardiac arrhythmias: pharmacological, electrical, and surgical techniques. In: Braunwald E, ed. Heart disease. Philadelphia: WB Saunders, 1988;621–657.

**Table 14.4**
**Pharmacokinetic Drug Interactions**

| | On Other Drugs | On Antiarrhythmic |
|---|---|---|
| Class IA | | |
| Quinidine | ↑ Digoxin | ↓ By phenobarbial |
| Procainamide | — | — |
| Disopyramide | — | ↓ By phenobarital, phenytoin, rifampicin |
| Class IB | | |
| Lidocaine | — | — |
| Mexiletine | ↑ Theophylline | ↓ By phenobarbital, phenytoin, rifamipicin |
| Class IC | | |
| Flecainide | ↑ Digoxin, propranolol | ↑ By cimitidine, propranolol, amiodarone<br>↑ By quinidine, cimetidine (but ↓'s metabolites and thus no ECG effect) |
| Propafenone | ↑ Digoxin, warfarin, propranolol, metoprolol | ↓ By rifampicin |
| Class III | | |
| Amiodarone | ↑ Warfarin[a], digoxin, quinidine, procainamide, disopyramide, mexiletine, propafenone | |
| Sotalol | — | — |
| Bretylium | — | — |
| Ibutilide | — | — |
| Class IV | | |
| Verapamil | ↑ Digoxin, metoprolol, carbamazepine, phenazone | ↓ By rifampicin and perhaps by cimitidine[b] |
| Diltiazem | ↑ Digoxin, cyclosporine, carbamazapine;<br>↓ Theophylline, propanolol | ↑ By cimitidine |
| Class V | | |
| Adenosine | — | ↑ By rifampicin, carbamazepine, dipyridamole.<br>↓ By methylxanthines, (theophylline) and quinidine |
| Digoxin | — | ↓ By bile acid binding resins, antacids, kaolin, pectate, erythromycin, tetracycline<br>↑ By quinidine verapamil, amiodarone |

**Table 14.4—*continued***
**Pharmacokinetic Drug Interactions**

| | On Other Drugs | On Antiarrhythmic |
|---|---|---|
| | | ↑ Somewhat propafenone, diltiazem, nifedipine, spironolactone, triamterine, indomethacin |

[a]Very important and requires close INR monitoring.
[b]Conflicting data.
Simpson RJ, Foster JR, Woelfel AK, Gettes LS. Management of atrial fibrillation and flutter. A reappraisal of digitalis therapy. Postgrad Med J 1986:79:241–253; Juhl RP, Summers RW, Guillory JK, et al. Effect of sulfasalazine on digoxin bioavailability. Clin Pharmacol Ther 1976:20:387–394; Klabunde RE. Dipyridamole inhibition of adenosine metabolism in human blood. Eur J Pharmacol 1983;16:21–26; Lee TH, Smith TW. Serum digoxin concentration and diagnosis of digitalis toxicity: current concepts. Clin Pharmacokinet 1983;8:279–285; Marcus FI, Huang SK. Digitalis. In: Hurst JW, Schlant RC, eds. The heart. 7th ed. New York: McGraw-Hill, 1990:1748–1761; Physicians Desk Reference. Montvale, NJ: Medical Economics Data Production, 1995; Meszaros J, Kelemen K, Kecskemeti V et al. Interaction between adenosine and antiarrrhythmic agents in atrial myocardium of guinea-pig. Arch Int Pharmacodyn Ther 1986;280:84–96. Tjandra Maga TB, van Hecken A, van Melle P, et al. Altered pharmacokinetics of oral flecainide by cimetidine. Br J Clin Pharmacol 1986;22:108.

## Class I Agents

Class I agents block sodium channels and therefore affect atrial, His-Purkinje, and ventricular tissues. They also suppress normal automaticity. All are negatively inotropic to varying degrees, but for some of the drugs this effect is mild and may be counterbalanced by afterload reducing properties (66). Hypotension may also occur (generally with intravenous but rarely with oral forms of these drugs) because of cardiac, α-adrenergic blocking (67), or direct vasodilating effects. Most drugs in this class are vagolytic.

Class I agents have been subdivided into A, B, and C subclasses based on specifics of sodium channel blockade. There are also differences in effects on action potential duration (and thus, $QT_c$ interval) (see Table 14.1).

### *Class IA Agents*

Class IA agents have intermediate potency between classes IB and IC in blocking sodium channels, slowing conduction, and prolonging action potential duration; currently used drugs are also anticholinergic. These agents have variable effects on ECG PR intervals (prolongation as a result of His-Purkinje effects and shortening because of anticholinergic properties) and prolong QRS duration and $QT_c$ intervals. Heart block is a possible complication of these drugs.

Class IA agents approved for use in the United States include quinidine, procainamide, and disopyramide. These agents are used in a wide spectrum of atrial and ventricular arrhythmias, but they can also provoke or exacerbate both bradyarrhythmias and tachyarrhythmias, including torsades de pointes. The drugs should be avoided in patients with baseline prolonged $QT_c$ intervals. Interestingly, they are also hypolipidemic (68).

Because of their vagolytic properties, all class IA agents (especially disopyramide) can cause distressing sinus tachycardia and be dangerous in patients with glaucoma or prostatism. However, anticholinergic effects can apparently be lessened by coexisting administration of sustained-release pyridostigmine, an anticholinesterase agent (69). The role of vagolytic properties in suppressing heart rate variability, a known predisposing factor to sudden death, has recently been of interest, (70).

Class IA agents are all negatively inotropic, which is a minimal problem with oral use, but heart failure and hypotension are important adverse effects with intravenous administration (at least for procainamide, the only agent extensively used intravenously) (71).

**Quinidine.** Quinidine, the d-isomer of quinine and the oldest specifically antiarrhythmic drug (1917), has protean uses for both for ventricular and atrial arrhythmias. The drug is available in oral form as a sulfate or gluconate (the latter more slowly absorbed); intramuscular and intravenous quinidine are rarely used. Quinidine has typical class IA properties and toxicity.

As indicated earlier, metaanalyses have shown that quinidine appears to increase mortality even in patients in whom it reduces arrhythmias, e.g., those with atrial fibrillation (Fig. 14.5*B*) (see also Chapter 15 for a more complete discussion of the use of quinidine in atrial fibrillation). These effects may be exacerbated by coexisting digoxin therapy and hypokalemia, e.g., during diuretic therapy. Quinidine has the longest history of use among antiarrhythmic agents and therefore the largest and most complete set of relevant data. Proarrhythmic adverse effects of other drugs may be similar to those of quinidine but sufficient data are not yet available for evaluation.

Other less profound adverse effects of quinidine, important because they may lead to complete or partial lack of patient compliance, include diarrhea, tinnitus and other manifestations of cinchonism, thrombocytopenia, fever, hepatitis, and anemia.

**Procainamide.** Procainamide has protean uses similar to those of quinidine for atrial and ventricular arrhythmias and a similar spectrum of cardiovascular adverse effects (72). It is used in oral (most commonly in sustained-release form every 6–8 hours) and intravenous preparations.

Procainamide is eliminated by the kidney but also metabolized (acetylated) by the liver into an active compound N-acetyl procainamide (NAPA). NAPA has class III properties (prolongation of action potential duration) and less sodium blocking action than the parent compound (73). Thus, it contributes more to torsades de pointes, especially at levels above 25–30 μg/L. However, NAPA does not contribute to procainamide-induced lupus (see below), which is less common in patients who are "fast acetylators" (more than half of the population) (74), i.e., those who rapidly and more completely convert procainamide to NAPA.

NAPA plays a role in oral but not in intravenous use of the drug and becomes more prominent relative to parent compound over time, especially in renal failure. Because NAPA and procainamide have different EP properties, antiarrhythmic effects may vary, depending on their relative levels. Although many clinicians add the levels of the two compounds in interpretation of serum levels, the situation is far more complex because of these differences.

Intravenous procainamide is commonly used for ventricular tachycardia (second to lidocaine) and for conversion of atrial fibrillation. In EP testing of patients with ventricular arrhythmias, procainamide is frequently used as an indicator drug for potential responsiveness to other agents. One study found that if procainamide prevented ventricular tachycardia induction, the probability that a single or combined class I regimen would be effective was 85% (20).

About one third of patients may have to discontinue procainamide because of adverse effects, the most important of which is the lupus syndrome. Drug-induced lupus is characterized by fever, arthralgias, arthritis, rash, and pericardial effusion but not renal involvement. Most patients on procainamide therapy develop anti-DNA antibodies (single strand), but only clinical lupus, rather than a positive test, is a reason for drug discontinuation. The syndrome clears on drug withdrawal (75). The drug may also cause leukopenia (increased with use of the sustained-released form), fever, and psychosis (76).

**Disopyramide.** Disopyramide is less often used than the other IA agents, although it has the same antiarrhythmic and toxic spectrum (77). In addition to its use in arrhythmias, disopyramide is used in hypertrophic obstructive cardiomyopathy. It is available in a sustained-release form that can be administered every 12 hours (78).

Among pharmacologic peculiarities of the drug is concentration-dependent protein binding (less at higher levels) that makes serum levels difficult to interpret and may cause greatly increased free drug with little increases in dose (79). Both the drug and its active metabolite (N-dealkyl disopyramide) are renally eliminated (80). D-disopyramide is not protein bound and has a higher renal clearance than the l-form (81). Compared with other IA agents, disopyramide has considerably more anticholinergic and myocardial depressant effects, both of which reside mainly in the R-(+)-enantiomer (81) and limit its use, especially in patients with glaucoma and prostatism. $QT_c$ prolongation appears to be mainly via the S-(−)-disopyramide. Hypoglycemia is another toxic effect of disopyramide.

### *Class IB Agents*

Class IB agents have modest effects on inward sodium current, and of all local anesthetic antiarrhythmic drugs, they exhibit the most prominent "use dependent" properties (see Table 14.1) (82), resulting in greater sodium blocking effects during rapid rates and depression of conduction only in ischemic but not in normal tissue ("ischemic zone selectivity") (83, 84).

Two class IB agents are now in use, lidocaine (long a mainstay of coronary care unit therapies) and mexiletine, a more recent (1985) oral lidocaine-like drug that is prescribed modestly. Both drugs are used almost exclusively for ventricular arrhythmias.

In many ways, class IB agents have a better cardiovascular profile than other antiarrhythmic drugs. They do not effect QRS or $QT_c$ intervals, do not cause torsades de pointes (for which they have been administered, although with modest success), and have few negative inotropic properties, especially with oral use. However, they may also increase the risk of mortality as do other class I drugs discussed earlier (43, 44, 52).

**Lidocaine.** Commonly used in several acute situations, most notably MI, lidocaine was first used as an antiarrhythmic drug in 1950. Over time, it has been suggested that lidocaine be administered prophylactically, either intramuscularly in the prehospital setting (dose 300–400 mg) (85) or intravenously. The metaanalysis data on mortality (53) (Fig. 14.5*C*) plus the fact that primary ventricular fibrillation is now unusual in patients with MI (86) have convinced experts of the inadvisability of this approach. Lidocaine is still appropriate treatment for monitored patients with ventricular arrhythmias (87) and is also occasionally used for arrhythmias associated with accessory pathways.

Lidocaine is metabolized by the liver with a high hepatic extraction ratio and thus extensive first-pass metabolism and low oral bioavailability and blood flow-related elimination (see Chapter 1). Therefore, the dose must be modified in low cardiac output states (Fig. 14.6) such as congestive heart failure or cardiogenic shock (88), common situations in which the drug is needed. The volume of distribution of lidocaine is also lowered in these states, necessitating reduction of the loading dose. In addition, the dose may need to be reduced after 24 hours of infusion because of an accumulated metabolite that interferes with elimination (89).

Serum levels of lidocaine are routinely monitored in the coronary care unit. Lidocaine is bound, however, to an acute phase reactant, α-1 acid glycoprotein, that rises in states in which lidocaine is likely to be administered (e.g., acute myocardial infarction) and that may lead to an increase in serum levels with no concomitant increase in effect.

Various approaches to lidocaine administration have been taken, all with the purpose of achieving and maintaining therapeutic blood levels quickly. A common method includes loading of 1–2 μg/kg at a rate of 20–50 μg/minute followed by a constant rate (maintenance) infusion of 1–4 mg/minute (or about 20–60 μg/kg/minute). Because serum levels may fall below therapeutic levels at 30–60 minutes with this method, other regimens of varying complexity have been suggested, as follows:

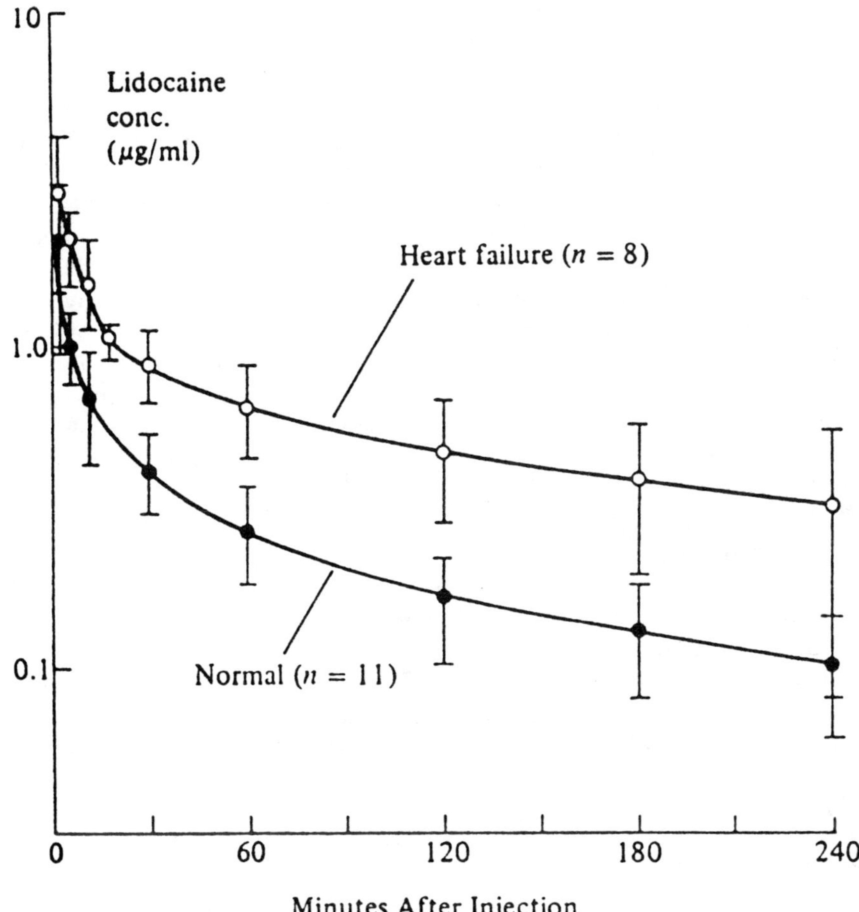


Figure 14.6 Drug levels after intravenous lidocaine administration in patients with and without congestive heart failure. The patients with heart failure have higher levels. Conc. = concentration. Reproduced with permission from Nies AS. Cardiovascular disorders. In: Melman KL, Morell HF, eds. Clinical pharmacology: basic principles in therapeutics. New York: McGraw Hill, 1972; 142–261.

1. 1–2 mg/kg of lidocaine at a rate of 20–50 mg/minute, followed by a second bolus of 0.5 mg/kg in 30 minutes
2. 1 mg/kg, followed by up to 2 doses of up to 1 mg/kg every 5 minutes if initial bolus ineffective (90)
3. exponential infusion of 75 mg, followed by a 5.33 mg/minute tapering to 2 mg/minute over 25 minutes (91)
4. 75 mg followed by 50 mg repeated three times (92)

Once steady-state is established, additional small boluses may be given if higher levels are needed quickly.

The most prominent toxic effects of lidocaine involve the central nervous system. Many patients taking the drug have subtle aberrations of the central nervous system. Drowsiness and dysarthria are common effects of the drug, but seizures are unusual. Bradycardia (both sinus node and heart block), hypotension (not uncommon), and congestive heart failure (rare) also may occur. Subcutaneous administration of lidocaine for local analgesia can also have systemic effects, especially in children (93).

**Mexiletine.** Mexiletine is an oral agent with EP and hemodynamic effects similar to those of lidocaine. It is approved for use against ventricular arrhythmias and, unlike other class IB agents, also has antiarrhythmic properties in supraventriclar tachycardias (SVTs). Although mexiletine is described as a "lidocaine-like" agent, the efficacy of lidocaine in an individual patient often is not predictive of that for mexiletine. Mexiletine is best used in combination with other drugs (94–96), often class IA agents for enhancement of refractory period-prolonging effects or β-blockers in ventricular arrhythmias (97).

Mexiletine is administered every 6–8 hours with food to modulate swings in serum levels and avoid toxicity at peak; such administration does not reduce overall bioavailability. It is eliminated mainly but not entirely by the liver to unknown active metabolites (98). Dosage may have to be reduced in patients with either hepatic or renal disease.

The most common adverse effects of mexiletine are tremor, dizziness, and visual disturbance, which diminish when the drug is administered with food to modify serum level peaks. Other adverse effects include nausea, bradycardia, and heart block (99). The drug has little organ toxicity (rare thrombocytopenia).

### *Class IC Agents*

Class IC agents are the most potent sodium channel blocking drugs and, therefore, also cause the greatest slowing of conduction. They greatly prolong QRS duration, which may also lengthen $QT_c$ intervals without prolonging action potential duration; $JT_c$ intervals, however, remain the same (100). The drugs are intense myocardial depressants and are vagolytic (70).

Class IC agents have been used against several atrial and ventricular arrhythmias, but enthusiasm for these agents has been dampened by the results of CAST (41, 42). Consequently, perhaps, three IC agents that were approved by the Food and Drug Administration—moricizine, encainide (both used in CAST), and indecainide—are not now marketed in the United States. Flecainide and propafenone are the two agents available in this category. Present usage is mainly, though not exclusively, for atrial arrhythmias. Ventricular and possibly atrial (32) proarrhythmias have occurred.

**Flecainide.** Flecainide was used initially for ventricular arrhythmias, but since the CAST results such use is rare and occurs only after electrophysiologic testing (101, 102). Flecainide is used mainly for atrial fibrillation (103) and in paroxysmal SVT (PSVT) in patients with accessory pathways (104). In patients with atrial arrhythmias retrospective data show that mortality does not appear to be increased by the drug (104, 105).

Flecainide is both excreted unchanged in the urine and metabolized by the liver into two potentially active compounds that are, however, at subactive serum levels. At initiation of treatment with flecainide, serum levels should be monitored and never allowed to exceed 1000 μg/L because of possible toxic effects (101). Dosage should not be increased more frequently than every 4 days. Both renal and congestive heart failure may prolong the half-life of the drug.

Adverse effects of flecainide may occur at any drug level and include proarrhythmia, which may be exercise induced (106), and onset or worsening of congestive heart failure. Flecainide also has neurologic adverse effects, namely dizziness and difficulties in visual accommodation (107). These neurologic complications tend to be transient and are generally dose and serum level related, although in individual patients they may occur at any drug level.

**Propafenone.** Propafenone is a class IC agent with interesting therapeutic and pharmacologic features. It has the electrophysiologic properties of IC agents and, to a lesser extent, those of β-blockers (108, 109) and calcium channel blockers (110). At the usual propafenone serum concentrations, its β-blocking properties are 25% those of a similar concentration of propranolol (109), and its calcium channel blocking properties are 1/75 those of verapamil (110). Propafenone is useful for a wide variety of arrhythmias, but its main attractiveness at present is for certain SVTs (111), especially atrial fibrillation and arrhythmias related to Wolff-Parkinson-White syndrome. For routine PSVT and ventricular arrhythmias, it is a second choice agent.

Propafenone pharmacokinetics are complex as is its use (112, 113). The drug undergoes extensive first-pass metabolism, but hepatic enzymes are saturable. Thus, serum levels depend on dose, especially important in drug loading. As dose increases from 150–300 to 400 mg, bioavailablity increases from 5–12% to 40–50% (113, 114) (Fig. 14.7). Serum levels with daily doses of 900 mg are 10 times those with doses of 300 mg.

Propafenone has important active metabolites (5-OH propafenone and the less potent N-delakyl propafenone) (Table 14.3) that have less β-blocking activity and longer half-lives than the parent compound (112, 115). Over time these active metabolites rise to progressively higher serum levels.

The half-life of the drug is highly variable (as would be expected given the kinetic complexities) at 2–32 hours (115), depending on hepatic blood flow and saturation of enzymes. Loading of patients takes 4–5 days. Some patients (approximately 7% of whites) are slow metabolizers of the drug and thus have higher levels of propafenone relative to metabolites (116,

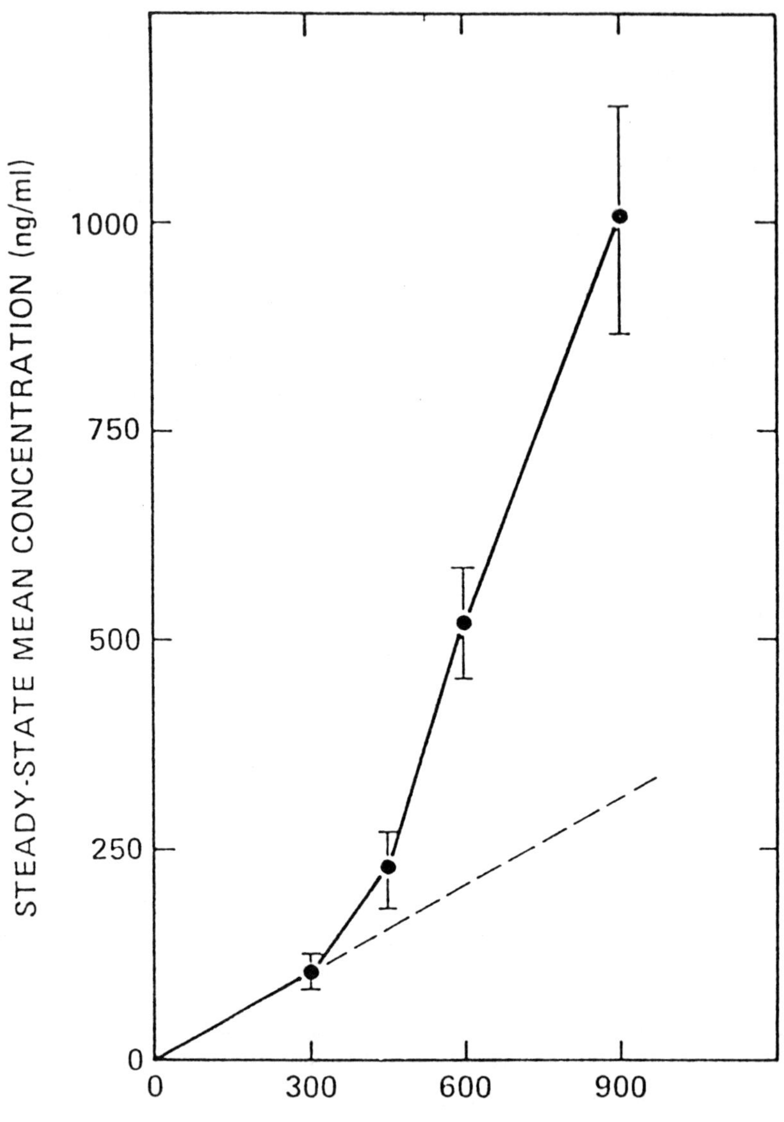


**Figure 14.7** Relationship of propafenone dosage (horizonal axis) to serum concentration (vertical axis). ***Dashed line*** indicates response if relationship was linear. As the dose exceeds 300 mg/day, propafenone concentration rises considerably in a nonlinear manner due to saturation of enzymes. See text for further discussion. Reproduced with permission from Connolly SJ, Kates RE, Lebsack CS, et al. Clinical pharmacology of propafenone. Circulation 1983;68:589–596.

117), whereas rapid metabolizers display increased propafenone levels on coadministration of drugs with food (for reasons unknown). Differences in metabolism among patients, however, are blunted because active metabolites are produced.

Thus, drug administration is difficult. The clinician must take into account saturable hepatic enzymes, hepatic flow, cardiac output, patient phenotype, duration of therapy and active metabolites that may blunt the pharmacodynamic consequences of kinetic peculiarities although their β-blocking properties are less. It is therefore necessary to carefully monitor both serum levels and dynamic effects especially during loading but also later (112).

Adverse effects of propafenone have been reported in 13–27% of patients (118), and 2.6–4.7% of them are cardiovascular related (including especially proarrhythmia and exacerbation of congestive heart failure) (117, 118). Besides the usual IC effects, the noncardiac adverse effects of propafenone are mild and include low level neurologic effects (dizziness, taste disturbance [both 8%], headache [5%], blurred vision, and paresthesias) and gastrointestinal disturbance (nausea and vomiting, anorexia, and constipation, 4%) (119). Exacerbation of asthma and other β-blocker type adverse effects may also occur, usually in the slow metabolizers.

Caution has been advised for all class IC agents since the CAST results, although propafenone itself was not used in CAST. It is logical that the β-blocking effects of propafenone (which would be expected to decrease mortality after MI) lessen the likelihood of similar results, but this remains to be proven in the clinic. Propafenone should be avoided in myasthenia gravis (120).

## Class II Agents

### *β-Adrenergic Blocking Agents*

β-Blockers have widespread cardiovascular use apart from arrhythmias and are discussed elsewhere in this book (Chapters 4 and 5). Three β-blockers are approved by the Food and Drug Administration for arrhythmias: propranolol, esmolol, and acebutalol. However, other β-blockers have also been used by practitioners for this purpose.

An important attribute of β-blockers is their ability to reduce both mortality after MI and reinfarction, a property that favors their use in ventricular arrhythmias. (Fig. 14.5*A*) (44). This attribute appears to be a class effect for all agents except those with intrinsic sympathomimetic activity (44). The proportion of mortality reduction resulting from antiarrhythmic effects compared with antiischemic or cardioprotective effects is unclear.

There are several uses of β-blockers in arrhythmias. They can be used for long-term preventive treatment of PSVT; acute treatment of PSVT (intravenously), although β-blockers are no longer first-line drugs; and slowing of the ventricular response in atrial fibrillation, for which β-blockers are effective both at rest and (unlike digoxin) during exercise. Acutely esmolol is administered for this purpose. However, β-blockers do not prevent recurrences of atrial fibrillation and may, in fact, foster them. For ventricular premature complexes, β-blockers are at times effective and preferred by some (in those uncommon instances when treatment is advised) because of comparisons of the CAST study (41, 42) with studies showing that β-blockers reduce mortality post-MI trial (44) (Fig. 14.5*A*). In ventricular tachycardia or fibrillation the drugs are used both after EP testing (often combination with class I agents) and empirically. In a study noted earlier, patients given metoprolol empirically had arrhythmia-free survival rates similar to those undergoing EP drug testing (22). These findings add justification to the use of β-blockers in life-threatening ventricular arrhythmias. β-Blockers are first line drugs in congenital (but not acquired) long QT syndrome where beta blockers are a first line drug and have been found to decrease mortality (12, 121).

## Class III Agents

In the current state of knowledge about antiarrhythmic drugs, class III agents are a favored group. Because of promising results with amiodarone after MI compared with the adverse mortality data for class I agents, there has been interest in expanding the use of current class III agents and developing new ones. However, these agents may be heterogeneous, with amiodarone, in particular, having unique features.

Amiodarone has been considered the prototype and sotalol, ibutilide, and bretylium, are the other US Food and Drug Administration approved class III agents. Other agents tested include sematilide, almokalant, and dofetilide. Cibenzoline, clofilium, and N-acetylprocainamide have at times been, but are no longer, considered promising class III drugs.

The fundamental electrophysiologic effect of class III agents (and the criterion for classification in this group) is prolongation of action potential duration (122, 123) and, therefore, of $QT_c$ intervals. This effect is mediated by either a diminution of outward potassium or an increase in slow inward sodium current. Drugs in this class prolong refractoriness in atrial, His-Purkinje, and ventricular tissue, as well as in accessory pathways in patients with preexcitation. They are effective against many atrial and ventricular arrhythmias but may also cause torsades de pointes (12, 39, 124).

Amiodarone is unique and different from all other class III drugs for several reasons. Its effects on action potential duration are more profound than those of other agents in not being associated with reverse use dependence (see section on Amiodarone). This may result from amiodarone having different effects on the potassium channel. Amiodarone has properties of all the classes (including I, II, and IV); it is less likely to cause torsades de pointes and is the one with favorable results in long-term mortality trials.

A metaanalysis of eight post-MI trials revealed a significant decrease in mortality with amiodarone (Fig. 14.5*A*) (44, 125). These include a recent Polish trial of patients ineligible to receive β-blockers (1-year mortality was 10.7% with placebo, 6.9% with amiodarone) (125) and the Basal Antiarrhythmic Study of Infarct Survival (BASIS) (1-year mortality was 13% with placebo, 10% with individualized antiarrhythmic therapy, 5% with amiodarone) (126). The mortality difference persisted after 6 years in the amiodarone group despite discontinuation of the drug at 1 year (127).

Results in patients with congestive heart failure have varied. In one study of patients with congestive heart failure and nonsustained ventricular tachycardia, amiodarone conferred no mortality benefit (128). In another study mortality was reduced (from 41 to 34%, $P = 0.024$) in patients with congestive heart failure independent of the presence of complex ventricular arrhythmias (129). It may be that amiodarone is beneficial in the nonischemic cardiomyopathy group.

Results with sotalol in patients after MI have been mixed. In an early trial there was a trend toward decreased morality with sotalol (130). More recently D-sotalol (the sotalol isomer in which its class III properties reside) was found by the Survival with Oral D-Sotalol (SWORD) trial to increase mortality after MI in patients with left ventricular dysfunction (not selected for arrhythmias) (2762 patients, mortality 3.9 versus 2.0%), just as did the CAST drugs (131). This study and the fact that certain other class III agents have been unsuccessful has left it an open question as to whether there are distinctive favorable properties residing in amiodarone or whether there is an overall favorable class III effect that may emerge in other drugs.

Regarding atrial arrhythmia, the data are clear. Amiodarone, sotalol, and ibutilide are all effective in atrial flutter and atrial fibrillation (although amiodarone is not at present approved by the US Food and Drug Administration for this purpose).

### *Amiodarone*

Amiodarone has been a controversial drug among experts as well as one of the most unusual in the cardiovascular arena. It was first developed as an antithyroid and antianginal agent, but its antiarrhythmic properties were later recognized and used. Amiodarone is highly effective but its range of adverse effects and its unusual pharmacology have made for a constantly shifting place among antiarrhythmic treatments.

Amiodarone prolongs action potential duration and effective refractory period (considerably) but does not exhibit "reverse use dependence" as do other class III agents. That is, it prolongs action potential duration as much or relatively more at fast compared to slow rates, obviously an advantage in treating tachyarrhythmias. In addition, amiodarone has mild class I effects (sodium channel blockade) (132), antithyroid, vagal muscarinic, β-blocking, and calcium channel blocking properties. An active metabolite, desethyl amiodarone, has greater sodium channel and conduction blocking properties than the parent compound (132).

Clinically, amiodarone slows sinus rate, prolongs AV nodal conduction and refractoriness, and prolongs PR, QRS, and especially Q-$T_c$ intervals (133). It has modest hemodynamic effects when given orally and has been used extensively in patients with poor myocardial function. With intravenous administration, however, the solubilizing agent polysorbate 80 (tween 80) causes both hypotension and myocardial depression (134).

Amiodarone's pharmacokinetic properties are also unique (see Table 14.3) and variable among subjects (135, 136). Tissue uptake, which is predominantly in tissue with high fat content, is extensive and slow because of the enormous volume of distribution (more than 5000 L/kg); α and β half-lives are 3–21 hours and 14–53 days, (Fig. 14.8), respectively (137), though significant (but not final) electrophysiologic effects occur early. After initiation of treatment (whether oral or intravenous) there is a dip in serum level over the first months or longer and tissue redistribution, during which recurrent arrhythmias may occur; however, these do not necessarily signal long term failure. High loading doses may (138) or may not (139) eliminate the problem.

As the parent compound is hepatically transformed over time, desethylamiodarone, which has a longer half-life, plays a greater role (140). After several months it can be expected to approach (60–80%) or occasionally exceed the level of the parent compound in serum and to exceed it in all tissues except adipose. In addition, with time, tissue levels of drug rise relative to those in serum, leading to greater effect (and toxicity) at somewhat lower serum levels.

Amiodarone is eliminated by hepatic transformation with some enterhepatic circulation and virtually no renal elimination. After discontinuation of treatment it can take 4–6 months or longer for the drug to be completely removed from the body (135–137, 141). Because of the unusual kinetics, predicting long-term efficacy of amiodarone by EP testing is difficult. After much controversy on this topic, the recommendation is that the EP study for drug evaluation should be performed at least 10–14 days after initiation of oral drug (still, however, too early for the steady-state) and that partial effectiveness (i.e., need for more aggressive stimulation protocol to initiate ventricular tachycardia and a slower ventricular tachycardia rate on drug) appears to be at least somewhat predictive of efficacy (22, 142).

Amiodarone is front line therapy for hemodynamically significant ventricular tachycardia or ventricular fibrillation (its only uses approved by the US Food and Drug Administration at present) to improve survival (143, 144) as well as to reduce arrhythmic discharges in patients with implantable cardioverter defibrillators (145). At the time of this writing, apart from the post-MI trials noted earlier, only observational data justify amiodarone use in these situations, although data are soon to emerge from several randomized studies.

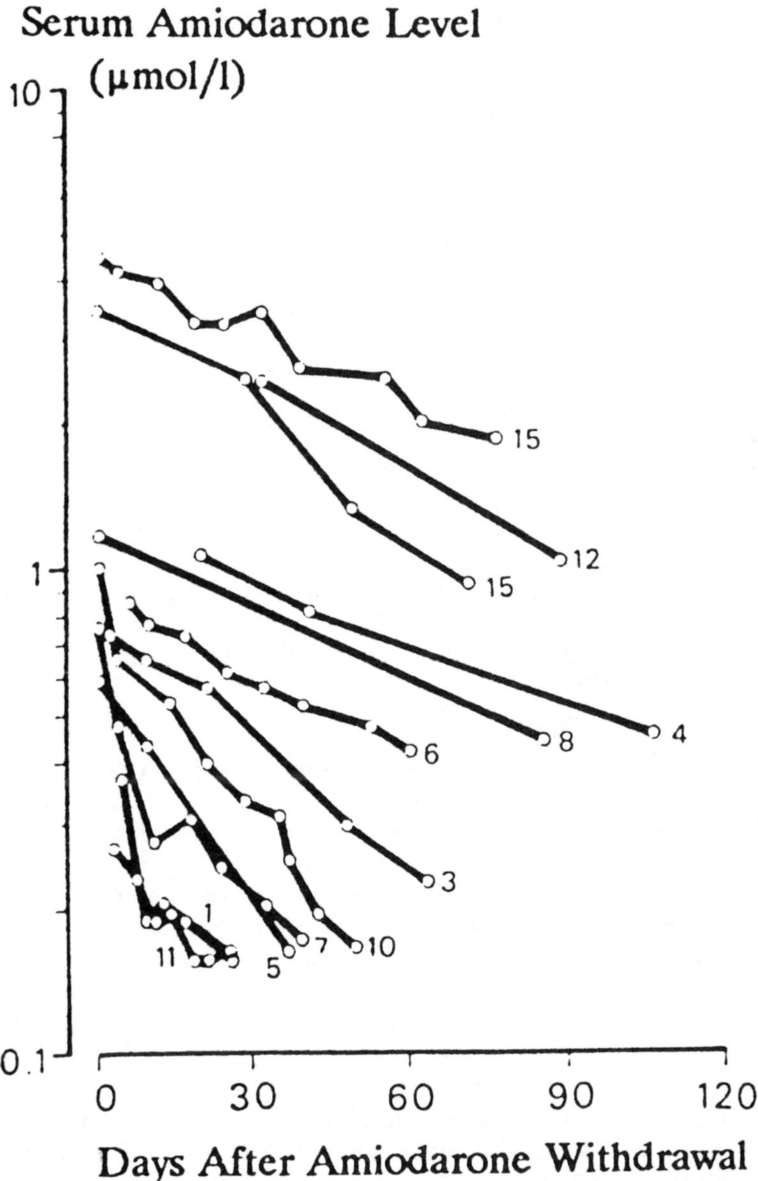


Figure 14.8 Decline in serum amiodarone levels after withdrawal from steady-state (12 evaluations in 11 patients). Numbers refer to individual patients in the original study. There is a slow but variable decline in amiodarone levels, with a mean half-life of 41 ± 19 days. Reproduced with permission from Staubli M, Burchard J, Gateazzi RL, et al. Serum concentrations of amiodarone during long-term therapy in relation to dose efficacy and toxicity. Eur J Clin Pharmacol 1983;24:485–494.

Although not approved by the US Food and Drug Administration for this purpose, amiodarone also has proven efficacy in atrial fibrillation and flutter (146, 147) and in arrhythmias caused by preexcitation, even at doses of less than 200 mg/day; however, catheter ablation has largely superceded the latter use. Although amiodarone has been used in other SVTs (147) and ventricular premature complexes, it has not been advocated in either situation because of toxicity. The drug has also been used empirically in hypertrophic cardiomyopathy. Intravenous amiodarone is useful for ventricular arrhythmias (it has been used in cardiac arrest situations in spite of its unusual kinetics), and it had been found to be effective for conversion of atrial fibrillation (148).

The following dosage regimens of amiodarone have been suggested (149, 150):

1. Oral: 800–1600 mg/day for 1–3 weeks followed by 800 mg/day for 2–4 weeks followed by 600 mg for 4–8 weeks; after this, maintenance of 200–400 mg/day
2. High oral dose: 50 mg/kg for days 1–3, 30 mg/kg for days 4 and 5, and 300–400 mg twice daily for days 6–10. This regimen was found more effective in one (138) but not another (139) study
3. Intravenous:
   (a) 5–10 mg/kg over 20–30 minutes followed by 1 g/day for several days; additional doses of 1–3 mg/kg may be given.
   (b) 2.0–2.5 mg/minute for 12 hours followed by 0.7 mg/minute for the next 36 hours

Amiodarone use is limited by its toxicity, which is largely dose related. Reports from Europe, where lower doses were used, have generally noted lower rates of toxicity than in the United States (137). However, as more experience with the drug accumulates in the United States, pulmonary and other severe toxicities seem to be declining.

Pulmonary toxicity, which is unlikely at doses of 400 mg/day or less (151), begins with a reversible lipoidal pneumonia that progresses to pulmonary fibrosis (152). Pulmonary function tests display a reduced diffusing capacity, and gallium scans are positive for inflammation. Corticosteroids are advised therapeutically as is drug discontinuation. Early recognition is crucial. Postoperative acute respiratory distress syndrome may also occur with the drug (153).

Amiodarone blocks the deiodination of $T_4$ to $T_3$ and also decreases the cellular link of $T_3$ with its nuclear receptor. As a result, thyroid-stimulating hormone (TSH), $T_4$, and $rT_3$ are increased and $T_3$ is moderately decreased (154). Hypothyroidism may result because of the increased amounts of iodine released (it is more likely in renal failure, which otherwise has no effect on amiodarone elimination) (155, 156). Hyperthyroidism may also occur because of iodine load in sensitive patients (156). Chemical diagnosis of hypothyroidism or hyperthyroidism (both of which have been treated with potassium perchlorate) (157) is difficult to make because the drug distorts thyroid function tests even when it does not have a metabolic effect. However, in amiodarone-induced hypothyroidism more substantial increases in TSH may occur.

Hepatic enzyme abnormalities may occur with amiodarone, mild elevations of which can be tolerated, and also rarely hepatic injury. Photosensitivity, slate blue discoloration, corneal microdeposits, anorexia, and constipation are common. Neurologic toxicity includes peripheral neuropathy and sleep disturbance. Testicular dysfunction may occur (158).

Cardiac toxicity includes sinus bradycardia (rarely severe and lethal) and worsening congestive heart failure. However, although amiodarone causes considerable prolongation of $QT_c$ intervals, torsades de pointes occurs in less than 1% of patients. In fact, when 31 patients with torsades de pointes and prolonged $QT_c$ intervals on various drugs were placed on amiodarone, neither a change in $QT_c$ interval nor torsade de pointes occurred (124). It has been postulated that torsades de pointes may be prevented by the calcium channel blocking effects of the drug. Figure 14.9 shows percentage of adverse effects in one series of patients on amiodarone therapy.

Because of the drug's enterohepatic circulation, cholestyramine has been suggested for toxicity (159), especially in drug overdoses. Among drug interactions (Table 14.4), interference with elimination of warfarin and digoxin mandate close observation of patients given these drugs.

### *Sotalol*

After many years of testing in the United States and use overseas, oral sotalol was approved by the US Food and Drug Administration in 1992. Sotalol exhibits β-blocking (class II) as well as class III effects. Its D-isomer has strictly class III properties (160).

Cardiovascular actions of sotalol reflect its combined class II and class III properties with β-blockade occurring at lower doses than do class III effects (161). Sotalol slows the sinus rate, prolongs AV conduction and refractoriness and therefore prolongs PR interval and causes modest $QT_c$ prolongation. It has no effect on duration of QRS complex (161).

Regarding myocardial contractility, the action potential duration–prolonging effects of sotalol (which allow entry of more calcium into the cell, promoting contractility) to some degree counteract the β-blocker–induced negative inotropy. In patients with depressed myocardium, however, sotalol can cause marked additional depression (162).

Sotalol is effective against both atrial and ventricular arrhythmias. For atrial fibrillation it is now considered a first-line drug with particular advantages (163). Sotalol is effective against ventricular arrhythmias (162, 164, 165); the ESVEM trial found that sotalol was more beneficial than several other agents (26) (however, see also SWORD trial, mentioned earlier) (131).

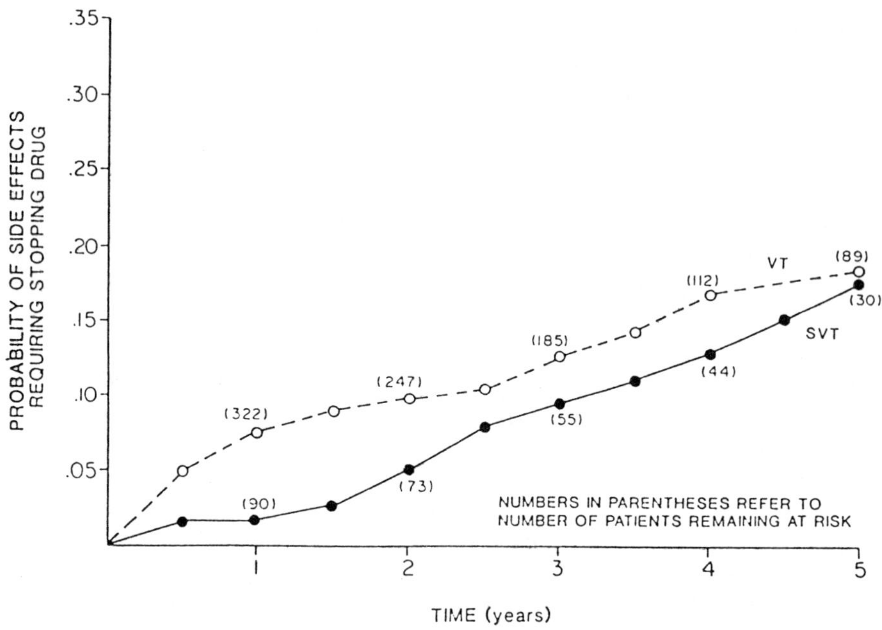


Figure 14.9 Probability of adverse effect requiring discontinuation of amiodarone in patients with ventricular tachycardia (VT, *dashed line*) and supraventricular tachycardia (SVT, *solid line*). Over 5 years about 15% of patients have to discontinue amiodarone. See text for further discussion. Reproduced with permission from Weinberg BA, Miles WM, Klein LS, et al. Five year follow-up of 589 patients treated with amiodarone. Am Heart J 1993;125:109–120.

The pharmacokinetics of sotalol are relatively straightforward (Table 14.3). The drug is eliminated by the kidney and has no active metabolites. Because of its relativity long half-life, dose increments should be made at intervals of 60 hours or more (166).

The adverse effect of greatest concern is torsades de pointes. In one study, proarrhythmia occurred in 4.3% of patients, with torsades de pointes in 1.9% (167). It has been stated that the maximum allowable $QT_c$ interval is 500 milliseconds and that considerable caution should be taken above this level (161), although torsades may occur at lower levels. A predisposing factor may be bradycardia because of the β-blocking actions of the drug. Congestive heart failure may be exacerbated (1.9%) and other adverse effects caused by β-blockade may still occur. Overall, about 16% of patients in randomized trials have discontinued sotalol because of toxic effects (167).

### *Ibutilide*

Ibutilide fumarate is the newest class II agent to be in clinical use. It was approved by the US Food and Drug Administration in 1995 as an intravenous drug with one purpose: rapid conversion of atrial fibrillation or flutter.

Ibutilide has reasonably selective class III electrophysiologic properties (168, 169). It prolongs action potential duration and refractory period in both atrium and ventricle, but this effect is mediated by enhancement of slow inward sodium rather than by diminution of potassium current, as with amiodarone. Ibutilide also slows the sinus rate but appears not to affect the action potential upstroke, inotropy, or hemodynamics. On the ECG it has no effect on QRS duration, prolongs $QT_c$ interval (up to 4 hours after infusion, directly related to serum concentration), and slows the rate.

Kinetics of ibutilide (169a) vary among patients. The β half-life averages about 6 hours, with a range of 2–12 hours. About 82% is excreted in urine, predominately as metabolites. Hepatic clearance is high (29 mL/minute/kg). There is one active metabolite (ω hydroxyibutilide), but it is present in very low concentrations.

In animal studies, ibutilide has been effective against both atrial and ventricular arrhythmias (168, 170). Its approval by the US Food and Drug Administration, however, is strictly for acute conversion of atrial fibrillation or flutter. (170a,b) In clinical trials (170b), arrhythmia was converted with one or two doses in 70% of those with atrial flutter and 43% of those with atrial fibrillation; conversion usually occurred within 30 minutes, but in some instances it took as long as 90 minutes. Success rate was higher than for either sotalol or procainamide, and most patients remained in sinus rhythm at 24 hours. These trials of the drug were conducted in adult patients who had atrial arrhythmias for less than 90 days in the absence of symptomatic congestive heart failure, recent myocardial infarction, or angina.

As perhaps expected, the main adverse effect of ibutilide, as with sotalol, is ventricular arrhythmia. In clinical trials (170a,b), 4.9% of patients developed nonsustained monomorphic ventricular tachycardia, 2.7% nonsustained polymorphic ventricular tachycardia, and 1.7% sustained polymorphic ventricular tachycardia that required electroconversion. The last generally occurred within 40 minutes but could take up to 3 hours after intravenous drug infusion and occurred with or without $QT_c$ prolongation. Caution and preparation are therefore advised in use of this drug. It should not be administered if potassium is below 4 mEq/dL or there is a baseline prolonged $QT_c$ interval. In addition, caution is also advised regarding concomitant administration of drugs with this property. No other drug interactions have been uncovered.

*Bretylium*

Bretylium is an antiarrhythmic drug with very limited (in fact essentially only one) use. It is generally placed in class III because it prolongs action potential duration (171) and refractoriness, but it is not at all clear whether this property is related to antiarrhythmic effects.

Besides primary electrophysiologic effects, bretylium also affects the sympathetic nervous system. On administration, it causes a sympathetic discharge with various consequences, including at times proarrhythmia (generally isolated ventricular premature complexes) and then a sympathetic depletion with its set of consequences, especially hypotension.

The one use of bretylium is in acute treatment of ventricular tachycardia or fibrillation after failure of lidocaine therapy. In this situation, a 5-mg/kg loading dose is administered quickly. Additional doses may be given as tolerated, with hypotension the limiting feature. A time delay may occur between administration and effect because of delayed uptake of the drug in the myocardium. Maintenance dose is 1–4 mg/minute, and therapeutic effects occur over a wide range of serum levels (172) (see also Chapter 17).

Adverse effects of bretylium include hypotension (the main feature limiting its use), nausea, and vomiting, as well as proarrhythmia (ventricular premature complexes) and hypertension during the initial sympathetic discharge.

## Class IV Agents

### *Calcium Channel Blockers*

The two calcium channel blockers approved for antiarrhythmic use in the United States are verapamil and diltiazem. Verapamil and diltiazem depress automaticity in the sinus node and both automaticity and conduction in the AV node. They are also negatively inotropic and coronary and peripheral vasodilators. Thus, they tend to lower blood pressure, which in turn elicits a sympathetic response that has several potential consequences, including blunting of the drugs' direct bradycardic, hypotensive, and myocardial depressive effects. Tables 14.2 to 14.4 include information on dosage and pharmacology of diltiazem and verapamil. Both drugs undergo substantial hepatic first-pass metabolism (173, 174).

Diltiazem and verapamil are used to slow the ventricular response in atrial fibrillation (175). However, in atrial fibrillation associated with preexcitation, calcium channel blockers may accelerate the ventricular response possibly because of loss of retrograde concealed conduction in the AV node or sympathetic stimulation (176).

Intravenous verapamil and diltiazem are used to terminate acute PSVT but are second-line drugs to adenosine because of the latter's extremely short half-life. They may also be associated with self-limited ventricular arrhythmias (177). Verapamil has also been used orally in chronic PSVT. Calcium channel blockers are not useful in ventricular arrhythmias, because they tend to be detrimental in inducing hypotension, although they have been used in one uncommon form of exercise-induced ventricular tachycardia that may result from delayed afterdepolarizations (178).

Adverse effects of calcium channel blockers (which are additive to those of β-blockers) include AV nodal block, sinus bradycardia, hypotension, and congestive heart failure. Intravenous calcium chloride is the antidote for hypotension and isoproterenol for the bradycardia or heart block.

## Class V Agents

### *Adenosine*

Adenosine has one use in arrhythmias, i.e., acute treatment of PSVT, although it has also been used in pharmacologic stress testing. Adenosine slows sinus node rate and selectively blocks AV nodal conduction (179). It is also a coronary and peripheral vasodilator and, in patients with coronary artery disease, has the ability to induce a steal syndrome that is the basis of its use in pharmacologic stress testing. The drug prolongs PR interval but not QRS duration. Adenosine monophosphate, diphosphate, and triphosphate all have similar properties (180).

Adenosine is the drug of choice to terminate acute PSVT largely because of its half-life of 1–7 seconds (181). It can be used to distinguish PSVT with aberrant conduction or that arising because of accessory pathways from ventricular tachycardia. If the rhythm is reversed, PSVT is diagnosed (sensitivity 90%, specificity 94%, predictive accuracy 92%) (182). Occasionally, adenosine may terminate atrial flutter, ectopic atrial tachycardia, or exercise-induced ventricular tachycardia. The exercise-induced ventricular tachycardia and some AV nodal junctional tachycardias appear to be caused by cyclic AMP-mediated triggered activity (183).

Adenosine should not be given in atrial flutter or fibrillation (184) or ectopic atrial tachycardia. In Wolff-Parkinson-White syndrome it has occasionally caused atrial flutter or fibrillation. Ventricular premature complexes and atrial premature complexes may occur after adenosine use in PSVT. Adverse effects of the drug are transient and rarely important. The drug may cause flushing (18%), dyspnea (12%), chest tightness (7%), and rarely ischemia and AV block. All of these adverse effects usually reverse in less than 1 minute after discontinuation (182–184) but may be prolonged with dipyridamole, which antagonizes adenosine uptake. The methylxanthines inhibit or prevent adenosine action, whereas atropine has no effect on it.

### *Digoxin*

Digoxin has some uses in arrhythmias, specifically in PSVT and atrial fibrillation in which use is based mainly on parasympathomimetic effects and effects on atrial conduction. There is no justification for its use in ventricular arrhythmias, and use in congestive heart failure is discussed elsewhere (Chapter 11).

In acute treatment of PSVT, digoxin is a second-line drug to adenosine and verapamil. However, it has certain advantages in long-term use because it is generally well tolerated compared with other drugs. Digoxin has long been used to decrease episodes and control rate in atrial fibrillation; however, the drug not only does not diminish AF episodes, it may actually increase them (185). Use in atrial fibrillation resulting from Wolff-Parkinson-White syndrome is considered risky and generally contraindicated because the drug may shorten refractory periods in the accessory pathway and thereby increase ventricular response (to rarely cause ventricular fibrillation) (186).

For rate control in atrial fibrillation, although digoxin slows resting rate, it has less influence on exertional rate, probably because its primary mechanism of action is enhanced vagal tone, which is easily overcome by sympathetic discharge. Digoxin therapy also does not modify ventricular rates during paroxysmal atrial fibrillation, possibly because high sympathetic tone during episodes counteracts its effects (185). Pharmacologic information on digoxin is shown in Tables 14.2 to 14.4.

---

## REFERENCES


1. Vaughan-Williams EM. Classification of anti-arrhythmic drugs. In: Sandoe E, Flensted-Jansen E, Olesen KH, eds. Symposium on cardiac arrhythmias. Soderatalje, Sweden: AB Astra, 1970;449–472.
2. Vaughan-Williams EM. Classifying antiarrhythmic actions: by facts or speculation. J Clin Pharmacol 1992;32:964–977.
3. Vaughan-Williams EM. A classification of antiarrhythmic actions re-assessed after a decade of new drugs. J Clin Pharmacol 1984;24:129–147.
4. Janse MJ. Reentry rhythms. In: Fozzard HA, Haber E, Jennings RB, et al., eds. The heart and cardiovascular system. New York: Raven Press, 1986;1203–1238.
5. Allessie MA, Schalij MJ, Kirchhof CJ, et al: Experimental electrophysiology and arrhythmogenicity. Anisotropy and ventricular tachycardia. Eur Heart J 1989;10: E2–E8.
6. Mayer AG. Rhythmical pulsation in scyphomedusae. Publication 47 of the Carnegie Institution. Washington, DC: Carnegie Institute of Washington, 1906:1–62.
7. Mines GR. On dynamic equilibrium in the heart. J Physiol (Lond) 1914;46:349–382.
8. Schmidt FO, Erlanger J. Directional differences in the conduction of the impulse through heart muscle and their possible relation to extrasystolic and fibrillary contractions. Am J Physiol 1928:87;326–347.
9. Wit AL, Rosen MR, Hoffman BF: Electrophysiology and pharmacology of cardiac arrhythmias. I. Relationship of normal and abnormal electrical activity of cardiac fibers to the genesis of arrhythmia. B Reentry. Am Heart J 1974;88:664–806.
10. Katzung BG. Electrically induced automaticity in ventricular myocardium. Life Sci 1974;14:1133–1140.
11. Imanishi S, Surawicz B. Automatic activity in depolarized guinea pig ventricular myocardium: characteristics and mechanisms. Circ Res 1976;39:751–759.
12. Kupersmith J. Long QT syndrome. In: Singer I, Kupersmith J, eds. Clinical manual of electrophysiology. Baltimore: Williams & Wilkins, 1993;143–168.

13. Cranefield PF, Aronson R Cardiac arrhythmias: the role of triggered activity and other mechanisms. Mt. Kisco: Futura , 1988.
14. Kupersmith J. Antiarrhythmic drugs: specific agents. In: Singer I, Kupersmith J, eds. Clinical manual of electrophysiology. Baltimore: Williams & Wilkins, 1993;186–207.
15. Mason JW, Winkle RA. Accuracy of the ventricular tachycardia-induction study for predicting long-term efficacy and inefficacy of antiarrhythmic drugs. N Engl J Med 1980;303:1073–1077.
16. Swerdlow CD, Winkle RA, Mason JW. Determinants of survival in patients with ventricular tachyarrhythmias. N Engl J Med 1983;308:1436–1442.
17. Kastor JA, Horowitz LN, Harken AH, et al. Clinical electrophysiology of ventricular tachycardia. N Engl J Med 1981;304:1004–1020.
18. Wilber JD, Garan H, Kelly E, et al. Out-of-hospital cardiac arrest: role of electrophysiologic testing in the prediction of long-term outcome. N Engl J Med 1988;318: 19–24.
19. Morady F, Sledge C, Shen E, et al. Electrophysiologic testing in the management of patients with the W-P-W syndrome and atrial fibrillation. Am J Cardiol 1983;51: 1623–1628.
20. Waxman HL, Buxton AE, Sadowski LM, et al. The response to procainamide during electrophysiologic study for sustained ventricular tachyarrhythmias predicts the response to other medications. Circulation 1982;67:30–37.
21. Steinbeck G, Andersen D, Bach P, et al. A comparison of electrophysiologically guided antiarrhythmic drug therapy with beta-blocker therapy in patients with symptomatic, sustained ventricular tachyarrhythmias. N Engl J Med 1992;327: 987–992.
22. Horowitz L, Greenspan A, Spielman S, et al. Usefulness of electrophysiologic testing in evaluation of amiodarone therapy for sustained ventricular tachyarrhythmias associated with coronary heart disease. Am J Cardiol 1985;55:367–371.
23. Hindman MC, Last JH, Rosen KM. Wolff-Parkinson-White syndrome observed by portable monitoring. Ann Intern Med 1973;79:654–663.
24. Morganroth J, Anderson JL, Gentzkow GD. Classification by type of ventricular arrhythmia predicts frequency of adverse cardiac events from flecainide. J Am Coll Cardiol 1986;8:607–615.
25. Mason JW, ESVEM Investigators. A comparison of electrophysiologic testing with Holter monitoring to predict antiarrhythmic-drug efficacy for ventricular tachyarrhythmias. N Engl J Med 1993;329:445–451.
26. Mason JW, ESVEM. A comparison of seven antiarrhythmic drugs in patients with ventricular tachyarrhythmias. New Engl J Med 1993;329:452–458.
27. Klein RC, ESVEM Investigators. Comparative efficacy of sotalol and class I antiarrhythmic agents in patients with ventricular tachycardia or fibrillation: results of the Electrophysiology Study Versus Electrocardiographic Monitoring (ESVEM) trial. Eur Heart J 1993;14:78–84.
28. Greenspon AJ, Kidwell GA. The effects of antiarrhythmic drugs on the signal-averaged electrocardiogram in patients with malignant ventricular arrhythmias. Prog Cardiovasc Dis 1993;35:399–406.
29. Morganroth J, Goin JE. Quinidine-related mortality in the short-to-medium-term treatment of ventricular arrhythmias: a meta-analysis. Circulation 1991;84: 1977–1983.
30. Sager PT, Perlmutter RA, Rosenfeld LE, et al. Antiarrhythmic drug exacerbation of ventricular tachycardia inducibility during electrophysiologic study. Am Heart J 1992;123:926–933.
31. Velebit V, Podrid PJ, Lown B, et al. Aggravation and provocation of ventricular arrhythmias by antiarrhythmic drugs. Circulation 1982;65:886–894.
32. Feld GK, Chen PS, Nicod P, et al. Possible atrial proarrhythmic effects of Class IC antiarrhythmic drugs. Am J Cardiol 1990;66:378–383.
33. Falk RH, Leavitt JI. Digoxin for atrial fibrillation: a drug whose time has gone? Ann Intern Med 1991;114:573–575.
34. Shenasa M, Denkes S, Mahmud R, et al. Effect of verapamil on retrograde atrioventricular nodal conduction in the human heart. J Am Coll Cardiol 1983;3: 545–550.

35. Singh BN, Ellrodt G, Peter CT. Verapamil: a review of its pharmacologic properties and therapeutic uses. Drugs 1978;15:169–197.
36. Roden DM, Woosley RL, Primm RK. Incidence and clinical features of the quinidine-associated long QT syndrome: implications for patient care. Am Heart J 1986; 111:1088–1093.
37. Faber TS, Zehender M, VanDeLoo A, et al. Torsades de pointes complicating drug treatment of low-malignant forms of arrhythmia: four case reports. Clin Cardiol 1994;17:197–202.
38. Selzer A, Wray HW. Quinidine syncope: paroxysmal ventricular fibrillation occurring during treatment of chronic atrial arrhythmias. Circulation 1964;30:17–23.
39. Hii JTY, Wyse G, Gillis AM, et al. Precordial QT interval dispersion as a marker of torsades de pointes: disparate effects of class Ia antiarrhythmic drugs and amiodarone. Circulation 1992;86:1376–1382.
40. Chouty F, Funck-Brentano C, Landau JM, et al. Efficacite de fortes doses de lactate molaire par voie veineuse lors des intoxications au flecainide. Presse Med 1987; 16:808.
41. Echt DS, Liebson PR, Mitchenn LB, et al., CAST Investigators. Mortality and morbidity in patients receiving encainide, flecainide, or placebo. N Engl J Med 1991;324: 781–788.
42. Greene HL, Roden DM, Katz RJ, et al., the CAST Investigators. The cardiac arrhythmia suppression trial: first CAST . . . then CAST-II. J Am Coll Cardiol 1992;19:894–898.
43. IMPACT Research Group. International mexiletine and placebo antiarrhythmic coronary trial: I. Report on arrhythmia and other findings. J Am Coll Cardiol 1984;6:1148–1163.
44. Teo KK, Yusuf S, Furberg CD. Effects of prophylactic antiarrhythmic drug therapy in acute myocardial infarction. JAMA 1993;270:1589–1595.
45. Coplen SE, Antman EM, Berlin JA, et al. Efficacy and safety of quinidine therapy for maintenance of sinus rhythm after cardioversion: A meta-analysis of randomized control trials. Circulation 1990;82:1106–1111
46. Boissel JP, Wolf E, Gillet J, et al. Controlled trial of a long-acting sustained atrial fibrillation. Eur Heart J 1981;2:49–55.
47. Byrne-Quinn E, Wing AJ. Maintenance of sinus rhythm after DC reversion of atrial fibrillation: a double-blind controlled trial of quinidine bisulphate. Br Heart J 1970;32:370–376.
48. Hartel G, Vouhija A, Konttinen A, et al. Value of quinidine in maintenance of sinus rhythm after electric conversion of atrial fibrillation. Br Heart J 1970;32:57–60.
49. Hillstad L, Bjerkelund C, Dale J, et al. Quinidine in maintenance of sinus rhythm after electroconversion of chronic atrial fibrillation: a controlled clinical study. Br Heart J 1971;33:518–521.
50. Lloyd EA, Gersh BJ, Forman R. The efficacy of quinidine and disopyramide in the maintenance of sinus rhythm after electroconversion from atrial fibrillation. S Afr Med J 1984;65:367–369.
51. Sodermark T, Jonsson B, Olsson A, et al. Effect of quinidine on maintaining sinus rhythm after conversation of atrial fibrillation or flutter: a multicentre study from Stockholm. Br Heart J 1975;37:486–492.
52. Flaker GC, Blackshear JL, McBride R, et al., The Stroke Prevention in Atrial Fibrillation Investigators: Antiarrhythmic drug therapy and cardiac mortality in atrial fibrillation. J Am Coll Cardiol 1992;20:527–532.
53. Hine LK, Laird N, Hewitt P, et al. Meta-analytic evidence against prophylactic use of lidocaine in acute myocardial infarction. Arch Intern Med 1989;149:2694–2698.
54. Pitt A, Lipp H, Anderson ST. Lignocaine given prophylactically to patients with acute myocardial infarction. Lancet 1971;1:612–616.
55. Mogensen L. Ventricular tachyarrhythmias and lignocaine prophylaxis in acute myocardial infarction: a clinical and therapeutic study. Acta Med Scand 1970; 513(Suppl):1–80.
56. Chopra MP, Thadani U, Portal RW, et al. Lignocaine therapy for ventricular ectopic activity after acute myocardial infarction: a double blind trial. Br Med J 1971; 3:668–670.

57. Darby S, Cruickshank JC, Bennett MA, et al. Trial of combined intramuscular and intravenous lignocaine in prophylaxis of ventricular tachyarrhythmias. Lancet 1972;1:817–819.
58. Bennett MA, Wilner JM, Pentecost BL. Controlled trial of lignocaine in prophylaxis of ventricular arrhythmias complicating myocardial infarction. Lancet 1970;2: 909–911.
59. O'Brien KP, Taylor PM, Croxson RS: Prophylactic lignocaine in hospitalized patients with acute myocardial infarction. Med J Aust 1973;2(Suppl):36–37.
60. Kupersmith J. Antiarrhythmic drugs: changing concepts. Am J Cardiol 1976;38: 119–121 (Editorial).
61. Harrison DC. Antiarrhythmic drug classification: new science and practical applications. Am J Cardiol 1985;56:185–187.
62. Harrison DC. The Sicilian gambit: reasons for maintaining the present antiarrhythmic drug classification. Cardiovasc Res 1992;26:566–567.
63. Task Force of the Working Group on Arrhythmias of the European Society of Cardiology. The Sicilian gambit: a new approach to the classification of antiarrhythmic drugs based on their actions on arrhythmogenic mechanisms. Circulation 1991;84: 1831–1851.
64. Schwartz PJ, Zaza A. The Sicilian gambit revisited— theory and practice. Eur Heart J 1992;13:23–29.
65. Janse MJ. Putting the Sicilian gambit to the test. Eur Heart J 1992;13:30–37.
66. Gottlieb SS, Kukin ML, Medina N, et al. Comparative hemodynamic effects of procainamide, tocainide, and encainide in severe chronic heart failure. Circulation 1990;81:860–864.
67. Schmid PG, Nelson LD, Heistad DD, et al. Vascular effects of procainamide in the dog: predominance of the inhibitory effect on ganglionic transmission. Circ Res 1974;35:948–960.
68. Boden WE, Moss AJ, Oakes D. Hypolipidemic effect of type Ia antiarrhythmic agents in postinfarction patients. Circulation 1992;85:2039–2044.
69. Teichman SL, Ferrick A, Kim SG, et al. Disopyramide-pyridostigmine interactions, selective reversal of anticholinergic symptoms with preservation of anticholinergic effect. J Am Coll Cardiol 1987;10:633–641.
70. Zuanetti G, Latini R, Neilson JMM, et al., The Antiarrhythmic Drug Evaluation Group (ADEG). Heart rate variability in patients with ventricular arrhythmias: effect of antiarrhythmic drugs. Am Coll Cardiol 1991;17:604–612.
71. Miller RR, Hillard G, Lies JE, et al. Hemodynamic effects of procainamide in patients with acute myocardial infarction and comparison with lidocaine. Am J Med 1973;55:161–168.
72. Ellenbogen KA, Wood MA, Stambler BS: Procainamide: a perspective on its value and danger. Heart Dis Stroke 1993;2:473–476.
73. Dangman KH, Hoffman BF. In vivo and in vitro antiarrhythmic and arrhythmogenic effects of N-acetryl procainamide. J Pharmacol Exp Ther 1981;217:851–862.
74. Woosley RL, Drayer DE, Reidenberg MM, et al. Effect of actylator phenotype on the rate at which procainamide induces antinuclear antibodies and the lupus syndrome. N Engl J Med 1978;298:1157–1159.
75. Blomgren SE, Condemi JJ, Vaughan JH. Procainamide-induced lupus erythematosus-clinical and laboratory observations. Am J Med 1972;52:338–348.
76. McCrum ID, Guildry JR. Procainamide-induced psychosis. JAMA 1978;12: 1265–1266.
77. Podrid PJ, Kowey PR. Disopyramide: when is it justified? J Cardiovasc Med 1981;6:997–1007.
78. Karim A, Shubert EN, Burns TS, et al. Disopyramide plasma concentrations following single and multiple doses of the immediate-release and controlled-release capsules. Angiology 1983;34:375–392.
79. Mellin PFJ, Robert EW, Winkle RA, et al. The role of concentration-dependent plasma protein binding in disopramide disposition. J Pharmacokinet Biopharm 1979;7:29–46.
80. Aitio M, Mansury L, Tala E, et al. The effect of enzyme-induction on the metabolism of disopyramide in man. Br J Clin Pharmacol 1981;11:279–295.

81. Giacomini KM, Cox BM, Blaschke TF. Comparative anticholinergic potencies of R- and S-disopyramide in longitudinal muscle strips from guinea pig ileum. Life Sci 1980;27:1191.
82. Hille B. Local anesthetics: hydrophilic and hydrophobic pathways for the drug-receptor reaction. J Gen Physiol 1977;69:497–515.
83. Kupersmith J. Electrophysiologic and antiarrhythmic effects of lidocaine in canine acute myocardial ischemia. Am Heart J 1979;97:320–327.
84. Kupersmith J, Antman EM, Hoffman BF. In vivo electrophysiologic effects of lidocaine in canine acute myocardial infarction. Circ Res 1975;36:84.
85. Koster RW, Dunning AJ. Intramuscular lidocaine for prevention of lethal arrhythmias in the prehospitalization phase of acute myocardial infarction. N Engl Med 1985;313:1105–1110.
86. Antman EM, Berlin JA. Declining incidence of ventricular fibrillation in myocardial infarction: implications for the prophylactic use of lidocaine. Circulation 1992;86: 764–773.
87. Johnson RG, Goldberger AL, Thurer RL, et al. Lidocaine prophylaxis in coronary revascularization patients: A randomized, prospective trial. Soc Thoracic Surgeons 1993;55:1180–1184.
88. Nies AS. Cardiovascular disorders. In: Molmon KL, Morrelli HF, eds. Clinical pharmacology: Basic principles in therapeutics. New York: McGraw Hill, 1972:142–261.
89. LeLorier J, Grenon D, Latour Y, et al: Pharmacokinetics of lidocaine after prolonged intravenous infusions in uncomplicated myocardial infarction. Ann Intern Med 1977;87:700–702.
90. Nattel S, Zipes DP. Clinical pharmacology of old and new antiarrhythmic drugs. Cardiovas Res 1980;11:221–248.
91. Sefaldt RJ, Nattel S, Kreeft JH, et al. Lidocaine therapy with an exponentially declining infusion. Ann Intern Med 1984;101:632–634.
92. Wyman MG, Slaughter RL, Farolino DA, et al. Multiple bolus technique for lidocaine administration in acute ischemic heart disease. II. Treatment of refractory ventricular failure. J Am Coll Cardiol 1983;2:764–769.
93. Buckles DS, Knick B, Gillette PC. Subcutaneous lidocaine affects inducibility in programmed electrophysiology testing in children: a follow-up study. Am Heart J 1992;124:1241–1244.
94. Greenspan AM, Spielman SR, Webb CR, et al. Efficacy of combination therapy with mexiletine and a type IA agent for inducible ventricular tachyarrhythmias secondary to coronary artery disease. Am J Cardiol 1985;56:277–284.
95. Ujhelyi MR, O'Rangers EA, Fan C, et al. Antifibrillatory and electrophysiologic actions of morcizine alone and in combination with lidocaine: a prospective, randomized trial. Crit Care Med 1993;21:1577–1584.
96. Bonavita GJ, Pires LA, Wagshal AB, et al. Usefulness of oral quinidine-mexiletine combination therapy for sustained ventricular tachyarrhythmias as assessed by programmed electrical stimulation when quinidine monotherapy has failed. Am Heart J 1994;127:847–851.
97. Deedwania PC, Olukotun AY, Kupersmith J, et al. Beta blockers in combination with class I antiarrhythmic agents. Am J Cardiol 1987;60:21D–26D.
98. Campbell RWF: Mexiletine. N Engl J Med 1987;316:29–34.
99. Roos JC, Paalman ACA, Dunning AJ. Electrophysiological effects of mexiletine in man. Br Heart J 1976;38:1262–1271.
100. Estes NAM, Garan H, Ruskin JN. Electrophysiologic properties of flecainide acetate. Am J Cardiol 1984;53:26B.
101. Roden DM, Woosley RL. Medical intelligence drug therapy: flecainide. N Engl J Med 1986;315:36–41.
102. Malik R, Ellenbogen KA, Stambler BS, et al. Flecainide: its value and danger. Heart Dis Stroke 1994:85–89.
103. Anderson JL, Gilbert EM, Alpert BL, et al. Flecainide Supraventricular Tachycardia Study Group. Prevention of symptomatic recurrences of paroxysmal atrial fibrillation in patients initially tolerating antiarrhythmic therapy. Circulation 1989; 80:1557–1570.

104. Crozier I. Flecainide in the Wolff-Parkinson-White syndrome. Am J Cardiol 1992;70:26A–32A.
105. Pritchett ELC, Wilkinson WE. Mortality in patients treated with flecainide and encainide for supraventricular arrhythmias. Am J Cardiol 1991;67:976–980.
106. Morganroth J, Horowitz LN. Flecainide: its proarrhythmic effect and expected changes on the surface electrocardiogram. Am J Cardiol 1984;53:89B–94B.
107. Henthorn RW, Waldo AL, Anderson JL, et al. Flecainide acetate prevents recurrence of symptomatic paroxysmal supraventricular tachycardia. Circulation 1991; 83:119–125.
108. Malfatto G, Pessano P, Zaza A, et al. Experimental evidence for beta adrenergic blocking properties of propafenone and for their potential clinical relevance. Eur Heart J 1993;14:1253–1257.
109. Vaughan-Williams EM. Classification of the antiarrhythmic action of morcizine. J Clin Pharmacol 1991;31:216–221.
110. Dukes ID, Vaughan-Williams EM. The multiple modes of action of propafenone. Eur Heart J 1984;5:115–125.
111. Weiner P, Ganam R,Zidan F, et al. Clinical course of recent-onset atrial fibrillation treated with oral propafenone. Chest 1994;105:1013–1016.
112. Hii JTY, Duff HJ, Burgess ED. Clinical pharmacokinetics of propafenone. Clin Pharmacokinet 1991;21:1–10.
113. Shen EN, Sung RJ, Morady F, et al. Electrophysiologic and hemodynamic effects of intravenous propafenone in patients with recurrent ventricular tachycardia. J Am Coll Cardiol 1984;3:1291–1297.
114. Connolly SJ, Kates RE, Leback CS, et al. Clinical pharmacology of propafenone. Circulation 1983;68:681–684.
115. Siddoway LA, Thompson KA, McAllister CB, et al. Polymorphism of propafenone metabolism and disposition in man: clinical and pharmacokinetic consequences. Circulation 1987;75:785–791.
116. Kroemer HK, Turgeon J, Parker RA, et al. Flecainide enantiomers: disposition in human subjects and electrophysiologic actions in vitro. Clin Pharmacol Ther 1989;46:584–590.
117. Bryson HM, Palmer KJ, Langtry HD, et al. Propafenone: a reappraisal of its pharmacology, pharmacokinetics and therapeutic use in cardiac arrhythmias. Drugs 1993;45:85–130.
118. Ravid S, Podrid PJ, Novrit B. Safety of long-term propafenone therapy for cardiac arrhythmia—experience with 774 patients. J Electrophys 1987;1:580–590.
119. Singh BN, Kaplinsky E, Kirsten E, et al. and the Propafenone Multi-Center Research Group. Effects of propafenone on ventricular arrhythmias: double-blind, parallel, randomized, placebo-controlled dose-ranging study. Am Heart J 1988; 116:1542–1551.
120. D'Arcy PF. Drug reactions and interactions. Intl Pharmacy J 1990;4:244.
121. Moss AJ, Robinson J. Identification of high-risk population and clinical features of the idiopathic long Q-T syndrome. Circulation 1992;85:140–144.
122. Aomine M. Multiple electrophysiological actions of amiodarone on guinea pig heart. Naunym Schmiedebergs Arch Pharmacol 1988;338:589–599.
123. Singh BN. Controlling cardiac arrhythmias by lengthening repolarization: historical overview. Am J Cardiol 1993;72:18F–24F.
124. Hohnloser SH, Klingenheben T, Singh BN. Amiodarone-associated proarrhythmic effects: a review with special reference to torsades de points tachycardia. Ann Intern Med 1994;121:529–535.
125. Ceremuzynski L, Kleczar E, Krzeminska-Pakula MK, et al. Effect of amiodarone on mortality after myocardial infarction: a double-blind, placebo-controlled, pilot study. J Am Coll Cardiol 1992;20:1056–1062.
126. Burkhart F, Pfisterer M, Kiowski W, et al. Effect of antiarrhythmic therapy on mortality in survivors of myocardial infarction with asymptomatic complex ventricular arrhythmias: Basal Antiarrhythmic Study of Infarct Survival (BASIS). J Am Coll Cardiol 1990;16:1711–1718.
127. Pfisterer ME, Kiowski W, Brunner H, et al. Long-term benefit of 1-year amiodarone

treatment for persistent complex ventricular arrhythmias after myocardial infarction. Circulation 1993;87:309–311.
128. Singh S, Fletcher R, Fisher S, et al. Amiodarone in patients with congestive heart failure and asymptomatic ventricular arrhythmia. N Engl J Med 1995;333:77–82.
129. Doval H, Nul D, Grancelli H, et al. for Grupo de Estudio de la Sobrevida en la Insuficiencia Cardiaca en Argentina (GESICA). Randomised trial of low-dose amiodarone in severe congestive heart failure. Lancet 1994;344:493–498.
130. Julian DG, Jackson FS, Prescott RJ, et al. Controlled trial of sotalol for one year after myocardial infarction. Lancet 1982:1142–1147.
131. Waldo A, Camm A, de Ruyter H, et al., SWORD Investigators. Preliminary mortality results from the survival with oral D-Sotalol (SWORD) trial. J Am Coll Cardiol 1995;25:15A (Abstract).
132. Pallandi RT, Campbell TJ. Resting, and rate-dependent depression of $V_{max}$ of guinea-pig ventricular action potentials by amiodarone and desethylamiodarone. Br J Pharmacol 1987;92:97–103.
133. Ikeda N, Nademanee K, Kannan R, et al. Electrophysiologic effects of amiodarone: experimental and clinical observation relative to serum and tissue drug concentrations. Am Heart J 1984;108:890–898.
134. Munoz A, Karita P, Gallay P, et al. A randomized hemodynamic comparison of intravenous amiodarone with and without Tween 80. Eur Heart J 1988;9:142–148.
135. Pfeiffer A, Vidon N, Bovet M, et al. Intestinal absorption of amiodarone in man. J Clin Pharmacol 1990;30:615–620.
136. Roden DM. Pharmacokinetics of amiodarone: implications for drug therapy. Am J Cardiol 1993;72:45F–50F.
137. Gill J, Heel RC, Fitton A. Amiodarone: an overview of its pharmacological properties, and review of its therapeutic use in cardiac arrhythmias. Drugs 1992;43:69–110.
138. Evans SJL, Myers M, Zaher C, et al. High dose oral amiodarone loading: electrophysiologic effects and clinical tolerance. J Am Coll Cardiol 1992;19:169–173.
139. Kalbfleisch SJ, Williamson B, Man KC, et al. Prospective, randomized comparison of conventional and high dose loading regimens of amiodarone in the treatment of ventricular tachycardia. J Am Coll Cardil 1993;22:1723–1729.
140. Robinson K, Johnston A, Walker S, et al. Stability of plasma amiodarone levels during chronic oral therapy. Cardiovasc Drug Ther 1990;4:529–530.
141. Staubli M, Bircher J, Cateazzi RL, et al. Serum concentrations of amiodarone during long-term therapy, relation to dose, efficacy, and toxicity. Eur J Clin Pharmacol 1983;24:485–494.
142. Naccarelli GV, Fineberg NS, Zipes DP, et al. Amiodarone: risk factors for recurrence of symptomatic ventricular tachycardia identified at electrophysiologic study J Am Coll Cardiol 1985;6:814–821.
143. Burckhardt D. Clinical efficacy of long-term treatment with amiodarone for life-threatening arrhythmias. J Cardiovasc Pharmacol 1992;20:S59–S62.
144. Herre JM, Sauve MJ, Maloe P, et al. Long-term results of amiodarone therapy in patients with recurrent sustained ventricular tachycardia or ventricular fibrillation. J Am Coll Cardiol 1989;13:442–449.
145. Dolack GL, CASCADE Investigators. Clinical predictors of implantable cardioverter-defibrillator shocks (results of the CASCADE trial). Am J Cardiol 1994;73:237–241.
146. Chapman MJ, Moran JL, O'Fathartaigh MS, et al. Management of atrial tachyarrhythmias int he critically ill: A comparison of intravenous procainamide and amiodarone. Intensive Care Med 1993;19:48–52.
147. Kopelman HA, Horowitz LN. Efficacy and toxicity of amiodarone for the treatment of supraventricular tachyarrhythmias. Prog Cardiovasc Dis 1989;31:355–366.
148. Pilati G, Tiziano L, Trisolino G, et al. Amiodarone versus quinidine for conversio of recent onset atrial fibrillation to sinus rhythm. Current Ther Res 1991;49:140–146.
149. Zipes DP. Management of cardiac arrhythmias: pharmacological, electrical, and surgical techniques. In: Braunwald E, ed. Heart disease. Philadelphia: WB Saunders, 1988:621–657.
150. Wellens HF, Brugada P, Abdollah H, et al. A comparison of the electrophysiological effects of intravenous and oral amiodarone in the same patient. Circulation 1985;72:1064–1075.

151. Fraire AE, Guntupalli KK, Greenberg SD, et al. Amiodarone pulmonary toxicity: A multidisciplinary review of current status. South Med J 1993;86:67–77.
152. Sobel SM, Rakita L. Pneumonitis and pulmonary fibrosis associated with amiodarone treatment: A possible complication of a new antiarrhythmic drug. Circulation 1982;65:819–824.
153. Greenspon AJ, Kidwell GA, Hurley W, et al. Amiodarone-related postoperative adult respiratory distress syndrome. Circulation 1991;84:III407–III415.
154. Figge HL, Figge J. The effects of amiodarone on thyroid hormone function: a review of the physiology and clinical manifestations. J Clin Pharmacol 1990;30: 588–595.
155. Enia G, Costante G, Catalano C, et al. Severe hypothyroidism induced by amiodarone in a dialysis patient. Nephron 1987;46:206–207.
156. Chow CC, Cockram CS. Thyroid disorders induced by lithium and amiodarone: an overview. Adv Drug React Acute Poison Rev 1990;9:207–222.
157. Van Dam EWCM, Prummel MF, Wiersinga WM, et al. Treatment of amiodarone-induced hypothyroidism with potassium perchlorate. Netherlands J Med 1993; 41:21–24.
158. Dobs AS, Sarma PS, Guarnieri T, et al. Testicular dysfunction with amiodarone use. J Am Coll Cardiol 1991;18:1328–1332.
159. Nitsch J, Luderitz B. Letter to the editor. N Engl J Med 1990;317:452.
160. Hiromasa S, Coto H, Li ZY, et al. Dextrorotatory isomer of sotalol: electrophysiologic effects and interaction with verapamil. Am Heart J 1988;116:1552–1557.
161. Hohnloser SH, Woosley RL. Sotalol. N Engl J Med 1994;331:31–38.
162. Kehoe RF, MacNeil DJ, Zheutlin TA, et al. Safety and efficacy of oral sotalol for sustained ventricular tachyarrhythmias refractory to other antiarrhythmic agents. Am J Cardiol 193;72:56A–66A.
163. Antman EM, Beamer AD, Cantillon C, et al. Therapy of refractory symptomatic atrial fibrillation and atrial flutter: a staged care approach with new antiarrhythmic drugs. J Am Coll Cardiol 1990;15:698–707.
164. Young GD, Kerr CR, Mohama R, et al. Efficacy of sotalol guided by programmed electrical stimulation for sustained ventricular arrhythmias secondary to coronary artery disease. Am J Cardiol 1994;73:677–682.
165. Kuchar DL, Garan H, Venditti FJ, et al: Usefulness of sotalol in suppressing ventricular tachycardia or ventricular fibrillation in patients with healed myocardial infarcts. Am J Cardiol 1989;64:33–36.
166. Fitton A, Sorkin EM. Sotalol: an updated review of its pharmacological properties and therapeutic use in cardiac arrhythmias. Drugs 1993;46:678–719.
167. Soyka LF, Wirtz C, Spangenberg RB. Clinical safety profile of sotalol in patietns iwth arrhythmias. Am J Cardiol 1990;65;74A–81A.
168. Buchanon LV, Kabell G, Gibson JK. Acute intravenous conversion of canine atrial flutter: comparison of antiarrhythmic agents. J Cardiovasc Pharmacol 1995; 25: 539–544.
169. Lee KS. Ibutilide, a new compound with potent class III antiarrhythmic activity, activates a slow inward Na current in guinea pig ventricular cells. J Pharmacol Exp Ther 1992:262:99–108.
169a. Upjohn Company, Kalamazoo, Michigan, studies 0001, 0016 and 0022.
170. Buchanan LV, Kabell GG, Turcotte UM, et al. Effects of ibutilide on spontaneous and induced ventricular arrhythmias in 24-hour canine myocardial infarction: A comparative study with sotalol and encainide. J Cardiovasc Pharmacol 1992;19: 256–263.
170a. Bih-Fang Guo G, Ellenbogen KA, Wood MA, et al. Conversion of atrial flutter by ibutilide is associated with increased atrial cycle length variable. JACC 1996;27: 1083–1089.
170b. Upjohn Company, Kalamazoo, Michigan, studies 0003, 0014, 0015, 0019 and 0021.
171. Bigger JT Jr, Jaffee CC. The effect of bretylium tosylate on the electrophysiology: properties of ventricular muscle and Purkinje fibers. Am J Cardiol 1971;27:82–92.
172. Harrison DC, Meffin PJ, Winkle RA. Clinical pharmacokinetics of antiarrhythmic drugs. Prog Cardiovasc Dis 1977;20:217–242.
173. Kelly JG, O'Malley K. Clinical pharmacokinetics of calcium antagonists. Clin Pharmacokinet 1992;22:416–433.

174. O'Malley K, Cusack B, Kelly JG. Enzyme induction and first past metabolism in man: effects of aging. In: van Bezooijen CF, ed. Pharmacological, morphological and physiological aspects of liver aging. The Netherlands: Eurage, 1984:149–154.
175. Salerno DM, Dias VC, Kleiger RE, et al. Efficacy and safety of intravenous diltiazem for treatment of atrial fibrillation and atrial flutter. The Diltiazem-Atrial Fibrillation/Flutter Study Group. Am J Cardiol 1989;63:1046–1051.
176. Garratt C, Antoniou A, Ward D, et al. Misuse of verapamil in pre-excited atrial fibrillation. Lancet 1989;1:367–369.
177. Winters S, Schweitzer P, Kupersmith J, et al. Verapamil-induced polymorphic ventricular tachycardia. J Am Coll Cardiol 1985;6:257–259.
178. Palileo EV, Ashley WW, Swiryn S, et al. Exercise-provacable right ventriclar utflow tract tachycardia. Am Heart J 1982;104:185–193.
179. DiMarco JP, Miles W, Akhtar M, et al. Adenosine for paroxysmal supraventricular tachycardia: dose ranging and comparison with verapamil: assessment in placebo-controlled, multicentre trials. Ann Intern Med 1990;113:104–110.
180. Belardinelli L, Linden J, Berne RM. The cardiac effects of adenosine. Prog Cardiovasc Dis 1989;32:73–97.
181. Moser GH, Schrader J, Deussen A. Turnover of adenosine in plasma of human and dog blood. Am J Physiol 1989;256:C799–806.
182. Faulds D, Chrisp P, Buckley MMT: Adenosine: an evaluation of its use in cardiac diagnostic procedures, and in the treatment of paroxysmal supraventricular tachycardia. Drugs 1991;41:596–624.
183. Lemann BB, Belardinelli I, West GA, et al. Adenosine sensitive ventricular tachycardia: evident suggesting cyclic AMP-mediated triggered activity. Circulation 1986;74:270–280.
184. Malcolm AD, Garratt CJ, Camm AJ. The therapeutic and diagnostic cardiac electrophysiological uses of adenosine. Cardiovasc Drugs Ther 1993;7:139–147.
185. Falk RH, Knowlton AA, Bernard SA, et al. Digoxin for converting recent-onset atrial fibrillation to sinus rhythm. Ann Intern Med 1987;106:503–506.
186. Dreifus LS, Hiat R, Watanabe Y, et al. Ventricular fibrillation: a possible mechanism of sudden death in patients with Wolff-Parkinson-White syndrome. Circulation 1971;43:520–527.

CHAPTER 15

# Pharmacologic Therapy for Supraventricular Arrhythmias

Rodney H. Falk, MD, and Jack W. Kinch, MD

Supraventricular arrhythmias constitute a diverse group of disorders of rhythm whose management is greatly aided by precise recognition of the specific arrhythmia. With an understanding of the mechanisms responsible for the different forms of supraventricular tachycardia (SVT), the most appropriate therapy can be chosen. Conversely, an unexpected failure to respond to a therapy that has been targeted to a specific diagnosis may cause the clinician to reconsider that diagnosis.

There are three major mechanisms for supraventricular arrhythmias: enhanced automaticity, reentry, and triggered activity (see also Chapter 14) (1–3). Enhanced automaticity may be thought of as an increased rate of firing by a group of cardiac cells. The normal heart responds to stimuli arising from the sinus node but has a built-in "back-up" system so that atrial, nodal, His-Purkinje, and ventricular cells all have the propensity to function as a pacemaker (with decreasing rates and stability) if a higher pacemaker fails. Enhanced automaticity represents an exaggeration of these properties usually because of an intrinsic abnormality in the responsible tissue, external factors such as hypoxia or drug toxicity, or both.

Reentrant tachycardias are characterized by an electrical impulse that circles around an area of the heart and propagates to the remaining areas of the heart. Reentry may occur at many sites in the heart, but the most common sites for atrial arrhythmias are the atrium in atrial flutter, the atrioventricular (AV) node in AV nodal tachycardia, and the AV node and a bypass tract in Wolff-Parkinson-White (WPW) syndrome. Atrial fibrillation is also predominantly the result of a reentrant mechanism but, in this case, multiple reentrant circuits coexist and are constantly extinguishing and reforming. The response of reentrant arrhythmias to cardiac drugs depends on the site of reentry. Reentrant arrhythmias that include the AV node as part of the circuit are often easily terminated, whereas those located in the atrium are less responsive to drug therapy and may require nonpharmacologic treatments.

Triggered activity is the least common arrhythmia mechanism. The term *triggered activity* refers to impulse initiation that is caused by oscillations in membrane potential that follow the upstroke of an action potential (afterdepolarizations). If these afterpotentials achieve threshold values, a cardiac action potential is generated. Triggered activity is probably responsible for digoxin toxic arrhythmias, ventricular tachycardia with "structurally normal" hearts, and some ectopic atrial tachycardias (3).

The approach to therapy of supraventricular arrhythmias is twofold: termination of the acute episode and prevention of recurrence. In patients with atrial fibrillation additional considerations apply, specifically the need for anticoagulation and measures to control the ventricular response. This chapter considers the common supraventricular arrhythmias and the approach to their acute and long-term management.

## SPECIFIC ARRHYTHMIAS

The common specific arrhythmias and their management are described below. A schematic diagram of the mechanisms of these arrhythmias is shown in Figure 15.1.

### AV Nodal Tachycardia

#### *Mechanism*

AV nodal reentry is the most common regular tachycardia and is generally unassociated with underlying organic heart disease. It requires the participation of two pathways within the AV node—the so-called "slow" and "fast" pathways. Electrophysiologic evidence of dual AV nodal pathways can be shown in about 10% of subjects undergoing electrophysiologic studies for reasons other than SVT (4), although sustained SVT cannot be induced in every patient in whom these pathways exist. For sustained tachycardia to occur, a premature impulse must arrive at the AV node at a time when one of the pathways is refractory and the other is able to conduct. The impulse traverses the nonrefractory pathway and, on exiting, finds the other pathway now able to conduct. Conduction through this pathway in a retrograde direction permits perpetuation of the cycle.

The characteristics of dual AV nodal pathways are responsible for the surface electrocardiographic appearance of reentrant AV nodal tachycardia. The fast pathway has a greater conduction velocity but a longer refractory period than the slow pathway. Consequently, precipitation of a reentrant tachycardia by a critically timed atrial premature beat is likely to find the fast pathway refractory and thus to be conducted down the slow pathway, returning to the atrium retrogradely up the fast pathway. Because the ventricle is activated in the normal fashion through the His-Purkinje system, the QRS complex is usually normal, although occasionally a rate-related bundle branch block may occur (Fig. 15.2). The atrium is activated retrogradely, but the small size of the AV nodal reentrant circuit results in atrial activation that is virtually simultaneous with ventricular activation. This results in inverted P waves that are either hidden within the QRS complex or that are inscribed shortly after its terminal portion.

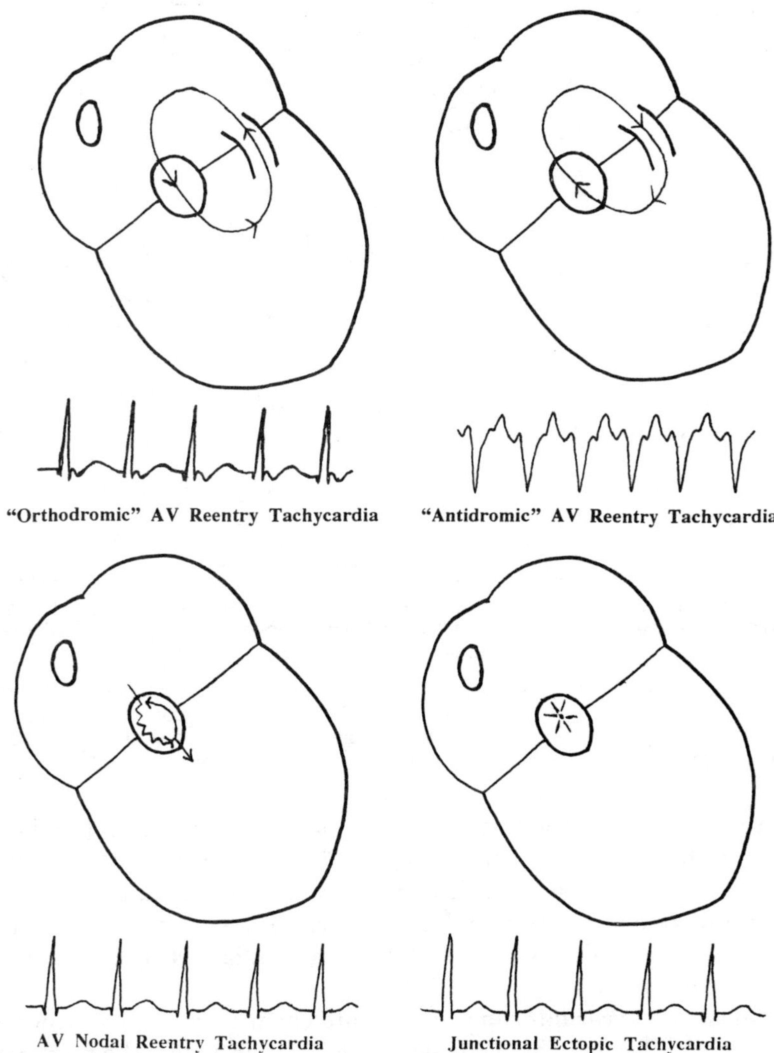


Figure 15.1 Diagrammatic representation of the mechanisms of various supraventricular tachycardias. The sinus node is represented as the small circle in the upper half of each figure, the atrioventricular (AV) node as the central circular structure, and a bypass tract as the two curved lines spanning the atria and ventricles. The schematic electrocardiograms underneath each diagram demonstrate typical features of each arrhythmia. In Figure 1*A*, the upper figures show two types of reentry involving bypass tracts: orthodromic, in which the AV node is the antegrade pathway and the bypass tract is the retrograde pathway, and antidromic, in which the converse is true. The lower left figure shows reentry within the AV node and the lower right an ectopic tachycardia.

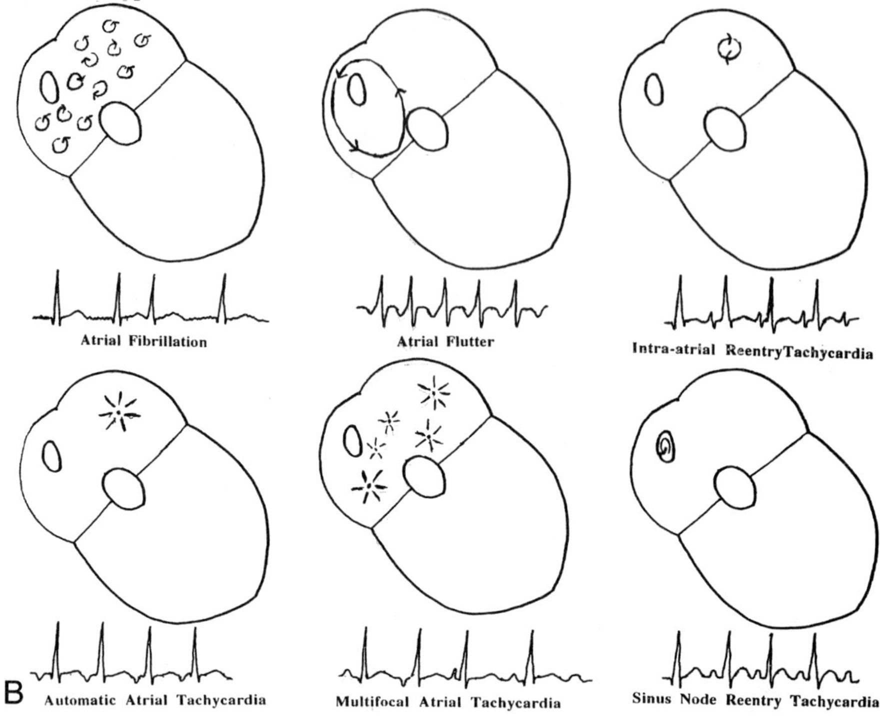


Figure 15.1 Figure 1*B* shows various arrhythmias, including atrial fibrillation (multiple reentrant pathways), atrial flutter (a form of intraatrial reentrant tachycardia), multifocal atrial tachycardia, and sinus node reentrant tachycardia. Some arrhythmias (e.g., ectopic atrial tachycardia) may have several mechanisms, only the predominant one of which is shown.

On rare occasions the fast pathway may have a shorter refractory period than the slow conducting pathway. The tachycardia is then initiated with either an atrial or ventricular premature beat and, because of the longer time taken for the impulse to return to the atrium, the P wave is seen long after the QRS complex. Such tachycardias are described as *long RP tachycardias.*

AV nodal tachycardias can be terminated by interruption of either limb of the circuit. Because the AV node is vagally innervated, the tachycardia may be terminated by carotid sinus massage or other vagal methods. Only when these fail is pharmacologic therapy needed.

*Symptoms*

Patients with AV nodal tachycardia are frequently young patients without evidence of structural heart disease. They usually present with rapid, regular palpitations experienced in the chest, neck, or both. Not infrequently, patients have a prolonged dull chest ache that does not indicate coexistent coronary disease. Tachycardia-related ST segment depression

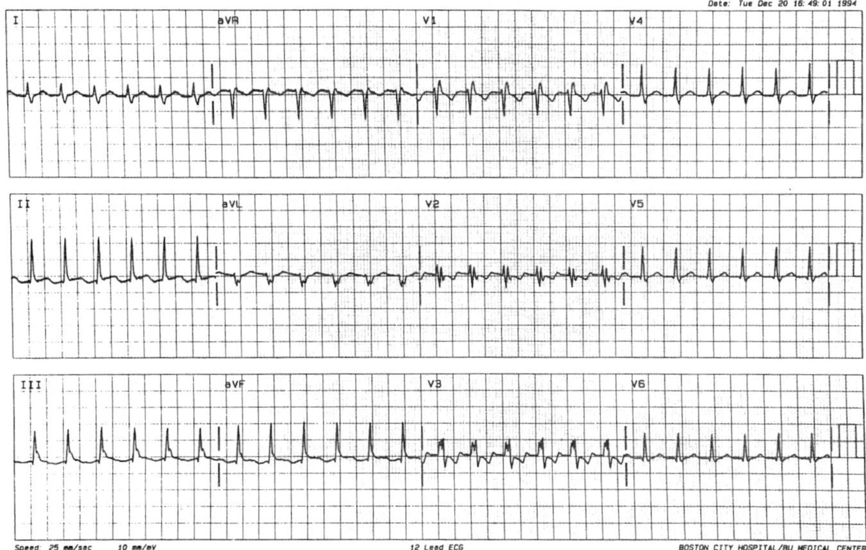


Figure 15.2 An example of atrioventricular-nodal tachycardia conducted with right bundle branch block aberration. P waves cannot be clearly discerned.

sometimes occurs on the electrocardiogram (ECG) but is rarely an indicator of coronary artery disease. Low blood pressure in a young patient with AV nodal tachycardia commonly represents a reading close to the patient's normal pressure and is rarely cause for concern.

### *Therapy*

Treatment of AV nodal tachycardia, as with all other sustained arrhythmias, can be divided into termination of the acute event and prevention of recurrence. Not all agents used for termination are effective for prevention, and the relative efficacy of a drug may differ when used for termination or prevention.

**Acute termination.** AV nodal tachycardia rarely produces severe hemodynamic compromise and thus there is adequate time for a careful assessment, including a good quality 12-lead ECG. Carotid sinus massage should be attempted initially. A differential effect of left-sided and right-sided pressure may be seen, and the opposite side of the neck should be massaged if pressure on the first side is ineffective. If carotid massage or a Valsalva maneuver fails to terminate the arrhythmia, intravenous therapy with either adenosine or a calcium channel blocker (verapamil or diltiazem) is indicated.

Adenosine has an extremely short half-life (less than 5 seconds) and high efficacy for terminating reentrant tachycardias using the AV node. It is the first-line drug and is administered as an initial rapid intravenous bolus of

6 mg. If the arrhythmia has not terminated within 1–2 minutes, a second bolus of 12 mg may be administered. Several trials have documented an 80–90% success rate using this dosing regimen (5–7). Adenosine is associated with side effects of chest discomfort and flushing or shortness of breath, but in keeping with its short half-life, these are short-lived.

Theophylline blocks the receptor responsible for adenosine's electrophysiologic effect. Therefore patients receiving theophylline are less sensitive to adenosine and may require higher doses. Carbamazepine and dipyridamole potentiate the effects of adenosine; thus, adenosine should be avoided in patients receiving these drugs (8). The termination of an SVT with adenosine has rarely been followed by the precipitation of polymorphic ventricular tachycardia (9). This side effect, although rare, mandates that the drug be given under ECG monitoring. Patients receiving class I antiarrhythmic drugs are theoretically at greater risk of post-adenosine torsades de pointes because the transient bradycardia provoked by the drug may predispose them to this arrhythmia.

If adenosine fails to terminate the tachycardia or if it is contraindicated, intravenous verapamil or diltiazem may be used. Before these agents are given, the ECG strip recorded during adenosine administration should be carefully examined. It may reveal a transient heart slowing that exposes ongoing P waves or flutter waves, indicating an initial misdiagnosis of the type of arrhythmia and the possible need for therapy other than calcium channel blocking agents (Fig. 15.3).

Verapamil is administered as an initial bolus of 5 mg. If the arrhythmia is not terminated after 5 minutes, a second dose of 10 mg may be given and repeated after 10 minutes (7, 10). Verapamil has a vasodilator effect that may provoke hypotension, particularly if the arrhythmia is not terminated. It has been suggested that the coadministration of calcium will reduce the likelihood of verapamil-induced hypotension. However, we have not found that symptomatic hypotension is a clinically significant factor in most patients with AV nodal tachycardia.

An alternative to verapamil therapy is a bolus injection (20 mg) of diltiazem (11). The efficacy for termination is similar to that of verapamil (70–80%), and diltiazem may have less of a negative inotropic effect (not a significant consideration in most patients with this arrhythmia). A second dose of diltiazem (25 mg) may be given after 10 minutes if the arrhythmia has not terminated. If either diltiazem or verapamil fails to terminate the arrhythmia, these agents may still slow conduction in the reentrant circuit. This may be recognized by a slight slowing of the tachycardia rate. Even if initially ineffective, carotid sinus massage following injection of these drugs may produce sufficient additional vagal stimulus to restore sinus rhythm.

If carotid massage fails, a further 6-mg dose of adenosine (followed if necessary by 12 mg) may be administered because the previously administered calcium channel blocker may have altered the AV node refractory

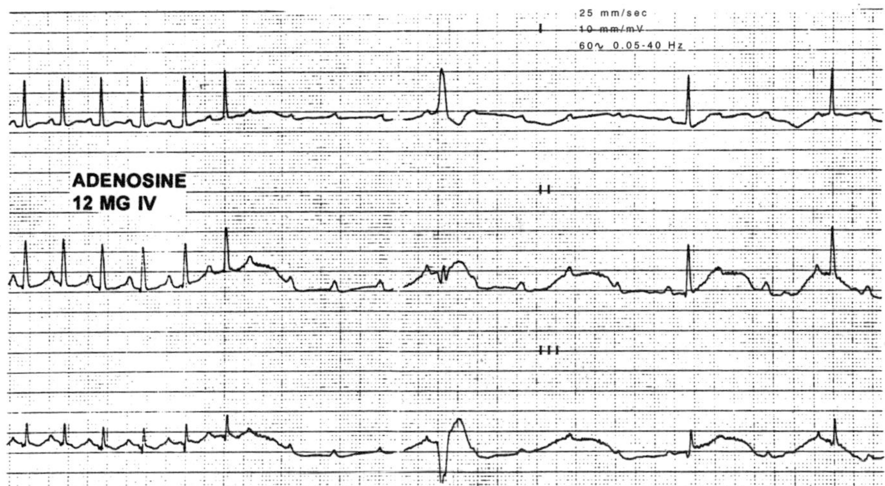


Figure 15.3 The effect of adenosine, 12 mg IV, in exposing P waves. Transient atrioventricular (AV) block (4.8 seconds) followed by 2:1 AV block reveals P waves at a rate similar to that of the original tachycardia. These P waves had the same morphology as the patient's sinus P waves and confirmed a sinus tachycardia, in this case secondary to severe pneumonia. (The slight slowing of the sinus rate is due to adenosine's effect on the sinus node.)(Courtesy of Dan Alford, MD.)

period enough to render a previously unsuccessful trial of adenosine successful. The ECG should be monitored carefully during this therapy because failure to terminate the arrhythmia may indicate that the initial diagnosis was incorrect and adenosine may transiently expose the correct underlying arrhythmia.

**Long-Term Therapy.** Before embarking on long-term treatment of AV nodal tachycardia, therapeutic choices should be discussed with the patient. Patients in whom episodes are infrequent may not wish to take daily medications and may be satisfied to seek acute termination for their spontaneous episodes. For patients with frequent episodes, radiofrequency catheter ablation of the slow pathway is an effective procedure with a cure rate of more than 90% in experienced hands (12, 13). Once a cure has been effected, drug therapy is no longer necessary. For patients wishing to try long-term drug therapy, β-blockade, diltiazem, or verapamil are effective agents. We prefer either verapamil (180–240 mg daily as a single slow release form or in divided doses) or diltiazem (180–240 mg daily) over β-blockers because the latter may cause considerable fatigue in young patients. High-dose digoxin (0.375–0.5 mg daily) in patients with normal renal function may also be effective and can be used alone as an adjunct to diltiazem. The dose of digoxin should be reduced when this agent is used in conjunction with verapamil, which increases digoxin levels.

If these agents are unsuccessful, flecainide (100–150 mg twice daily) (14) or propafenone (150–225 mg three times a day) may be effective (15). Care should be taken to avoid use of flecainide or propafenone in patients with coronary artery disease. Several other agents such as sotalol, quinidine, or disopyramide also may be effective, but they are rarely used for this indication.

## AV Tachycardia in Wolff-Parkinson-White Syndrome

### *Mechanism*

Patients with classic Wolff-Parkinson-White syndrome have an ECG during sinus rhythm that demonstrates a short PR interval and a delta wave. Tachycardia in a patient with Wolff-Parkinson-White syndrome is usually the result of a reentrant tachycardia proceeding anterogradely down the AV node and retrogradely up the bypass tract (Fig. 15.1*A*). This results in a narrow complex tachycardia. Because the pathway constituting the reentrant circuit includes the bypass tract, however, it is longer than that of an AV nodal tachycardia. This results in retrograde atrial activation slightly later than anterograde ventricular activation so that a retrograde P wave may be visible after the QRS complex.

### *Acute Therapy*

Orthodromic AV tachycardia using a bypass tract (Fig. 15.1*A*) may be indistinguishable from AV nodal tachycardia on the surface ECG. However, the approach to treatment of an acute episode is virtually identical in the two arrhythmias, because drugs that slow conduction in the AV node terminate orthodromic tachycardia. As with AV nodal tachycardia, vagal maneuvers should be tried first followed by bolus adenosine administration.

The use of intravenous calcium channel blockers in narrow complex AV tachycardia is controversial. However, the use of calcium channel blockers is absolutely contraindicated in preexcited atrial fibrillation. Because it is often unclear if a patient presenting for the first time with a narrow complex reentrant tachycardia has a bypass tract or has AV nodal tachycardia, we prefer adenosine as the first-line drug. If this drug fails, verapamil or diltiazem may be administered, as described above for AV nodal reentry. Even if the patient is known to have a bypass tract, a calcium channel blocker may be used for acute termination of a narrow-complex orthodromic tachycardia providing that the physician is aware of the rare complication of precipitating preexcited atrial fibrillation with a rapid ventricular response (16). A defibrillator should be immediately available in case this arrhythmia occurs and results in hemodynamic instability.

Once an episode of AV reentrant tachycardia has terminated, the ECG in sinus rhythm frequently shows a pattern of preexcitation, confirming the etiology of the narrow complex tachycardia (Fig. 15.4). If the anterograde refractory period is long, however, preexcitation may not occur (concealed bypass tract), or it may be intermittent.

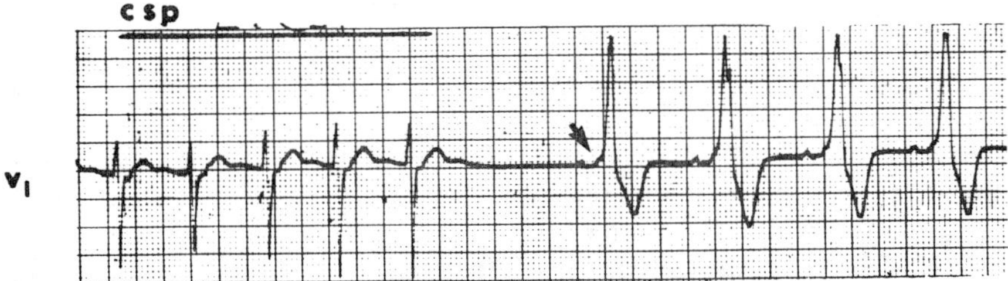


Figure 15.4 Termination of atrioventricular(AV) reentry tachycardia in the Wolff-Parkinson-White syndrome. The narrow complex tachycardia is abruptly terminated after carotid sinus pressure (csp). A delta wave (*arrow*) is now clearly seen, indicating that the tachycardia was an orthodromic AV reentrant arrhythmia.

### *Long-Term Therapy*

The introduction of radiofrequency ablation procedures has changed radically long-term therapy for patients with Wolff-Parkinson-White syndrome and recurrent tachycardia. In patients with frequent arrhythmias, electrophysiologic study with radiofrequency ablation of the accessory pathway is now the treatment of choice, with a success rate in excess of 80–85% (17, 18). Although we favor attempted bypass tract ablation in all patients with preexcitation and frequent symptomatic arrhythmia, a subgroup of patients exists for whom drug therapy (or no therapy) may be a reasonable alternative.

In an individual patient, if the arrhythmia is infrequent and invariably consists of a regular tachycardia, therapy may not be needed. If the patient is troubled by the tachycardia and ablation is not an option, several antiarrhythmic drugs may be of value. The class IC agents flecainide and propafenone may be particularly effective (19), but other drugs have been used, including β-blockers, sotalol, disopyramide, and amiodarone.

A less common, but more serious, complication of the Wolff-Parkinson-White syndrome is atrial fibrillation. Subjects with this syndrome are more prone to this arrhythmia than age-matched subjects in the general population, and the ventricular response may be extremely rapid, resulting in profound hypotension, syncope, or degeneration into ventricular fibrillation (20). Treatment of preexcited atrial fibrillation is discussed later in the section on atrial fibrillation.

## Atrial Tachycardias

There are two types of atrial tachycardia that differ in etiology and management: multifocal atrial tachycardia (MAT) and unifocal atrial tachycardia. The latter is usually simply referred to as atrial tachycardia. These two arrhythmias will be discussed separately.

### *Multifocal Atrial Tachycardia*

MAT is characterized by three or more P wave morphologies on the ECG with an atrial rate of 120 beats/minute or more. It is most commonly seen in patients with pulmonary disease, often during a deterioration in their respiratory state (21).

**Mechanisms.** The precise mechanism of MAT is unclear, but it appears to be caused by abnormal automaticity or triggered activity. Lin et al. (22) have shown that theophylline facilitates the development of spontaneous slow response action potentials in human atrial fibers as a result of triggered activity. This effect is blocked by diltiazem. Many patients with MAT also take theophylline, which although not a prerequisite for the development of this arrhythmia, may be a contributing factor together with hypoxia, electrolyte abnormalities, and an increased adrenergic state. It has been shown that MAT in patients receiving theophylline frequently resolves with theophylline withdrawal and recurs on rechallenge even when theophylline levels are therapeutic.

**Therapy.** The initial treatment of MAT is to correct, as far as possible, any electrolyte or metabolic abnormalities and, if possible, to withdraw drugs such as theophylline. Drug withdrawal is often difficult because patients with MAT commonly have severe pulmonary disease and are dependent on bronchodilators.

Although suppression of the ectopic foci is ideal, the major goal in treating MAT is reduction of the ventricular response to levels appropriate for the clinical state of the patient. A mild tachycardia (100–110 beats/minute) might be an appropriate response to the underlying disease in some of these patients; therefore, slowing heart rates to less than 100 beats/minute may not be desirable. Although MAT may be confused with atrial fibrillation on superficial inspection of the ECG, the ventricular rate rarely slows after digoxin administration. This may be partly because of a hyperadrenergic state associated with MAT that would counteract the primary vagotonic action of digoxin.

An early, uncontrolled trial in patients with MAT suggested that verapamil was an effective therapy (23). In a subsequent controlled trial, however, verapamil was effective only in four of nine patients (44%) compared with a 20% placebo response and a response in eight of nine patients receiving metoprolol (24). Although these results suggest that metoprolol was the most effective agent, efficacy was based on a reduction of ventricular rate to less than 100 beats/minute rather than resolution of the arrhythmia. In addition metoprolol is potentially dangerous in patients with a bronchospastic component to their underlying pulmonary disease.

We urge caution in attempting to treat patients with MAT. If the arrhythmia does not appear to be causing problems and the mean ventricular response is not excessive (e.g., it is less than 130 beats/minute), watchful waiting appears to be appropriate, together with correction of any underlying precipitating factors. Magnesium therapy may be tried because it is relatively harmless and has sometimes been successful (25). If the ventricular rate needs to be controlled, a calcium channel blocker should be tried first. Although verapamil has been recommended, a bolus dose of diltiazem in the range used for atrial fibrillation and flutter (20–25 mg) is equally appropriate, because if it is successful, it may be followed by an infusion of 5–15 mg/hour.

Isolated cases of control of MAT with flecainide or amiodarone have been reported, but these drugs should be used only in refractory, symptomatic cases after consideration of the appropriate risk:benefit ratio. These considerations include associated ischemic heart disease or heart failure as a contraindication to flecainide and severe pulmonary disease as a contraindication to amiodarone.

### *Atrial Tachycardia*

Atrial tachycardia is a rhythm arising from either atrium and is characterized by a uniform P wave morphology at a rate of 120–220 beats/minute with a different morphology from that seen in sinus rhythm. Short bursts of atrial tachycardia (fewer than 10 beats) are not uncommon in normal subjects, whereas sustained runs of atrial tachycardia are frequently associated with organic heart disease (26). Incessant atrial tachycardia, defined as an arrhythmia occurring for 12 or more hours a day, may occur in the absence of overt structural disease and may result in a tachycardia-mediated cardiomyopathy (27, 28). Atrial tachycardia with block is a classic arrhythmia associated with digoxin toxicity, although it may occur without digoxin in patients with significant cardiac disease.

**Mechanisms.** Sustained atrial tachycardia is uncommon compared with other supraventricular arrhythmias, occurring in only 7% of a large series (26). Careful electrophysiologic studies have indicated that most cases are the result of atrial reentry or an automatic focus. An occasional case may be caused by triggered activity. The differential diagnosis includes sinus tachycardia, sinus node reentry, and atrial flutter with a slow atrial rate. Atrial flutter may show the more typical sawtooth pattern in the inferior leads. Sinus tachycardia and sinus node reentry often can be distinguished from atrial tachycardia because they have a P wave morphology that is identical to that in sinus rhythm. In patients in whom the atrial focus is close to the sinus node, it may be difficult to differentiate atrial tachycardia from sinus tachycardia because the change in P wave morphology with onset of atrial tachycardia may be subtle. However, physiologic sinus tachycardia manifests a decreasing PR interval as the heart rate increases, whereas the PR interval increases in atrial tachycardia. This is because sinus tachycardia, unlike atrial tachycardia, is sympathetically mediated and associated with sympathetic effects on the AV node.

**Therapy.** Because of the variety of mechanisms and underlying cardiac diseases associated with atrial tachycardia, coupled with its relative infrequency, no adequately controlled trial of therapy has been reported.

Electrolyte abnormalities should be sought and corrected in all patients. If digoxin toxicity is suspected as a cause of atrial tachycardia, the drug should be withdrawn. Digoxin-specific antibodies are rarely indicated unless there is coexistent ventricular tachycardia or high-degree AV block (29).

A prolonged episode of paroxysmal atrial tachycardia may sometimes be terminated by intravenous verapamil or propranolol. The efficacy of adenosine in paroxysmal atrial tachycardia is unclear. Some investigators have found it to be rarely effective, whereas others have found it to terminate atrial tachycardia in more than 70% of cases (30, 31). The varying response to adenosine may reflect the different electrophysiologic mechanisms of tachycardia in the patients reported. Even if adenosine fails to terminate the tachycardia, it may be helpful in identifying an atrial origin of an unclear arrhythmia by transient exposure of atrial activity during induction of AV block.

If acute termination fails, therapy can be aimed at controlling the ventricular rate with calcium channel blockers, β-blockers (contraindicated in the presence of associated heart failure), or digoxin (if digoxin toxicity is not a possible cause). In the absence of controlled trials, long-term pharmacologic control of the arrhythmia is empiric. Incessant atrial tachycardia rarely responds to drug therapy, but repeated long episodes of paroxysmal atrial tachycardia may be successfully suppressed. Several antiarrhythmic drugs have been reported to be successful in individual cases, but flecainide, and possibly propafenone, appear to be most promising (32). The use of these class IC agents should, however, be limited to patients without documented or suspected coronary artery disease. Amiodarone may also be effective in some cases (33).

Although enhanced automaticity may be the mechanism in a significant proportion of cases of atrial tachycardia, electrical cardioversion can be attempted in patients with hemodynamic compromise or in whom the diagnosis is uncertain. It is effective in patients with an intraatrial reentrant mechanism for the arrhythmia or in whom a slow atrial flutter exists as the result of a markedly diseased atrium (Fig. 15.5). Electrical cardioversion should not be attempted in patients with suspected digoxin toxicity because ventricular arrhythmias may be provoked.

**Long-Term Therapy.** Frequent or prolonged recurrences of paroxysmal atrial tachycardia may produce troublesome symptoms. Oral forms of β-blockers or calcium channel blockers are less effective in preventing recurrences than are the intravenous forms in terminating atrial tachycardia. Class IC agents may be successful.

If drug therapy is not tolerated or fails, radiofrequency ablation of atrial tachycardia may be successful. The technique requires careful mapping of multiple atrial sites; the published experience with both children and adults is, however, small (26). In skilled hands, the success rate exceeds

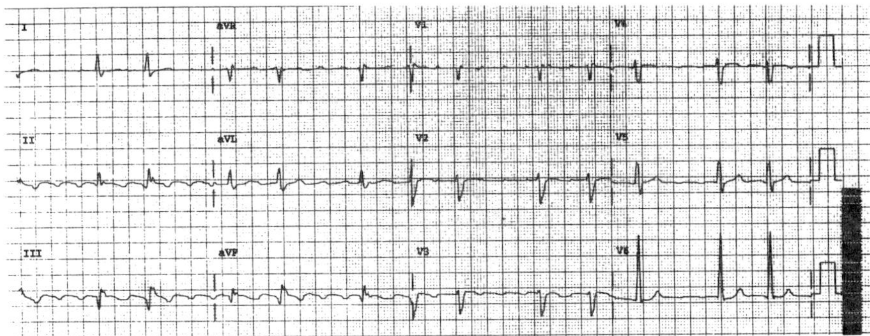


Figure 15.5 "Slow" atrial flutter with variable block. Inverted P waves are present in the inferior leads at a rate of 210 beats per minute. It is difficult to distinguish between an atrial tachycardia and an atrial flutter with a relatively slow atrial rate, but electrical cardioversion in this patient was successful at 50 J, suggesting a reentrant mechanism.

70% (26, 30, 31). If catheter ablation of the focus is not feasible and drug therapy is unsuccessful, radiofrequency AV nodal ablation or modification is an effective alternative to control the ventricular response. Surgical ablation has also been successful for patients with incessant atrial tachycardia and left ventricular dysfunction. Control of the ventricular rate by ablation of the atrial tachycardia or AV nodal ablation frequently results in improvement of the impaired ejection fraction (27, 28).

## Atrial Flutter

### *Mechanism*

Atrial flutter is a reentrant rhythm, although its anatomic circuit is much larger than those in the arrhythmias discussed so far. Mapping studies in animals and humans have shown that the most common mechanism is a reentrant circuit in the right atrium (Fig. 15.1*B*) (34, 35). Although right-sided or left-sided cardiac disease is almost invariably present in patients with atrial flutter, the presence of a fixed anatomic obstacle appears to be a prerequisite for the large flutter circuit. The inferior vena cava commonly delineates a part of the reentry circuit, although the tricuspid valve annulus often also plays a role. The circuit itself does not necessarily include both atria. Although the left atrium may be an integral part of the flutter cycle, it may frequently be a "bystander" that is activated from the right atrium (34–36).

The electrocardiographic diagnosis of typical atrial flutter is characterized by flutter waves with a sawtooth appearance in the inferior leads that occur at a rate of 280–320 beats/minute. This is commonly associated with 2:1 AV block with a regular ventricular response of 140–160 beats/minute or with variable block. In patients with 2:1 AV block, flutter waves may be obscured by the QRS-T complexes, making it difficult to distinguish between flutter and other supraventricular rhythms. The most common differential diagnoses are sinus tachycardia and AV nodal or AV reentrant tachycardia. Sinus tachycardia rarely approaches 150 beats/minute in resting patients unless they are seriously ill. The monotonous regularity of the ventricular response of flutter with 2:1 AV block contrasts with the slight, but usually apparent, variation in rate with sinus tachycardia. Occasionally, the skilled observer may be able to show rapid regular pulsations in the jugular venous pulse representing the atrial contraction and occurring at a rate double that of the ventricular response. Although carotid massage or adenosine treatment usually fail in terminating atrial flutter, both are valuable in transiently increasing AV block and showing flutter waves.

### *Treatment of Atrial Flutter*

Sustained atrial flutter is a difficult arrhythmia to terminate with drugs. The same agents used for termination of atrial fibrillation (see below) are used in atrial flutter but generally with less success. An exception may be the new class III agent ibutilide, which appears to be more successful in treating an acute episode of flutter than of atrial fibrillation (data on file, Upjohn Company, Kalamazoo, Michigan). As with all arrhythmias, the initial aim is to assess the stability of the patient and to determine the need for urgent therapy. Most patients seem to tolerate atrial flutter relatively well, although occasionally a patient with poor cardiac function may need prompt termination of arrhythmia. Under these circumstances electrical cardioversion is the treatment of choice and has a high success rate.

Correction of any electrolyte abnormality is a precursor to any therapy. Because atrial flutter is common in patients with chronic obstructive pulmonary disease, serum levels of theophylline should also be assessed in patients receiving these drugs.

The acute therapy of an episode of atrial flutter is twofold: control of the ventricular response and termination of the arrhythmia. Digoxin is less effective in slowing the ventricular response to atrial flutter than it is in atrial fibrillation, even when sympathetic tone is not excessive and even if the drug is given in high doses. This is most likely because 2:1 AV block in atrial flutter is a simple function of the refractory period of the AV node, whereas the ventricular response to atrial fibrillation is more complex, because it is affected by factors such as concealed AV nodal conduction. Therapy for acute termination of atrial flutter is similar to that for atrial fibrillation; however, certain differences exist. Most drugs used for terminating atrial flutter other than ibutilide are less effective in that situation than for terminating atrial fibrillation. A further problem of drug therapy for atrial flutter is the propensity of many atrial arrhythmic agents to slow the atrial rate and thereby increase the possibility of 1:1 AV nodal conduction.

The prevention of episodes of atrial flutter is similar to the prevention of those of atrial fibrillation. For patients in whom recurrent atrial flutter cannot be prevented, AV nodal ablation with pacemaker implantation is an option if the ventricular rate is difficult to control. Successful ablation of flutter itself has also been reported and obviates the necessity for cardiac pacing (37).

## Atrial Fibrillation

Atrial fibrillation is the most common sustained arrhythmia. It is characterized by rapid irregular atrial rhythm on the ECG with a random ventricular response. As with other supraventricular arrhythmias, therapy can be divided into treatment of acute and chronic episodes. However, atrial fibrillation differs from the other rhythm disturbances in that therapy is frequently focused on control of heart rate rather than termination of arrhythmia. Prevention of thromboembolism is also a major consideration. Anticoagulation is dealt with elsewhere in this volume (see Chapters 9 and 10) and will not be discussed in detail here.

### *Treatment of the Acute Episode*

**Mechanisms.** Atrial fibrillation is a reentrant arrhythmia characterized by multiple reentrant circuits in the atria (Fig. 15.1*B*). The size of the individual circuits varies and may be influenced by changes in autonomic tone and by drug effect.

Atrial fibrillation may be paroxysmal or sustained. No uniform definition exists for these two terms, but paroxysmal atrial fibrillation can be defined as an episode that terminates spontaneously. Episodes lasting more than 1 week generally tend to persist and require pharmacologic or direct current termination unless an underlying, treatable condition (e.g., hyperthyroidism) exists.

The high spontaneous conversion of recent-onset atrial fibrillation (defined as a duration of 7 days or less) makes the assessment of trials of therapy difficult unless a placebo-control design is used (38, 39).

The aim of therapy in the patient presenting with recent-onset atrial fibrillation is control of heart rate and, in selected cases, termination of the rhythm. Although it presents a small risk, thromboembolism is always a possibility, even in recent-onset atrial fibrillation. Although no controlled data exist, it is common practice to administer an anticoagulant to any patient who has had the arrhythmia for more than 3 days before cardioversion is attempted. For arrhythmias of shorter duration, cardioversion can usually be safely carried out without anticoagulation, although cases of thromboembolism occurring within hours of arrhythmia onset have been reported.

**Termination.** Clinical assessment of the patient with recent-onset atrial fibrillation should focus on the presence of symptoms. The urgency with which to treat an acute episode depends on the severity of the symptoms associated with the arrhythmia. The loss of atrial kick and rapid ventricular response may precipitate heart failure even in patients with normal systolic ventricular function if ventricular hypertrophy exists. Angina may occur in patients with ischemic heart disease. In many patients symptoms may be limited to palpitations that cause minimal discomfort.

About 40–50% of episodes of recent-onset atrial fibrillation spontaneously terminate without therapy. Because digoxin is frequently prescribed for new-onset atrial fibrillation, the high spontaneous conversion rate led to the belief that it is effective in terminating atrial fibrillation. However, a double blind study of digoxin for atrial fibrillation of less than 1 week's duration showed an equal conversion rate in digoxin-treated patients and those given placebo, and also showed that the effect of digoxin in slowing the heart rate takes several hours (38).

A reasonable approach is therefore to initially slow the ventricular response and observe the patient for 12–24 hours to see if spontaneous conversion occurs. Unless contraindicated, intravenous heparin may be prescribed to permit flexibility in timing electrical cardioversion should spontaneous or pharmacologic conversion fail. If mitral stenosis is suspected, an echocardiogram should be obtained before pharmacologic conversion is attempted because the presence of mitral stenosis mandates adequate anticoagulation prior to restoration of sinus rhythm even if the duration of arrhythmia is short.

In the absence of spontaneous conversion, patients with a short duration of nonanticoagulated atrial fibrillation (3 days or less) can be either electrically cardioverted without an antiarrhythmic agent or treated with antiarrhythmic drugs followed by electrical cardioversion if necessary. Quinidine (200 mg followed by 400 mg 1–2 hours later), disopyramide (300 mg), or flecainide (300 mg) as single doses often may restore a normal rhythm within a few hours (39–42). If sinus rhythm is not restored, additional doses may be given (quinidine sulfate, 200–300 mg; disopyramide, 150 mg; or flecainide, 100 mg) and electrical cardioversion performed if the patient remains in atrial fibrillation. Another regimen that has been used is intravenous procainamide, 100 mg every 5 minutes until conversion or hypotension occurs or a total of 1000 mg is administered.

Ideally, an adequate number of doses of the chosen drug should be given to obtain therapeutic levels at the time of electrical cardioversion. For drugs that have a long half-life, such as sotalol or flecainide, it may take 3–4 days (43, 44). However, it is not clear that therapeutic levels of antiarrhythmic agents facilitate electrical cardioversion of atrial fibrillation, and it is acceptable to electrically terminate the arrhythmia before a steady state is reached.

The decision to prescribe or continue antiarrhythmic therapy after spontaneous electrical or pharmacologic cardioversion depends on several factors. Because it is not known if a single episode of atrial fibrillation will recur, we prefer not to prescribe long-term antiarrhythmic drugs after the first episode of arrhythmia but to follow such a patient without therapy.

However, if the patient has cardiac pathology that favors the recurrence of symptomatic atrial fibrillation (e.g., mitral stenosis or hypertrophic cardiomyopathy) or has symptoms of heart failure or angina with the initial episode, an antiarrhythmic drug may be prescribed. The choice of drug depends on physician preference and follows the same reasoning as that used after electrical cardioversion for sustained atrial fibrillation.

*Atrial Fibrillation of Uncertain or Prolonged Duration*

Most patients with newly diagnosed atrial fibrillation are uncertain of the precise onset of their arrhythmia or have delayed seeking medical treatment for several days. In these patients anticoagulation may be necessary before cardioversion is attempted; therefore, control of heart rate is of greater importance. The use of transesophageal echocardiography to exclude atrial thrombi is valuable in these patients if cardioversion is being considered. However, postcardioversion atrial stunning may occur and still necessitates pericardioversion and postcardioversion anticoagulant therapy (45, 46).

*Acute Heart Rate Control*

The untreated patient presenting with atrial fibrillation most commonly has a ventricular rate of 110–150 beats/minute, although even in the absence of preexcitation or thyrotoxicosis, the ventricular response may briefly surge as high as 200 beats/minute. The urgency of ventricular rate control depends on symptoms associated with the tachycardia. In a few patients (those with hemodynamic compromise or clear electrocardiographic changes of ischemia), restoration of sinus rhythm by urgent cardioversion is indicated. These patients usually have very recent-onset arrhythmia, but even if the duration is unknown, rapid correction of arrhythmia takes preference over consideration of anticoagulation. Patients whose arrhythmia is either an incidental finding or is causing minimal discomfort with no other clinical abnormality, however, may need only digoxin for rate control. The maximum effect of digoxin on ventricular rate may not be seen for several hours even when adequate doses are given (38, 47). This delay is usually not significant in minimally symptomatic patients. Digoxin may be administered orally with a loading dose of 1.0–1.5 mg over the first 24 hours or as intravenous bolus (47).

Once the small group of patients needing urgent cardioversion has been excluded and the group needing least urgent attention is identified, there remains a sizeable percentage of patients in whom digoxin is likely to be ineffective because of a high sympathetic tone (e.g., fever, thyrotoxicosis, acute hypoxia) or in whom a more rapid control of ventricular rate is desired. Intravenous verapamil or diltiazem, or an intravenous β-blocker (esmolol or propranolol) is effective in these patients (48, 49). The doses of these drugs are listed in Table 15.1. Generally, calcium channel blockers are a better choice in this situation because their use avoids the possibility

**Table 15.1**
**Effective Agents for Slowing Ventricular Rate in Atrial Fibrillation[a]**

| Drug | Acute Dose | Maintenance dose | Comments |
|---|---|---|---|
| Digoxin | 1.0–1.5 mg i.v.or p.o. over 24 h in increments of 0.25–0.5 mg | 0.125–0.5 mg daily | Loading takes several hours to slow the rate and can be avoided if no urgency. Minimally effective during exercise, fever, and other high catecholamine states. Caution in elderly patients or those with renal impairment |
| Propranolol | 1–5 mg i.v. (1 mg q 2 min) | 10–120 mg t.i.d. | Extreme caution in patients with congestive heart failure. May be adequate long-term therapy b.i.d. |
| Esmolol | 0.5 mg/kg/min i.v. | 0.05–0.2 mg/kg/min i.v. | Very short half-life. Only available intravenously. Hypotension common |
| Verapamil | 5–10 mg i.v. over 2–3 min; repeat 5–10 mg 30 min later if required. Maintenance infusion rate is not well documented | 40–120 mg t.i.d. daily or 120–240 mg of the slow-release form once or b.i.d. | May be synergistic with digoxin but also increases digoxin levels. Peripheral edema may mimic congestive heart failure |
| Diltiazem | 20 mg or 0.25 mg/kg i.v. over 2 min, followed if necessary by 25 mg or 0.35 mg/kg i.v. 15 minutes later. Maintenance infusion of 5–15 mg/h thereafter | 60–120 mg t.i.d. or single dose 120–300 mg slow-release form once daily | Synergistic with digoxin; no significant effects on digoxin levels. May cause ankle edema |

[a]In the absence of preexcitation.
b.i.d. = twice a day; h = hour; min = minute; p.o. = by mouth; q = every; t.i.d. = three times a day.

of precipitating bronchospasm in susceptible patients. Diltiazem has an advantage over verapamil because it may be administered easily as an infusion after bolus injection (48) and is well tolerated acutely even in the presence of severe heart failure (50). Intravenous β-blockade is preferred when atrial fibrillation complicates acute myocardial infarction or thyrotoxicosis.

Once heart rate control has been achieved, it may be maintained by the use of oral digoxin, β-blockade, or calcium channel blockers in the doses listed in Table 15.1. For the patient in whom heart rate control during atrial fibrillation is a temporary measure until restoration of sinus rhythm, a detailed evaluation during daily activities is not necessary, but for those in whom sustained atrial fibrillation with rate control is the long-term plan, a more careful assessment may be valuable.

### *Suggested Approach to Long-Term Heart Rate Control*

There is no uniform approach to heart rate control in sustained atrial fibrillation; thus, symptoms, urgency, and long-term goals should be assessed. The following is one approach to reaching decisions about appropriate therapy.

Digoxin therapy remains the mainstay of monotherapy for sustained atrial fibrillation in most asymptomatic patients. The dose necessary to achieve an adequate resting heart rate is often more than the standard daily dose (0.25 mg), particularly in young patients with normal renal function. In some patients the vagal effects of digoxin may be easily overcome with exercise or other adrenergic input to cause disproportionate rate increases. Routine digoxin levels are not valuable in assessing adequate dose but may be helpful if the heart rate is uncontrolled or when toxicity is clinically suspected.

Generally Holter monitoring or exercise testing to determine adequacy of rate control are unnecessary in the asymptomatic, relatively sedentary older patient with a resting rate less than 90 beats/minute. In younger, more active patients with chronic atrial fibrillation, particularly those with reduced exercise tolerance, Holter monitoring is useful in determining the range of heart rate throughout the day (Fig. 15.6). Often symptoms attributed to underlying heart disease (particularly mitral valve disease) are found to be associated with disproportionate tachycardia at low levels of exertion; the addition of another negative chronotropic agent may improve patient well-being. Treadmill exercise testing is useful for assessing the efficacy of treatment in patients in whom Holter monitoring has revealed excessive periods of disproportionate tachycardia during daily activity.

The addition of a calcium channel blocking agent to digoxin is the treatment of choice if digoxin alone fails to control symptoms related to excessive tachycardia. In contrast to β-blockers (51), calcium channel blockers have shown a modest increase in exercise tolerance when prescribed for heart rate control in atrial fibrillation in some trials (52, 53). Although there are no published data on the efficacy of the slow-release preparations of verapamil or diltiazem for rate control in chronic atrial fibrillation, personal experience suggests that a good response may be anticipated with either agent. If verapamil is chosen over diltiazem, the patient should be carefully monitored for evidence of digoxin toxicity. Serum digoxin levels should be measured before and approximately 7–10 days after the institution of therapy with appropriate dose adjustments as required.

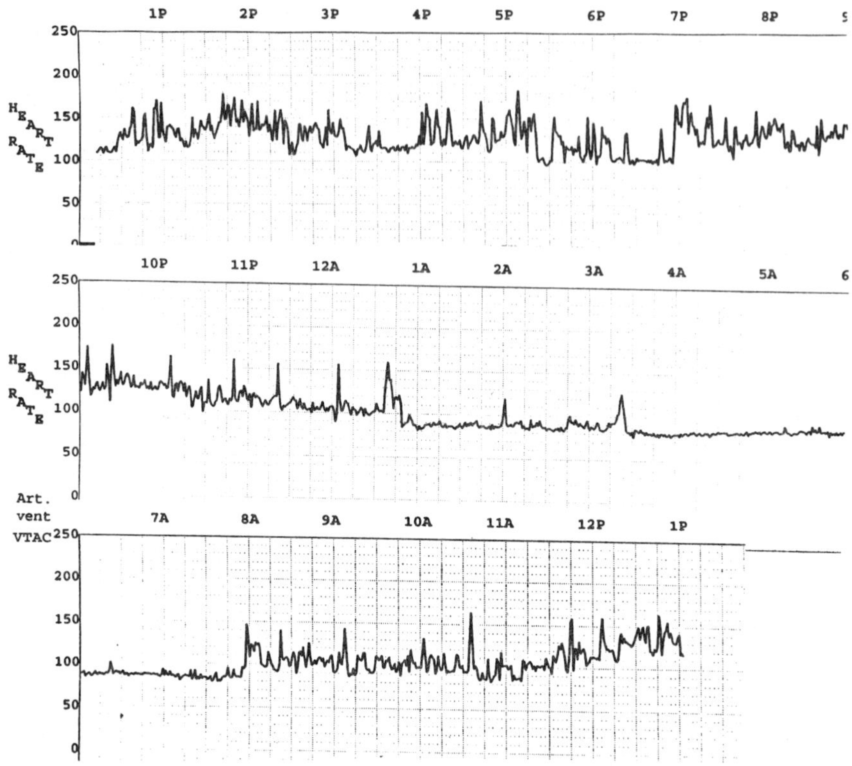


Figure 15.6 A 24-hour heart rate trend from a 50-year-old patient with incidentally noted atrial fibrillation and a history of hypertension. The heart rate exceeds 110 beats per minute during the day, with peaks as high as 185 beats during daily activities. Note that the rate falls and smoothes during sleep (1 am–8 am). This patient had an ejection fraction of 40% and was initially believed to have atrial fibrillation secondary to a cardiomyopathy. However, electrical cardioversion and maintenance of sinus rhythm with disopyramide resulted in normalization of left ventricular function, suggesting a tachycardia-medicated cardiomyopathy.

Although trials of β-blockers do not seem to indicate a significant effect of therapy on exercise duration (and some have shown a decrease in exercise tolerance), the doses used were rarely individually titrated and may have been too high, resulting in excessive heart rate slowing in many patients. In addition, maximal exercise tolerance is a poor indicator of drug efficacy, because most patients do not routinely perform vigorous exertion and require therapy only for symptoms such as palpitations. An example of the discrepant benefit of β-blockade on patient well-being and exercise tolerance was shown in a study in which 50% of patients experienced symptomatic relief when timolol was added to digoxin, despite the failure to prolong exercise duration (54). Presumably this was because of the blunting of heart rate at lower levels of exertion. β-Blockers therefore may have a role in selected patients with atrial fibrillation and may be added to digoxin if the rate is poorly controlled. This is particularly so in anxious patients with symptomatic palpitations, in whom only a small dose (propranolol, 10 mg twice daily) may be required. β-Blockers should be considered first-line therapy in patients in whom angina coexists with atrial fibrillation.

An issue related to the optimal dose of either β-blockers or calcium channel blockers is the dosing interval used for short-acting preparations of propranolol, diltiazem, and verapamil. In clinical trials these drugs have been prescribed three times daily, frequently in conjunction with digoxin. However, nocturnal heart rates during atrial fibrillation are generally low and frequently associated with ventricular pauses (55). Thus, an evening dose of medication appears not to be necessary for rate control. When short-acting agents are used for this purpose, it is appropriate to prescribe only a morning and a midday dose and to confirm the efficacy of this regimen with Holter monitoring.

*Heart Rate Control in Paroxysmal Atrial Fibrillation*

Patients with paroxysmal atrial fibrillation often are troubled by palpitations, particularly at the onset of the arrhythmia. Symptomatic episodes of atrial fibrillation have been found to have a higher mean heart rate than asymptomatic episodes. This suggests that heart rate control might be valuable in reducing symptoms, although the abolition of symptoms in paroxysmal atrial fibrillation does not necessarily abolish the arrhythmia.

Long-term digoxin therapy is often prescribed in patients with paroxysmal atrial fibrillation to maintain a slower ventricular rate should a paroxysm occur. Digoxin is chosen because of its documented efficacy in slowing heart rate in recent-onset atrial fibrillation and for maintaining a controlled resting ventricular response in sustained atrial fibrillation. Although controlled data are sparse, review of the available literature suggests that digoxin fails to adequately control heart rate at the onset of a paroxysm of atrial fibrillation. Thus, in a group of patients who experienced an episode of paroxysmal atrial fibrillation during Holter monitoring, the mean ventricular response at the onset of atrial fibrillation was not statistically different between those taking digoxin (140 ± 25 beats/minute) and those not (134 ± 22 beats/minute) (56). Furthermore, serum digoxin levels did not correlate with the ventricular response. Observations from placebo arms of controlled trials of quinidine and flecainide in preventing atrial fibrillation also suggest that patients receiving digoxin do not have better ventricular rate control than those not receiving the drug (57, 58).

The apparent failure of digoxin to prevent excessive tachycardia at the onset of a paroxysm may be related either to sympathetic nervous system triggering of some episodes of atrial fibrillation or to sympathetic activation triggered by the sudden change in stroke volume produced by the arrhythmia. Either mechanism would result in a rapid heart rate similar to the effect of physical exercise in sustained atrial fibrillation.

Recently the Controlled Randomized Atrial Fibrillation Trial (CRAFT) investigators reexamined the efficacy of digoxin in paroxysmal atrial fibrillation and reported conflicting data (59, 60). Thirty-five patients with documented paroxysms of atrial fibrillation were randomly assigned to receive digoxin (0.25–0.5 mg daily, adjusted to blood levels) or placebo in a blinded crossover fashion. Digoxin modestly increased the time to the first attack (59). However, despite a small decrease in symptomatic attacks, analysis of Holter monitor recordings in 31 of the 35 patients failed to show any significant reduction either in the frequency or amount of atrial fibrillation or in the mean and maximum heart rate during the arrhythmia (60). It is therefore feasible that digoxin has a modest effect in reducing symptomatic episodes of atrial fibrillation in some patients without affecting the overall prevalence of arrhythmia; however, definitive conclusions regarding its symptomatic effect and effect on heart rate await the final results of this study.

Diltiazem, verapamil, or β-blocking agents may effectively slow the heart rate during a paroxysm of arrhythmia (61). Neither class of drug has any documented antiarrhythmic effect for paroxysmal atrial fibrillation but their long-term use may decrease symptomatic recurrences. Alternatively low-dose propranolol or other β-blockers may be given at the onset of a paroxysm to decrease the surge in sympathetic tone often associated with the arrhythmia. The use of β-blockers in this fashion may lessen the duration of the patient's symptoms.

Some agents that are used for maintenance of sinus rhythm also show negative chronotropic effects when a patient reverts to atrial fibrillation. These include sotalol, amiodarone, propafenone, and flecainide. Although not useful as primary agents for heart rate control in atrial fibrillation, their negative chronotropic effect may make them favorable choices for maintenance of sinus rhythm when the likelihood of recurrence of atrial fibrillation is high.

### *Antiarrhythmic Therapy*

Electrical cardioversion of sustained atrial fibrillation is a simple and highly effective procedure. Antiarrhythmic therapy is frequently prescribed after the procedure because of a high incidence of reversion to atrial fibrillation in untreated patients. Although several drugs are effective in the maintenance of sinus rhythm, no agent is perfect. The decision to use a particular drug should depend upon the side effect profile and the characteristics of the patient being treated. We believe that antiarrhythmic therapy is not required for all patients and that an individualized approach to therapy is preferred. Furthermore, the duration of therapy is unclear, i.e., should it be lifelong or limited to a few months? Although there is no definitive answer to these questions, an examination of the current knowledge may help establish guidelines.

It is well recognized that atrial fibrillation may be precipitated by transient noncardiac factors in susceptible subjects. These include infection, thyrotoxicosis, hypoxia, and alcohol. Several acute cardiac conditions such as acute myocardial infarction, pericarditis, and exacerbation of heart failure may also provoke the arrhythmia. Frequently, correction of noncardiac precipitating factors results in spontaneous reversion and, even in those patients with sustained arrhythmia who still require cardioversion, the correction of the initiating factor may result in a greater likelihood of continued sinus rhythm.

Data regarding the incidence of reversion to atrial fibrillation after cardioversion in the absence of antiarrhythmic drugs can be gleaned from trials using a placebo arm. These results must be interpreted with caution because inclusion of patients with prior episodes of drug failure may favor the selection of a group at higher risk of reversion. In a series of 95 patients undergoing cardioversion without antiarrhythmic therapy, only 30% were still in sinus rhythm at 3 months and 23% at 1 year (62). This 12-month figure is similar to the 25% reported in the placebo arms in a retrospective meta-analysis of several trials comparing quinidine with placebo (63). Attempts to define characteristics of patients remaining in sinus rhythm are not very successful at accurately defining such a group, but success is lower in patients with a long duration of arrhythmia or significant atrial enlargement.

When antiarrhythmic drugs are used, sinus rhythm may be maintained at 1 year in 50–60% of patients. The increased success, however, must be measured against the cost and side effects of therapy. Only two agents, quinidine and flecainide, are approved by the Food and Drug Administration for maintenance of sinus rhythm; a third (propafenone) will shortly be approved. Other drugs are effective and have been used with reasonable success. The various agents and their advantages and disadvantages are outlined in Table 15.2. It is not possible to recommend a "best agent" because individual patients respond differently in terms of both efficacy and development of side effects. Furthermore, studies directly comparing individual drugs are infrequent and data derived from studies of individual agents are rarely comparable because of population differences such as underlying heart disease, atrial fibrillation duration. and the number of previous drug trials failed. Nevertheless a schema based on ventricular function, symptoms, and age is a reasonable approach.

The efficacy of an agent may also depend on route of administration and dosage; assessment of efficacy may differ depending on the end point studied. Thus, an agent may show a different efficacy for terminating recent-onset atrial fibrillation compared with terminating chronic arrhythmia, and differ again in its ability to maintain sinus rhythm after electrical car-

**Table 15.2**
**Drugs Used for Restoration and Maintenance of Sinus Rhythm in Patients with Atrial Fibrillation**

| Drug | Dose | Concomitant Rate Slowing Effect[a] | Interaction with Digoxin | Major Side Effects |
|---|---|---|---|---|
| Quinidine | 200–300 mg q.i.d. (sulfate) or 324–648 mg b.i.d. or t.i.d. (gluconate) | No | Yes | Diarrhea, fever, hepatitis, torsades de pointes (not dose related) |
| Procainamide | 500–1000 mg q 6 h | No | No | Lupus, conduction disturbance, agranulocytosis, torsades de pointes |
| Disopyramide | 150 mg q 6 h or 300 mg b.i.d. (controlled release) | No | No | Dry mouth, heart failure, hypoglycemia, torsades de pointes |
| Sotalol | 80–160 mg b.i.d. | Yes | No | Excessive bradycardia, torsades de pointes (dose-related risk) |
| Flecainide | 100–150 mg b.i.d. | Insignificant | Yes (minor) | CHF, flutter with 1:1 AV conduction, ventricular proarrhythmia |
| Propafenone | 150–300 mg t.i.d. | Mild | Yes | Taste disturbance, CHF, flutter with 1:1 AV conduction, ventricular proarrhythmia |
| Amiodarone | 600 mg daily for 1–2 wk, then 400 mg daily for 3–4 wk Maintenance of 100–200 mg daily | Yes | Yes | Pulmonary fibrosis, thyroid disturbance, hepatotoxicity, skin discoloration |

[a]"Concomitant rate slowing effect" refers to the effect on the ventricular response if a patient reverts to atrial fibrillation. Doses represent the most commonly used range; for further detail see text.
AV = atrioventricular; b.i.d. = twice a day; CHF = congestive heart failure; q = every; q.i.d. = four times a day; t.i.d. = three times a day; wk = weeks.

dioversion. The ability of a drug to control ventricular response at the time of reversion from sinus rhythm to atrial fibrillation may also be an important factor in some patients in whom rapid rate leads to an acute clinical deterioration. With these factors in mind the following outlines of drug therapy are presented. Details of the individual agents, their mechanism of action and side-effects are given in Chapter 14 and are only considered here where particularly relevant to supraventricular arrhythmias.

**Quinidine.** Of all the antiarrhythmic drugs available, quinidine has been used the longest and is possibly still the most popular in the United States. Several early studies showed the efficacy of quinidine for maintaining sinus rhythm. A metaanalysis of randomized studies indicated a 50% prevalence of sinus rhythm after 12 months of therapy compared with 25% in patients given placebo (63). However, quinidine may have the greatest side effect profile of atrial antiarrhythmic drugs. Up to 30% of patients prescribed quinidine have intolerable side effects, the most common being diarrhea that occurs early during therapy. Torsades de pointes occurs in 1–2% of patients, and sudden death (presumably because of torsades) can occur in up to 50% of those experiencing torsades. The metaanalyses of quinidine use from both randomized (63) and nonrandomized (64) trials showed an excess mortality related to the drug, suggesting that it should be used with great caution. Although most deaths were not sudden, all sudden deaths occurred in quinidine-treated patients. The risk of torsades with quinidine can be minimized by maintaining serum potassium levels at or above 4 mEq/L. Magnesium replacement should also be considered in patients receiving diuretics. Although torsades is predominantly preceded by QT prolongation on the ECG, most patients with QT prolongation do not develop the arrhythmia. The precise parameters at which QT prolongation significantly increases the risk of torsades have not been well defined. Recently it has been suggested that lead-to-lead variability of QT interval may predict the risk of torsades better than absolute or heart rate corrected QT duration (65, 66). We believe that the high incidence of noncardiac side effects produced by quinidine coupled with its potential for producing torsades de pointes, relegate it to a second-line drug for treatment of atrial fibrillation.

**Procainamide.** Procainamide is the only arrhythmic agent available in both intravenous and oral forms that is widely used for atrial arrhythmia in the United States (intravenous preparations of propafenone, flecainide, and disopyramide are available elsewhere; ibutilide is available only in intravenous form; and amiodarone is approved for ventricular fibrillation and hypotensive ventricular tachycardia). Procainamide may be useful in terminating and preventing recurrence of atrial fibrillation, particularly in hospitalized patients unable to take oral medication.

In limited clinical trials, oral procainamide has been shown to be better than no therapy for maintenance of sinus rhythm after cardioversion. This agent was also approximately as effective as quinidine in a group of patients with rheumatic heart disease (67). The chronic side effects of procainamide, particularly its lupus-like effect, make it an uninviting choice for long-term therapy.

**Disopyramide.** Disopyramide is a reasonable agent for the maintenance of sinus rhythm in patients without significant systolic dysfunction. In older men, especially those with prostatic hypertrophy, it may cause acute urinary retention and its anticholinergic side effects may be troublesome. Although disopyramide is a class IA agent, torsades de pointes has uncommonly been reported as a side effect (68). In placebo-controlled studies, disopyramide has been shown to be effective for the maintenance of sinus rhythm after electrical cardioversion (69, 70) and for terminating atrial fibrillation in patients with preexcitation (71).

**Flecainide.** Flecainide is an effective agent for preventing recurrence of paroxysmal atrial fibrillation, preventing recurrence of arrhythmia after cardioversion, and terminating recent-onset arrhythmia.

In patients with atrial fibrillation of 7 days' duration or less, a single 300-mg oral dose of flecainide successfully converted 20 of 22 (91%) patients to sinus rhythm within 8 hours compared with a success rate of 37% with intravenous amiodarone and 48% with placebo (72). (By 24 hours, 89% of the amiodarone patients had converted to sinus rhythm.) Intravenous flecainide is available in Europe and has also been shown to successfully terminate atrial fibrillation (73).

As noted, flecainide is useful in the treatment of paroxysmal atrial fibrillation. In a double-blind trial of 48 patients who had failed an average of 3.8 atrial antiarrhythmic agents, 31% of patients treated with flecainide were arrhythmia-free during the 8-week study period compared with only 9% receiving placebo (74). Although this indicates a high recurrence rate even with flecainide, the time to first attack and the time interval between attacks was considerably lengthened by this drug, which is an important consideration in patients with frequent troublesome palpitations.

A major drawback to the use of flecainide is concern about the results of the Cardiac Arrhythmias Suppression Trial (CAST) study (75). In this study, patients treated with flecainide or encainide for postmyocardial infarction premature ventricular beats had a significantly increased mortality compared with patients who received placebo. Although the precise mechanisms for the increase in mortality are unknown, flecainide treatment should be avoided for atrial arrhythmias in patients with a prior myocardial infarction and probably in those with angina but no prior infarct. Compromised ventricular function is another contraindication to use of this drug.

**Propafenone.** Propafenone is a class IC agent with efficacy similar to, or slightly less than that of, flecainide for maintaining sinus rhythm and converting atrial fibrillation (76, 77). Propafenone has a mild β-blocking action and may be better than flecainide in controlling the ventricular response when atrial fibrillation recurs. Properties of propafenone suggest that its potential for adverse effects in patients with coronary artery disease may be similar to that of flecainide. Thus, as with flecainide, this drug should be used with extreme caution in patients with prior myocardial infarction or active ischemia and in patients with diminished ventricular function.

**Amiodarone.** Amiodarone is a potent antiarrhythmic drug with proven efficacy in a broad spectrum of ventricular and supraventricular arrhythmias. It has mild β-blocking and calcium channel blocking effects as well as class III properties (78). In the United States, initial trials of amiodarone concentrated on patients with ventricular arrhythmias in whom high doses (800–1200 mg daily) were found to be associated with reasonable efficacy but significant drug toxicity. Several published studies of amiodarone for the treatment of atrial fibrillation using daily doses of 200–400 mg (79) showed an efficacy for sinus rhythm maintenance that may exceed that of other agents. In one study, the actuarial rate of maintenance of sinus rhythm among 91 patients with atrial fibrillation (44 chronic, 47 paroxysmal) treated with a mean dose of 277 ± 102 mg amiodarone daily was 87% at 1 year and 80% at 2 years (80). Likelihood of recurrence was greater in the paroxysmal group compared with those treated after cardioversion. In a comparative study with quinidine, 79% of amiodarone-treated patients remained in sinus rhythm 6 months after cardioversion compared with 26% of patients receiving quinidine (81).

The toxic effects of amiodarone include abnormalities of thyroid function, hepatic dysfunction, and peripheral neuropathy, but pulmonary fibrosis is the most feared side effect, causing many physicians to avoid amiodarone. Published data indicate that clinical pulmonary toxicity is uncommon at doses of 200 mg daily (82, 83). This was confirmed in a report of a large series of patients treated with amiodarone in which no cases of pulmonary toxicity were observed when the drug was prescribed at a daily dose of 300 mg or less (84). Although individual cases of pulmonary toxicity with low-dose amiodarone have been reported, this drug offers a useful and underutilized option for managing patients with atrial fibrillation. It is especially reasonable to use amiodarone as a first-line drug in patients in whom the onset of atrial fibrillation is associated with severe symptoms or in elderly subjects in whom a daily pill is easily remembered and for whom the cumulative effect of low-dose therapy over many years is unlikely to be of concern.

Intravenous amiodarone is approved in the United States for the treatment of malignant ventricular arrhythmias, but it is also effective in the management of atrial fibrillation. Cowan and colleagues (85) administered the drug to a group of patients with atrial fibrillation after suspected myocardial infarction in a dose of 7 mg/kg over 30 minutes followed by an infusion over 23 hours to a total of 1500 mg. After 4 hours of therapy, 13 of

18 patients randomized to this therapy had reverted to sinus rhythm, compared with 5 of 16 receiving digoxin. Amiodarone slowed the ventricular rate by about 30 beats/minute after 1 hour compared with 6 beats/minute in the digoxin group. A similar conversion and rate-slowing effect has been found by other investigators (86).

At present we would not recommend intravenous amiodarone as the initial treatment of atrial fibrillation or flutter, either in an attempt to convert the arrhythmia or to slow the heart rate, but it may be a useful agent when other drugs have failed and the arrhythmia is clinically troublesome.

Since the drug has the highest propensity for provoking torsades de pointes in patients with a history of heart failure (a group at high risk of recurrent arrhythmia), it should be avoided in this population. It may be of value in patients in whom long-term antiarrhythmic therapy is not being considered and may be most valuable for the treatment of atrial flutter.

**Sotalol.** Racemic (d- and l-) sotalol is a class III antiarrhythmic agent with β-blocking properties. In a multicenter, randomized study, 80–160 mg sotalol twice daily was found to be as effective as slow release quinidine sulfate (600 mg twice daily) for the maintenance of sinus rhythm after electrical cardioversion (57). Sotalol-treated patients relapsing into atrial fibrillation were less symptomatic than quinidine-treated patients, probably because of the slower ventricular rate.

Doses of sotalol of up to 480 mg twice daily were found to have equal efficacy with propafenone for preventing recurrence of arrhythmia in patients with either paroxysmal atrial fibrillation or after cardioversion for sustained atrial fibrillation (87). Two patients on sotalol therapy died suddenly; both had normal ejection fractions, and torsades de pointes was the documented cause of death in one. Because sotalol has a dose-related risk of causing torsades de pointes, we would not recommend prescribing such high doses for atrial fibrillation. We generally prescribe 80–120 mg twice daily and, occasionally, 160 mg twice a day. The dextro-isomer of sotalol (d-sotalol) is almost devoid of β-blocking properties and may be better tolerated in patients with reactive airway disease. Similar to certain class IC agents, it has been found to increase mortality postmyocardial infarction (see Chapter 14). Studies of its efficacy in atrial fibrillation are limited (88), but they suggest that it has an efficacy similar to that of the racemic formulation. d-Sotalol is not available in the United States.

**Ibutilide.** Recently the United States Food and Drug Administration approved intravenous ibutilide for the treatment of atrial fibrillation or flutter of recent onset (defined as up to 90 days' duration). This pure class III agent is available only in intravenous form and thus cannot be used to maintain sinus rhythm after pharmacologic or electrical cardioversion. In patients weighing 60 kg or more, 1 mg of ibutilide is administered over 10 minutes with continuous electrocardiographic monitoring of the QT interval. If the arrhythmia persists for 10 minutes after the infusion ends, a second 1-mg dose of ibutilide may be administered. For patients weighing less than 60 kg, the recommended dose is 0.01 mg/kg (0.1 mL/kg) repeated once if the arrhythmia fails to convert.

The major side effect of ibutilide is the provocation of torsades de pointes. Before the drug is used, predisposing factors for this arrhythmia should be sought and corrected. Specifically, the serum potassium level should be equal to or more than 4.0 mEq/L and the drug should be avoided in patients already receiving antiarrhythmic agents or other drugs (e.g., certain antidepressants or phenothiazines that prolong the QT interval). The risk of torsades de pointes with ibutilide was 4.4% in clinical trials. Approximately one-third of those who experienced torsades (1.7% of all patients treated) had a sustained episode. In patients with a history of congestive heart failure, the incidence of sustained torsades was 5.4%. The presence of hepatic or renal impairment seems to have little effect on the toxicity of this agent.

Because of the lack of an oral form and the propensity for proarrhythmia, the role of ibutilide in the treatment of atrial fibrillation or flutter is not well defined. In clinical trials (data on file, Upjohn Company, Kalamazoo, Michigan) the conversion rate for an arrhythmia lasting less than 30 days was 42% for atrial fibrillation and 50% for flutter. The rates fell to 16% and 31%, respectively, for arrhythmia lasting 31–90 days.

### *Treatment of Atrial Fibrillation in Wolff-Parkinson-White Syndrome*

Patients with the Wolff-Parkinson-White syndrome have an increased risk of atrial fibrillation. The exact prevalence of this arrhythmia is unknown, but in tertiary care centers from 10–35% of patients requiring therapy for preexcitation have experienced atrial fibrillation (89). This figure greatly exceeds that of an unselected population with the electrocardiographic manifestations of Wolff-Parkinson-White syndrome because most of these patients are asymptomatic and have no documented arrhythmia (90).

The ventricular response to atrial fibrillation in Wolff-Parkinson-White syndrome depends on properties of both the AV node and the accessory pathway. Electrocardiographic recordings during spontaneous atrial fibrillation often show narrow complexes representing conduction through the AV node and wide complexes of slightly varying morphology resulting from the varying degrees of fusion between beats arising from ventricular depolarization with the accessory pathway and the AV node. Although the shortest preexcited RR interval during atrial fibrillation correlates with the anterograde refractory period of the accessory pathway, this interval is shortened by heightened sympathetic tone and possibly lengthened by retrograde concealed conduction into the accessory pathway from impulses conducted via the AV node.

Clinical assessment of the patient during an acute episode of atrial fibrillation associated with the Wolff-Parkinson-White syndrome is critical for appropriate therapy. If hemodynamic impairment exists, urgent electrical cardioversion is required. In a stable patient intravenous procainamide is the drug of choice in the United States, but intravenous flecainide, propafenone, or disopyramide (none of which are available in the United States) have also shown efficacy.

Digoxin is ineffective in this situation and may provoke ventricular fibrillation by shortening the anterograde refractory period of the accessory pathway. Intravenous verapamil has also been associated with hemodynamic collapse and ventricular fibrillation (91). Although the mechanisms of deterioration after verapamil are complex, they probably include vasodilation, negative inotropy, and a decrease of retrograde concealed conduction into the bypass tract; these all tend to accelerate the ventricular rate. β-Blockers are also ineffective and, rarely, may result in ventricular rate acceleration (92). Although generally safe, lidocaine shows inconsistent effects on accessory pathway conduction, occasionally causing hemodynamic deterioration (93).

Long-term drug therapy in patients with one or more episodes of atrial fibrillation has been successful using several antifibrillatory agents, most of which also prolong the anterograde refractory period of the accessory pathway. The class IC agents, flecainide and propafenone, may be particularly effective in totally abolishing anterograde conduction. Amiodarone is a highly effective agent, but its use in the young population, even at low doses, raises concern about long-term toxicity.

Surgical interruption of the bypass tract is an effective technique that has been replaced by radiofrequency catheter ablation. After surgery the incidence of atrial fibrillation is considerably decreased, thus supplying further evidence that the accessory pathway plays a role in its genesis. Presumably a similar phenomenon will be seen after catheter ablation. The safety and high success rate of radiofrequency catheter ablation when performed by practitioners skilled in its use makes this the procedure of choice for patients with preexcited episodes of atrial fibrillation. Successful ablation is a cure obviating the necessity for either long-term drug therapy or thoracotomy. Drug or surgical therapy are available for the occasional patient who refuses catheter ablation or in whom the location of the bypass tract or tracts renders the procedure unsuccessful.

### *Atrial Fibrillation or Flutter After Cardiac Surgery*

Atrial arrhythmias commonly occur after cardiac surgery. Studies in patients undergoing coronary artery bypass grafting (CABG) have failed consistently to identify predisposing factors other than age and have shown that the incidence of arrhythmia increases from approximately 15%

in patients less than 65 years to 30% in those 65 years and older (94). Although atrial arrhythmias are usually transient and self-limiting, hemodynamic deterioration may occur, and an association with postoperative stroke has been recognized (95).

Lack of therapy with β-blockade (either preoperative or postoperative) is associated with postoperative arrhythmia. A metaanalysis of 24 studies of drug therapy to prevent post-CABG atrial fibrillation demonstrated a significant reduction in postoperative atrial fibrillation in patients treated with a variety of β-blockers (96). The antifibrillatory effects of β-blockade are unlikely to represent an antiischemic effect because postoperative atrial fibrillation is not more common in inadequately revascularized patients, and it is not usually associated with electrocardiographic evidence of ischemia. Furthermore, verapamil is ineffective in preventing post-CABG atrial fibrillation despite being an effective antiischemic agent. It is therefore likely that the antiarrhythmic action of β-blockers is mediated by their antiadrenergic properties, which block sympathetic nervous system triggering of atrial arrhythmias in the vulnerable postoperative heart. Digoxin has no obvious effect in preventing postoperative atrial fibrillation (96).

Although the most effective therapy for postoperative atrial arrhythmias is their prevention by perioperative β-blockade, many patients with ischemic heart disease are unable to tolerate this therapy because of obstructive pulmonary disease or severe ventricular dysfunction, and even those receiving β-blockade are not completely protected from postoperative atrial arrhythmia. Early in the postoperative period, atrial flutter is common and may be terminated by rapid atrial pacing using the temporary wires routinely placed by most surgeons (97). By the third or fourth postoperative day, however, atrial flutter is less common and fibrillation becomes the predominant arrhythmia. In many patients, the arrhythmia is brief and does not require treatment; when it occurs with a relatively well-controlled ventricular response and no symptoms, the need for therapy is unclear. If control of heart rate is poor, intravenous diltiazem or verapamil may be given; metoprolol or propranolol may also be considered unless contraindicated by the presence of obstructive airway disease. For termination of an arrhythmia that has persisted for 12 hours or more, intravenous procainamide or oral antiarrhythmic agents may be given. Once sinus rhythm is restored, antiarrhythmic therapy need not necessarily be continued after hospital discharge (unless the patient has a history of atrial fibrillation or mitral valve disease), although many surgeons do so until the first postoperative visit.

Several small trials of prophylactic antiarrhythmic agents initiated preoperatively have been reported, but the cost and risk:benefit ratio of widespread prophylactic antiarrhythmic use for this indication seem to offer more risk than benefit.

## PROARRHYTHMIC EFFECTS OF ATRIAL ANTIARRHYTHMIC AGENTS

A major concern in using antiarrhythmic agents in patients with supraventricular arrhythmias is the risk of aggravation or provocation of serious arrhythmias. The risk factors for proarrhythmia in patients being treated for ventricular arrhythmias are well recognized. However, the risk:benefit ratio of drug therapy in supraventricular arrhythmia differs from that of ventricular tachycardia or fibrillation. In the latter conditions, a small but fatal proarrhythmic response may be offset by a marked reduction in sudden death rate, leading to a favorable risk:benefit ratio. The same proarrhythmic response with a drug used for atrial arrhythmias may be totally unacceptable if the benefit is simply improvement in palpitations or cosmetic improvement of the ECG. However, the incidence varies with the agent and dose used, and proarrhythmia is more likely to occur in patients with underlying structural heart disease (e.g., myocardial infarction or congestive heart failure) and with the use of various antiarrhythmics. Proarrhythmia may be seen with all antiarrhythmic drugs and in any patient; the major types are described below.

### Torsades de pointes

Polymorphic ventricular tachycardia associated with prolongation of the QT interval (torsades de pointes) is perhaps the most widely recognized arrhythmia associated with use of antiarrhythmic drugs in atrial fibrillation (98). Unlike monomorphic ventricular tachycardia, torsades de pointes is not uncommon in patients with a normal or near-normal ventricle, although it probably occurs more frequently when underlying heart disease exists (99).

Almost all antiarrhythmic agents have been reported to cause torsades, but the arrhythmia is most commonly associated with class IA antiarrhythmics such as quinidine, procainamide, and disopyramide. Because quinidine is the drug most frequently used for the prevention of atrial fibrillation in the United States, the risks for torsades with this drug are best known.

In a metaanalysis of six randomized controlled trials of quinidine prophylaxis conducted between 1970 and 1984, Coplen and colleagues found an unadjusted total mortality rate of 2.9% for quinidine-treated patients (12 of 413) compared with 0.8% (3 of 387) in the control groups—a threefold increase (63). However, these figures represent all modes of death, and the precise cause of death was documented in only 7 of the 12 quinidine-treated patients, and only 3 of these deaths were sudden. Thus, it is possible that much of quinidine's apparent association with excess mortality was coincidental and related to its use in sicker patients. If all sudden deaths are assumed to be caused by ventricular arrhythmia, the overall prevalence of fatal arrhythmia in the quinidine group (including two additional nonfatal cardiac arrests) was 1.2% (1.5% if an unclassified death was arrhythmic) compared with 0% in the control group.

Quinidine-induced torsades have several predisposing factors, including bradycardia, hypokalemia, and drug-induced QT prolongation (100). It has been estimated that quinidine use carries a minimum annual risk for the development of torsades de pointes of 1.5%, with almost all cases occurring within 48 hours of initiation of drug therapy. Quinidine-induced torsades is not dose related, and it has even been suggested that low serum levels of the drug may be more likely to provoke torsades than higher levels (101). Most cases have been reported to occur after conversion of atrial fibrillation to sinus rhythm, possibly because the heart rate is slower than during atrial fibrillation. The association of torsades with bradycardia suggests that the widespread practice of observing patients during the initiation of drug therapy but discharging them shortly after electrical cardioversion may miss a significant proportion of cases of torsades occurring during the night after cardioversion.

Both procainamide and disopyramide are effective for preventing atrial fibrillation and both have been associated with the provocation of torsades (68, 102), but no study has attempted to determine the prevalence of this arrhythmia. As with quinidine-induced torsades, hypokalemia is considered to be a major precipitating factor. Although quinidine-associated torsades is not related to drug levels and may occur at subtherapeutic doses, procainamide-induced torsades may be more common in patients with elevated levels of N-acetylprocainamide, the first metabolite of procainamide (102, 103).

Several reports have documented the risk for torsades with sotalol (104, 105). Unlike the QT prolongation seen with quinidine that may occur at low serum levels, prolongation of QT interval caused by sotalol is primarily concentration-dependent, and sotalol overdose is commonly complicated by torsades (106). The incidence of sotalol-induced torsades ranges from approximately 0.5% in patients receiving doses of 160 mg daily to 5.8% in patients receiving more than 640 mg a day (107). As with the class IA agents, sotalol-induced torsades is aggravated by hypokalemia. The combination of sotalol and a diuretic in a single tablet was implicated as a serious risk factor for this arrhythmia in patients receiving therapy for hypertension (104). The β-blocking properties of sotalol do not seem to be protective and may further increase the risk for torsades in susceptible patients by producing a relative or absolute bradycardia.

Most of the antiarrhythmic agents used to treat SVT have been described as causing torsades de pointes, but this arrhythmia is uncommon with amiodarone (108) (which has also been used successfully to suppress torsades) (98). It is also rarely seen with the class IC agents, which have minimal effects on the QT interval.

### Monomorphic Ventricular Tachycardia and Fibrillation

Patients with atrial fibrillation associated with ventricular dysfunction may have concomitant ventricular arrhythmias, and provocation of sustained ventricular arrhythmia by drug treatment of atrial fibrillation is probably a function of the underlying myocardial disease. Reports of drug-induced ventricular tachycardia or fibrillation in patients treated for atrial fibrillation are rare, presumably because many controlled trials exclude patients with clinically significant ventricular dysfunction.

The class IC agents, which have been implicated in increasing the risk of sudden death when used after myocardial infarction, have a good safety profile for the treatment of atrial fibrillation. However, a small series of cases suggested that, in the setting of chronic atrial fibrillation, the use of flecainide may cause life-threatening, wide complex tachycardia during vigorous exertion even in patients without clinically insignificant ventricular dysfunction (109). A similar event has been reported in a patient with previous myocardial infarction receiving flecainide for paroxysmal atrial fibrillation (110). In these cases it is possible that the rapid and irregular ventricular rate during atrial fibrillation, combined with both the use-dependent properties of the class IC agents and the high levels of circulating catecholamine during exercise, may have resulted in a minimally diseased ventricle to produce a substrate suitable for sustained ventricular arrhythmia.

## Drug-Induced Acceleration of Ventricular Response During Atrial Arrhythmias

The ventricular response to atrial fibrillation, atrial flutter, and atrial tachycardia is determined by the refractory period of the AV node, the degree of concealed conduction within the node, and the level of autonomic tone. Alteration of one or more of these factors by antiarrhythmic agents, or the conversion of fibrillation to flutter, may result in an increased ventricular rate that may occasionally be dramatic and be associated with adverse hemodynamic consequences.

Quinidine-induced acceleration of ventricular rate is widely recognized and warrants some discussion because of the widespread practice among cardiologists of prescribing digoxin in conjunction with quinidine whenever the latter is used to prevent recurrent atrial fibrillation (this is done in the belief that recurrence will occur at a slower ventricular rate). This recommendation was first made more than half a century ago, at a time when very high dose quinidine sulfate (3200 mg daily) was frequently used to pharmacologically revert atrial fibrillation to sinus rhythm (111, 112). At these doses, atrial fibrillation was converted (at least transiently) to atrial flutter in more than 75% of therapeutic trials, and quinidine-induced slowing of the flutter rate permitted 1:1 conduction in 4–5% of patients (113). Quinidine-induced flutter appears to be less common with currently used doses of 800–1200 mg daily and is now a rare complication.

There are no convincing data to suggest that atrial fibrillation occurring in a quinidine-treated patient will be conducted with an excessive ventricular response or that digoxin will slow this response. In a comparative trial of quinidine or sotalol for maintenance of sinus rhythm after direct current cardioversion of atrial fibrillation, Jull-Möller et al. (87) noted that the heart rate in patients receiving quinidine who relapsed into atrial fibrillation increased by a mean of 29 beats/minute (from 80 to 109 beats/minute) and did not differ among patients receiving concomitant digoxin and those not receiving it. A relatively slow ventricular rate during relapse to atrial fibrillation is probably caused by concealed AV nodal anterograde conduction of the fibrillation waves. Concealed conduction is absent if flutter occurs, potentially resulting in 1:1 AV conduction if the flutter rate has been slowed by quinidine. To prevent a rapid ventricular response, it is preferable to prescribe either a β-blocking drug or a calcium channel blocking agent in conjunction with quinidine for any patient in whom atrial flutter has been documented because digoxin may have little effect.

Disopyramide and procainamide have been associated with an accelerated ventricular response during atrial flutter and therefore may cause a paradoxical heart rate increase if atrial fibrillation converts to flutter during therapy. The negative inotropic effect of disopyramide in conjunction with a rapid ventricular response may be particularly harmful.

The class IC agents flecainide and propafenone may organize and slow the rate of atrial fibrillation and convert it to atrial flutter with a slow enough atrial rate for 1:1 AV conduction to occur. When this happens, the rapid ventricular response is often associated with frequency-dependent slowing of intraventricular conduction resulting in an ECG that may be confused with ventricular tachycardia. Murdock and colleagues noted the occurrence of atrial flutter in 14 of 82 patients treated with propafenone for atrial fibrillation, 3 of whom developed 1:1 AV conduction with ventricular rates of 200–275 beats/minute and QRS widths up to 160 milliseconds (114). A similar phenomenon has been observed during therapy with flecainide.

The overall incidence of the transformation of atrial fibrillation to flutter with class IC agents appears to be in the range of 3.5–5% (115). Because significant hemodynamic compromise may occur if the onset of flutter is associated with an increased ventricular response, it has been suggested that concomitant β-blocking agents, digoxin, or calcium channel blockers also should be prescribed when class IC agents are used to treat atrial fibrillation, particularly if atrial flutter has occurred previously. The safety of verapamil combined with flecainide has been shown in a small, selected series of patients (116), but caution is warranted in patients with reduced ventricular function because of the potential for substantial additive negative inotropic effects. Further studies are needed before the value of this combination can be accurately assessed.

Digoxin, in combination with flecainide or propafenone, has a modest effect in controlling the ventricular rate during exercise in patients with atrial fibrillation (117, 118), but there is no firm evidence that its use will be adequate to prevent 1:1 AV conduction should atrial flutter occur. Similar to verapamil, β-blocking agents are potentially negatively inotropic agents when used in conjunction with class IC agents, although this combination is probably safe in patients with normal ventricular function. In selected patients, β-blockers have been shown to be effective in preventing the ventricular proarrhythmic effects of flecainide and to be well tolerated despite a reduced ejection fraction (119).

## SUMMARY

The treatment of supraventricular arrhythmias is a rapidly changing field. This chapter has concentrated on drug therapy, but catheter ablation techniques are rapidly becoming first-line therapy for specific arrhythmias, particularly those associated with preexcitation. Although we believe that pharmacologic therapy will remain the mainstay of treatment for most patients with supraventricular arrhythmias, such therapy requires an individualized approach that is tailored to the symptoms of the patient. Despite the wide variety of pharmacologic agents available for long-term treatment of supraventricular arrhythmias, the small risk of serious proarrhythmic effects must always be weighed against the benefits of arrhythmia control, particularly in patients with infrequent, minimally symptomatic arrhythmias.

---

## REFERENCES


1. Gilmour RF Jr. Enhanced automaticity. In: Podrid PJ, Kowey PR, eds. Cardiac arrhythmia, mechanisms, diagnosis and management. Baltimore: Williams & Wilkins, 1995:78–87
2. Wathen MS, Klein GJ, Yee R, et al. Classification and terminology of supraventricular tachycardia. Cardiol Clin 1993;11:109–120.
3. Wit AL, Rosen MR. Afterdepolarizations and triggered activity: distinction from automaticity as an arrhythmogenic mechanism. In: Fozzard HA, Haber E, Jennings RB, et al., eds. The heart and cardiovascular system. Scientific foundations. New York: Raven Press, 1991:2113–2163.
4 Denes P, Wu D, Dhingra RC, et al. Dual atrioventricular nodal pathways—a common electrophysiological response. Br Heart J 1979;37:1069–1076.
5. DiMarco JP, Sellers TD, Berne RM, et al. Adenosine: electrophysiologic effects and therapeutic use for terminating paroxysmal supraventricular tachycardia. Circulation 1983;68:1254–1263.
6. DiMarco JP, Miles W, Akhtar M, et al. Adenosine for paroxysmal supraventricular tachycardia: dose ranging and comparison with verapamil in placebo-controlled, multicenter trials. Ann Intern Med 1990;113:104–110.
7. Garratt C, Linker N, Griffith M, et al. Comparison of adenosine and verapamil for termination of paroxysmal junctional tachycardia. Am J Cardiol 1989;64:1310–1316.
8. Watt AH, Bernard MS, Webster J, et al. Intravenous adenosine in the treatment of supraventricular tachycardia: a dose-ranging study and interaction with dipyridamole. Br J Clin Pharmacol 1986;21:227–230.
9. Wesley RC Jr., Turnquest P. Torsades de pointes after intravenous adenosine in the presence of prolonged QT syndrome. Am Heart J 1992;123:794–796.

10. Heng MK, Singh BN, Roche AHG, et al. Effects of intravenous verapamil on cardiac arrhythmias and on the electrocardiogram. Am Heart J 1975;90:487–498.
11. Dougherty AM, Jackman WM, Naccarrelli GV, et al. Acute conversion of paroxysmal supraventricular tachycardia with intravenous diltiazem. Am J Cardiol 1992; 70:587.
12. Wu D, Yeh SJ, Wang CC, et al. Nature of dual atrioventricular node pathways and the tachycardia circuit as defined by radiofrequency ablation technique. J Am Coll Cardiol 1992;20:884–895.
13. Lee MA, Morady F, Kadish A, et al. Catheter modification of the atrioventricular junction with radiofrequency energy for control of atrioventricular nodal reentry tachycardia. Circulation 1991;83:827–835.
14. Henthorn RW, Waldo AL, Anderson JL, et al., and the Flecainide Supraventricular Tachycardia Study Group. Flecainide acetate prevents recurrence of symptomatic proxysmal supraventricular tachycardia. Circulation 1991;83:119–125.
15. Pritchett ELC, McCarthy EA, Wilkinson WE. Propafenone treatment of symptomatic paroxysmal supraventricular arrhythmias. A randomized placebo-controlled, cross-over trial in patients tolerating oral therapy. Ann Intern Med 1991;114:542.
16. Garrett C, Ward D, Camm AJ. Degeneration of junctional tachycardia pre-excited atrial fibrillation after intravenous verapamil. Lancet 1989;2:219.
17. Jackman WM, Wang X, Friday KJ, et al. Catheter ablation of accessory atrioventricular pathways (Wolff-Parkinson-White syndrome) by radiofrequency current. N Engl J Med 1991;324:1605–1611.
18. Lesh MD, Van Hare GF, Schamp DJ, et al. Curative percutaneous catheter ablation using radiofrequency energy for accessory pathways in all locations: results in 100 consecutive patients. J Am Coll Cardiol 1992;19:1303–1309.
19. Ludmer PL, McGowan NE, Antman EM, et al. Efficacy of propafenone in Wolff-Parkinson-White syndrome: electrophysiologic findings and long-term followup. J Am Coll Cardiol 1987;9:1357–1363.
20. Klein GJ, Bashore TM, Sellers TD, et al. Ventricular fibrillation in the Wolff-Parkinson-White syndrome. N Engl J Med 1979;301:1080–1085.
21. Kastor J. Multifocal atrial tachycardia. N Engl J Med 1990;322:1713–1717.
22. Lin C, Chuang I, Cheng K, et al. Arrhythmogenic effects of theophylline in human atrial tissue. Int J Cardiol 1987;17:289–297.
23. Levine J, Michael J, Guarnieri T. Treatment of multifocal atrial tachycardia with verapamil. N Engl J Med 1985;312:21–25.
24. Arsura E, Lefkin A, Scher D, et al. A randomized, double-blind, placebo-controlled study of verapamil and metoprolol in treatment of multifocal atrial tachycardia. Am J Med 1988;85:519–524.
25. Iseri L, Fairshter R, Hardemann J, et al. Magnesium and potassium therapy in multifocal atrial tachycardia. Am Heart J 1985;110:789–794.
26. Wellens HJJ. Atrial tachycardia. How important is the mechanism? Circulation 1994;90:1576–1577.
27. Packer DL, Bardy GH, Worley SJ, et al. Tachycardia-induced cardiomyopathy: a reversible form of left ventricular dysfunction. Am J Cardiol 1986;57:562–570.
28. Gillette PC, Smith RT, Garson A, et al. Chronic supraventricular tachycardia: a curable cause of congestive cardiomyopathy. JAMA 1985;253:391–392.
29. Marchlinski FE, Hook BG, Callans DJ. Which cardiac disturbances should be treated with digoxin immune Fab (ovine) antibody? Am J Emerg Med 1991;9(Suppl 1):24.
30. Engelstein ED, Lippman N, Stein KM, et al. Mechanisms and specific effects of adenosine on atrial tachycardia. Circulation 1994;89:2645–2654.
31. Chen SA, Chiang CE, Yang CJ, et al. Sustained atrial tachycardia in adult patients: electrophysiological characteristics, pharmacologic response, possible mechanisms, and effects of radiofrequency ablation. Circulation 1994;90:1262–1278.
32. Creamer J, Nathan A, Camm A. Successful treatment of atrial tachycardias with flecainide acetate. Br Heart J 1985;53:164–166.
33. Kouvaras G, Cokkinos D. Halal G, et al. The effective treatment of multifocal atrial tachycardia with amiodarone. Jpn Heart J 1989;30:301–312.

34. Cosio FG, Arrubas F, Palacios J, et al. Fragmented electrograms and continuous electrical activity in atrial flutter. Am J Cardiol 1986;57:1309–1314.
35. Olshansky B, Okumura K, Henthorn RW, et al. Characterization of double potentials in human atrial flutter: studies during transient entrainment. J Am Coll Cardiol 1990;15:833–841.
36. Klein GJ, Guiraudon GM, Sharma AD, et al. Demonstrations of macroreentry and feasibility of operative therapy in the common type of atrial flutter. Am J Cardiol 1986;57:587–591.
37. Feld GK, Fleck P, Cheng P-S, et al. Radiofrequency catheter ablation for the treatment of human type I atrial flutter. Identification of a critical zone in the reentrant circuit by endocardial mapping techniques. Circulation 1992;86:1233–1240.
38. Falk RH, Knowlton AA, Bernard SA, et al. Digoxin for converting recent-onset atrial fibrillation to sinus rhythm. A randomized double-blinded trial. Ann Intern Med 1987;106:503–506.
39. Botto GH, Broffoni T, Bernasconi G, et al. Effect of single loading oral propafenone or digoxin in recent onset atrial fibrillation: conversion to sinus rhythm and modulation of ventricular rate. A randomized, placebo controlled study. J Am Coll Cardiol 1995;25(Suppl A):66A (Abstract).
40. Margolis B, DeSilva RA, Lown B. Episodic drug treatment in the management of paroxysmal arrhythmias. Am J Cardiol 1980;45:621 (Abstract) 626.
41. Capucci A, Boriani G, Botto L. Oral loading with propafenone in recent onset atrial fibrillation: a controlled evaluation on 240 patients. J Am Coll Cardiol 1995;25(Suppl A):219A.
42. Fujiki A, Yoshida S, Tani M, et al. Efficacy of class IA antiarrhythmic drugs in converting atrial fibrillation unassociated with organic heart disease and their relationship to atrial electrophysiologic characteristics. Am J Cardiol 1994;74:282–283.
43. Conard GJ, Ober RE. Metabolism of flecainide. Am J Cardiol 1984;53:41B–51B.
44. Antonaccio MJ, Gomoll A. Pharmacologic basis of the antiarrhythmic and hemodynamic effects of sotalol. Am J Cardiol 1993;72:27A.
45. Black IW, Fatkin D, Sager KB, et al. Exclusion of atrial thrombus by transesophageal echocardiography does not preclude embolism after cardioversion of atrial fibrillation. Circulation 1994;89:2509–2513.
46. Manning WJ, Silverman DI, Keighley CS, et al. Transesophageal echo facilitated early cardioversion for patients with new onset atrial fibrillation. A 4 year experience. Circulation 1995;90(Suppl I):I-21 (Abstract).
47. Roberts SA, Diaz C, Nolan PE, et al. Effectiveness and costs of digoxin for atrial fibrillation and flutter. Am J Cardiol 1993;72:567–573.
48. Salerno DM, Dias VC, Kleiger RE, et al. Efficacy and safety of intravenous diltiazem for treatment of atrial fibrillation and atrial flutter. The diltiazem-atrial fibrillation/flutter study group. Am J Cardiol 1989;63:1046–1051.
49. Abrams J, Allen J, Allin D, et al. Efficacy and safety of esmolol versus propranolol in the treatment of supraventricular tachyarrhythmias. A multicenter double-blind clinical trial. Am Heart J 1985;110:913–922.
50. Heywood TJ, Graham JT, Marais GE, et al. Effects of intravenous diltiazem on rapid atrial fibrillation accompanied by congestive heart failure. Am J Cardiol 1991; 67:1150.
51. Atwood JE, Sullivan M, Forbes S, et al. Effects of beta-adrenergic blockade on exercise performance in patients with chronic atrial fibrillation. J Am Coll Cardiol 1987;10:314–320.
52. Lundstrom T, Ryden L. Ventricular rate control and exercise performance in chronic atrial fibrillation: effects of diltiazem and verapamil. J Am Coll Cardiol 1990; 16:86–90.
53. Lang R, Klein H, Segni E, et al. Verapamil improves exercise capacity in chronic atrial fibrillation: double-blind crossover study. Am Heart J 1983;105:820–824.
54. David D, Segni E, Klen HO, et al. Inefficiency of digitalis in the control of heart rate in patients with chronic atrial fibrillation: beneficial effect of an added beta-adrenergic blocking agent. Am J Cardiol 1979;44:1378–1382.

55. Pitcher DW, Papouchado M, James MA, et al. Twenty-four hour ambulatory electrocardiography in patients with chronic atrial fibrillation. Br. Med J 1986;292:594.
56. Rawles JM, Metcalf MJ, Jennings K. Time of occurrence, duration and ventricular rate for paroxysmal atrial fibrillation on the effect of digoxin. Br Heart J 1990; 63:225–227.
57. Jull-Möller S, Edvardsson N, Rehngvist-Alzlberg N. Sotalol versus quinidine for the maintenance of sinus rhythm after direct current conversion of atrial fibrillation. Circulation 1990;82:1932–1939.
58. Anderson JL, Gilbert EM, Alpert BL, et al. Prevention of symptomatic recurences of paroxysmal atrial fibrillation in patients initially tolerating antiarrhythmic therapy. A multicenter, double-blind, crossover study of flecainide and placebo with transtelephonic monitoring. Circulation 1989;80:1557–1570.
59. Murgatroyd FD, Curzen NP, Aldergather J, et al. Clinical features and drug therapy in patients with paroxysmal atrial fibrillation: results from the CRAFT multicenter registry. J Am Coll Cardiol 1993;21(Suppl A):380A (Abstract).
60. Murgatroyd FD, Xie B, Gibson SM, et al. The effects of digoxin in patients with paroxysmal atrial fibrillation: analysis of Holter data from the CRAFT-1 trial. J Am Coll Cardiol 1993;21(Suppl A):203A (Abstract).
61. Murgatroyd FD, O'Farrell DM, Foran JP, et al. A multicenter double-blind crossover comparison of disopyramide, atenolol and placebo for symptomatic paroxysmal atrial fibrillation. J Am Coll Cardiol 1995;25(Suppl A):231A (Abstract).
62. Lundstrom T, Ryden L. Chronic atrial fibrillation. Long term results of direct current conversion. Acta Med Scand 1988:223:53–59.
63. Coplen SE, Antman FM, Berlin JA, et al. Efficacy and safety of quinidine therapy for maintenance of sinus rhythm after cardioversion. Circulation 1990;82:1106–1116.
64. Reimold SC, Chalmers TC, Berlin JA, et al. Assessment of the efficacy and safety of antiarrhythmic therapy for chronic atrial fibrillation: observations on the role of trial design and implications of drug-related mortality. Am Heart J 1992;124:924–932.
65. Day CP, McComb JM, Campbell RWF. QT dispersion: an indication of arrhythmia risk in patients with long QT intervals. Br Heart J 1990;63:342–344.
66. Hohnloser SH, Baedeker F, Van de Loo A. Quinidine or sotalol-induced changes in QT-dispersion during pharmacological conversion therapy of atrial fibrillation. Link to proarrhythmia as assessed in a prospective, randomized trial. J Am Coll Cardiol 1995;25(Suppl A):66A (Abstract).
67. Szekely P, Sideris DA, Batson GA. Maintenance of sinus rhythm after atrial fibrillation. Br Heart J 1969;82:1011.
68. Riccioni N, Castiglioni M, Bartolomei C. Disopyramide-induced QT prolongation and ventricular tachyarrhythmia. Am Heart J 1983;105:870–871.
69. Karlson BW, Torstensson I, Abjorn C, et al. Disopyramide in the maintenance of sinus rhythm after electroversion of atrial fibrillation —a placebo controlled one year follow-up study. Eur Heart J 1988;9:284–290.
70. Woo KS, Kong SM. Disopyramide and quinidine in maintenance of sinus rhythm after electroversion—a controlled study. Hong Kong Cardiol Soc 1979;6:137.
71. Fujimura O, Klein GJ, Sharma AD, et al. Acute effect of disopyramide on atrial fibrillation in the Wolff-Parkinson-White syndrome. J Am Coll Cardiol 1989;13: 113–117.
72. Capucci A, Lenzi T, Borian G, et al. Effectiveness of loading oral flecainide for converting recent-onset atrial fibrillation to sinus rhythm in patients without organic heart disease or with only systemic hypertension. Am J Cardiol 1992;70:69–72.
73. Suttorp MJ, Kingma JH, Lie AHL, et al. Intravenous flecainide versus verapamil for acute cardioversion of paroxysmal atrial fibrillation or flutter to snus rhythm. Am J Cardiol 1989;63:693–696.
74. Anderson JA, Gilbert EM, Alpert BL, et al. Prevention of symptomatic recurrences of paroxysmal atrial fibrillation in patients initially tolerating antiarrhythmic therapy: a multicenter, double-blind, crossover study of flecainide and placebo with transtelephonic monitoring. Circulation 1989;80:1557–1570.

75. CAST Investigators. Preliminary report: effect of encainide and flecainide on mortality in a randomized trial of arrhythmia suppression after myocardial infarction. N Engl J Med 1989;321:406–412.
76. Antman EM, Beamer AD, Cautillon C, et al. Long-term oral propafenone therapy for suppression of refractory symptomatic atrial fibrillation and atrial flutter. J Am Coll Cardiol 1988;12:1005–1011.
77. Pritchett ELC, McCarthy EA, Wilkinson WE. Propafenone treatment of symptomatic paroxysmal supraventricular arrhythmias. A randomized, placebo-controlled, crossover trial in patients tolerating oral therapy. Ann Intern Med 1991;114:539–544.
78. Singh BN, Venkatesh N, Nadamanee K, et al. The historical development, cellular electrophysiology and pharmacology of amiodarone. Prog Cardiovasc Dis 1989;31:249–280.
79. Middlekauf HR, Wiener I, Saxon LA, et al. Low-dose amiodarone for atrial fibrillation? Time for a prospective study? Ann Intern Med 1992;116:1017–1020.
80. Chuun S, Sager P, Stevenson W, et al. Amiodarone is highly effective in maintaining normal sinus rhythm in refractory atrial fibrillation/flutter. J Am Coll Cardiol 1993;21:203A (Abstract).
81. Vitolo F, Tronci M, Larovere MT, et al. Amiodarone versus quinidine in the prophylaxis of atrial fibrillation. Cardiology 1981;36:431–444.
82. Doval HC, Nui DR, Grancelli HO, et al. Randomized trial of low-dose amiodarone in severe congestive heart failure (GESICA).
83. Pfisterer ME, Kiowski W, Brunner H, et al. Long-term benefit of 1 year amiodarone treatment for persistent complex ventricular arrhythmia after myocardial infarction. Circulation 1993;87:309–311.
84. Dunsman RE, Stanton MS, Miles WM, et al. Clinical features of amiodarone-induced pulmonary toxicity. Circulation 1990;82:51–59.
85. Cowan JC, Gardiner P, Reid DS, et al. A comparison of amiodarone and digoxin in the treatment of atrial fibrillation complicating suspected acute myocardial infarction. J Cardiovasc Pharmacol 1986;8:252–256.
86. Hou ZY, Chang MS, Chen CY, et al. Acute treatment of recent-onset atrial fibrillation and flutter with a tailored dosing regimen of intravenous amiodarone. A randomized, dixogin-controlled study. Eur Heart J 1995;16:521–528.
87. Reimold SC, Cantillon CO, Friedman PL, et al. Propafenone versus sotalol for suppression of recurrent symptomatic atrial fibrillation. Am J Cardiol 1993;71:558–563.
88. Sahar DI, Raffel JA, Bigger JT Jr, et al. Efficacy, safety and tolerance of d-sotalol in patients with refractory supraventicular tachyarrhythmias. Am Heart J 1989;117:562–568.
89. Wellens HJ, Smeets JL, Rodriquez LM, et al. Atrial fibrillation in Wolff-Parkinson-White syndrome. In: Falk RH, Podrid PH, eds. Atrial fibrillation, mechanisms and management. New York: Raven Press, 1992:333–344.
90. Klein GJ, Prystowsky EN, Yee R, et al. Asymptomatic Wolff-Parkinson-White—should we intervene? Circulation 1989;80:1902–1905.
91. Gulambussein S, Ko P, Klein GJ. Ventricular fibrillation following verapamil in the Wolff-Parkinson-White syndrome. Am Heart J 1983;106:145–147.
92. Morady F, DiCarlo LA Jr, Baerman JM, et al. Effect of propranolol on ventricular rate during atrial fibrillation in the Wolff-Parkinson-White syndrome. PACE Pacing Clin Electrophysiol 1987;10:492–496.
93. Akhtar M, Gilbert CJ, Shenasa M. Effect of lidocaine on atrioventricular response via the accessory pathway in patients with Wolff-Parkinson-White syndrome. Circulation 1981;63:435–441.
94. Fuller JA, Adams GC, Buxton B. Atrial fibrillation after coronary artery bypass grafting: is it a disorder of the elderly? J Thorac Cardiovasc Surg 1989;97:821–825.
95. Roffman JA, Feldman A. Digoxin and propranolol in the prophylaxis of supraventricular tachydysrhythmias after coronary artery bypass surgery. Ann Thorac Surg 1981;31:496–501.
96. Andrews TC, Reimold SC, Berlin JA, et al. Prevention of supraventricular arrhythmias after coronary artery bypass surgery. Circulation 1991;84(Suppl III):236–244.

97. Waldo AL, MacLean WAH, Karp RB, et al. Entrainment and interruption of atrial flutter with atrial pacing: studies in man following open heart surgery. Circulation 1977;56:737–745.
98. Nguyen PT, Scheinman MM, Seger J. Polymorphous ventricular tachycardia: clinical characterization, therapy and the QT interval. Circulation 1986;74:340–349.
99. Kupersmith J. Long QT syndrome. In: Singer I, Kupersmith J, eds. Clinical man ual of electrophysiology. Baltimore: Williams & Wilkins, 1993:143–168.
100. Roden DM, Woosley RL, Primm RK. Incidence and clinical features of the quinidine-associated long QT syndrome: implications for patient care. Am Heart J 1986;111:1088–1093.
101. Roden DM, Hoffman BF. Action potential prolongation and induction of abnormal automaticity by low quinidine concentrations in canine Purkinje fibers. Relation to potassium and cycle length. Circ Res 1985;56:857–867.
102. Herre JM, Thompson JA. Polymorphic ventricular tachycardia and ventricular fibrillation due to N-acetyl procainamide. Am Heart J 1985;55:227–228.
103. Stratmann HG, Walter KE, Kennedy HL. Torsades de pointes associated with elevated N-acetyl procainamide levels. Am Heart J 1985;109:375–376.
104. McKibbin JK, Pocock W, Barlow JM, et al. Sotalol, hypokalemia, syncope and torsade de pointes. Br Heart J 1984;51:157–162.
105. Neuvonen PJ, Elonen E, Vuorenmaa T, et al. Prolonged Q-T interval and severe tachyarrhythmias, common features of sotalol intoxication. Eur J Clin Pharmacol 1981;20:85–89.
106. Wang T, Bergstrand RH, Thompson KA, et al. Concentration dependent pharmacologic properties of sotalol. Am J Cardiol 1986;57:1160–1165.
107. Betapace (Sotalol). Physician's Desk Reference 1995. Montvale NJ: Medical Economics, 610-614.
108. Brown MA, Smith WM, Lubbe WF, et al. Amiodarone-induced torsades de pointes. Eur Heart J 1986;7:234–239.
109. Falk RH. Flecainide-induced ventricular tachycardia and fibrillation in patients treated for atrial fibrillation. Ann Intern Med 1989;111:107–111.
110. Wang YS, Scheinman MM, Chien WW, et al. Patients with supraventricular tachycardia presenting with aborted sudden death: incidence, mechanism and long-term follow-up. J Am Coll Cardiol 1991;18:1711–1719.
111. London F, Howell M. Atrial flutter: 1 to 1 conduction during treatment with quinidine and digitalis. Am Heart J 1954;48:152–156.
112. Tandowsky RM, Oyster JM, Silverglade A. The combined use of lanatoside C and quinidine sulphate in the abolition of auricular flutter. Am Heart J 1946;32: 617–633.
113. Cheng TO. Atrial flutter during quinidine therapy of atrial fibrillation. Am Heart J 1956;52:273–289.
114. Murdock CJ, Kyles AE, Yeung-Lai-Wa JA, et al. Atrial flutter in patients treated for atrial fibrillation with propafenone. Am J Cardiol 1990;66:755–777.
115. Marcus FI. The hazards of using type IC antiarrhythmic drugs for the treatment of paroxysmal atrial fibrillation. Am J Cardiol 1990;66:366–367.
116. Van Gelder IC, Crijn HJ, Van Gilst WH, et al. Efficacy and safety of flecainide acetate in the maintenance of sinus rhythm after electrical cardioversion of chronic atrial fibrillation or atrial flutter. Am J Cardiol 1989;64:1317–1321.
117. Timm CT, Knowlton AA, Battinelli NJ, et al. Flecainide for heart rate control in atrial fibrillation. J Am Coll Cardiol 1989;13:164 (Abstract).
118. Capucci A, Boriani G, Botto G, et al. Effects of propafenone plus digoxin on ventricular rate during atrial fibrillation. A randomized study. J Am Coll Cardiol 1995;25(Suppl A):220A (Abstract).
119. Myerburg RJ, Kessler KM, Cox MM, et al. Reversal of proarrhythmic effects of flecainide acetate and encainide hydrochloride by propranolol. Circulation 1989;80: 1571–1579.

CHAPTER 16

# Management of Ventricular Arrhythmias

Frank I. Marcus, MD

Ventricular arrhythmias encompass a wide spectrum of rhythm disorders ranging from occasional premature ventricular beats to ventricular fibrillation. Intermediate forms consist of complex ventricular arrhythmias defined as multiformed pairs or couplets, nonsustained ventricular tachycardia consisting of brief runs of greater than three consecutive premature ventricular beats at a rate of 100 beats/minute or more, and sustained monomorphic ventricular tachycardia that is variably defined as lasting for 15–30 seconds.

There are marked individual variations in the patient's perception of ventricular arrhythmias. Some individuals are aware of each ventricular premature beat (VPB), often described as a transient sinking feeling followed by a thump that represents the post-VPB beat. The VPB may invoke a cough or simply be described as an uncomfortable feeling in the chest. The more sustained the arrhythmia, the faster the rate of the ventricular tachycardia, and the poorer the left ventricular function the more symptomatic are the patients.

Sustained ventricular tachycardia at a rate of 100–110 beats/minute may not immediately cause symptoms even if the patient has poor left ventricular function. However, if the arrhythmia is sustained over hours or days it may provoke congestive heart failure. In contrast, patients with normal left ventricular function who have ventricular tachycardia twice this rate may complain only of lightheadedness or weakness. Contrary to general belief, even ventricular fibrillation can be transient and self-terminating. This phenomenon is commonly seen, for example, during induction of ventricular fibrillation at the time of implantation and testing of an implanted cardioverter defibrillator.

## DIFFERENTIAL DIAGNOSIS OF VENTRICULAR ARRHYTHMIAS

It is beyond the scope of this chapter to provide a detailed discussion of the differential diagnosis of a wide QRS complex tachycardia. There are several characteristics, however, that are useful in differentiating supraventricular beats conducted slowly or aberrantly from VPBs.

This distinction is relatively easy for single wide QRS complexes during sinus rhythm. When premature atrial beats are conducted aberrantly, evidence of premature atrial activity or a P wave preceding this wide QRS complex can usually be found. The P wave may distort the previous T wave. When the PP interval is measured before and after the wide complex beat, it is different from that before the premature beat because the premature atrial beat transiently suppresses the sinus activity. In contrast, VPBs seldom disturb the sinus rhythm; thus the PP interval occurs "on time" after the wide premature QRS complex. It is much more difficult to distinguish between beats conducted with aberrancy and VPBs , and in fact, such a distinction is generally unreliable when the underlying rhythm is atrial fibrillation (1).

The distinction between supraventricular tachycardia (SVT) that is conducted aberrantly with a wide QRS complex versus ventricular tachycardia follows similar principles as discussed for the differential diagnosis of premature beats. SVT with aberrancy that has the pattern of a regular wide QRS complex tachycardia usually starts with a premature atrial beat. It is helpful to have a multichannel electrocardiographic (ECG) recording to identify atrial activity. In patients with ventricular tachycardia one specifically looks for atrioventricular (AV) dissociation with atrial activity considerably slower than the ventricular rate. The best leads to recognize atrial activity are leads II, V1, and V2.

Although there are specific morphologic criteria to differentiate SVT with aberrancy from ventricular tachycardia (2–4), the clinical history can be most useful. For example, the first appearance of a sustained arrhythmia after a recent or remote myocardial infarction makes it likely that the arrhythmia is ventricular tachycardia. If the tachycardia has a wide QRS complex, it should be considered to be ventricular tachycardia unless there is a history of prior sustained supraventricular arrhythmias. This principle is useful because aberrantly conducted SVT is very difficult to distinguish from ventricular tachycardia and to assume the latter may be safer.

Adenosine is a relatively safe pharmacologic agent for the differential diagnosis of a wide QRS complex tachycardia (5, 6). Except for unusual forms of ventricular tachycardia, adenosine does not terminate ventricular tachycardia, whereas it is almost always effective in stopping SVT provided that it involves the sinus node or one of the pathways that uses the AV node. Intraatrial reentrant arrhythmias such as atrial flutter, atrial fibrillation, or atrial tachycardia are usually not terminated by adenosine. However, by its effect on the AV node, it can block impulse transmission between the atrium and the ventricle and thereby slow the ventricular response and unmask atrial activity such as atrial flutter. Adenosine is usually administered rapidly as a bolus followed by a saline flush because the concentration of drug in the heart must be high to achieve the desired effect. The use of smaller than recommended doses of adenosine such as 1 or

3 mg is suggested when adenosine is used in patients taking β-blocking or calcium channel blocking drugs. Under these circumstances adenosine may cause long pauses that may last for many seconds because of marked depression of sinus node or AV nodal function by this combination of the drugs. Adenosine is safer than verapamil to elucidate the mechanism of wide QRS complex tachycardia because the effect of adenosine is fleeting, lasting less than 1 minute, whereas the negative inotropic and hypotensive effects of verapamil are prolonged and can cause hemodynamic deterioration, particularly if the arrhythmia is caused by ventricular tachycardia. In turn, this can lead to hypotension and ventricular fibrillation. (See also Chapter 14 for general discussion of adenosine and Chapter 15 for discussion of its use in atrial arrhythmias.)

## MANAGEMENT OF VENTRICULAR ARRHYTHMIAS

### General Considerations

Ventricular arrhythmias are treated because they are symptomatic or to prevent sustained ventricular tachycardia or ventricular fibrillation. The management of asymptomatic ventricular arrhythmias changed once it was recognized that antiarrhythmic drugs, particularly those in the Vaughan-Williams Class I, have a risk of inducing fatal arrhythmias (see Chapter 14). In addition, none of the antiarrhythmic drugs except the β-blocking drugs which are listed under a Class II category, have been shown to decrease arrhythmic death. The lower mortality associated with β-blocker use has been shown in patients after myocardial infarction. Even then it is not clear whether the mechanism of the reduction in sudden arrhythmic death associated with β-blockers is caused by its antiarrhythmic effect per se. The decrease in mortality in the β-Blocker in Heart Attack Trial (BHAT) occurred equally in those patients who had frequent VPBs before drug administration and in those who did not (7).

In normal healthy subjects 10–30 years of age, the incidence of ventricular tachycardia is defined as three or more consecutive VPBs and ranges from 1–3% as detected by 24-hour ambulatory ECG recordings (8). The prevalence of VPBs, couplets, and ventricular tachycardia increases with age. Ventricular couplets were observed during 24-hour ambulatory ECG recording in 11%, and ventricular tachycardia of 3–13 beats in 4% of a group of healthy elderly people aged 60–85 years (9). In an elderly population that included patients with cardiac disease, ventricular tachycardia was found in 10.3% of men (10). The prevalence of frequent VPBs (15 or more VPBs/hour) in combination with transient ventricular tachycardia was higher in those with an abnormal left ventricular ejection fraction.

Because ventricular arrhythmias are common, particularly in the elderly and in patients with cardiac disease, are they simply a marker for the presence of heart disease? Are they associated with an increased mortality, and if so, under what circumstances? Does treatment with antiarrhythmic drugs or with nonpharmacologic therapy such as implantation of a defibrillator decrease mortality in patients with serious ventricular arrhythmias? The data to answer these questions are as yet incomplete.

The benefit of treatment of ventricular arrhythmias is clear when it results in the immediate termination of sustained ventricular tachycardia. Under these circumstances the period of drug administration is circumscribed and side effects can be observed and are usually manageable. Treatment to prevent recurrence of sustained ventricular arrhythmias is more difficult because the frequency of recurrences may be unpredictable. In addition, the methods available to determine antiarrhythmic drug efficacy (e.g., suppression of ambient ectopy as assessed by ambulatory monitoring in a controlled hospital environment or prevention of an induced sustained ventricular arrhythmia by provocative electrical stimulation of a sedated patient in the electrophysiologic laboratory) are imperfect at best. These methods of evaluating antiarrhythmic drugs cannot reproduce on the arrhythmogenic substrate the effects of daily stress and extraordinary events that are common during life. Thus, assessment of antiarrhythmic drug efficacy using either of the above methods is associated with a rate of arrhythmia recurrence over 4 years as high as a 60% even when the in-hospital assessment is predictive of drug efficacy (11)!

These considerations that relate to treatment of arrhythmias should not be interpreted as a negative approach to the management of ventricular arrhythmias. Rather, they should be viewed as a realistic assessment of the limitations of current knowledge. Nevertheless the clinician who is confronted with a patient who has asymptomatic or symptomatic ventricular arrhythmias must act on this incomplete database. Because the risk:benefit ratio for treatment of ventricular arrhythmias may be partly determined by the presence and severity of the cardiac condition, the treatment of ventricular arrhythmias is categorized using these criteria.

## Ventricular Arrhythmias in the Absence of Heart Disease

It was previously noted that VPBs are common in healthy individuals without heart disease and that nonsustained ventricular tachycardia is an infrequent finding that increases with age. VPBs may be discovered on a routine ECG or may be symptomatic. Patient evaluation usually includes 24-hour ambulatory ECG monitoring, exercise testing, and evaluation of both left and right ventricular size and function, usually by echocardiography. Transient ventricular arrhythmias in patients who have no organic heart disease are appropriately termed "benign" because their presence does not have any adverse long-term prognostic significance.

In the patient who has sustained monomorphic ventricular tachycardia and a normal echocardiographic examination, the ECG pattern of the ventricular tachycardia should be observed carefully. There are certain ECG patterns that are now recognized as being caused by specific entities that are treatable either by β-blocking or calcium channel blocking drugs, or by radiofrequency ablation. For example, if the QRS complex during tachycardia has a left bundle branch block morphology with an inferior frontal plane axis, this arrhythmia may arise from the right ventricular outflow tract (12, 13). Exercise testing and isoproterenol infusion with incremental atrial or ventricular pacing are the most common laboratory methods for initiating this tachycardia. It can be terminated with adenosine, verapamil, β-blockers, or vagal maneuvers. Oral drug therapies include β-blockers, calcium channel blockers, and class IC drugs such as flecainide or propafenone. Radiofrequency ablation of the ventricular tachycardia has been curative in many patients.

Another form of monomorphic ventricular tachycardia that is sensitive to verapamil has also been described. The ECG morphology is usually that of right bundle branch block with left axis deviation (14). This tachycardia can usually be initiated with extra stimuli. During programmed stimulation, verapamil terminates the tachycardia and prevents reinitiation; however, adenosine, lidocaine, and procainamide have no effect. These observations suggest that the mechanism for the tachycardia may be calcium channel–mediated reentry. The tachycardia originates in the left ventricle, typically in the region of the left posterior fascicle. Long-term therapy with verapamil may prevent the sustained tachycardia. Radiofrequency ablation of the arrhythmogenic site is usually effective.

In patients with no history of heart disease who have ventricular arrhythmias of left bundle branch block morphology, it is important for the echocardiographer to focus on the right ventricle to verify that it is not enlarged and that there are no contraction abnormalities. These VPBs may be the clue to the diagnosis of an unusual condition called *arrhythmogenic right ventricular dysplasia* (ARVD). Figure 16.1 shows an example of an ECG in a patient with this disorder. In ARVD the left ventricle is usually normal. The disease process consists of fatty replacement and infiltration between right ventricular muscle fibers, and this forms the substrate for reentrant tachycardias (15). In patients with ARVD, sotalol and amiodarone have been found to be the most effective antiarrhythmic drugs in suppressing nonsustained or sustained ventricular arrhythmias arising from the right ventricle.

## Ventricular Arrhythmias After Acute Myocardial Infarction

About 10 days after a myocardial infarction, 15–25% of patients have 10 or more VPBs per hour (16). In this subgroup, mortality rates are two to four times higher than those in patients with lower VPB frequency. In addition, pairs or runs of VPBs are associated with death independent of VPB frequency. Transient ventricular tachycardia defined as 3 or more consecutive VPBs at a rate of more than 100 beats/minute recorded on a predischarge

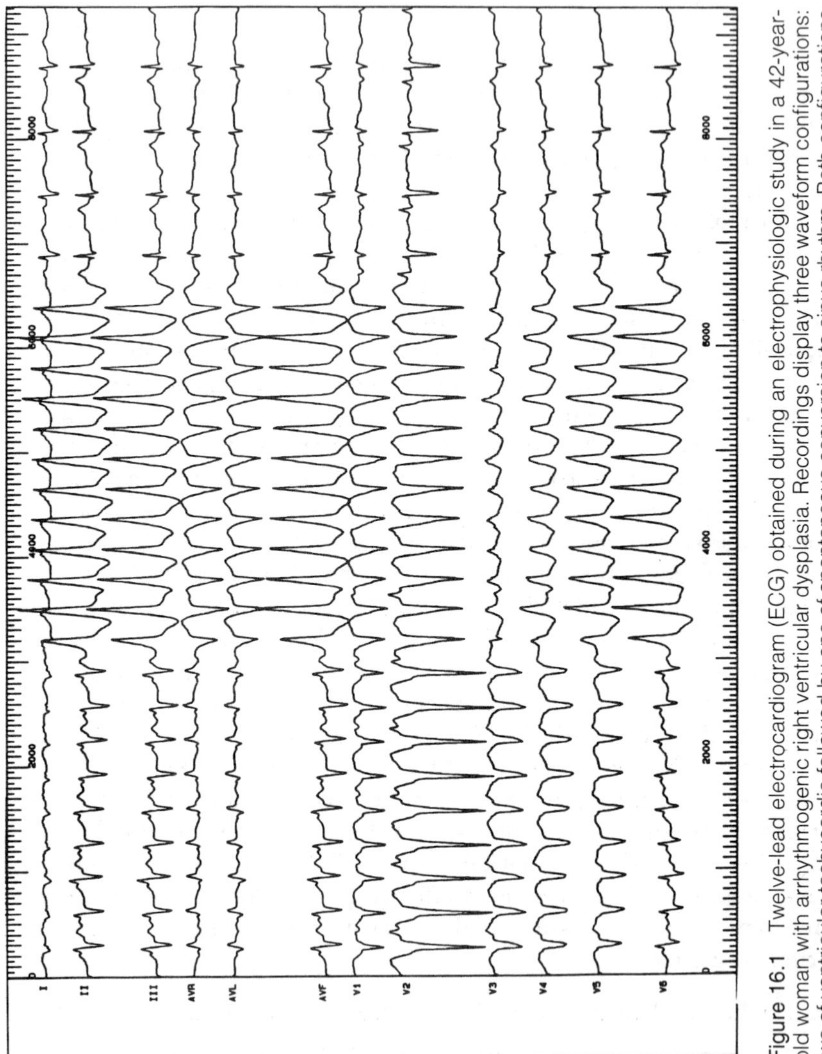


Figure 16.1 Twelve-lead electrocardiogram (ECG) obtained during an electrophysiologic study in a 42-year-old woman with arrhythmogenic right ventricular dysplasia. Recordings display three waveform configurations: two of ventricular tachycardia followed by one of spontaneous conversion to sinus rhythm. Both configurations of the tachycardia have left bundle branch morphology. The initial morphology (on the left) is a superior axis suggesting that it originates from the inferior right ventricle. The second tachycardia morphology displays an inferior axis (center), suggesting origin in the right ventricular outflow tract. These tracings illustrate that there may be several areas of arrythmogenic foci. On the right, the waveform during sinus rhythm displays the typical T-wave inversion in the right pericordial leads, $V_1$-$V_4$ of this syndrome.

24-hour ECG monitor has a strong relation to subsequent mortality (odds ratio, 4:2) but occurs in only about 12% of patients. These ventricular arrhythmias are a risk indicator for subsequent mortality independent of associated left ventricular dysfunction (16).

Because ventricular arrhythmias after myocardial infarction have been found to be an independent risk factor, it was reasonable to assume that VPBs, singly or in runs, could trigger ventricular tachycardia or ventricular fibrillation and that suppression of ventricular ectopy would decrease the mortality in the first few years after a myocardial infarction. Treatment with β-blocking drugs blunts the rise in VPB frequency noted after myocardial infarction (17). Long-term therapy with β-blocking drugs after a myocardial infarction is associated with a reduction in the rate of sudden death (presumably arrhythmic). For example, timolol reduced the incidence of sudden death by 71% (38 deaths among 939 patients given placebo versus 11 deaths among 945 patients given timolol; $P < 0.001$) (18). However, this decrease in the sudden death rate is not tightly linked to the suppression of ventricular ectopic beats. Because β-blocking drugs have only moderate antiectopic activity the post–mycardial infarction trials with β-blocking drugs did not resolve the question of whether supressing VPBs and repetitive forms would decrease mortality in those patients who had these arrhythmias and who survived a myocardial infarction.

In 1987 the Cardiac Arrhythmia Pilot Study (CAPS) was undertaken to address this question (19). CAPS was designed to determine whether frequent or repetitive ventricular arrhythmias after myocardial infarction could be suppressed with a drug strategy that incorporated dose ranging and changing drugs. The class IC drugs encainide and flecainide as well as moricizine, a drug with some characteristics of a class IC drug, were selected because of their recognized effectiveness in suppressing ventricular ectopy. Their use was also known to be associated with low incidence of adverse effects. This preliminary study confirmed that these drugs were effective in suppressing ambient ectopy with a low incidence of adverse noncardiac effects (19). Therefore, the second phase of this study was launched and was called the Cardiac Arrhythmia Suppression Trial (CAST). This randomized, placebo-controlled, double-blind, multicenter clinical trial was designed to determine if suppression of ventricular arrhythmias after myocardial infarction with antiarrhythmic drugs would reduce arrhythmic death (20). The patients consisted of survivors of myocardial infarction aged less than 80 years who had 6 or more VPBs an hour on a 24-hour ECG obtained between 6 days and 2 years after myocardial infarction. The primary end point was arrhythmic death or cardiac arrest. The study was stopped in 1989 because of compelling evidence that encainide and flecainide increased the death rate compared to placebo (21) (Table 16.1).

The study design was changed to include patients with an increased risk of arrhythmic death by limiting enrollment to those with a left ventricular

**Table 16.1**
**Results of Treatment in the Cardiac Arrhythmia Suppression Trial**

| | Placebo | Eucainide/Flecainide | Odds Ratio |
|---|---|---|---|
| Patients | 725 | 730 | |
| Follow-up | 10 (months) | 10 (months) | |
| Sudden cardiac death | 9 (1.2%) | 33 (4.5%) | 3.2 (1.7–5.9) |
| Other cardiac death | 6 (0.8%) | 14 (1.9%) | 2.2 (0.9–5.4) |
| Noncardiac/unclassified | 7 (0.9%) | 9 (1.2%) | |
| Total number of deaths or cardiac arrests | 22 (3.0%) | 56 (7.6%) | 2.5 (1.6–3.9) |

ejection fraction of 40% or less who had their infarction 6–90 days before enrollment. The inclusion criteria were broadened to include asymptomatic ventricular runs exceeding 15 beats at a rate of 120 beats/minute or more lasting up to 30 seconds. The trial was continued with patients randomized between placebo and moricizine. The trial was subsequently discontinued because there was no apparent difference in mortality between those receiving placebo and moricizine-treated patients (22). The results of the CAST study indicate that suppression of ventricular arrhythmias after myocardial infarction with class IC antiarrhythmic drugs does not improve survival and actually is associated with an increased risk of arrhythmic death.

The results of the CAST study should not be generalized to all antiarrhythmic drugs, although metaanalysis of other class I antiarrhythmic drugs after myocardial infarction is consistent with the results of CAST (23). The CAST results also cannot be generalized to other situations such as patients who do not have ischemic heart disease, patients who have sustained ventricular tachycardia, or patients resuscitated from cardiac arrest.

Observations from the CAPS study provided insight regarding patient characteristics that were predictive of VPB suppression. In patients treated with encainide or flecainide, arrhythmia was more frequently suppressed in those who had not had a myocardial infarction prior to the index infarction and in patients with a higher ejection fraction or in those of younger age (24). Also, patients with greater cardiac damage were less likely to respond to antiarrhythmic drugs.

In the CAST study patients were not entered in the randomized drug trial phase to double-blind therapy primarily because of a lack of suppression of VPBs or adverse effects during titration. These patients were older and had a lower left ventricular ejection fraction; they also used digitalis, diuretics, and antihypertensive drugs to a greater extent (25).

It is possible that antiarrhythmic drugs with different electrophysiologic actions such as amiodarone, a class III agent, may have favorable effects on mortality in cardiac arrest in patients after myocardial infarction with frequent or complex ventricular ectopy (26). Preliminary results from the Canadian Amiodarone Myocardial Infarction Trial (CAMIAT) are encouraging (27). In this pilot study there was a trend toward a lower mortality associated with suppression of ventricular ectopy in the amiodarone-treated patients. The Basel Antiarrhythmic Study of Infarct Survival (BASIS) trial randomized patients to placebo or amiodarone treatment 1–3 days before hospital discharge after myocardial infarction (28). They had frequent multiform or repetitive ventricular arrhythmias (Lown class 3 or 4b) in 2 or more of 24 hours of ECG recording. In this small study (n = 198) survival was significantly better in amiodarone-treated patients than in those taking placebo. In addition, arrhythmic events (sudden death and sustained ventricular tachycardia and fibrillation) were significantly reduced by amiodarone. Complex (Lown class above 3) arrhythmias were significantly reduced in the amiodarone- treated group compared with controls. The European Myocardial Infarction Amiodarone Trial (EMIAT) is currently evaluating the role of amiodarone after myocardial infarction in patients with a left ventricular ejection fraction of less than 40%. However, this study is not testing the VPB suppression hypothesis; although 24-hour ECG recordings are being obtained, the results do not constitute part of the inclusion criteria. Furthermore, follow-up ECG recordings are not being done routinely. The above data suggest that the VPB suppression hypothesis may still have some validity when amiodarone is used. However, results obtained with amiodarone may not be generalized to other class III antiarrhythmic drugs because amiodarone is a unique compound with many different electrophysiologic and metabolic effects. Prophylactic therapy with the class III agent oral d-sotalol in a post–myocardial infarction population with left ventricular dysfunction resulted in a significantly increased mortality (29).

Based on current data, there is no therapeutic indication for obtaining a routine ambulatory ECG recording in patients who do not have symptomatic ventricular arrhythmias after myocardial infarction. In fact, it is best to avoid doing so because the clinician may be tempted to prescribe antiarrhythmic drugs if frequent ventricular ectopy or nonsustained ventricular tachycardia is discovered. β-Adrenergic blocking drugs should be used after myocardial infarction regardless of whether ventricular arrhythmias are present. For patients with symptomatic nonsustained ventricular tachycardia after myocardial infarction, amiodarone appears to be safe and effective, although the results of the large scale trials discussed earlier could possibly change these recommendations. Class IC and probably IA drugs should not be used for the treatment of asymptomatic ventricular ectopy within the first year after myocardial infarction.

The widespread use of thrombolytic therapy appears to result in fewer post–myocardial infarction patients with nonsustained ventricular tachycardia, but there is probably no decrease in the prevalence of frequent

VPBs (more than 10 VPBs per hour) (30). Furthermore, frequent VPBs remain a significant predictor of total as well as sudden death mortality even after the use of thrombolytic agents (30). Nevertheless there also appears to be a marked decrease in the prevalence of symptomatic sustained ventricular tachycardia after myocardial infarction in the fibrinolytic era (31).

## Ventricular Arrhythmias in Patients with Heart Failure

Frequent VPBs are common in patients with congestive heart failure, and between 28 and 80% of patients with cardiac failure have transient ventricular tachycardia (32). Although the prognostic significance of VPBs alone in these patients is still unclear, patients with heart failure who have transient ventricular tachycardia have an increased risk of cardiac mortality and sudden cardiac death. For example, in the Veterans Administration Cooperative Trial VHeFT II, which compared the outcome of 804 patients with left ventricular ejection fraction less than 45% randomized to enalapril or hydralazine and (n-)isosorbide dinitrate treatment, couplets were noted in 56–60% of patients and ventricular tachycardia of 3 or more consecutive beats in 7–29%. Ventricular tachycardia recorded at 3 months, 1 year, and 2 years predicted a significantly higher mortality during the subsequent year (33). Patients with more than 10 VPBs per hour had a higher mortality in the first 18 months than those with either no VPBs or fewer than 10 VPBs per hour. VPB frequency is correlated with severe left ventricular dysfunction such as a left ventricular ejection fraction less than 20% and increasing age. In the captopril-digoxin multicenter study, frequency of VPB and frequency of ventricular tachycardia were univariate predictors of total mortality (34). Couplets and ventricular tachycardia frequency were also significant univariate predictors of sudden cardiac death.

Because ventricular tachycardia and couplets, and possibly VPB frequency, predict increased mortality in heart failure, it could be hypothesized that a decrease in ventricular ectopy would be associated with a decrease in mortality rate, particularly of sudden cardiac death. This correlation has been observed in patients treated with angiotensin-converting enzyme (ACE) inhibitors but not in patients treated with antiarrhythmic drugs (33). In the VHeFT II trial there was a 49% reduction in sudden cardiac death at 2 years in the enalapril-treated group compared with the patients who received hydralazine-isosorbide dinitrate. This decrease was associated with a reduction in the prevalence of ventricular tachycardia and a decrease in the emergence of new episodes of ventricular tachycardia (Fig. 16.2). This effect was not associated with a preferential improvement in left ventricular function because left ventricular ejection fraction improved more in patients in the hydralazine isosorbide dinitrate arm than in the enalapril arm.

Suppression of VPBs with class I antiarrhythmic drugs does not appear to decrease the risk of sudden cardiac death in patients with heart failure.

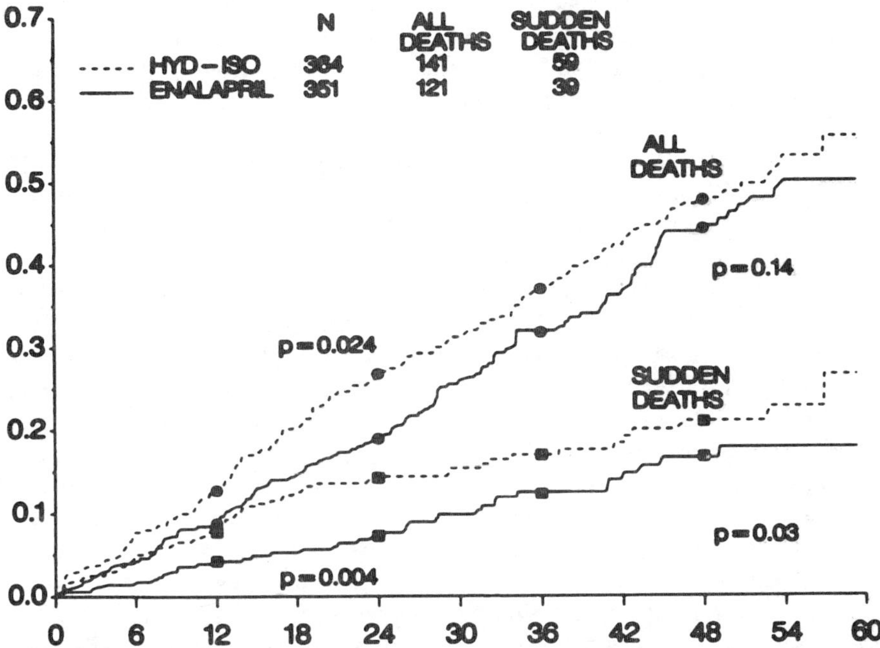


Figure16.2 Cumulative mortality in VHeFT II study patients with baseline ambulatory electrocardiograms (ECGs) (n=715). Cumulative mortality at 2 years for this subset of patients was similar to that in the overall trial. Over a 5-year period, sudden death was significantly different between the hydralazine-isosorbide (HYD-ISO) and enalapril (*P*=0.03) groups, accounting also for the overall difference between these two therapies. In addition, the reduction in sudden death paralleled the reduction in ventricular tachycardia prevalence in the enalapril group. At 2 years (a predetermined end point) both overall mortality (*P*=0.024) and sudden death (*P*=0.004) were significantly decreased in the enalapril-treated patients. Reproduced with permission of the American Heart Association, Inc., from Fletcher RD, Guillermo BC, Johnson G, et al. Enalapril decreases prevalence of ventricular tachycardia in patients with chronic congestive heart failure. Circulation 1993; 87(Suppl VI):VI-49–VI-55.

Several trials, however, have reported a trend toward decreasing mortality in patients with heart failure treated with amiodarone, although two recently reported large trials have had dissimilar results. In a multicenter trial conducted in Argentina (Grupo de Estudio de la Sobrevida en la Insuficiencia Cardiaca en Argentina; GESICA), 516 patients with advanced heart failure who had a mean left ventricular ejection fraction of 20% were randomized to amiodarone, 300 mg/day, or standard treatment (35). A 24-hour ambulatory ECG was performed before amiodarone treatment began. This showed that 71% of the patients had VPBs exceeding 10 beats/hour and 33% had transient ventricular tachycardia. Treatment with amiodarone was associated with a 27% reduction in 2-year total mortality. There was a similar trend toward decreased sudden death and death caused by progressive heart failure in the amiodarone-treated patients.

This decrease in mortality was independent of the presence of transient ventricular tachycardia. In contrast, the Veterans Administration Cooperative Study compared patients treated with amiodarone, 400 mg/day, to those given placebo in a randomized double-blind trial in 674 patients with congestive heart failure (New York Heart Association class III or IV), left ventricular dilatation, left ventricular ejection fraction 40% or less, and 10 or more VPBs per hour (36). Amiodarone significantly suppressed frequency of arrhythmia , but there was no significant difference in all cause mortality between the treatment groups.

Based on results of these two studies, one can conclude that amiodarone does not increase mortality in patients with congestive heart failure. It is possible that, in selected groups yet to be defined, this drug may decrease mortality. The VPB suppression hypothesis has not been substantiated in patients with congestive heart failure even with the marked decrease in ventricular ectopy associated with amiodarone treatment. Therefore if a patient presents with congestive heart failure and has frequent VPBs and even runs of asymptomatic nonsustained ventricular tachycardia, the clinician should avoid suppressing these VPBs with antiarrhythmic drugs. Treatment of ventricular arrhythmias cannot be disregarded if a patient with heart failure has transient symptomatic ventricular tachycardia, e.g., 8–20 consecutive beats at a rate of 150–200 beats/minute. In this situation treatment with amiodarone appears to be rational, although there are no definitive data to indicate that sudden cardiac death will be prevented in these patients.

## Ventricular Arrhythmias in Patients with Hypertrophic Cardiomyopathy

Cardiac death, presumably arrhythmic, occurs in patients with hypertrophic cardiomyopathy at an annual rate of 2–4% in referral centers (37). Sudden death is most common in affected children and young adults aged between 10 and 35 years. Hypertrophic cardiomyopathy is the most common cause of unexpected death in competitive athletes. The mechanism of sudden death in this condition encompasses the spectrum of paroxysmal atrial fibrillation initiating fibrillation, ventricular arrhythmias, and ischemia. In children and adolescents who have been resuscitated from cardiac arrest, the presence of transient ventricular tachycardia on ambulatory monitoring is uncommon. Thus, ambulatory ECG monitoring does not appear to be a useful prognostic test to evaluate patients at high risk for sudden cardiac death in this age group. In the adult with hypertrophic cardiomyopathy, transient ventricular tachycardia, often at a slow rate, can be found in about 25% of patients. Transient ventricular tachycardia on ambulatory ECG monitoring is the single best marker of high risk. Although its positive predictive value is only approximately 22%, the absence of this finding has a 97% negative predictive value (38, 39). Because transient ventricular tachycardia carries a sevenfold increase in the incidence of sudden death and the positive predictive value of this finding is low, other means are needed to identify patients with transient ventricular tachycardia who are at risk of sudden cardiac death. Thus, findings on the ambulatory ECG alone are not adequate to stratify patients with hypertrophic cardiomyopathy into a high risk subgroup to determine further treatment strategies for preventing sudden cardiac death. Preliminary data indicate that patients with hypertrophic cardiomyopathy who are at risk of sudden death have increased fractionation of paced right ventricular electrograms (indicating increased dispersion in homogeneity of intraventricular conduction) determined at electrophysiologic study (40). This may create the conditions necessary for sustained arrhythmogenesis.

Treatment of asymptomatic patients with transient ventricular tachycardia with amiodarone is controversial. In patients with hypertrophic cardiomyopathy who have transient ventricular tachycardia or frequent VPBs it is rational to treat with β-blocking drugs. This class of drugs may have several beneficial effects, including a decrease in left ventricular outflow tract gradient, decrease in ischemic potential, and a modest decrease in ventricular ectopy. With the exception of disopyramide, class I antiarrhythmic drugs are generally avoided. Type III antiarrhythmic drugs such as amiodarone or sotalol can also be used to treat ventricular arrhythmias in this population.

## Ventricular Arrhythmias in Patients with Valvular Heart Disease

Mitral valve prolapse is a common condition, particularly in women. Patients with mitral valve prolapse have not been shown to have an excess of complex ventricular arrhythmias compared with a control population (41). Significant mitral regurgitation is associated with frequent VPBs and transient ventricular tachycardia. Mortality in patients with mitral valve prolapse is determined by the degree of left ventricular dysfunction rather than the presence of ventricular tachycardia per se. Patients with mitral valve prolapse who have symptomatic ventricular arrhythmias are usually treated with β-blocking drugs to decrease both the frequency of ventricular ectopy and the symptoms related to VPBs. A minority of patients with mitral valve prolapse suffer arrhythmic death (41), and it is not clear how to identify these patients. Risk factors that have been proposed to identify patients susceptible to arrhythmic death include redundancy of the mitral valve leaflets on echocardiogram, severity of mitral regurgitation, inferolateral ST segment changes, and prolonged QT interval. A history of unexplained syncope or familial history of sudden cardiac death is an indication for treatment with β-blocking drugs.

Complex ventricular ectopy is common in patients with mitral regurgitation, aortic stenosis, or aortic regurgitation. In these conditions, the presence and severity of the arrhythmias relate to the degree of left ventricular dysfunction. Some clinicians recommend valve repair or replacement if there has been an increase in ventricular ectopy, especially if an impairment of left ventricular function exists. There are insufficient data to indicate clearly that transient ventricular tachycardia is an independent adverse prognostic factor related to sudden cardiac death in patients with valvular heart disease (42).

## Management of Patients who Have Sustained Ventricular Tachycardia or Have Been Resuscitated from Cardiac Arrest

Management of patients who have sustained ventricular tachycardia or have been resuscitated from cardiac arrest is a controversial area. Marked changes in the management of such patients have evolved over the past 7 years. There has also been a trend toward implantation of implantable cardioverter defibrillators, particularly because these devices now can be implanted without thoracotomy. Until recently, these serious arrhythmias were managed with antiarrhythmic drugs evaluated by either their effect on suppression of ventricular ectopy or their effect in preventing inducibility of a sustained ventricular arrhythmia during electrophysiologic studies.

In 1982 Graboys and colleagues published their results describing a large number of patients with sustained ventricular tachycardia or survivors of cardiac arrest. They used ambulatory ECG to evaluate antiarrhythmic drug efficacy (43). Their data indicated that protection against sudden cardiac death could be achieved by suppression of ventricular arrhythmias using ambulatory ECG monitoring. Their approach consisted of a short control monitoring period, followed by ECG monitoring for 3–5 hours after administration of a single, large oral dose of an antiarrhythmic drug. If the drug suppressed runs of ventricular tachycardia and was tolerated, a 24-hour ECG recording was obtained while the patient received maintenance doses of the drug. Exercise testing was also performed to verify suppression of ventricular ectopy during exertion. Their criteria for efficacy was total elimination of transient ventricular tachycardia and R on T beats and reduction of more than 90% of pairs and more than 50% of VPBs. Two antiarrhythmic drugs were usually used to provide a "so-called fail safe program of drug protection" (43). During an average follow-up of 29.6 months, 6 of 98 patients in whom an antiarrhythmic drug was predicted to be effective died (annual mortality, 2.3%). In contrast, of the 25 patients in whom the drug did not abolish ventricular ectopy to the required extent, there were 17 sudden deaths. The initial presentation of the arrhythmia as ventricular tachycardia or ventricular fibrillation was not a determinant of mortality. Subsequently, the authors reported that there was a decreased chance of suppressing ventricular tachycardia with antiarrhythmic drugs if a markedly diminished left ventricular ejection fraction existed or if a high density of ventricular tachycardia was present on the baseline ambulatory ECG monitoring. In a later publication, they stated that control of ventricular arrhythmias did not significantly improve survival when the left ventricular ejection fraction was less than 30% (44).

The initial encouraging results for the use of ambulatory ECG monitoring to guide antiarrhythmic drug efficacy was a major impetus to compare this method with that of electrophysiologic testing to determine the most accurate predictor of drug efficacy. This was the aim of a multicenter trial supported by the National Institutes of Health, Electrophysiological Study versus Electrocardiographic Monitoring (ESVEM), for selection of antiarrhythmic treatment of ventricular arrhythmias. Between 1985 and 1991, 2103 patients with sustained ventricular tachycardia, aborted sudden cardiac death or unmonitored syncope with inducible ventricular tachycardia were screened for enrollment (Fig. 16.3) To qualify for inclusion in the study, patients had to have ventricular tachycardia or ventricular fibrillation induced twice at electrophysiologic study, and have an average of more than 10 VPBs per hour over 48 hours of ambulatory ECG monitoring. A total of 486 patients were randomized, 242 to the electrophysiologic study limb and 244 to the ambulatory monitoring limb. Patients received up to six drugs in random order until one was predicted to be effective by suppression of inducible arrhythmias in the electrophysiologic study group or by suppression of VPBs in the ambulatory ECG group. The patients were then followed for a 6-year period for recurrence of arrhythmia or death (45).

No significant difference was found in predicting recurrence of arrhythmia or mortality by either method. However, ambulatory ECG monitoring identified an antiarrhythmic drug predicted to be effective more often than did electrophysiologic study in these patients. The probability of recurrence of arrhythmia after a prediction of drug efficacy by either method was significantly lower for patients treated with sotalol than for patients treated with other antiarrhythmic drugs (45). The results of this study, however, apply only to patients who met the enrollment criteria. This is a very specific group and does not include most patients with sustained ventricular tachycardia or cardiac arrest. It is not known if the ESVEM results apply to patients who have this density of VPBs who are not inducible or to patients who are inducible and who do not have the required degree of VPBs.

ESVEM has evoked considerable controversy relating to the criteria for assessment by electrophysiologic study and ambulatory ECG monitoring. Both criteria were criticized for not being sufficiently rigorous, particularly because there was a high recurrence rate of ventricular arrhythmias in both groups. This recurrence rate of 37±3% in 1 year was lower (21±4%) in patients treated with sotalol. The 1-year arrhythmic death rate was relatively low for both groups together (10±2%) and still lower for patients treated with sotalol (6±3%). These differences persisted at the end of 4

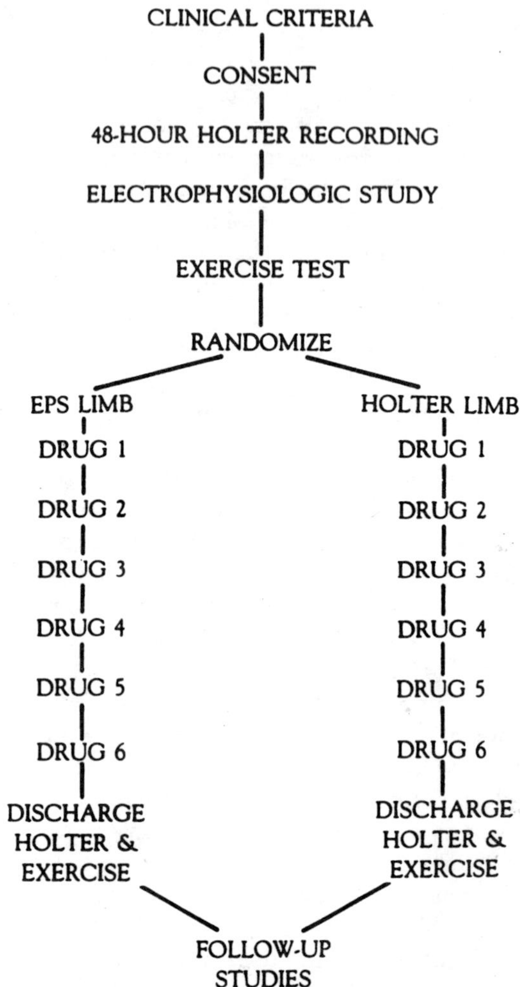


Figure 16.3 Schematic depiction of the design of the Electrophysiologic Study Versus Electrocardiographic Monitoring (ESVEM) trial. Patients fulfilling entry criteria had to give consent, then meet specific eligibility criteria by Holter monitoring and subsequently by electrophysiologic study. They were then randomly allocated to undergo assessment of up to six antiarrhythmic drugs by either electrophysiologic study (EPS limb) or electrocardiographic monitoring and exercise testing (Holter limb). An exercise test was performed before drug assessment and before follow-up in patients receiving a drug that was predicted to be effective in suppressing arrhythmia. An additional Holter monitor study was obtained at the time of discharge in both limbs but was not used to assess efficacy. Reproduced with permission of the American Heart Association, Inc., from The ESVEM Trial: electrophysiologic study versus electrocardiographic monitoring for selection of antiarrhythmic therapy of ventricular tachyarrhythmias. Circulation 1989; 79:1354–1360.

years. Retrospective analyses of the ESVEM data base have shown that the major outcome criteria of the study would not be altered by selection of a more rigorous criteria for efficacy prediction by electrophysiologic study (three versus two extra stimuli) or by demanding a higher degree of suppression of ventricular ectopy. Patients who were treated with an antiarrhythmic drug that prevented inducible ventricular tachycardia or fibrillation were found to have a similar recurrence rate of ventricular arrhythmias regardless of whether their ambient ventricular ectopy was suppressed on 24-hour ambulatory ECG monitoring (46).

Because there was no placebo group in the ESVEM study and the arrhythmia recurrence rate was high, it is not known whether the results would be similar if patients were treated empirically with an antiarrhythmic drug that was well tolerated and did not cause proarrhythmia. Also, because sotalol has β-blocking effects, it is not known if a β-blocking drug that does not have class III antiarrhythmic properties would be as effective. Of the 296 patients treated with an antiarrhythmic drug that was predicted to be effective, it was found that there was a lower recurrence rate in patients who had not failed an antiarrhythmic drug before enrollment (11). In addition, it was observed that a decreased left ventricular ejection fraction as a continuous variable was an independent predictor of arrhythmia recurrence when all 486 randomized patients were studied (47). Thus, it is not clear if arrhythmia recurrence and arrhythmic death are more importantly related to variables other than suppression of VPBs by ambulatory ECG or by prevention of induction of arrhythmia by electrophysiologic study.

The results of the ESVEM trial in conjunction with data from numerous other studies indicate that there is a low accuracy in predicting arrhythmia recurrence using currently available methods in the high-risk population that has sustained ventricular tachycardia or has been resuscitated from sudden cardiac death. In addition, the worse the left ventricular function, the less chance there is of finding a drug that is predicted to be effective, and there is an increased incidence of adverse cardiovascular effects in patients with poor left ventricular function. The data of Lampert and colleagues suggest that control of a ventricular arrhythmia does not significantly improve outcome in patients with left ventricular ejection fraction less than 30% (44). Therefore, therapy with automatic defibrillators may be a superior strategy in this patient group with poor left ventricular function. This hypothesis, however, needs to be verified and is being tested in several large-scale trials. Thus, the best approach to management of patients with serious or life-threatening ventricular arrhythmias is not known (48).

Factors that may contribute to the arrhythmia must be identified and corrected before antiarrhythmic drug therapy is begun. These include hypokalemia (even if mild, e.g., a potassium level of less than 4.0 mEq/L) or hypomagnesemia. Ischemia as a trigger for cardiac arrest should be investigated using clinical history, coronary angiography (when indicated), and exercise treadmill testing to elucidate ischemic symptoms. If a myocardial scar is absent, it is possible that correction of ischemia by angioplasty or coronary artery bypass graft surgery may prevent recurrence of the arrhythmia. Ischemia is less likely as the only explanation for serious arrhythmia when a previous infarction or an identifiable myocardial scar that serves as a substrate for the arrhythmia exists. Many advocate repeat electrophysiologic testing after recovery from coronary artery revascularization if the clinical arrhythmia is induced before revascularization. The optimal treatment in addition to coronary artery bypass graft surgery for patients who have sudden cardiac arrest and inducible polymorphic ventricular tachycardia with critical coronary artery stenosis remains undetermined (49, 50). Specifically, the selection of patients in this category who may benefit from an automatic defibrillator is still controversial.

It is not known whether empiric amiodarone therapy or placement of an implantable cardioverter defibrillator (ICD) is more effective in preventing arrhythmic death or decreasing total mortality. Randomized trials are now underway to address questions regarding ICD therapy. Many patients with ICDs require antiarrhythmic therapy (usually amiodarone) to suppress frequent device discharges. In patients who have serious ventricular arrhythmias but good left ventricular function, total mortality and sudden death mortality appear to be low. The Conventional Antiarrhythmic versus Amiodarone in Survivors of Cardiac Arrest Drug Evaluation (CASCADE) results indicate that empiric treatment with amiodarone appears to be associated with a lower risk of cardiac mortality in patients resuscitated from cardiac arrest compared with other conventional antiarrhythmic drugs guided by electrophysiologic testing and ambulatory ECG recordings (51). On the other hand, many electrophysiologists consider the ICD first-line therapy, especially because the endocardial (transvenous) device has come into use.

## RADIOFREQUENCY ABLATION OF VENTRICULAR TACHYCARDIA

Catheter ablation for treatment of ventricular tachycardia in patients with coronary artery disease has had limited success (52) and is not widely used. This may be because the size of the lesion made with radiofrequency energy using an electrode with a 4-mm tip is limited to the area under the electrode and because the depth of the lesion is usually 3–5 mm in normal tissue. In the scarred tissue of patients with coronary disease, the average size of the lesion is unknown but is probably more shallow. In addition, mapping has not been sufficiently precise in locating the critical zone of this macro reentrant circuit. Other methods are now being explored to make deeper lesions using other forms of energy such as microwave or ultrasound. Another approach that is being tested is cooling of the electrode tip using saline irrigation to allow more power to be delivered and therefore deeper lesions to be made. It is anticipated that with improved technology, particularly to perform more precise mapping and to create larger lesions, many patients with ventricular tachycardia resulting from coronary artery disease will be able to undergo a curative ablative procedure in the near future.

Several unusual forms of ventricular tachycardia can be cured by ablation (53). These include patients who have a focal tachycardia originating from the right ventricular outflow tract and verapamil-sensitive tachycardia (described previously in the section on ventricular arrhythmias in the absence of heart disease). In addition, patients with bundle branch reentrant tachycardia can be treated by ablation of the right bundle.

*Acknowledgments*

The author gratefully acknowledges the expert secretarial assistance of Ms. E. Makler and thanks Dr. Philip Serlin for review of the manuscript.

## REFERENCES

1. Chaudry II. Ramsaran EK, Spodick DH. Observations on the reliability of the Ashman phenomenon. Am Heart J 1994;128:205–209.
2. Akhtar M, Shenasa M, Jazayeri M, et al. Wide complex tachycardia. Reappraisal of a common clinical problem. Ann Intern Med 1988;109:905–912.
3. Wellens HJJ, Bar FW, Vanagt EJ. The differentiation between ventricular tachycardia and supraventricular tachycardia with aberrant conduction: the value of the 12-lead electrocardiogram . In: Wellens HJJ, Kulbertus HE, eds. What's new in electrocardiography. Boston: Martinus Nijhoff, 1981:184–192.
4. Antunes E, Brugada J, Steurer G, et al. The differential diagnosis of a regular tachycardia with a wide QRS complex on the 12-lead ECG: ventricular tachycardia, supraventricular tachycardia with aberrant intraventricular conduction, and supraventricular tachycardia with anterograde conduction over an accessory pathway. PACE 1994;17:1515–1524.
5. Sharma AD, Klein GJ, Yee R. Intravenous adenosine triphosphate during wide QRS tachycardia:safety, therapeutic efficacy, and diagnostic utility. Am J Med 1990;88: 337–343.
6. Griffith MJ, Ward DE, Linker NJ, et al. Adenosine in the diagnosis of broad complex tachycardia. Lancet 1988;1:672–675.
7. Friedman LM, Byington RP, Capone RJ, et al. Effect of propranolol in patients with myocardial infarction and ventricular arrhythmia. J Am Coll Cardiol 1986;7:1–8.
8. Bjerregaard P. Continuous ambulatory electrocardiography in healthy adult subjects over a 24 hour period. Danish Med Bull 1984;31:282–297.
9. Fleg JL, Kennedy HL. Long-term prognostic significance of ambulatory electrocardiographic findings in apparently healthy subjects >60 years of age. Am J Cardiol 1992;70:748–751.
10. Manolio TP, Furberg CD, Rautaharju PM. Cardiac arrhythmias on 24 hour ambulatory electrocardiography in older women and men. The cardiovascular health study. J Am Coll Cardiol 1984;23:916–925.
11. Mason JW for the Electrophysiologic Study versus Electrocardiographic Monitoring Investigators. A comparison of electrophysiological testing with Holter monitoring to predict antiarrhythmic-drug efficacy for ventricular tachycardias. N Engl J Med 1993;329:445–451.

12. Ritchie AH, Kerr CR, Qi A, et al. Nonsustained ventricular tachycardia arising from the right ventricular outflow tract. Am J Cardiol 1989;64:594–598
13. Mont L, Seixas T, Brugada P, et al. The electrocardiographic, clinical and electrophysiological spectrum of idiopathic monomorphic ventricular tachycardia. Am Heart J 1992;124:746–753.
14. Gaita F, Giustetto C, LeClercq J-F, et al. Idiopathic verapamil-responsive left ventricular tachycardia: clinical characteristics and long-term follow-up of 33 patients. Eur Heart J 1994;15:1252–1260.
15. Marcus FI, Fontaine G. Arrhythmogenic right ventricular dysplasia/cardiomyopathy. A review. PACE 1995;18:1298–1314.
16. Moss AJ, Bigger JT, Odoroff CL. Postinfarction risk stratification. Prog Cardiovasc Dis 1987;29:389–412.
17. Lichstein E, Morganroth J, Harris R, for the BHAT Study Group. Effect of propranolol on ventricular arrhythmia. The beta-blocker heart attack trial experience. Circulation 1983;67(suppl 1):I5–I10.
18. The Norwegian Multicenter Study Group. Timolol-induced reduction in mortality and reinfarction in patients surviving acute myocardial infarction. N Engl J Med 1981;304:801–807.
19. The CAPS Investigators. Effects of encainide, flecainide, imipramine and moricizine on ventricular arrhythmias during the year after acute myocardial infarction: CAPS. Am J Cardiol 1988;61:501–509.
20. Bigger JT. Clinical aspects of trial design: What can we expect from the cardiac arrhythmia suppression trial? Cardiovasc Drugs Ther 1990;4:657–664.
21. The Cardiac Arrhythmia Trial (CAST) Investigators. Increased mortality due to encainide or flecainide in a randomized trial of arrhythmia suppression after myocardial infarction. N Engl J Med 1989;321:406–412.
22. The Cardiac Arrhythmia Suppression Trial II Investigators. Effect of the antiarrhythmic agent moricizine on survival after myocardial infarction. N Engl J Med 1992;327:227–233.
23. Teo KK, Yusuf S, Furberg CD. Effects of prophylactic antiarrhythmic drug therapy in acute myocardial infarction. JAMA 1993;270:1589–1595.
24. Anderson JL, Hallstrom AP, Griffith LS, et al. Relation of baseline characteristics to suppression of ventricular arrhythmias during placebo and active antiarrhythmic therapy in patients after myocardial infarction. Circulation 1989;79:610–619.
25. Wyse DG, Hallstrom A, McBride R, et al. Events in the Cardiac Arrhythmia Suppression Trial (CAST). Mortality in patients surviving open label titration but not randomized to double-blind therapy. J Am Coll Cardiol 1991;18:20–28.
26. Nademanee K, Singh BN, Stevenson WG, et al. Amiodarone and post-MI patients. Circulation 1993;88:764–774.
27. Cairns JA, Connolly SJ, Gent M, et al. Post-myocardial infarction mortality in patients with ventricular premature depolarizations: Canadian Amiodarone Myocardial Infarction Arrhythmia Trial pilot study. Circulation 1991;84:550–557.
28. Burkart F, Pfisterer M, Kiowski W, et al. with the technical assistance of Jordi H. Effect of antiarrhythmic therapy on mortality in survivors of myocardial infarction with asymptomatic complex ventricular arrhythmias: Basel Antiarrhythmic Study of Infarct Survival (BASIS). J Am Coll Cardiol 1990;16:1711–1718.
29. Waldo AL, Camm AJ, de Ruyter H, et al., SWORD Investigators. Preliminary mortality results from the survival with oral D-sotalol (SWORD) trial. J Am Coll Cardiol 1995;25:15A (Abstract).
30. Maggioni AP, Zuanetti G, Franzosi MG, et al. Prevalence and prognostic significance of ventricular arrhythmias after acute myocardial infarction in the fibrinolytic era. GISSI-2 results. Circulation 1993;87:312–322.
31. Andresen D, Steinbeck G, Dissmann R, et al. Decreasing risk of symptomatic sustained ventricular tachycardia in myocardial infarction patients. J Am Coll Cardiol 1995;25:314A (Abstract).
32. Deedwania PC. Ventricular arrhythmias in heart failure: to treat or not to treat? Cardiol Clin 1994;12:137–154.

33. Fletcher RD, Cintron GB, Johnson G, et al. Enalapril decreases prevalence of ventricular tachycardia in patients with chronic congestive heart failure. Circulation 1993;87(Suppl VI):49–55.
34. Gradman A, Deedwania P, Cody R, for the Captopril-Digoxin Study Group. Predictors of total mortality and sudden death in mild-to-moderate heart failure. J Am Coll Cardiol 1989;14:564–570.
35. Doval HC, Nul DR, Grancelli HO, et al., for Grupo de Estudio de la Sobrevida en la Insuficiencia Cardiaca en Argentina (GESICA). Randomised trial of low-dose amiodarone in severe congestive heart failure. Lancet 1994;344:493–498.
36. Singh SN, Fletcher RD, Fisher SG, et al. Results of the congestive heart failure survival trial of antiarrhythmic therapy. Circulation 1994;90:I-546 (Abstract).
37. Stewart JT, McKenna WJ. Hypertrophic cardiomyopathy: treatment of arrhythmias. Cardiovasc Drug Ther 1994;8:95–99.
38. Spirito P, Rapezzi C, Autore C, et al. Prognosis of asymptomatic patients with hypertrophic cardiomyopathy and nonsustained ventricular tachycardia. Circulation 1994; 90:2743–2747.
39. McKenna WJ, Sadoul N, Slade AKB, et al. The prognostic significance of nonsustained ventricular tachycardia in hypertrophic cardiomyopathy. Circulation 1994; 90:315–317 (Editorial).
40. Saumarez RC, Camm AJ, Panagos A, et al. Ventricular fibrillation in hypertrophic cardiomyopathy is associated with increased fractionation of paced right ventricular electrograms. Circulation 1992;86:467–474.
41. Hauer RNW, Wilde AAM. Mitral valve prolapse. In: Zipes DP, Jalife J, eds. Cardiac electrophysiology from cell to bedside. 2nd ed. Philadelphia: W.B. Saunders, 1995: 833–837.
42. Kinder C, Tamburro P, Kopp D, et al. The clinical significance of nonsustained ventricular tachycardia: current perspectives. PACE 1994;17:637–664.
43. Graboys TB, Lown B, Podrid P, et al. Long term survival of patients with malignant ventricular arrhythmias treated with antiarrhythmic drugs. Am J Cardiol 1982; 50:437–443.
44. Lampert S, Lown B, Graboys TB, et al. Determinants of survival in patients with malignant ventricular arrhythmias associated with coronary artery disease. Am J Cardiol 1988;61:791–797.
45. Mason JW, for the Electrophysiologic Study versus Electrocardiographic Monitoring Investigators. A comparison of seven antiarrhythmic drugs in patients with ventricular tachycardias. N Engl J Med 1993;329:452–458.
46. Reiter MJ, Mann DE, Reiffel JE, et al. and the ESVEM Investigators. Significance and incidence of concordance of drug efficacy predictions by Holter monitoring and electrophysiological study in the ESVEM study. Circulation 1995;91:1988-1995.
47. Caruso AC, Hahn EA, Marcus FI for the ESVEM Investigators. Predictors of arrhythmic death and cardiac arrest in the ESVEM study. Circulation 1993;88:606 (Abstract).
48. Zipes DP. Are implantable cardioverter-defibrillators better than conventional antiarrhythmic drugs for survivors of cardiac arrest? Circulation 1995;91:2115–2117 (Editorial).
49. Natale A, Jasbir SRA, Kathi A, et al. Ventricular fibrillation and polymorphic ventricular tachycardia with critical coronary artery stenosis: does bypass surgery suffice? J Cardiovasc Electrophysiol 1994;5:988–994.
50. Epstein AE. When is bypass surgery enough? The answer is still uncertain. J Cardiovasc Electrophysiol 1994;5:995–998.
51. The CASCADE Investigators. Randomized antiarrhythmic drug therapy in survivors of cardiac arrest (the CASCADE study). Am J Cardiol 1993;72:280–287.
52. Kim YH, Sosa-Suarez G, Trouton TG, et al. Treatment of ventricular tachycardia by transcatheter radiofrequency ablation in patients with ischemic heart disease. Circulation 1994;89:1094–1102.
53. Manolis AS, Wang PJ, Estes NAM. Radiofrequency catheter ablation for cardiac tachyarrhythmias. Ann Intern Med 1994;121:452–461.

CHAPTER 17

# Drugs in Cardiopulmonary Resuscitation

Karl B. Kern, MD, and Gordon A. Ewy, MD

Cardiopulmonary resuscitation (CPR) is intended to restore circulation after unexpected respiratory or circulatory arrest. It must be emphasized, however, that external chest compression and assisted ventilation, even when applied immediately and optimally, is merely temporizing therapy that provides a modicum of circulatory support, retarding the process of cellular death until definitive therapy (usually defibrillation) can be applied (1).

Nevertheless, the importance of prompt initiation of basic life support efforts through early use of CPR is now well recognized (2–6). In communities where large numbers of lay persons have been trained in basic CPR and where emergency medical services are rapidly available, survival rates from out-of-hospital sudden death induced by ventricular fibrillation are as high as 30–40% when prompt bystander CPR is followed in less than 8 minutes by definitive therapy (3–6). The initiation of CPR by a bystander, even when defibrillation is delayed, can result in improved survival compared with circumstances in which no such attempt is made (Table 17.1). Unfortunately, because of fear of transmitted disease and lack of training and other resources, CPR is initiated by bystanders in only 15–20% of out-of-hospital cardiac arrests. In an effort to increase bystander CPR, there is increased interest and research in "no ventilation," or chest compression, only CPR (7).

Over the past two decades several approaches and techniques have been attempted to improve survival after cardiac arrest. Numerous new techniques and variations of old techniques have been devised with this goal in mind (8–22). Of most interest are open chest cardiac massage (21, 23), interposed abdominal compression (24), and active compression-decompression CPR (25). It is likely, however, that none of these new methods will be better than standard high-impulse manual chest compression.

No matter which technique proves to be the most effective, pharmacologic therapy remains an important component of advanced cardiac life support.

## RATIONALE FOR DRUG THERAPY DURING CPR

Appropriate drug therapy can increase the effectiveness of prolonged CPR. The objectives of drug therapy during CPR are to augment arterial

**Table 17.1**
**Time to Initiation of Therapy and Subsequent Survival in Cardiac Arrest**

| | Defibrillation (min) | | |
|---|---|---|---|
| | <8 | 8–16 | >16 |
| CPR <4 min | 43% | 19% | 10% |
| CPR 4–8 min | 27% | 19% | 6% |
| CPR >8 min | — | 7% | 0% |

CPR = cardiopulmonary resuscitation; min = minute.
Reproduced with permission from Eisenberg MS, Bergner L, Hallstrom AP. Cardiac resuscitation in the community. JAMA 1979;241:1905–1907.

blood pressure and thereby coronary perfusion pressure, to improve forward blood flow, to improve the metabolic milieu associated with cardiac arrest, and to stabilize the cardiac rhythm.

Forward blood flow during CPR varies but rarely exceeds 25% of normal (26–31). Efforts to improve forward blood flow during CPR have included volume administration (32, 33) and the use of vasoconstricting agents (34–41). Volume is sometimes useful, particularly for subjects in whom rapid manual chest compression is used or in whom hypovolemia is known to be present (42). Vasoconstriction of the peripheral vasculature does not uniformly enhance blood flow to all vascular beds. Flow to certain organs may actually diminish, but blood flow to vital organs, the central nervous system, and the myocardium is increased by vasoconstriction in conjunction with closed or open chest CPR techniques (43, 44).

Cessation of ventilation and circulation results in marked tissue acid-base disturbances. In the absence of adequate tissue perfusion, anaerobic metabolism results in the production of lactic acid and other metabolites that can cause severe acidosis and cellular dysfunction. Attempts to retard and compensate for these processes have been made by using supplemental oxygen and metabolic buffers such as sodium bicarbonate. The limitation of metabolic buffers such as sodium bicarbonate are discussed later in this chapter.

Stabilization of the cardiac rhythm is an important step during CPR and in the postresuscitation period. Ventricular fibrillation is treated with defibrillation countershock. However, if refibrillation occurs, antiarrhythmic drug therapy may be helpful. Antiarrhythmic therapy has been advocated not only to decrease the defibrillation threshold during ventricular fibrillation but also to increase the fibrillation threshold once sinus rhythm is restored. When high-dose epinephrine or repeated doses of epinephrine has been used and ventricular tachycardia or recurrent ventricular fibrillation recurs, β-adrenergic blocking drugs may be life saving because they block the adverse β-adrenergic effects of epinephrine without blocking the beneficial α-agonist or peripheral vasoconstrictive effects. If hemodynamically compromising bradycardia is the cause of cardiac arrest or the result of CPR effects, drugs such as atropine or epinephrine can be effective.

## BASIC PHARMACOKINETIC PRINCIPLES DURING CPR

Cardiac arrest and subsequent CPR may result in major alterations in the pharmacokinetics of a drug. These changes include the volume of distribution of the drug and its elimination; therefore, the concentration of the drug may be markedly altered. The markedly diminished circulation seen even with effective CPR produces a dramatic decrease in the effective volume within which a drug is distributed (Fig. 17.1). Less impressive decreases in the volume of drug distribution have been documented in other conditions in which effective circulation is compromised, such as advanced congestive heart failure (Fig. 17.1). When studying lidocaine pharmacokinetics during CPR, Chow and associates found that the volume of distribution was only 8% of normal (45). Similar changes were found in lidocaine clearance, which was reduced to 10% of normal. These alterations resulted in an 8 to 10 fold increase in the arterial concentration of lidocaine when standard dosing schemes were used during CPR (45, 46).

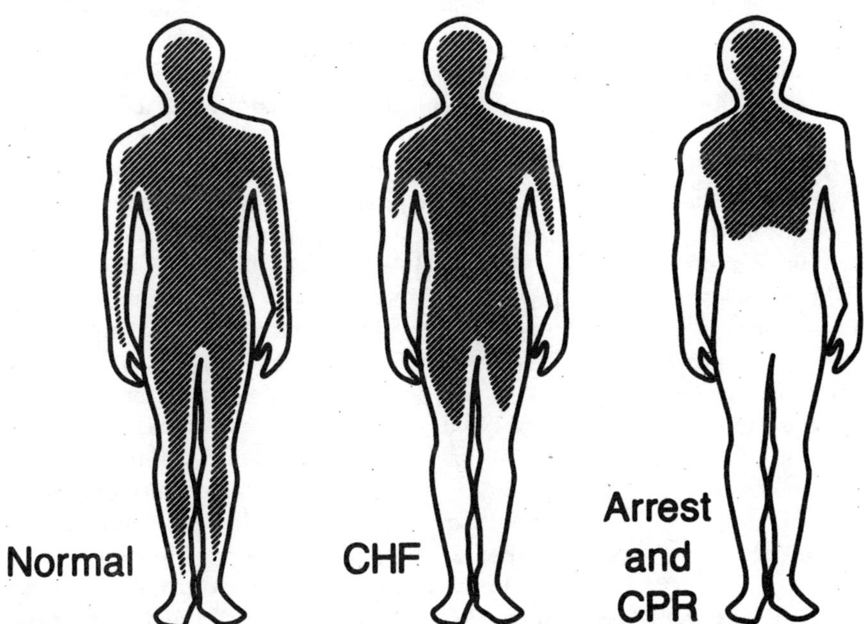


Figure 17.1 The effective volume of distribution decreases dramatically with cardiac arrest and accompanying cardiopulmonary resuscitation. Hence, drug doses must be appropriately altered. CHF = congestive heart failure; CPR = cardiopulmonary resuscitation.

The effect of CPR on drug metabolism is not well defined. Blood flow to the liver and kidneys is markedly compromised during CPR such that blood flow to some organs is less than 2% of normal (31, 44). Thus, hepatic and renal metabolism of drugs during CPR is markedly diminished. After restoration of blood flow after successful resuscitation, drug metabolism may increase, but hepatic and renal injury resulting from ischemia or reperfusion injury may impair drug metabolism even after spontaneous circulation is restored.

## ADMINISTRATION OF DRUGS DURING CPR

The establishment of intravenous access for drug administration is an important aspect of advanced cardiac life support (26). However, administration of critically important drugs should not be delayed for placement of an intravenous access because effective alternative routes exist.

Peripheral intravenous injections result in a significant delay in drug distribution even when effective CPR is being performed (47, 48). Furthermore, peak drug levels are lower when peripheral sites are used for drug injection (47, 49). Because of the impaired circulation during CPR, central line injections are more effective. Peripheral venous cannulation can be used to administer drugs during CPR; despite the disadvantages, is often easier, results in fewer serious complications, and usually does not disrupt ongoing CPR efforts (26). When peripheral venous injection sites are used, the drugs should be given by rapid bolus followed by 20-mL bolus of fluid and, if possible, the elevation of the extremity to ensure a more rapid and complete delivery of the drug into the central circulation. The distal veins in the hands, wrists, and feet should not be used because of the marked diminution of peripheral blood flow during CPR (26). If circulation is not rapidly restored after initial drug administration via a peripheral line, a central line should be placed (26). The central circulation can be entered through an internal jugular site or a subclavian site. Increased risk of complications is associated with placement of central lines, especially if the patient is to receive thrombolytic therapy. "Even one unsuccessful central line attempt is a strong relative contraindication to initiation of thrombolysis" (48).

Finding an intravenous access may be difficult in many patients, including those in shock, infants and children, obese patients, intravenous drug abusers, and those with numerous previous vascular cutdowns. Intracardiac injections are feasible but should not be routinely performed because of potential complications. Attempted transchest intracardiac injections can result in pneumothorax, hemothorax, tamponade, myocardial or coronary laceration, or intramural injections. In all instances, external chest compressions and ventilations must be temporarily interrupted during intracardiac injections. The consensus from the 1992 American Heart Association's quinquennial guidelines was to reserve intracardiac administration of drugs for situations in which neither an intravenous nor an endotracheal route is available (26). Intracardiac administration should be used only during open cardiac massage or when all other routes of administration are unavailable (26).

The endotracheal tube provides an alternative route for drug administration in cardiac emergencies (50–54). Endotracheal drug administration during CPR was initially described by Pearson and Redding in 1967 (50) and was popularized in the 1980s by Roberts, Greenberg, and others (51–54). Epinephrine given endotracheally is rapidly absorbed, with peak blood concentrations occurring within 15 seconds; paradoxically, the effects last longer than they do with intravenous administration. Because metabolism of the drug is the same after intravenous or endotracheal administration, the endotracheal route must provide a depot for continued delayed release. Other drugs that have been shown to be well absorbed via the endotracheal route include atropine, lidocaine (55), propranolol (56), nalozone, and diazepam (for status epilepticus) (57). Calcium chloride and norepinephrine should not be administered via the endotracheal tube because these drugs cause pulmonary damage. Sodium bicarbonate has not been studied but will probably not be practical because of the large volume of fluid necessary for an effective dose. Isoproterenol is not reliably administered endotracheally (56).

Because all endotracheally administered drugs have an extended duration of action of two to five times that of drugs administered intravenously (58, 59), repeated doses should be administered with this in mind. The volume of endotracheal drug should not be excessive so that pulmonary complications can be avoided. Some studies suggest that 1:1 dilution of the drug in sterile normal saline is appropriate (60). Sterile normal saline appears to be an appropriate dilutant because of its isotonicity (61), but more rapid absorption has been reported with distilled water (62). Sterile water has, however, a more negative effect on arterial oxygenation (26). Endotracheal drugs need not be administered deep into the lungs for optimal absorption (63). The medication should be given forcefully to get a spray effect, with the catheter tip beyond the endotracheal tube. Forceful manual hyperventilation following endotracheal administration is essential to ensure bilateral and optimal distal delivery of the endotracheally administered drug (63). Therefore, endotracheal administration of all drugs should be followed by a short period of hyperventilation (about five inflations with a breathing bag). Drugs administered endotracheally have a potential for toxicity, as do those administered intravenously.

The current recommendation is that epinephrine, lidocaine, and atropine can be administered endotracheally (26). Medications "should be administered at 2.0–2.5 times the recommended intravenous dose and should be diluted in 10 mL of normal saline" (26).

The endotracheal administration of drugs may be especially valuable in the prehospital setting where paramedics are skilled in performance of rapid endotracheal intubation and the patient's state or field conditions may preclude efficient intravenous access.

## DRUGS USED IN CPR

### Adrenergic Agonists

No drugs have been proved to be more useful during CPR than adrenergic agonists, and no adrenergic agonist has been shown to be superior to epinephrine; thus, epinephrine continues to be the drug of choice. The primary benefit of epinephrine during CPR is its ability to cause α-adrenergic receptor stimulation producing peripheral vasoconstriction (34–41). Table 17.2 summarizes the classic work of Redding and Pearson showing the relative effectiveness of various catecholamines during anoxic cardiac arrest and CPR (34–41). The importance of α-receptor stimulation in the successful treatment of cardiac arrest is obvious. Table 17.3 summarizes the results of the coadministration of epinephrine with an α-adrenergic blocker, a β-adrenergic blocker, both, or neither (36, 37). The importance of the α-agonist effect and the lack of an important β-agonist effect is apparent. As shown in Table 17.4, high-dose dopamine, producing peripheral vasoconstriction, is as effective as epinephrine. However, dobutamine, a catecholamine whose dominant action is to stimulate the heart, is ineffec-

**Table 17.2**
**Catecholamines in Cardiopulmonary Resuscitation (Fibrillatory Arrest)**

| Drug | Circulation Restored |
|---|---|
| Epinephrine (α,β) | 10/10 |
| Phenylephrine (α) | 9/10 |
| Isoproterenol (β) | 0/10 |
| Saline control | 1/10 |

Reproduced with permission from Redding JS, Pearson JW. Evaluation of drugs for cardiac resuscitation. Anesthesiology 1963;24:203–207.

**Table 17.3**
**Results of Administration of Epinephrine with an α-Adrenergic Blocker**

| Drug | Circulation Restored |
|---|---|
| Epinephrine + α-blocker | 0/8 |
| Epinephrine + β-blocker | 6/8 |
| Epinephrine + α- and β-blocker | 0/8 |
| Epinephrine | 7/8 |

Reproduced with permission from Otto CW, Yakaitis RW, Blitt CD. Mechanism of action of epinephrine in resuscitation from asphyxial arrest. Crit Care Med 1981;9:364–365.

**Table 17.4**
**Catecholamines in Cardiopulmonary Resuscitation (Fibrillatory Arrest)**

| Drug | Survival |
|---|---|
| Dopamine, 40 mg | 9/10 |
| Dobutamine, 50 mg | 2/10 |
| Epinephrine, 1 mg | 10/10 |
| Saline | 3/10 |

Data from Otto CW, Yakaitis RW, Redding JS, et al. Mechanism of action of epinephrine in resuscitation from asphyxial arrest. Crit Care Med 1981;9:366.

tive (37). Through vasoconstriction, particularly of the peripheral vasculature, central aortic diastolic and coronary perfusion pressures rise. Increasing the aortic diastolic and coronary perfusion pressures during CPR results in improved myocardial blood flow and survival (43, 44). Every incremental increase in myocardial perfusion pressure, defined as aortic diastolic pressure minus simultaneous right atrial diastolic pressure, (Fig. 17.2) results in a corresponding incremental increase in myocardial blood flow. This important relationship during CPR has been documented in numerous experimental laboratories (29, 43, 44, 64). Increases in both coronary perfusion pressure and left ventricular blood flow result in improved resuscitation outcome (43, 44).

Is epinephrine the optimal α-adrenergic agonist for use during CPR? Concern about possible detrimental effects of β-agonist or stimulation from mixed agonists such as epinephrine has resulted in increased interest in "pure" α-agents (65–67). Theoretically, pure α-agonists should have several advantages. In some studies, pure α-agonists are less successful in stimulating myocardial oxygen consumption than agents with β-adrenergic properties (65, 67). Less myocardial oxygen consumption during the period of low flow associated with CPR could result in a less severe ischemic insult.

To date, no pure α-adrenergic agonist has been shown in an experimental animal to be superior to epinephrine in restoring spontaneous circulation or for neurologic benefit after treatment of cardiac arrest (68, 69). As noted, epinephrine increases coronary blood flow but may not improve the balance between myocardial oxygen supply and demand during CPR. Ditchey and Slinker postulated that an α-adrenergic vasoconstrictor administered with a β-adrenergic blocker might be optimal because cardiac arrest evokes such a dramatic endogenous catecholamine response (70). They measured coronary perfusion pressure and myocardial adenosine 5′-triphosphate (ATP) levels. Coronary perfusion pressures remained higher for a longer duration and myocardial ATP levels were higher with the combination of phenylephrine and propranolol (70). This study found that the balance between myocardial oxygen supply and demand during CPR was

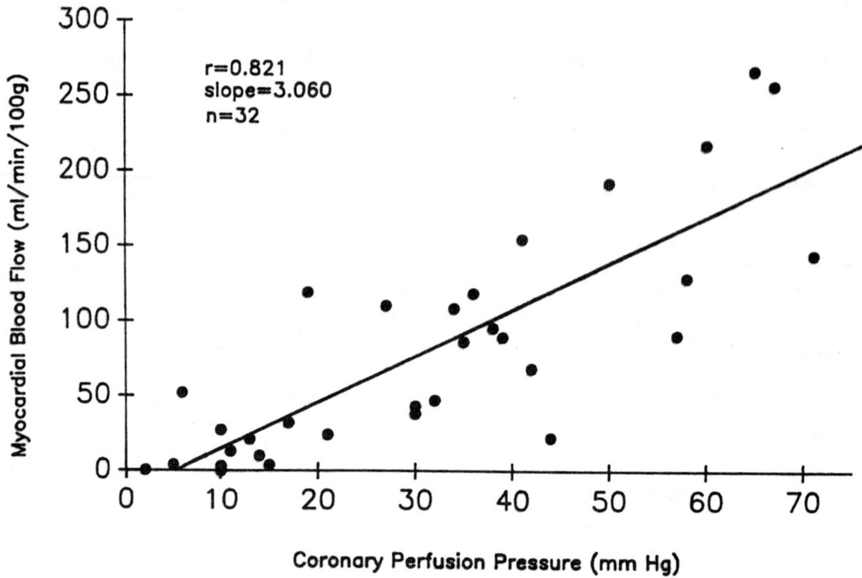


Figure 17.2 The relationship between myocardial perfusion pressure and myocardial blood flow during cardiopulmonary resuscitation (CPR) is apparent. The higher the CPR-generated myocardial perfusion pressure, the greater the resulting left ventricular blood flow.

improved by use of a combination of phenylephrine (a pure α-agonist) and propranolol (a β-blocker) but not by use of large doses of epinephrine or phenylephrine alone (70). Further studies, including survival studies, are needed before this combination can be recommended in humans.

Several clinical trials have now compared epinephrine with other more selective α-agonists. Silfast and coworkers randomized 65 cardiac arrest patients to either 0.5 mg of epinephrine or 1 mg of phenylepinephrine (71). Initial resuscitation success was similar in both groups (10 of 36 with epinephrine versus 9 of 29 with phenylepinephrine). Turner and colleagues studying patients with electromechanical dissociation found no difference in resuscitation or survival rates between patients treated with epinephrine (1 mg) and those treated with methoxamine (10 mg) (72). In another clinical series, Olson and colleagues found that epinephrine (0.5 mg) was more effective for successful defibrillation (40 versus 28%; $P < 0.03$) and initial resuscitation (39 versus 18%; $P < 0.02$) than methoxamine (10 mg) (73). Long-term survival, however, did not differ between the two treatment groups (73). Because pure α-agonists have not been shown to be superior to epinephrine and because of the wide clinical experience with epinephrine during cardiac arrest, epinephrine remains the drug of choice in patients with cardiac arrest. However, as noted, the combination of an α-agonist plus a β-blocker or epinephrine plus a β-blocker may be best.

### *Epinephrine Dose*

The optimal dosing regimen for adrenergic agonists during CPR has recently been questioned. The 1986 American Heart Association Standards and Guidelines state that 0.5–1.0 mg of epinephrine should be given every 5 minutes during CPR (22). This dosing schedule appears to have originated from animal experiments done in 1906 (74). Crile found this dose effective in improving resuscitation results but did not attempt dose-response experiments. Brown and coworkers have shown that the original dose of approximately 0.2 mg/kg is effective in raising aortic pressure, coronary perfusion pressure, and regional myocardial and cerebral blood flow during CPR, whereas the extrapolated clinically recommended dose of 0.02 mg/kg (1 mg for a person of 50–75 kg) has no effect on hemodynamics or blood flow during resuscitation efforts (75, 76).

The first report of a clinical dose-response study using epinephrine appeared in 1989 (77). Gonzalez and Ornato reported on 10 patients who suffered out-of-hospital cardiac arrest. Instruments were inserted for intraarterial pressure monitoring, then the patients were studied during CPR for their response to three different doses of epinephrine (1 mg, 3 mg, and 5 mg). The results are shown in Table 17.5. The 5-mg dose produced the highest arterial pressures and, in fact, the one patient who responded with successful return of spontaneous circulation did so after the 5 mg dose. This patient gradually became hypotensive, however, and died.

Several anecdotal reports and one clinical series followed that either advocated or denounced high-dose epinephrine therapy for the treatment of cardiac arrest. Warwick found a reduction in immediate survival rates in patients treated with high-dose epinephrine compared with previous historical controls treated with more standard doses (78). Kosgrove and Paradis, however, reported on two patients who responded to boluses of 4 or 5 mg after failing to respond to 1-mg doses of epinephrine (79). An additional anecdotal report of seven pediatric patients indicated that six of the seven children responded to high-dose epinephrine administration after failing to respond to standard doses (80).

**Table 17.5**
**Evidence of a Dose-Response Curve with Epinephrine**

| | CPR-Generated Arterial Pressure (mm Hg) | |
|---|---|---|
| Epinephrine | Systolic | Diastolic |
| 1 mg | 69±7 | 27±3 |
| 3 mg | 74±8 | 25±4 |
| 5 mg | 85±8 | 36±6 |

Reproduced with permission from Gonzalez ER, Ornato JP, Garnett AR, et al. Dose-dependent vasopressor response to epinephrine during CPR in human beings. Ann Emerg Med 1989;18:920–926.

Callaham (81) studied epinephrine at doses of 1 mg (standard dose) and 15 mg (high dose) and norepinephrine, 11 mg, in 928 cardiac arrests. There were 762 patients enrolled in the study. Ventricular fibrillation occurred in 23% of the patients. The average patient age was 68 years and 69% were men; 58% of the arrests were witnessed, and bystander CPR was begun in 31%. Return of spontaneous circulation occurred in 116 patients, 104 patients were admitted to the hospital, and 48 patients were discharged alive (Table 17.6). A limitation of this study is that of the 48 survivors, 35 had early defibrillation only. Therefore, only 13 surviving patients were given the study drug. With three different rhythms and three groups, the study drug had only one or two patients survive in each group.

Brown (82) directed a multicenter trial randomizing standard-dose epinephrine (0.02 mg/kg) with high-dose epinephrine (0.2 mg/kg). This study had 1262 patients and no difference in survival was found (Table 17.7). Stiell and colleagues (83) had similar results with 650 patients treated both in the prehospital environment and in the hospital (Table 17.8).

Thus, in randomized trials higher doses of epinephrine in adults failed to increase survival at 1 hour or at hospital discharge and also failed to improve neurologic status even though there was an increase in the number of patients with return of spontaneous circulation. High-dose epinephrine did not cause an increase in side effects. The problem with all of these studies, however, is that most patients survived before the study drug was given.

It is possible that high-dose epinephrine might be beneficial in pulseless electrical activity or in asystole; however, data are insufficient for forming any conclusion except that no improvement in survival has been seen. Therefore, the 1992 guidelines for CPR (26) state that high doses of epinephrine may be used. Alternative regimens include high-dose epinephrine (7–10 mg/kg every 3–5 minutes), intermediate-dose epinephrine (2–5 mg every 3–5 minutes), or escalating doses of epinephrine (i.e., 1 mg followed by 3 mg followed by 5 mg, each 3 minutes apart).

**Table 17.6**
**Comparison of High-Dose Epinephrine, Standard-Dose Epinephrine, and Norepinephrine in Treatment of Prehospital Cardiac Arrest**

| | HDE | NE | SDE | Significance |
|---|---|---|---|---|
| Return of spontaneous circulation | | | | |
| Hospital admission | 18% | 13% | 10% | $P<0.02$ (HDE vs SDE) |
| Hospital discharge | 2% | 3% | 1% | |

HDE = high-dose epinephrine (15 mg); NE = norepinephrine (11 mg); SDE = standard-dose epinephrine (1 mg).

Reprinted with permission from Callaham M, Madsen CD, Barton CW, et al. A randomized clinical trial of high-dose epinephrine and norepinephrine vs standard-dose epinephrine in prehospital cardiac arrest. JAMA 1992;268:2667–2672.

**Table 17.7**
**Comparison of High-Dose Epinephrine and Standard-Dose Epinephrine in Treatment of Prehospital Arrest**

| | HDE | SDE | Significance |
|---|---|---|---|
| Return of spontaneous circulation | 34.0% | 29.9% | $P = 0.13$ |
| Admitted to hospital | 22.0% | 20.6% | |
| Discharged alive | 4.6% | 4.2% | |

HDE = high-dose epinephrine (0.2 mg/kg); SDE = standard-dose epinephrine (0.02 mg/kg).
Reprinted with permission from Brown CG, Martin DR, Pepe PE, et al. A comparison of standard-dose and high-dose epinephrine in cardiac arrest outside the hospital. N Engl J Med 1992;327:1051–1055.

**Table 17.8**
**Comparison of High-Dose Epinephrine and Standard-Dose Epinephrine in Treatment of Prehospital Cardiac Arrest**

| | HDE | SDE |
|---|---|---|
| Return of spontaneous circulation | 17.7% | 22.8% |
| Discharged alive | 3.2% | 4.8% |

HDE = high-dose epinephrine (up to 5 doses of 7 mg); SDE = standard-dose epinephrine (up to 5 doses of 1 mg).
Reproduced with permission from Stiell IG, Herbert PC, Weitzman BN, et al. High-dose epinephrine in adult cardiac arrest. N Engl J Med 1992;327:1045–1050.

The 1992 guideline states that a high dose of epinephrine (5 mg or approximately 0.1 mg/kg) should be considered only after the 1-mg dose has failed (26). If high-dose epinephrine is used, serious consideration must be given to the concomitant administration of intravenous β-adrenergic blockers. Our experimental studies suggest that high-dose epinephrine is deleterious, resulting in excessive tachycardia and early coronary care era deaths (84).

## Sodium Bicarbonate

The use of sodium bicarbonate has been controversial. As a result, the enthusiasm for the use of buffers to combat the systemic acidemia associated with the poor perfusing state of cardiac arrest and CPR has waned during the last several years. Reversing earlier stands, the recommendation of the 1985 consensus for CPR guideline was that "bicarbonate should be used, if at all, only after more proven interventions such as defibrillation, cardiac compression, support of ventilation including intubation, and pharmacologic therapies such as epinephrine and antiarrhythmics have been employed" (22).

It is now recognized that, during the first 15–20 minutes of cardiac arrest and subsequent CPR, acid-base disturbances almost inevitably reflect the adequacy of ventilation. Typically, before the institution of artificial ventilation, hypercapnia results in respiratory acidosis. However, as soon as efforts are begun to artificially ventilate, it is common for the arterial partial pressure of carbon dioxide to fall to levels below normal, resulting in a respiratory alkalosis in the arterial blood. Rarely does metabolic acidosis become a concern until after 15–20 minutes of cardiac arrest and CPR. Therefore, ventilation may be the key to early acid-base control during CPR. There is little need for organic buffers, such as sodium bicarbonate, during the early phases of resuscitation efforts.

Several potentially adverse effects from the administration of sodium bicarbonate during CPR have been suggested. These include shifting the oxyhemoglobin saturation curve to the left (thereby inhibiting the release of oxygen from the hemoglobin molecule), creating a hyperosmolar state secondary to the osmolar load associated with large quantities of sodium bicarbonate administration (85), production of a paradoxical central nervous system acidosis (86, 87), and possibly impairment of myocardial oxygen consumption (88, 89).

Most importantly, the majority of available data fails to show that organic buffer use during CPR enhances survival (90–92). Studies have been uniformly hampered by small patient numbers, allowing for the possibility that a potential benefit from sodium bicarbonate could be undetected secondary to a large beta or type II statistical error. An exception to these studies is that of Sanders and associates, who showed that concurrent use of sodium bicarbonate and volume loading was crucial in improving resuscitation outcomes with rapid manual chest compression CPR (42).

The American Heart Association's Guidelines state that sodium bicarbonate may be beneficial in patients with preexisting acidosis or hyperkalemia, but they strongly caution its routine use: "however its use early during a code sequence should be predicated on a clearly defined diagnosis. When bicarbonate is used, 1 mEq/kg should be given as the initial dose and no more than half this dose given every 10 minutes thereafter" (26). Even this advice is difficult to translate into clinical practice because of the recent debate regarding whether arterial or mixed venous blood samples are best for determining the need for systemic buffer therapy (93).

Bicarbonate is probably helpful in cases of known preexisting bicarbonate-responsive acidosis or overdose of tricyclic antidepressants and to alkalinize the urine in other drug overdoses. Sodium bicarbonate may be helpful in patients with prolonged arrests or upon return of a pulse after prolonged arrest; however, the evidence for benefit is only possible and not proven.

## Calcium Chloride

Calcium plays an important role in myocardial contractile performance and impulse formation. In experimental preparations, the administration of calcium can increase ventricular contractility and automaticity and prolong systole. Because of these effects, calcium was thought to be a potentially useful agent in treating certain cardiac arrest circumstances, including electromechanical dissociation and asystole.

The benefit of calcium in improving the outcome of cardiac arrest has been more difficult to verify. Without question, calcium can be a lifesaving drug in some cardiac arrest conditions, e.g., if hyperkalemia is the cause of cardiac arrest, appropriate therapy includes the administration of intravenous calcium chloride. However, administration of one ampule (10 mL) of 10% calcium chloride can result in life-threatening (although transient) hypercalcemia (94). Finally no evidence exists that calcium improves the outcomes of patients suffering electromechanical dissociation or asystole (95–97).

Accordingly, the revised American Heart Association Guidelines no longer recommend use of calcium chloride for treating electromechanical dissociation and asystole. The exceptions are hyperkalemia, hypocalcemia (e.g., after multiple blood transfusions), or calcium channel blockade toxicity. When necessary, calcium chloride can be given in a dose of 2 mL of a 10% solution (2–4 mg/kg) and repeated at 10-minute intervals (26).

## Antiarrhythmic Drug Therapy

Lidocaine and bretylium have been included in cardiac arrest treatment protocols for decades. Their role includes the prevention of ventricular tachyarrhythmias, the termination of such arrhythmias, and the prevention of recurrent arrhythmias. Few workers will argue the benefit of suppressing significant ventricular ectopy, particularly ventricular tachycardia, after successful defibrillation from cardiac arrest. It is unclear if bretylium can terminate ventricular fibrillation without concurrent electrical therapy. Anecdotal reports of chemical defibrillation with bretylium have been difficult to verify in the laboratory (98).

Lidocaine has been shown to increase the ventricular fibrillation threshold and to reverse the fall in this threshold associated with myocardial ischemia (99). This desirable effect makes lidocaine attractive for use after successful restoration of a supraventricular rhythm. However, lidocaine may also raise the defibrillation threshold, making defibrillation more difficult during ventricular fibrillation (100).

Bretylium tosylate is a quaternary ammonium compound used to treat resistant ventricular tachycardia and fibrillation unresponsive to defibrillation, epinephrine, and lidocaine. Its actions are complex and include a release of catecholamines initially followed by a postganglioma adrenergic blocking action that frequently induces hypotension (26), and also an increase in the ventricular fibrillation threshold, especially during acute ischemia (101). Its effect on the defibrillation threshold is controversial. Tacker and associates found that bretylium lowers the defibrillation threshold (102), but Koo noted that the defibrillation threshold is increased after the administration of bretylium (103). Hanyok and coworkers showed that a combination of lidocaine and bretylium had the rapid and prolonged effect of increasing the ventricular fibrillation threshold (104). One distinct disadvantage of bretylium is its potential for lowering systemic blood pressure during acute administration (105).

Several clinical trials have compared lidocaine and bretylium during cardiac arrest. Harrison and associates reported that lidocaine did not improve the rate of successful defibrillation in a nonrandomized, retrospective study (106). Nowak and coworkers compared bretylium with placebo to test its effect on the success of resuscitation and found that 35% of patients with either ventricular fibrillation or asystole survived after receiving the active compound whereas only 6% survived after receiving placebo (107). However, careful scrutiny of this study reveals that, if only patients with documented ventricular fibrillation are analyzed, no difference is seen. Haynes and associates performed a randomized, controlled trial of bretylium and lidocaine therapy in out-of-hospital ventricular fibrillation (108). Chemical defibrillation was not observed, and no difference in either successful defibrillation or resuscitation was seen among the 146 study patients. Olson and coworkers have recently confirmed this lack of significant advantage for either agent (109).

In reviewing the data concerning the equivalence of bretylium and lidocaine in improving resuscitation outcomes and noting the hemodynamic advantages of lidocaine, the American Heart Association Standards and Guidelines Committee in 1986 changed its previous recommendation and indicated that lidocaine is the drug of choice for the treatment of all ventricular arrhythmias, including ventricular fibrillation (22). In refractory ventricular fibrillation, 5 mg/kg of bretylium tosylate is given intravenously as a bolus followed by electrical defibrillation. If ventricular fibrillation persists, the dose can be increased to 10 mg/kg and repeated every 5 minutes to a maximal dose of 30–35 mg/kg (26).

## Atropine Sulfate

Atropine is often used during bradycardiac-asystolic cardiac arrest. The parasympatholytic action of atropine is well described, and its use in hemodynamically compromising sinus bradycardia and atrioventricular nodal block is well established. The effectiveness of atropine in infranodal block or asystole, however, is less certain. Several clinical trials have failed to show a significant impact of atropine in successfully treating asystolic cardiac arrest (110, 111). The key to success in all forms of cardiac arrest is early restoration of adequate myocardial and cerebral blood flow. Current schemes for treatment of asystolic-bradycardiac arrests emphasize the use of epinephrine both for peripheral vasoconstriction (raising perfusion pressures to the myocardium and cerebrum) and for its chronotrophic effect. Atropine is recommended as a second-line agent after epinephrine. The recommended dose of atropine is 1 mg intravenously, and this dose should be repeated every 5 minutes if asystole persists (22).

### Aminophylline

Adenosine may have a role in treating asystole, and therefore, aminophylline may also play a role. Viskin and associates reported that 11 of 15 patients with asystole or bradycardiac pulseless electrical activity who had failed epinephrine and atropine therapy, responded to the rapid intravenous infusion of 250 mg of aminophylline. Only one patient survived to discharge (112). Because aminophylline can antagonize adenosine, their report was of interest, but this report has not been confirmed by others.

## DRUGS TO PREVENT POSTRESUSCITATION SYNDROMES

Increasing concern about neurologic function after successful resuscitation has led to attempts to find therapeutic agents capable of lessening central nervous system injury from global ischemia and subsequent reperfusion. Experiments from the 1960s suggest that barbiturates could lower cerebral metabolism, thereby prolonging a tolerable period of hypoxia before neurologic damage ensued. Bleyart and associates showed impressive neurologic benefits from thiopental after coma was induced by global ischemic brain injury in a monkey model (113). However, a subsequent large clinical trial could not show any neurologic advantage using thiopental in survivors of cardiac arrest (114). Barbiturates are now occasionally used in treating increased intracranial pressure, but they are not routinely given after successful resuscitation.

The elucidation of central nervous system reperfusion injury has led to attempts to find drugs capable of preventing neurologic damage occurring both during and after resuscitation. Calcium channel antagonists have been suggested as possible agents in this regard (115–117). Nimodipine is a calcium channel antagonist that has, in some models, produced an improvement in cerebral blood flow following global ischemia (118); however, in other experimental studies it has failed to improve neurologic outcome (119). Preliminary results from a randomized double-blind clinical trial of nimodipine failed to show any neurologic benefit in patients treated within 30 minutes of successful resuscitation. Retrospective analysis of these data suggested that in 50 patients for whom advanced life support was delayed longer than 10 minutes, nimodipine improved both survival and neurologic function (120). Further randomized trials of nimodipine in this subgroup of patients are in progress.

An understanding of the role of free radicals in tissue injury following reperfusion has also led to numerous attempts to improve neurologic function following cardiac arrest and resuscitation with antioxidants or other free radical scavengers. Experimental results are encouraging (121–124), but no clinical trials have yet been completed.

## Myocardial Stunning After Cardiac Arrest

The myocardium suffers a significant insult during cardiac arrest and subsequent CPR. A cardiovascular postresuscitation syndrome has been reported by investigators at the University of Pittsburgh. Cerchiari and colleagues studied myocardial filling pressures and cardiac output before and after cardiac arrest in a canine model (125). Three different groups were studied varying the time of untreated cardiac arrest before CPR. Group 1 had 7.5 minutes of untreated arrest before resuscitation; Group 2, 10 minutes; and Group 3, 12.5 minutes. Central venous pressure, pulmonary artery pressures including pulmonary occlusive wedge pressure, and cardiac outputs were all measured before and after CPR. Right atrial pressure rose in all three groups at 30 minutes after resuscitation but returned to baseline within 1 hour. Pulmonary capillary occlusive pressure increased at 30 minutes after resuscitation and returned to normal within 1 hour except in the group that underwent the most prolonged period of untreated ventricular fibrillation. In this group it remained abnormal for the first 6 hours after CPR. Cardiac index fell in all three groups and remained depressed for 6 hours, except in the 12.5-minute group, in which it remained depressed for 72 hours (125). Tang and coworkers showed both systolic and diastolic dysfunction following resuscitation using an isolated rat heart with a Langendorf preparation (126). After a 4-minute period of untreated ventricular fibrillation with an additional 5 minutes of precordial compression, myocardial dysfunction was documented at 2 minutes and 20 minutes postresuscitation. Pressure volume relationships showed compromise in systolic contraction and diastolic compliance at 20 minutes postresuscitation (126).

We have recently shown the occurance of myocardial stunning (127). In an in vivo porcine model of cardiac arrest, progression of left ventricular systolic and diastolic dysfunction was found during the first 6 hours after successful cardiac resuscitation with complete resolution of this myocardial dysfunction by 48 hours (127, 128).

### CONCLUSIONS

In the early moments of cardiac arrest, medications take second place to basic chest compression, ventilation, and defibrillation. Thereafter, drug therapy is a vital part of CPR efforts. The proven efficacy of epinephrine in improving both myocardial and cerebral blood flow during CPR makes it the drug of choice in cardiac arrest. Sodium bicarbonate administration is best reserved for hyperkalemic arrests or documented severe metabolic acidemias that are not responsive to hyperventilation. Presently, there is little role for calcium, atropine, or aminophylline in the treatment of cardiac arrest.

## REFERENCES

1. Liberthson RR, Nagel EL, Hirschman JC, et al. Prehospital ventricular defibrillation. N Engl J Med 1974;291:317–321.
2. Copley DP, Mantle JA, Rogers WJ, et al. Improved outcome for prehospital cardiopulmonary collapse with resuscitation by bystanders. Circulation 1977;56: 901–905.
3. Thompson RG, Hallstrom AP, Cobb LA. Bystander initiated cardiopulmonary resuscitation in the management of ventricular fibrillation. Ann Intern Med 1979;90: 737–740.
4. Eisenberg MS, Bergner L, Hallstrom AP. Cardiac resuscitation in the community. JAMA 1979;241:1905–1907.
5. Cobb LA, Werner JA, Trobaugh GB, et al. Sudden cardiac death: I. A decade's experience with out-of-hospital resuscitation. Mod Concepts Cardiovasc Dis 1980;49: 31–36.
6. Eisenberg MS, Hallstrom AP, Bergner L. Long-term survival after out-of-hospital cardiac arrest. N Engl J Med 1982;306:1340–1343.
7. Bert RA, Kern KB, Sanders AB, et al. Bystander cardiopulmonary resuscitation. Is ventilation necesary? Circulation 1993;88:1907–1915.
8. Criley JM, Blaufuss AH, Kissel GL. Cough-induced cardiac compression. JAMA 1976;236:1246–1250.
9. Criley JM. Cough CPR. In: Schluger J, Lyons AF, eds. CPR and emergency cardiac care: looking to the future. New York: EM Books, 1980;47.
10. Chandra N, Rudikoff M, Tsitlik J, et al. Augmentation of carotid blood flow during cardiopulmonary resuscitation (CPR) in the dog by simultaneous compression and ventilation with high airway pressure. Am J Cardiol 1979;43:422 (Abstract).
11. Chandra N, Rudikoff M, Weisfeldt ML. Simultaneous chest compression and ventilation at high airway pressure during cardiopulmonary resuscitation. Lancet 1980; 1:175–178.
12. Niemann JT, Rosborough JP, Niskanen RA, et al. Mechanical "cough" cardiopulmonary resuscitation during cardiac arrest in dogs. Am J Cardiol 1985;55:199–204.
13. Halperin HR, Guerci AD, Chandra N, et al. Vest inflation without simultaneous ventilation during cardiac arrest in dogs: improved survival from prolonged cardiopulmonary resuscitation. Circulation 1986;74:1407–1415.
14. Kern KB, Carter AB, Showen RL, et al. Comparison of mechanical techniques of cardiopulmonary resuscitation: survival and neurologic outcome in dogs. Am J Emerg Med 1987;5:190–195.
15. Maier GW, Tyson GS, Olsen CO, et al. The physiology of external cardiac massage: high impulse cardiopulmonary resuscitation, Circulation 1984;70:86–101.
16. Feneley MP, Maier GW, Kern KB, et al. Influence of compression rate on initial success of resuscitation and 24-hour survival after prolonged manual cardiopulmonary resuscitation in dogs. Circulation 1988;77:240–250.
17. Kern KB, Carter AB, Showen RL, et al. Twenty-four hour survival in a canine model comparing three methods of manual cardiopulmonary resuscitation. J Am Coll Cardiol 1986;7:859–867.
18. Ralston SH, Babbs CF, Niebauer MJ, et al. Cardiopulmonary resuscitation with interposed abdominal compression in dogs. Anesth Analg 1982;61:645–651.
19. Voorhees WD, Niebauer MJ, Babbs CF. Improved oxygen delivery during cardiopulmonary resuscitation with interposed abdominal compression. Ann Emerg Med 1983;12:128–135.
20. Del Guercio LRM, Feins NR, Cohn JD, et al. Comparison of blood flow during external and internal cardiac massage in man. Circulation 1965;31(Suppl I):171.
21. Kern KB, Sanders AB, Badylak SF, et al. Long-term survival with open-chest cardiac massage after ineffective closed-chest compression in a canine preparation. Circulation 1987;75:498–503.

22. The 1985 National Conference on Cardiopulmonary Resuscitation and Emergency Cardiac Care. Standards and guidelines for cardiopulmonary resuscitation (CPR) and emergency cardiac care (ECC). JAMA 1986;255:2905–2932.
23. Sanders AB, Kern KB, Ewy GA, et al. Improved resuscitation from cardiac arrest with open-chest Massage. Ann Emerg Med 1984; 13:672–675.
24. Sack JB, Kesselbrenner MB, Bregman D. Survival from in-hospital cardiac arrest with interposed abdominal counterpulsation during cardiopulmonary resuscitation. JAMA 1992;267:379–385.
25. Redberg RF, Tucker KJ, Cohen TJ, et al. Physiology of blood flow during cardiopulmonary resuscitation. A transesophageal echocardiographic study. Circulation 1993;88:534–542.
26. Emergency Cardiac Care Committee and Subcommittee, American Heart Association. Guidelines for cardiopulmonary resuscitation and emergency cardiac care. JAMA 1992;268:2172–2302
27. Byrne D, Pass HI, Neely WA, et al. External versus internal cardiac massage in normal and chronically ischemic dogs. Am Surg 1980;46:657–662.
28. Luce JM, Ross BK, O'Quin RJ, et al. Regional blood flow during cardiopulmonary resuscitation in dogs using simultaneous and nonsimultaneous compression and ventilation. Circulation 1983;67:258–265.
29. Halperin HR, Tsitlik J, Guerci AD, et al. Determinants of blood flow to vital organs during cardiopulmonary resuscitation. Circulation 1986;73:539–550.
30. Bellamy RF, DeGuzman LR, Pedersen DC. Coronary blood flow during cardiopulmonary resuscitation in swine. Circulation 1984;69:174–180.
31. Taylor RB, Brown CG, Bridges T, et al. A model for regional blood flow measurements during cardiopulmonary resuscitation in a swine model. Resuscitation 1988; 16:107–118.
32. Ditchey RV, Lindenfeld J. Potential adverse effects of volume loading on perfusion of vital organs during closed-chest resuscitation. Circulation 1984;69:181–189.
33. Voorhees WD, Ralston SH, Kouglas C, et al. Fluid loading with whole blood or Ringer's lactate solution during CPR in dogs. Resuscitation 1987;15:113–123.
34. Redding JS, Pearson JW. Evaluation of drugs for cardiac resuscitation. Anesthesiology 1963;24:203–207.
35. Pearson JW, Redding JS. Peripheral vascular tone on cardiac resuscitation. Anesth Analg 1965;44:746–752.
36. Redding JS, Pearson JW. Resuscitation from ventricular fibrillation. Drug therapy. JAMA 1968;203:255–260.
37. Yakaitis RW, Otto CW, Blitt CD. Relative importance of alpha and beta adrenergic receptors during resuscitation. Crit Care Med 1981;7:293–296.
38. Holmes HR, Babbs CF, Voorhees WD, et al. Influence of adrenergic drugs upon vital organ perfusion during CPR. Crit Care Med 1980;8:137–140.
39. Otto CW, Yakaitis RW, Redding RW, et al. Mechanism of action of epinephrine in resuscitation from asphyxial arrest. Crit Care Med 1981;9:364–365.
40. Redding JS, Haynes RR, Thomas JD. Drug therapy in resuscitation from electromechanical dissociation. Crit Care Med 1983;11:681–684.
41. Sanders AB, Ewy GA, Taft TW. Prognostic and therapeutic importance of the aortic diastolic pressure in resuscitation from cardiac arrest. Crit Care Med 1984;12:871–873.
42. Sanders AB, Kern KB, Fonken S, et al. The role of bicarbonate and fluid loading in improving resuscitation from prolonged cardiac arrest with rapid manual chest compression CPR. Ann Emerg Med 1990;19:1–7.
43. Ralston SH, Voorhees WD, Babbs CF. Intra-pulmonary epinephrine during prolonged cardiopulmonary resuscitation: improved regional flow and resuscitation in dogs. Ann Emerg Med 1984;13:79–86.
44. Michael JR, Guerci AD, Koehler RC, et al. Mechanisms by which epinephrine augments cerebral and myocardial perfusion during cardiopulmonary resuscitation in dogs. Circulation 1984;69:822–835.
45. Chow MSS, Ronfeld RA, Hamilton RA, et al. Effect of external cardiopulmonary resuscitation on lidocaine pharmacokinetics in dogs. J Pharmacol Exp Ther 1983; 224:531–537.

46. Chow MSS, Ronfeld RA, Ruffett D, et al. Lidocaine pharmacokinetics during cardiac arrest and external cardiopulmonary resuscitation. Am Heart J 1981;102:799–801.
47. Kuhn GJ, White BC, Swetnam RE, et al. Peripheral vs central circulation times during CPR: a pilot study. Ann Emerg Med 1981;10:417–419.
48. Hedges JR, Barsan WG, Doan LA, et al. Central versus peripheral intravenous routes in cardiopulmonary resuscitation. Am Emerg Med 1984;2:385–390.
49. Barsan WG, Levy RC, Weir H. Lidocaine levels during CPR: differences after peripheral venous, central venous, and intracardiac injections. Ann Emerg Med 1981;10:73–78.
50. Redding JS, Asuncion JS, Pearson JW. Effective routes of drug administration during cardiac arrest. Anesth Analg 1967;46:253–258.
51. Roberts JR, Greenberg MI, Knaub MA, et al. Blood levels following intravenous and endotracheal epinephrine administration. J Am Coll Emerg Phys 1979;8:53–56.
52. Roberts JR, Greenberg MI, Baskin SI. Endotracheal epinephrine in cardiorespiratory collapse. J Am Coll Emerg Phys 1979;8:515–519.
53. Greenberg MI, Roberts JR, Baskin SI. Endotracheal naloxone reversal of morphine-induced respiratory depression in rabbits. Ann Emerg Med 1980;9:289–292.
54. Greenberg MI, Roberts JR, Krusz JC, et al. Endotracheal epinephrine in a canine anaphylactic shock model. J Am Coll Emerg Phys 1979;8:500–503.
55. Ward JT. Endotracheal drug therapy. Am J Emerg Med 1983;1:71–82.
56. Scott B, Martin GF, Matchett J, et al. Canine cardiovascular responses to endotracheally and intravenously administered atropine, isoproterenol, and propranolol. Ann Emerg Med 1987;16:1–10.
57. Barsan WG, Ward JT, Otten EJ. Blood levels of diazepam after endotracheal administration in dogs. Ann Emerg Med 1982;11:242–247.
58. Roberts JR, Greenberg MI, Knaub M, et al. Comparison of the pharmacological effects of epinephrine administered by the intravenous and endotracheal routes. J Am Coll Emerg Phys 1978;7:260–264.
59. Elam JO. The interpulmonary route for CPR drugs In: Safar P, Elam JO, eds. Advances in cardiopulmonary resuscitation. New York: Springer-Verlag, 1977:132.
60. Mace SE. The effect of dilution on plasma lidocaine levels with endotracheal administration. Ann Emerg Med 1987;16:522–526.
61. Greenberg MI, Baskin SI, Kaplan AM, et al. Effects of endotracheally administered distilled water and normal saline on the arterial blood gases of dogs. Ann Emerg Med 1982;11:600–604.
62. Pearson JW, Redding JS. Epinephrine in cardiac resuscitation. Am Heart J 1963; 66:210–214.
63. Greenberg MI, Spivey WH. Comparison of deep and shallow endotracheal administration of dionosil in dogs and effect of manual hyperventilation Ann Emerg Med 1985;14:209–212.
64. Linder KH, Ahnefeld FW, Schurmann W, et al. Effects of epinephrine and norepinephrine on myocardial oxygen delivery and consumption during cardiopulmonary resuscitation. Chest 1990;97:1458–1462.
65. Livesay JJ, Follette D, Fey KH, et al. Optimizing myocardial supply/demand balance with adrenergic drugs during cardiopulmonary resuscitation. J Thorac Cardiovasc Surg 1978;76:244–251.
66. Ditchey RV. High dose epinephrine does not improve the balance between myocardial oxygen supply and demand during cardiopulmonary resuscitation in dogs. J Am Coll Cardiol 1984;3:596 (Abstract).
67. Kern KB, Lancaster LD, Goldman S, et al. The effect of coronary artery lesions on the relationship between coronary artery perfusion pressure and myocardial blood flow during cardiopulmonary resuscitation in pigs. Am Heart J 1990;120:324–333.
68. Brillman JA, Sanders AB, Otto CW, et al. Outcome of resuscitation from fibrillatory arrest using epinephrine and phenylephrine in dogs. Crit Care Med 1985;13: 912–913.
69. Brown CG, Katz SE, Werman HA, et al. The effect of epinephrine versus methoxamine on regional myocardial blood flow and defibrillation rates following a prolonged cardiorespiratory arrest in a swine model. Am J Emerg Med 1987;5:362–369.

70. Ditchey RV, Slinker BK. Phenylephrine plus propranolol improves the balance between myocardial oxygen supply and demand during experimental cardiopulmonary resuscitation. Am Heart J 1994;127:324–330
71. Silfvast T, Saarnivaara L, Kinnunen A, et al. Comparison of adrenaline and phenylephrine in out-of-hospital cardiopulmonary resuscitation. Acta Anaesth Scand 1985; 29:610–613.
72. Turner LM, Parsons M, Luetkemeyer RC, et al. A comparison of epinephrine and methoxamine for resuscitation from electromechanical dissociation in human beings. Ann Emerg Med 1988;17:443–449.
73. Olson DW, Thakur R, Stueven HA, et al. Randomized study of epinephrine versus methoxamine in prehospital ventricular fibrillation. Ann Emerg Med 1989;18: 250–253.
74. Crile G, Dolley DT. Experimental research into resuscitation of dogs killed by anesthetics and asphyxia. J Exp Med 1906;8:713–725.
75. Brown CG, Werman HA, Davis EA, et al. Comparative effect of graded doses of epinephrine on regional brain blood flow during CPR in a swine model. Ann Emerg Med 1986;15:1138–1144.
76. Brown CG, Taylor RB, Werman HA, et al. Effect of standard doses of epinephrine on myocardial oxygen delivery and utilization during cardiopulmonary resuscitation. Crit Care Med 1988;16:536–539.
77. Gonzalez ER, Ornato JP, Garnett AR, et al. Dose-dependent vasopressor response to epinephrine during CPR in human beings. Ann Emerg Med 1989;18:920–926.
78. Marwick TH, Siskind V, Case C, et al. Adverse effect of early high-dose adrenaline on outcome of ventricular fibrillation. Lancet 1988;2:66–68.
79. Koscove EM, Paradis NA. Successful resuscitation from cardiac arrest using high-dose epinephrine therapy. JAMA 1988;259:3031–3034.
80. Goetting MG, Paradis NA. High dose epinephrine in refractory pediatric cardiac arrest. Crit Care Med 1989;17:1258–1262.
81. Callaham M, Madsen CD, Barton CW, et al. A randomized clinical trial of high-dose epinephrine and norepinephrine vs standard-dose epinephrine in prehospital cardiac arrest. JAMA 1992;268:2667–2672.
82. Brown CG, Martin DR, Pepe PE, et al. A comparison of standard-dose and high-dose epinephrine in cardiac arrest outside the hospital. N Engl J Med 1992;327: 1051–1055.
83. Stiell IG, Herbert PC, Weitzman BN, et al. High-dose epinephrine in adult cardiac arrest. N Engl J Med 1992;327:1045–1050.
84. Berg RA, Otto CW, Kern KB, et al. High-dose epinephrine results in greater early mortality after resuscitation from prolonged cardiac arrest in pigs: a prospective, randomized study. Crit Care Med 1994;22:282–290.
85. Bishop RL, Weisfeldt ML. Sodium bicarbonate administration during cardiac arrest. Effect on arterial pH $PCO_2$, and osmolality. JAMA 1976;235:506–509.
86. Berenyi KJ, Wolk M, Killip T, et al. Cerebrospinal fluid acidosis complicating therapy of experimental cardiopulmonary arrest. Circulation 1975;52:319–324.
87. Sanders AB, Otto CW, Kern KB, et al. Acid-base balance in a canine model of cardiac arrest. Ann Emerg Med 1988;17:667–671.
88. Bersin RM, Arieff AI. Improved hemodynamic function during hypoxia with carbicarb, a new agent for the management of acidosis. Circulation1988;77:227–233.
89. Bersin RM, Chatterjee K, Arieff AL. Metabolic and hemodynamic consequences of sodium bicarbonate administration in patients with heart disease. Am J Med 1989;87:7–14.
90. Telivuo L, Maamies T, Siltanem P, et al. Comparison of alkalizing agents in resuscitation of the heart after ventricular fibrillation. Ann Chir Gymaecol Fenn 1968; 57:221–224.
91. Minuck M, Shama GP. Comparison of THAM and sodium bicarbonate in resuscitation of the heart after ventricular fibrillation in dogs. Anesth Analg 1977;56:38–45.
92. Guerci AD, Chandra N, Johnson E, et al. Failure of sodium bicarbonate to improve resuscitation from ventricular fibrillation in dogs. Circulation 1986;74(Suppl IV):75.
93. Weil MH, Rackow EC, Trevino R, et al. Difference in acid-base state between venous and arterial blood during CPR. N Engl J Med 1986;315:153–156.

94. Mattar JA, Weil MH, Shubin H, et al. Cardiac arrest in the critically ill. Am J Med 1974;56:162–168.
95. Stueven H, Thompson BM, Aprahamian C, et al. Use of calcium in prehospital cardiac arrest. Ann Emerg Med 1983;12:136–139.
96. Stueven HA, Thompson BM, Aprahamian C, et al. Calcium chloride: reassessment of use in asystole. Ann Emerg Med 1984;13:820–822.
97. Harrison EE, Amey BD. Use of calcium in electromechanical dissociation. Ann Emerg Med 1984;13:844–845.
98. Sanna G, Arcidiacono R. Chemical ventricular defibrillation of the human heart with bretylium tosylate. Am J Cardiol 1973;32:982–987.
99. Spear JF, Moore EN, Gerstenblith G, et al. Effect of lidocaine on the ventricular fibrillation threshold in the dog during acute ischemia and premature ventricular contraction. Circulation 1972;46:65–73.
100. Babbs CF, Yim GK, Whistler SJ, et al. Elevation of ventricular defibrillation threshold in dogs by antiarrhythmic drugs. Am Heart J 1979;98:345–350.
101. Bacaner MB, Schreinemachers D. Bretylium tosylate for suppression of ventricular fibrillation after experimental myocardial infarction. Nature 1968;220: 494–496.
102. Tacker WA Jr., Niebauer MJ, Babbs CF, et al. The effect of newer antiarrhythmia drugs on defibrillation threshold. Crit Care Med 1980;8:177–180.
103. Koo CC, Allen JD, Pantridge JF. Lack of effect of bretylium tosylate on electrical ventricular defibrillation in a controlled study. Cardiovasc Res 1984;18:762–767.
104. Hanyok JJ, Chow MSS, Kluger J, et al. Antifibrillatory effects of high dose bretylium and a lidocaine-bretylium combination during cardiopulmonary resuscitation. Crit Care Med 1988;16:691–694.
105. Cooper JA, Frieden J. Bretylium tosylate. Am Heart J 1971;82:703–706.
106. Harrison EE. Lidocaine in prehospital countershock refractory ventricular fibrillation. Ann Emerg Med 1981;10:420–423.
107. Nowak RM, Bodnar TJ, Droned S, et al. Bretylium tosylate as initial treatment for cardiopulmonary arrest: randomized comparison with placebo. Ann Emerg Med 1981;10:404–407.
108. Haynes RE, Chinn TL, Copass MK, et al. Comparison of bretylium tosylate and lidocaine in management of out of hospital ventricular fibrillation: a randomized clinical trial. Am J Cardiol 1981;48:353–356.
109. Olson DW, Thompson BM, Darin JC, et al. A randomized comparison study of bretylium tosylate and lidocaine in resuscitation of patients from out-of-hospital ventricular fibrillation in a paramedic system. Ann Emerg Med 1984;13:807–810.
110. Myerburg RJ, Estes D, Zaman L, et al. Outcome of resuscitation from bradyarrhythmic or asystolic prehospital cardiac arrest. J Am Coll Cardiol 1984;4: 1118–1122.
111. Stueven HA, Tonsfeldt DJ, Thompson BM, et al. Atropine in asystole: human studies. Ann Emerg Med 1984;13:815–817.
112. Viskin S, Belhassen B, Roth A, et al. Aminophylline for brady asystolic cardiac arrest refractory to atropine and epinephrine. Ann Intern Med 1993;118:270–281.
113. Bleyaert AL, Nemoto EM, Safar P, et al. Thiopental amelioration of brain damage after global ischemia in monkeys. Anesthesia 1978;49:390–398.
114. Brain Resuscitation Clinical Trial I Study Group. Randomized clinical study of thiopental loading in comatose cardiac arrest survivors. N Engl J Med 1986;314: 397–403.
115. de Garavilla L, Babbs CF, Borowitz JL. Effect of diltiazem on brain calcium content following ischemia and reperfusion in a rat circulatory arrest model. Ann Emerg Med 1984;13:385 (Abstract).
116. White BC, Winegar CD, Wilson RF, et al. Calcium blockers in cerebral resuscitation. J Trauma 1983;23:788–794.
117. Vaagenes P, Cantadore R, Safar P, et al. Effect of lidoflazine on neurologic outcome after cardiac arrest in dogs. Anaesthsia 1983;59:100 (Abstract).
118. Steen PA, Newberg LA, Milde JH, et al. Nimodipine improves cerebral blood flow and neurologic recovery after complete cerebral ischemia in the dog. J Cerebral Blood Flow Metab 1983;3:38–43.

119. Tateishi A, Fleischer JE, Drummond JC, et al. Nimodipine does not improve neurologic outcome after 14 minutes of cardiac arrest in cats. Stroke 1989;20: 1044–1050.
120. Roine RO, Kaste M, Nikki P, et al. Randomized double-blind trial of nimodipine in out-of-hospital resuscitation. J Am Coll Cardiol 1990;15:28A.
121. Itoh T, Kawakami M, Yamauchi Y, et al. Effect of allopurinol on ischemia and reperfusion-induced cerebral injury in spontaneously hypertensive rats. Stroke 1986;17:1284–1287.
122. Meyer FB, Sundt TM, Yanagihara T, et al. Focal cerebral ischemia: pathophysiologic mechanisms and rationale for future avenues of treatment. Mayo Clin Proc 1987;62:35–55.
123. Myers ML, Bolli R, Lekich RF, et al. Enhancement of recovery of myocardial function by oxygen free-radical scavengers after reversible regional ischemia. Circulation 1985;72:915–921.
124. Przyklenk K, Kloner RA. Superoxide dismutase plus catalase improve contractile function in the canine model of "stunned myocardium." Circ Res 1986;58:148–156.
125. Cerchiari EL, Safar P, Klein E, et al. Cardiovascular function in neurologic outcome after cardiac arrest in dogs. The cardiovascular post-resuscitation syndrome. Resuscitation 1993;25:9–33.
126. Tang W, Neil MH, Sun S, et al. Progressive myocardial dysfunction after cardiac resuscitation. Crit Care Med 1993;21:1046–1050.
127. Kern KB, Hilwig RW, Fenster PE, et al. Myocardial dysfunction following successful resuscitation. Circulation 1993;88(Suppl):I-225 (Abstract).
128. Kern KB, Rhee KH, Raya TE, et al. Global myocardial stunning following successful resuscitation from cardiac arrest. Circulation 1994;90 (Suppl):I-5 (Abstract).

# INDEX

Page numbers in *italics* refer to figures and chemical structures; those followed by the letter "t" refer to tables.